Mosby's Textbook for

NURSING
ASSISTANTS

CONGRATULATIONS!

You now have access to Mosby's Assistive Personnel MERLIN Website!

Here's how to get there and what you'll find:

sign on at: http://www.mosby.com/MAPS/NsgAstTextbook/

A Website just for you as you use the new 5th edition of
Mosby's Textbook for Nursing Assistants

what you will find: Whether you're a student, an instructor, or a clinician, you'll find information just for you. Things like:

- Content Updates
- Links to Related Products
- Author Information
- Links to Related Websites
- Information Exchange
  . . . and more

Mosby's Electronic Resource Links & Information Network

Sheila A. Sorrentino, RN, PhD
Curriculum and Health Care Consultant
Normal, Illinois

Mosby's Textbook for
NURSING
ASSISTANTS

Fifth Edition
With 898 Illustrations

Mosby

An Imprint of Elsevier Science

St. Louis   London   Philadelphia   Sydney   Toronto

An Imprint of Elsevier Science

Editor-in-Chief: *Sally Schrefer*
Senior Editor: *Susan R. Epstein*
Associate Developmental Editor: *Maria Broeker*
Project Manager: *John Rogers*
Project Specialists: *Betty Hazelwood and Kathleen L. Teal*
Designer: *Kathi Gosche*

Fifth Edition
Copyright © 2000, 1996, 1992, 1987, 1984 by Mosby, Inc.

Mosby, Inc.
An Imprint of Elsevier Science
11830 Westline Industrial Drive
St Louis, Missouri 63146

Printed in the United States of America

ISBN: 0-323-00924-7 (sc) 0-323-00923-9 (hc)

02 03 GW/KPT 9 8 7 6 5 4

To my parents

For all that they have done for me
and for so many others

Sheila A. Sorrentino

Sheila A. Sorrentino

Sheila A. Sorrentino is currently a curriculum and health care consultant focusing on career ladder nursing programs and effective partnering with assistive personnel in hospitals, long-term care centers, and home care agencies. She has been instrumental in the development and approval of CNA-PN-ADN programs in the Illinois community college system and has taught in nursing assistant, practical nursing, associate degree, bachelor's degree, and master's degree nursing programs. Sheila's career includes experiences as a nursing assistant, staff nurse, charge nurse, head nurse, nursing educator, assistant dean and dean, and consultant. A Mosby author since 1982, Sheila has written several textbooks for nursing assistants and other assistive personnel. She was also involved in the development of a series of skills videos for nursing assistants that won the 1992 International Medical Films Award on caregiving.

Sheila has a bachelor of science degree in nursing, a master of arts degree in education, a master of science degree in community nursing, and a PhD in higher education administration. She is a member and the former chair of the Central Illinois Higher Education Health Care Task Force, is a member of Sigma Theta Tau, and serves on of the Iowa-Illinois Safety Council Board of Directors. In 1998 she received an alumni achievement award from Lewis University for outstanding leadership and dedication in nursing education.

REVIEWERS

Elizabeth Burns, RN, BSN, NMCC
Nurse Manager/Case Manager
Bonell Good Samaritan Center
Greeley, Colorado

Judy Kramer, RN, BSN, BS
San Clemente, California

Susan Lewsen, RN, BSN, MA
Director
Utah Health Technology Certification Center
Kaysville, Utah

Rebecca Rastkar, RN, CFNP
Certified Family Nurse Practitioner
University of Missouri Hospital and Clinics
Columbia, Missouri

Zee Sala, PT
Manager of Rehabilitation Services
Bonell Good Samaritan Center
Greeley, Colorado

Ginny Scribner, RN, BSN, RNC
Consultant
Staff Development Resource
Seattle, Washington

Dorothy Witmer, RN, BSN, MS, EdD
Consultant/Owner
Healthcare Education and Training
Boise, Idaho

ACKNOWLEDGMENTS

Textbooks are written and published by the combined efforts of many people. The planning, manuscript development, review, design, and production processes involve the insights, talents, and contributions of many individuals. I am especially grateful to:

Carol Miller (former Employment Specialist) and Gail Scoates (Director of Home Care) at OSF St. Joseph Medical Center in Bloomington, Illinois, for providing resources and information.

Bernie Gorek, co-author of *Mosby's Textbook for Long-Term Care Assistants* (3rd edition), for her insights, advice, and friendship.

Sandra Sorrentino Bookhout for helping me prepare for art and photography.

Rick Brady of Riva, Maryland, photographer and friend, for his wonderful photography.

The staff at the following agencies for their cooperation and assistance during photography sessions:

- Anne Arundel Medical Center, Annapolis, Maryland
- Pleasant Living Rehabilitation and Skilled Nursing Center, Edgewater, Maryland.
- Providence Hospital, Washington, D.C.
- Bowie Health Center, Bowie, Maryland
- South County Senior Center, Edgewater, Maryland
- Anne Arundel Community College, Arnold, Maryland

The artists at Graphic World, Inc. in St. Louis, Missouri, for their talented work.

Elizabeth Burns, Judy Kramer, Susan Lewsen, Rebecca Rastkar, Zee Sala, Ginny Scribner, and Dorothy Witmer for reviewing the manuscript and for their candor and suggestions. They have contributed to the thoroughness and accuracy of this book.

The people at Mosby, especially Suzi Epstein, Maria Broeker, Graquel Hutchinson, and the members of John Rogers' production team—Betty Hazelwood, Kathy Teal, and Kathi Gosche. In her role as editor, Suzi gave guidance and support and kept the project on track. Maria Broeker handled numerous details and manuscript needs. What would I do without Maria? And Graquel provided clerical and secretarial assistance. Betty Hazelwood, again amazing as a copy editor, made the process fun and painless. Her attention to detail enhanced the quality of this book. Kathy Teal again produced an excellent page layout making the proofreading and production process easy and pleasant. She is a joy to work with. And Kathi Gosche created another unique and colorful book and cover design. She made the book distinctive from the rest.

And to all those who contributed to this effort in any way, I am sincerely grateful.

Sheila A. Sorrentino

PREFACE TO THE INSTRUCTOR

Mosby's Textbook for Nursing Assistants is intended to prepare students to function in the traditional nursing assistant role in nursing centers, hospitals, and home care agencies. Like previous editions, this textbook serves the needs of students and instructors in educational programs taught in community colleges, technical schools, high schools, hospitals, nursing centers, and other agencies. It is also a resource for nursing assistants employed in clinical and home settings.

I believe that an ethical and legal imperative exists to provide individuals with the necessary education and training for safe, effective, and sensitive functioning as a nursing assistant. Focusing on nursing assistant skills and functions, safety, and the psychosocial approach to patient and resident care, the book emphasizes the needs of individuals across the life span, from infancy through old age. Sensitivity to the individual as a person with dignity and value is central to the essence of this book. I believe that students must appreciate the individual as a person with a past, a present, and a future. In every chapter, caring, understanding the person's rights, and respect for patients and residents as individuals with dignity and value are important attitudes and values conveyed to the student.

Also critical to safe and effective functioning is the need to understand the legalities of the role and delegation principles. Because nursing centers, hospitals, and home agencies vary in their use of nursing assistants, the responsibilities and limitations of nursing assistants are emphasized throughout the book and specifically in Chapter 2, which focuses on the ethical and legal aspects of the role. The nursing assistant role also is predicated on a positive work ethic. This concept also is integrated throughout the book with specific workplace behaviors addressed in Chapter 3.

ORGANIZATIONAL STRATEGIES AND VALUES

The concepts and principles related to safety, sensitivity to the individual as a person, ethical and legal aspects, and work ethics serve as the guiding framework for this book. Additional organizational strategies and values include:

- The need for nursing assistants to be aware of and understand their work environment and the individuals in that environment.

- Safe functioning within the legal limits of the nursing assistant role while recognizing that such limits vary among states.
- Respect for the person as a physical, social, psychological, and spiritual being with basic needs and protected rights.
- The importance of personal choice and dignity of person.
- Recognizing the role of cultural heritage in health and illness practices.
- That understanding body structure and function and normal growth and development are helpful for developing desirable attitudes toward individuals and for the safe and competent performance of nursing skills.
- That learning proceeds from the simple to the complex. Concepts and procedures integral to other activities and functions (safety, body mechanics, medical asepsis) are presented early as are those skills basic to the nursing assistant role. More complex content and skills follow.
- That the nursing process is the basis for planning and delivering nursing care and that nursing assistants must follow the person's care plan.

CONTENT ISSUES

Various factors were considered in deciding content issues:

- Minimum standards of the Omnibus Budget Reconciliation Act of 1987
- Various state curricula and training requirements
- Practice trends relating to restraints, subacute care, and advanced roles for assistive personnel
- The changing clientele in nursing centers, hospitals, and home care agencies resulting from managed care
- The special needs of children and older persons
- Cultural influences
- Work settings
- The need for a positive work ethic

These issues were accommodated through reorganization, additional content, and with special features and design elements. Reorganization involved eliminating the Special Procedures and Treatments chapter and the Home Health Care Assistant chapter in the fourth edition and integrating the respective content in new or existing chapters. For example,

- IV therapy content was moved to Chapter 18: Nutrition and Fluids.
- Content on oxygen therapy and collecting sputum specimens was moved to the new Chapter 27: Oxygen Needs.
- Suctioning is presented in Chapter 25: Wound Care and in Chapter 27: Oxygen Needs.
- Vaginal irrigation content was moved to Chapter 24: The Person Having Surgery.

The old Home Health Care Assistant chapter was not comprehensive, and content was often repeated from early chapters. To provide a more thorough and relevant treatment of home care, the home care content was expanded and integrated throughout the book in special *Focus on Home Care boxes.*

New and expanded chapter content and procedures include:

- History and trends related to nursing assistants
- Nurse practice acts
- Delegation principles: who can delegate, the delegation process, the nursing assistant's role in delegation
- Abuse: elderly abuse, child abuse, and domestic abuse
- Work ethics **(new chapter):** personal health, hygiene, and appearance; getting a job (what employers look for, job applications, the job interview, accepting a job); preparing for work (childcare and transportation); on the job (attendance, your attitude, gossip, confidentiality, personal hygiene and appearance, speech and language, courtesies, personal matters, meals and breaks, job safety, planning and organizing your work); harassment; resigning from a job; losing a job
- Dealing with conflict
- Dealing with the angry person
- The immune system
- Safety measures for infants and children
- Safety measures for preventing falls, burns, poisoning, and suffocation
- Restraints: reasons for use, physical and chemical restraints, complications, risks, restraint alternatives, safety guidelines
- Handling hazardous substances
- Workplace violence
- Risk management
- Home safety
- Aseptic measures
- Surgical asepsis: principles and practices; donning and removing sterile gloves
- Urinary drainage systems

- Medical nutrition therapy for diabetes mellitus
- Calorie counts
- Enteral nutrition: routes, formulas, scheduled and continuous feedings, preventing aspiration, observations, comfort measures
- IV therapy: sites, equipment, flow rate, safety measures, signs and symptoms of complications
- Preventing orthostatic hypotension
- Wound care **(new chapter):** types of wounds, pressure ulcers, circulatory ulcers, wound healing, dressings, binders, the person's basic needs
- Oxygen needs **(new chapter):** factors affecting oxygen needs, hypoxia, abnormal respirations, assisting with assessment and diagnostic testing (including pulse oximetry and collecting sputum specimens), promoting oxygenation (positioning, coughing and deep breathing, incentive spirometry), assisting with oxygen therapy, artificial airways (tracheostomies, tracheostomy care), suctioning the airway (routes, safety measures, oropharyngeal suctioning); mechanical ventilation; and chest tubes
- Early warning signs of dementia
- Permanent and temporary dementias
- Types and causes of dementia
- Delirium and depression
- Signs of Alzheimer's disease and the additional behaviors of screaming, abnormal sexual behaviors, repetitive behaviors
- Development disabilities **(new chapter):** mental retardation, Down syndrome, cerebral palsy, autism, epilepsy, spina bifida, hydrocephalus
- Consumer Product Safety Commission's Safety Guide for new and used nursery equipment
- Care of the mother
- Signs and symptoms of postpartum complications
- Anaphylactic shock
- New procedures:
  - Donning and Removing Sterile Gloves
  - Changing a Leg Bag to a Drainage Bag
  - Testing Urine With Reagent Strips
  - Changing an Ostomy Pouch
  - Measuring Height: The Person in Bed or a Wheelchair
  - Applying a Dry, Nonsterile Dressing
  - Using a Pulse Oximeter
  - Setting Up for Oxygen Administration

FEATURES AND DESIGN

As always, producing a readable, user friendly, and inviting book for nursing assistant students was of paramount importance. To achieve this goal, several features and design elements from previous editions were retained and new ones added to enhance the learning process (see Student Preface, p. xv).

- *Illustrations*—the book contains more than 898 full-color photographs and line art. With the exception of borrowed illustrations, this edition features all new line art and photographs.
- *Key terms with definitions*—appear at the beginning of each chapter.
- *Key terms in bold print*—are throughout the text. The definition is presented in narrative of the text. Unlike other books, students do not have to turn to the margin for the definition, return to the text, and then try to understand the context of the term in the text.
- *Boxes and tables*—are used to list principles, guidelines, signs and symptoms, nursing measures, and other information. The boxes and tables are presented in an efficient way for instructors to highlight content and provide useful study guides for students.
- *Bullets*—are used for listed items rather than numbering.
- *Icons*—in section headings alert the reader to an associated procedure. Procedure boxes contain the same icon. **(New!)**
- *Pre-Procedure, Procedure, and Post-Procedure sections*—differentiate procedure sections. Color gradients also differentiate the sections.
- *Quality of Life*—section in the procedure boxes reminds the student to knock before entering the room, address the person by name, and introduce oneself by name and title. **(New!)**
- *NNAAP™ Skill*—appears in the procedure box title bar for skills included in the National Nurse Aide Assessment Program **(New!)***
- *Caring About Culture boxes*—are intended to help

the student learn to appreciate the importance of cultural diversity and how culture influences health and illness practices. **(New!)**
- *Focus on Children boxes*—provide age-specific information about the needs, considerations, and special circumstances of children. This feature is useful in meeting age-specific training requirements of the Joint Commission on Accreditation of Healthcare Organizations. **(New!)**
- *Focus on Older Persons boxes*—provide age-specific information about the needs, considerations, and special circumstances of older persons. This feature is useful in meeting age-specific training requirements of the Joint Commission on Accreditation of Healthcare Organizations. **(New!)**
- *Focus on Home Care boxes*—highlight information necessary for safe functioning in the home setting. **(New!)**
- *Focus on Long-Term Care boxes*—highlight information unique to the long-term care setting. Such information includes requirements of the Omnibus Budget Reconciliation Act of 1987 (OBRA). **(New!)**
- *Review questions*—are found at the end of each chapter. They are followed by the page number where the answers are listed.

I hope that this book will serve you and your students well. My intent is to provide you and your students with the information needed to teach and learn safe and effective care during this time of dynamic change in health care.

Sheila A. Sorrentino, RN, BSN, MA, MSN, PhD

---

*NNAAP™ is a registered trademark of ASI and the National Council of State Boards of Nursing.

STUDENT PREFACE

This book was designed for you. It was designed to help you learn. The book is a useful resource as you gain experience and expand your knowledge.

This preface gives some study guidelines and helps you use the book. When given a reading assignment, do you read from the first page to the last page without stopping? How much do you remember? You will learn more if you use a study system. A useful study system has these steps:

- Survey or preview
- Question
- Read and record
- Recite and review

PREVIEW

Before you start a reading assignment, preview or survey the assignment. This gives you an idea of what the assignment covers. It also helps you recall what you already know about the subject. Carefully look over the assignment. Preview the chapter title, headings, subheadings, and terms or ideas in bold print or italics. Also survey the objectives, key terms, first paragraph, boxes, and the review questions at the end of the chapter. Previewing takes only a few minutes. Remember, previewing helps you become familiar with the material.

QUESTION

After previewing, you need to form questions to answer while you read. Questions should relate to what might be asked on a test or how the information applies to giving care. Use the title, headings, and subheadings to form questions. Avoid questions that have one-word answers. Questions that begin with what, how, or why are helpful. While reading, you may find that a question does not help you study. If so, just change the question. Remember, questioning sets a purpose for reading. So changing a question only makes this step more useful.

READ AND RECORD

Reading is the next step. Reading is more productive after determining what you already know and what you need to learn. Read to find answers to your questions. The purpose of reading is to:

- Gain new information
- Connect the new information to what you know already

Break the assignment into smaller parts. Then answer your questions as you read each part. Also, mark important information. The information can be marked by underlining, highlighting, or making notes. Underlining and highlighting remind you what you need to learn. You need to go back and review the marked parts later. Making notes results in more immediate learning. When making notes, you write down important information in the margins or in a notebook. Use words and summary statements that will jog your memory about the material.

After reading the assignment, you need to remember the information. To remember the material, you must work with the information. This step involves organizing information into a study guide. Study guides have many forms. Diagrams or charts help show relationships or steps in a process. Much of the information in this text is organized in this manner to help you learn. Note taking in outline format is also very useful. The following is a sample outline.

I. Main heading
  a. Second level
  b. Second level
    1. Third level
    2. Third level
II. Main heading

RECITE AND REVIEW

Finally, recite and review. Use your notes and the study guides. Answer the questions you formed earlier. Also answer any other questions that came up during the reading and the review questions at the end of the chapter. Answer all questions out loud (recite).

Reviewing is more about *when* to study rather than *what* to study. You already determined what to study during the preview, question, and reading steps. The best times to review the material are right after the first study session, one week later, and regularly before a quiz or test, midterm, or final exam.

I hope you enjoy learning and your work. You and your work are important. You and the care you give may be bright spots in a person's day. This book was designed also to help you study. Special design features are described on the next pages.

Objectives tell what is presented in the chapter and what you will learn.

Key terms are the important words and phrases in the chapter. Definitions are given for each term. The key terms introduce you to the chapter content. They are also useful study guides.

Bolded type is used to highlight the key terms in the text. You again see the key term and read its definition. This helps reinforce your learning.

Color illustrations and photographs visually present a key idea, concept, or procedure step. They help you apply and remember the written material.

OBJECTIVES

Define the key terms listed in this chapter
Explain the purpose and rules of using good body mechanics
Identify comfort and safety measures for lifting, turning, and moving persons in bed
Know the basic bed positions
Explain the purpose of a transfer belt
Explain why good body alignment and position changes are important
Identify the comfort and safety measures for positioning persons in bed
Position persons in the basic bed positions and in a chair
Perform the procedures described in this chapter

KEY TERMS

base of support The area on which an object rests

body alignment The way in which body parts are aligned with one another; posture

body mechanics Using the body in an efficient and careful way

dorsal recumbent position The back-lying or supine position

Fowler's position A semisitting position; the head of the bed is elevated 45 to 60 degrees

friction The rubbing of one surface against another

gait belt A transfer or safety belt

lateral position The side-lying position

logrolling Turning the person as a unit, in alignment, with one motion

posture The way in which body parts are aligned with one another; body alignment

prone position Lying on the abdomen with the head turned to one side

safety belt A transfer belt or gait belt

shearing When skin sticks to a surface and muscles slide in the direction the body is moving

side-lying position The lateral position

Sims' position A left side-lying position in which the upper leg is sharply flexed so that it is not on the lower leg and the lower arm is behind the person

supine position The back-lying or dorsal recumbent position

transfer belt A belt used to hold onto a person during a transfer or when walking with the person; a gait belt or safety belt

You will turn and reposition patients and residents in bed. You also transfer them to and from chairs, wheelchairs, and stretchers. During these and other activities, you must use your body correctly. This protects you and the person from injury.

Box 11-1 contains a review of the structure and function of the musculoskeletal system. For more detailed information, see Chapter 6.

BODY MECHANICS

Body mechanics means using the body in an efficient and careful way. It involves good posture and balance and using the strongest and largest muscles for work. Fatigue, muscle strain, and injury can result from improper use and positioning of the body during activity or rest. You must focus on the person's and your

Mosby's Textbook for Nursing Assistants   **304**

42

Fig. 11-16 Turning the person away from you.   Fig. 11-17 Turning the person toward you.

Icons in the headings alert you to an associated procedure. Procedure boxes contain the same icon.

Procedures are written in a step-by-step format. They are divided into pre-procedure, procedure, and post-procedure sections for easy studying.

Focus on Older Persons boxes provide age-specific information about the needs, considerations, and special circumstances of older persons.

NNAAP™ in the procedure title bar alerts you to those skills that are part of the National Nurse Aide Assessment Program (NNAAP™). The NNAAP skills identified in this textbook may be evaluated in part or in full on the NNAAP™ Skills Evaluation.

Quality of Life in the procedure boxes reminds you to knock before entering the room, to call the person by name, and to introduce yourself by name and title. These simple courtesies show respect for the person.

Boxes and tables contain important rules, principles, guidelines, signs and symptoms, nursing measures, and other information in a list format. They identify important information and are useful study guides for reviewing.

Caring About Culture boxes contain information to help you learn about the various practices of other cultures.

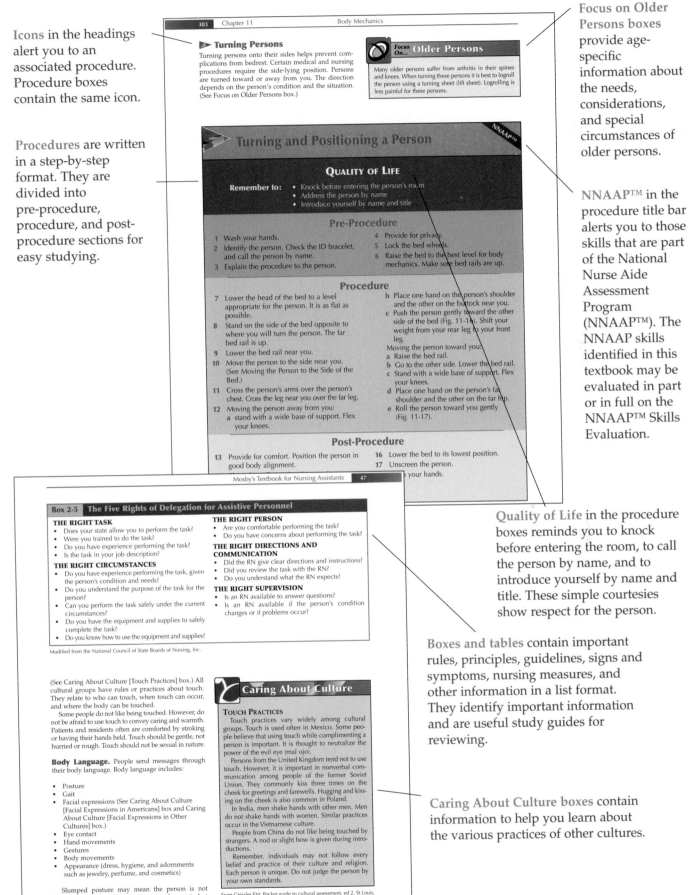

303 Chapter 11 Body Mechanics

► Turning Persons

Turning persons onto their sides helps prevent complications from bedrest. Certain medical and nursing procedures require the side-lying position. Persons are turned toward or away from you. The direction depends on the person's condition and the situation. (See Focus on Older Persons box.)

Focus On... Older Persons

Many older persons suffer from arthritis in their spines and knees. When turning these persons it is best to logroll the person using a turning sheet (lift sheet). Logrolling is less painful for these persons.

Turning and Positioning a Person

QUALITY OF LIFE

Remember to:
- Knock before entering the person's room
- Address the person by name
- Introduce yourself by name and title

Pre-Procedure

1. Wash your hands.
2. Identify the person. Check the ID bracelet, and call the person by name.
3. Explain the procedure to the person.
4. Provide for privacy.
5. Lock the bed wheels.
6. Raise the bed to the best level for body mechanics. Make sure bed rails are up.

Procedure

7. Lower the head of the bed to a level appropriate for the person. It is as flat as possible.
8. Stand on the side of the bed opposite to where you will turn the person. The far bed rail is up.
9. Lower the bed rail near you.
10. Move the person to the side near you. (See Moving the Person to the Side of the Bed.)
11. Cross the person's arms over the person's chest. Cross the leg near you over the far leg.
12. Moving the person away from you:
    a stand with a wide base of support. Flex your knees.

b Place one hand on the person's shoulder and the other on the buttock near you.
c Push the person gently toward the other side of the bed (Fig. 11-16). Shift your weight from your rear leg to your front leg.
Moving the person toward you:
a Raise the bed rail.
b Go to the other side. Lower the bed rail.
c Stand with a wide base of support. Flex your knees.
d Place one hand on the person's far shoulder and the other on the far hip.
e Roll the person toward you gently (Fig. 11-17).

Post-Procedure

13. Provide for comfort. Position the person in good body alignment.
16. Lower the bed to its lowest position.
17. Unscreen the person.
   ...h your hands.

Mosby's Textbook for Nursing Assistants 47

Box 2-5 The Five Rights of Delegation for Assistive Personnel

THE RIGHT TASK
- Does your state allow you to perform the task?
- Were you trained to do the task?
- Do you have experience performing the task?
- Is the task in your job description?

THE RIGHT CIRCUMSTANCES
- Do you have experience performing the task, given the person's condition and needs?
- Do you understand the purpose of the task for the person?
- Can you perform the task safely under the current circumstances?
- Do you have the equipment and supplies to safely complete the task?
- Do you know how to use the equipment and supplies?

THE RIGHT PERSON
- Are you comfortable performing the task?
- Do you have concerns about performing the task?

THE RIGHT DIRECTIONS AND COMMUNICATION
- Did the RN give clear directions and instructions?
- Did you review the task with the RN?
- Do you understand what the RN expects?

THE RIGHT SUPERVISION
- Is an RN available to answer questions?
- Is an RN available if the person's condition changes or if problems occur?

Modified from the National Council of State Boards of Nursing, Inc.

(See Caring About Culture [Touch Practices] box.) All cultural groups have rules or practices about touch. They relate to who can touch, when touch can occur, and where the body can be touched.

Some people do not like being touched. However, do not be afraid to use touch to convey caring and warmth. Patients and residents often are comforted by stroking or having their hands held. Touch should be gentle, not hurried or rough. Touch should not be sexual in nature.

Body Language. People send messages through their body language. Body language includes:

- Posture
- Gait
- Facial expressions (See Caring About Culture [Facial Expressions in Americans] box and Caring About Culture [Facial Expressions in Other Cultures] box.)
- Eye contact
- Hand movements
- Gestures
- Body movements
- Appearance (dress, hygiene, and adornments such as jewelry, perfume, and cosmetics)

Slumped posture may mean the person is not happy or feeling well. A person may deny pain but protects the affected body part by standing, lying, or sitting in a certain way. People send many other messages with body language.

You also send messages by the way you act and move. Your facial expressions and how you stand, sit, walk, and look at a person all send messages.

Caring About Culture

TOUCH PRACTICES
Touch practices vary widely among cultural groups. Touch is used often in Mexico. Some people believe that using touch while complimenting a person is important. It is thought to neutralize the power of the evil eye (mal ojo).

Persons from the United Kingdom tend not to use touch. However, it is important in nonverbal communication among people of the former Soviet Union. They commonly kiss three times on the cheek for greetings and farewells. Hugging and kissing on the cheek is also common in Poland.

In India, men shake hands with other men. Men do not shake hands with women. Similar practices occur in the Vietnamese culture.

People from China do not like being touched by strangers. A nod or slight bow is given during introductions.

Remember, individuals may not follow every belief and practice of their culture and religion. Each person is unique. Do not judge the person by your own standards.

From Geissler EM: Pocket guide to cultural assessment, ed 2, St Louis, 1998, Mosby.

Focus on Children boxes provide age-specific information about the needs, considerations, and special circumstances of children.

Focus on Long-Term Care boxes highlight information unique to the long-term care setting. Such information includes requirements of the Omnibus Budget Reconciliation Act of 1987 (OBRA).

Focus on Home Care boxes highlight information necessary for safe functioning in the home setting.

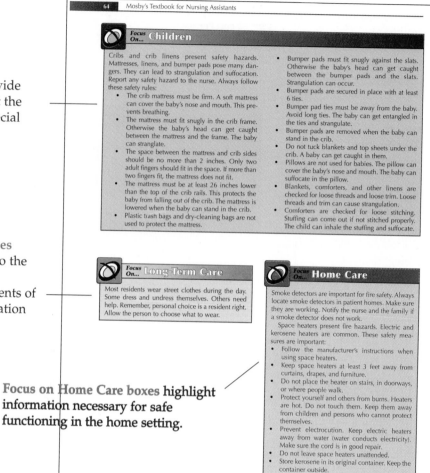

64   Mosby's Textbook for Nursing Assistants

Focus On... Children

Cribs and crib linens present safety hazards. Mattresses, linens, and bumper pads pose many dangers. They can lead to strangulation and suffocation. Report any safety hazard to the nurse. Always follow these safety rules:

- The crib mattress must be firm. A soft mattress can cover the baby's nose and mouth. This prevents breathing.
- The mattress must fit snugly in the crib frame. Otherwise the baby's head can get caught between the mattress and the frame. The baby can strangle.
- The space between the mattress and crib sides should be no more than 2 inches. Only two adult fingers should fit in the space. If more than two fingers fit, the mattress does not fit.
- The mattress must be at least 26 inches lower than the top of the crib rails. This protects the baby from falling out of the crib. The mattress is lowered when the baby can stand in the crib.
- Plastic trash bags and dry-cleaning bags are not used to protect the mattress.

- Bumper pads must fit snugly against the slats. Otherwise the baby's head can get caught between the bumper pads and the slats. Strangulation can occur.
- Bumper pads are secured in place with at least 6 ties.
- Bumper pad ties must be away from the baby. Avoid long ties. The baby can get entangled in the ties and strangulate.
- Bumper pads are removed when the baby can stand in the crib.
- Do not tuck blankets and top sheets under the crib. A baby can get caught in them.
- Pillows are not used for babies. The pillow can cover the baby's nose and mouth. The baby can suffocate in the pillow.
- Blankets, comforters, and other linens are checked for loose threads and loose trim. Loose threads and trim can cause strangulation.
- Comforters are checked for loose stitching. Stuffing can come out if not stitched properly. The child can inhale the stuffing and suffocate.

Focus On... Long-Term Care

Most residents wear street clothes during the day. Some dress and undress themselves. Others need help. Remember, personal choice is a resident right. Allow the person to choose what to wear.

Focus On... Home Care

Smoke detectors are important for fire safety. Always locate smoke detectors in patient homes. Make sure they are working. Notify the nurse and the family if a smoke detector does not work.

Space heaters present fire hazards. Electric and kerosene heaters are common. These safety measures are important:

- Follow the manufacturer's instructions when using space heaters.
- Keep space heaters at least 3 feet away from curtains, drapes, and furniture.
- Do not place the heater on stairs, in doorways, or where people walk.
- Protect yourself and others from burns. Heaters are hot. Do not touch them. Keep them away from children and persons who cannot protect themselves.
- Prevent electrocution. Keep electric heaters away from water (water conducts electricity). Make sure the cord is in good repair.
- Do not leave space heaters unattended.
- Store kerosene in its original container. Keep the container outside.

Review questions are a useful study guide. They help you to review what you have learned. They can also be used when studying for a test or the competency evaluation. Answers are given at the back of the book beginning on p. 833.

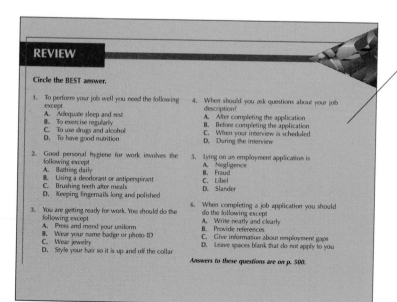

REVIEW

Circle the BEST answer.

1. To perform your job well you need the following except
   A. Adequate sleep and rest
   B. To exercise regularly
   C. To use drugs and alcohol
   D. To have good nutrition

2. Good personal hygiene for work involves the following except
   A. Bathing daily
   B. Using a deodorant or antiperspirant
   C. Brushing teeth after meals
   D. Keeping fingernails long and polished

3. You are getting ready for work. You should do the following except
   A. Press and mend your uniform
   B. Wear your name badge or photo ID
   C. Wear jewelry
   D. Style your hair so it is up and off the collar

4. When should you ask questions about your job description?
   A. After completing the application
   B. Before completing the application
   C. When your interview is scheduled
   D. During the interview

5. Lying on an employment application is
   A. Negligence
   B. Fraud
   C. Libel
   D. Slander

6. When completing a job application you should do the following except
   A. Write neatly and clearly
   B. Provide references
   C. Give information about employment gaps
   D. Leave spaces blank that do not apply to you

Answers to these questions are on p. 500.

CONTENTS

Mosby's Textbook for

NURSING
ASSISTANTS

INTRODUCTION TO HEALTH CARE AGENCIES

Define the key terms listed in this chapter

Explain the purposes and services of health care agencies

Identify the members of the health team and the nursing team

Describe the nursing service department

Know the differences between RNs, LPNs/LVNs, and nursing assistants

Explain how nursing assistants are members of the nursing team

Describe four nursing care patterns

Describe the programs that pay for health care

KEY TERMS

acute illness A sudden illness from which a person is expected to recover

assistive personnel A broad term applied to nursing staff who assist nurses in giving care

case management A nursing care pattern; a case manager (an RN) coordinates a person's care from admission through discharge and into the home setting

chronic illness An on-going illness, slow or gradual in onset, for which there is no known cure; the illness can be controlled and complications prevented

functional nursing A nursing care pattern that focuses on tasks and jobs; nursing personnel have specific tasks to do

health team Staff members who work together to provide health care

hospice A health care agency or program for persons who are dying

licensed practical nurse (LPN) An individual who completed a 1-year nursing program and passed a state licensing examination; called licensed vocational nurse (LVN) in some states

nursing assistant An individual who gives basic nursing care under the supervision of an RN or LPN/LVN

nursing team Individuals who provide nursing care—RNs, LPNs/LVNs, and nursing assistants

patient-focused care A nursing care pattern; hospital services are moved from departments to the bedside

primary nursing A nursing care pattern; an RN is responsible for patients' total care

registered nurse (RN) An individual who studied nursing for 2, 3, or 4 years and passed a state licensing examination

team nursing A nursing care pattern; the team leader (an RN) delegates the care of specific persons to RNs and LPNs/LVNs and delegates nursing tasks to nursing assistants

terminal illness An illness or injury for which there is no reasonable expectation of recovery

The many types of health care agencies include hospitals, long-term care centers, and home care agencies. Mental health hospitals, community centers, adult day care centers, hospices, doctors' offices, clinics, homes for persons with mental retardation, and centers for disabled persons are other health care agencies. There are also centers for drug and alcohol treatment and crisis centers for rape, abuse, suicide, and other mental health emergencies.

The people working in these agencies have special talents, knowledge, and skills. All work to meet the person's needs. The *person* is the focus of care.

HEALTH CARE AGENCIES

Health care agencies offer services to persons needing health care. The many services range from the simple to the complex. Some offer only one type of service.

PURPOSE

Health care agencies are concerned with health promotion, disease prevention, the detection and treatment of disease, and rehabilitation.

- *Health promotion* includes physical and mental health. The goal is to reduce the risk of illness. Health is promoted by teaching and counseling people about healthy living. This includes diet, exercise, changing unhealthy habits, and the warning signs and symptoms of illness. Ill persons are taught how to manage and cope with their diseases.
- *Disease prevention* involves identifying the risk factors and early warning signs of disease. Measures are taken to reduce the risk factors and prevent the disease. Simple life-style changes can prevent major health problems. For example, high blood pressure is noted during Mr. Parson's physical examination. High blood pressure can lead to heart attacks and brain attacks (strokes). Mr. Parsons has to exercise and change his diet to lower his blood pressure. Immunizations are another example. They prevent many infectious diseases such as polio, measles, mumps, smallpox, and hepatitis.
- *Detection and treatment of disease* are done by diagnostic testing, physical examinations, surgery, emergency care, and drugs. Treatment often involves respiratory therapy, physical therapy, and occupational therapy. Nursing is involved by observing signs and symptoms, giving care, and carrying out treatment measures ordered by the doctor.
- *Rehabilitation* (or restorative care) helps persons return to their highest possible level of physical and psychological functioning. It starts when the person first seeks health care. Rehabilitation helps persons learn or relearn the skills needed to live, work, and enjoy life. Maintaining function is also an important part of rehabilitation. The person also is assisted with making needed changes at home.

Many agencies provide work-based learning experiences for students. Students study to become nurses, doctors, x-ray and laboratory technicians, dietitians, or nursing assistants. These students also assist in health promotion, disease prevention, disease detection and treatment, and rehabilitation.

These purposes are all related. For example, Mr. Parsons goes to an emergency room with severe chest pain and difficulty breathing. After an examination and laboratory tests, the doctor makes the diagnosis of heart attack. Mr. Parsons is admitted to the hospital for treatment. During treatment, he is given health teaching and counseling about the causes of a heart attack and about changing habits. He is taught the importance of not smoking, eating a low-fat diet, and exercise. The teaching and counseling are done to promote health and to prevent another heart attack. Mr. Parsons is probably afraid of dying and worried about not leading an active life. A rehabilitation program is planned that begins activity slowly. Activity may progress to walking, jogging, or swimming. More teaching and counseling focus on diet, drugs, lifestyle, and activity. Mr. Parsons and his family are encouraged to talk about their fears and concerns and are given help in learning to cope. Thus a successful rehabilitation program helps promote the person's health and may prevent another heart attack.

TYPES OF AGENCIES

Nursing assistants work in many settings. Some work in doctors' offices. Most work in the following agencies.

Hospitals. Hospital services include emergency care, surgery, nursing care, x-ray procedures and treatments, and laboratory testing. Services also include respiratory therapy, physical therapy, occupational therapy, and speech therapy. People of all ages need hospital care. They go to have babies, for mental health problems, to have surgery, to heal broken bones, to diagnose and treat medical problems, or to die. Persons can have acute, terminal, or chronic illnesses:

- **Acute illness** begins suddenly. The person is expected to recover.
- **Chronic illness** is an on-going illness that often begins slowly and has no cure. With treatment, the illness can be controlled and complications prevented.
- **Terminal illness** eventually results in death (Chapter 37).

Some hospital stays are very short—less than 24 hours. Others last days, weeks, or months depending on the person's condition and illness. Outpatient services are common. The person needs hospital services but does not stay 24 hours. Some surgeries, diagnostic procedures, and therapies do not require 24-hour stays.

Subacute Care Agencies. Hospital stays are shorter than in the past because of changes in insurance coverage. A person does not need hospital care but is too sick to go home. The person's condition is stable. However, the person still needs medical care or rehabilitation. The person's needs fall between hospital care and long-term care. The person's care requires the use of complex equipment and care measures.

Subacute care has a strong focus on rehabilitation. Common programs include:

- *Ventilator weaning.* The person requires a mechanical ventilator for breathing (see Chapter 27). The goal is for the person to be able to breathe without the ventilator.
- *Pulmonary rehabilitation.* For example, the person has a tracheostomy (see Chapter 27). If the tracheostomy is temporary, the goal is for the person to breathe without it. If the tracheostomy is permanent, the person learns how to manage and care for it.
- *Wound management.* The person has chronic wounds from surgery or trauma (see Chapter 25). Wound healing is the goal.
- *Neurological rehabilitation.* The person had a brain attack (stroke) or has another neurological disease or injury (see Chapter 30).
- *Orthopedic rehabilitation.* The person had joint replacement surgery. Persons with some bone, joint, or muscle injuries or diseases may require subacute care.
- *Complex medical care.* The person has a complex heart, kidney, digestive, or other disorder. Cancer patients receiving chemotherapy and AIDS patients may require complex medical care (see Chapter 30).

Subacute care units are found in hospitals and long-term care centers. Separate agencies for subacute care are growing in number. Persons needing subacute care may fully recover. Others may need long-term care someday.

Long-Term Care Centers. Long-term care centers (nursing homes, nursing facilities, nursing centers) provide services to persons who cannot care for themselves at home but who do not need hospital care. These agencies provide medical, nursing, dietary, rec-reational, rehabilitative, and social services.

Persons in long-term care centers are called residents, not patients. They are residents because the center is their temporary or permanent home. Most residents are older, with chronic diseases, poor nutrition, or poor health. Long-term care centers are designed to meet the special needs of older persons (Fig. 1-1).

Not all residents are old. Some residents are permanently disabled from birth defects, accidents, or diseases. People often are discharged from hospitals while still sick or still recovering from surgery (see Paying for Health Care). Home care is an option for some. Others need long-term care. Some residents recover and return home; others need nursing care until death. *(See Focus on Long-term Care boxes throughout this book.)*

Fig. 1-1 Room in a long-term care center.

Mental Health Agencies. Mental health centers or hospitals care for and treat persons with mental illnesses. Some persons have difficulty dealing with events in life. Others are dangerous to themselves or others because of how they think and behave. Outpatient treatment is common. Some persons need hospital care for a short time or for life.

Home Care Agencies. Home care agencies provide care for persons in their homes. Public health departments, private businesses, and hospitals provide home care services. Services range from health teaching and supervision to bedside nursing care. Some older persons and persons who are dying often need home care. Besides nursing care, home care agencies may provide physical therapy, rehabilitation, and food services. Home care and the role of the nursing assistant are featured in *Focus on Home Care* boxes throughout this book.

Hospices. A **hospice** is a health care agency or program for persons who are dying. The physical, emotional, social, and spiritual needs of the person and family are provided for in a setting that allows much freedom. The person and family have much control over the person's quality of life. Children and pets usually can visit at any time. Family and friends can take part in giving care. Hospice care is provided by hospitals, long-term care centers, and home care agencies.

Health Care Systems. A health care system involves health care agencies joining together as one provider of care. The system usually includes one or more hospitals, long-term care centers, home care agencies, hospice settings, and doctors (Fig. 1-2, p. 4). Ambulance services and medical supply stores for home care are common. The system may serve a community or a large region.

| Box 1-1 | **Using a Health Care System** |

Dr. Moore practices in the health care system that owns Mercy Hospital. The hospital has a subacute unit and operates LifeCare Ambulance Service, a home care agency, and a medical supply store. Lakeside Nursing Center also is part of the system.

June Adams, age 78, sees Dr. Moore in his office. She complains of tightness in her chest, dizziness, and a "pounding heartbeat." Dr. Moore admits her to Mercy Hospital. He asks Dr. Gills, another Mercy Hospital doctor and a heart specialist (cardiologist), to take over her care. While in the hospital she has a heart attack. A few days later she has a brain attack (stroke) and cannot move the left side of her body. She is given needed medical care. When her condition is stable, she is transferred to the subacute unit.

After several days in the subacute unit, Mrs. Adams has the choice of having home care or going to a nursing center. She wants to go home. Her sister and her son and his wife want to help care for her. A nurse tells them about the need for a hospital bed, bedside commode, bedpan, wheelchair, and other equipment and supplies. They rent some items and buy others at the medical supply store owned by Mercy Hospital.

The nurse arranges for Mrs. Adams to be transported home by LifeCare Ambulance Service. The nurse also works with Mercy Hospital's home care agency to provide home care services.

Mrs. Adams is at home. Every day a nursing assistant comes to bathe her and assist with other hygiene and grooming needs. A nurse visits three times a week. The nurse and nursing assistant work for Mercy Hospital's home care agency.

A month later Mrs. Adams has another brain attack. She is taken to Mercy Hospital by LifeCare Ambulance Service. After an 8-day hospital stay, she is transferred to the subacute unit for rehabilitation. The second brain attack has caused more disabilities. Dr. Gills advises Mrs. Adams and her family that home care may be difficult. He suggests nursing home care. Mrs. Adams and her family discuss the matter and agree with the need for a nursing home. The nurse then arranges for Mrs. Adams to be admitted to Lakeside Nursing Center. She is transferred there by LifeCare Ambulance Service.

Fig. 1-2 The hospital and doctors' offices are part of a health care system. *(Courtesy Anne Arundel Health System Inc., Annapolis, Md.)*

A health care system intends to serve all health care needs. A person entering the system is referred to other system providers as needed (Box 1-1).

ORGANIZATION

An agency has a governing body called the *board of trustees.* The board makes policies for the agency to ensure that it gives good, safe care at the lowest possible cost. An administrator manages the agency and reports directly to the board. Directors or department heads are responsible for specific areas. Figure 1-3 is a sample organizational chart.

The Health Team. The **health team** involves staff members whose skills and knowledge are directed to the person's total care (Table 1-1, pp. 5-6). Their goal is to provide quality care. Health team members work together to meet the person's needs. The person is the focus of the health care team (Fig. 1-4, p. 7).

Many staff members are involved in the care of one person. Coordinated care is important. A registered nurse (RN) usually coordinates the person's care.

Nursing Service. Nursing service is a major department. The director of nursing (DON) is an RN. (Other titles include vice president of nursing and vice president of patient services.) Usually a bachelor's or master's degree is required for the position. The DON is responsible for the entire nursing staff. This includes the activities involved in giving safe nursing care. Nurse managers (also RNs) assist the director in managing and carrying out the department's functions.

Nurse managers are responsible for a work shift or nursing area. Hospital nursing areas include surgical nursing units, medical nursing units, intensive care units, maternity departments, pediatric units, operating and recovery rooms, an emergency department, and a mental health nursing unit. Nurse managers are responsible for all nursing care and the actions of nursing staff in their areas.

Each nursing area has RNs. They provide nursing care and supervise the work of LPNs/LVNs and

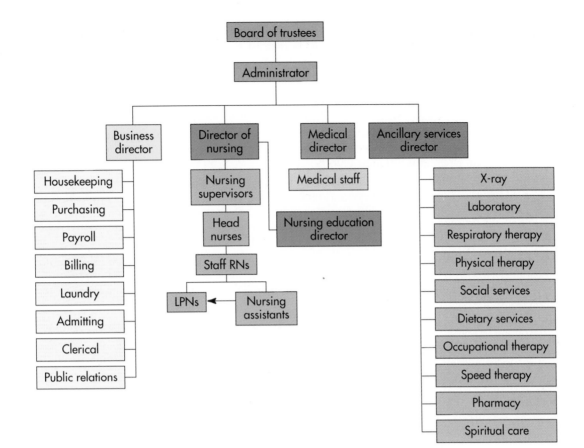

Fig. 1-3 The organizational chart of a health care agency.

Table 1-1	Health Team Members	
Title	**Description**	**Credentials**
Activities director	Assesses, plans, and implements recreational needs	Required training varies with state and/or employer; ranges from no training to bachelor's degree
Assistive personnel	Assist RNs and LPNs/LVNs in giving nursing care; must be supervised by a nurse	Must meet federal and state training requirements to work in long-term care and in some agencies; regulated training forthcoming in some states
Audiologist	Tests hearing; prescribes hearing aids; works with hearing-impaired persons	Master's degree in audiology, 1 year of supervised employment, and a national examination
Cleric (clergyman; clergywoman)	Assists persons with their spiritual needs	Priest, minister, rabbi, sister (nun), deacon, or other cleric with pastoral training
Dietitian	Assesses and plans for nutritional needs; teaches individuals and families about good nutrition, food selection, and preparation	Bachelor's degree; registered dietitian (RD) must pass a national registration examination; some states require licensure
Licensed practical/ vocational nurse (LPN/LVN)	Provides direct patient and resident care, including the administration of medications, under the direction of an RN	Graduate of a state-approved program (usually 1 year in length) and state licensure

Continued

Table 1-1	Health Team Members—cont'd	
Title	**Description**	**Credentials**
Medical laboratory technician (MLT)	Collects samples and performs laboratory tests on blood, urine, and other body fluids, secretions, and excretions	Graduate of a 2-year program and national certifying examination; state licensure may be required
Medical records technician	Maintains medical records; transcribes medical reports, files records, completes required reports	Graduate of a two-year program; takes the national accredited record technician (ART) examination
Medical technologist (MT)	Performs complicated laboratory tests on blood, urine, and other body fluids, secretions, and excretions; organizes, supervises, and performs diagnostic analyses; supervises MLTs	Bachelor's degree in medical technology; national certification examination; licensure required in some states
Occupational therapist (OT)	Assists persons to learn or retain skills needed to perform activities of daily living; designs adaptive equipment for activities of daily living	Bachelor's degree in occupational therapy and national certification; licensure required in some states
Pharmacist	Fills medication orders written by a doctor; monitors and evaluates drug interactions; consults with doctors and nurses about drug actions and interactions	Bachelor's degree in pharmacy and state licensure
Physical therapist (PT)	Assists persons with musculoskeletal problems; focuses on restoring function and preventing disability from illness or injury	Bachelor's degree in physical therapy and state licensure
Physician (doctor)	Diagnoses and treats diseases and injuries	Medical school graduate, residency, and national board examination; state licensure
Podiatrist	Prevents, diagnoses, and treats foot disorders	Doctor of Podiatric Medicine (DPM); state and/or national certification
Radiographer/ radiologic technologist	Takes x-rays and processes film for viewing	Graduate of an accredited program and national registry examination
Registered nurse (RN)	Assesses, makes nursing diagnoses, plans, implements, and evaluates nursing care; supervises LPNs/LVNs and assistive personnel	Graduate of a state-approved program with an associate degree, diploma, or bachelor's degree; state licensure
Respiratory therapist	Assists in treatment of lung and heart disorders; gives respiratory treatments and therapies	Graduation from a 1- or 2-year program and certification by National Board of Respiratory Therapy
Social worker	Helps persons and families with social, emotional, and environmental issues affecting illness and recovery; coordinates community agencies to assist persons and families	Bachelor's or master's degree in social work
Speech-language pathologist	Evaluates speech and language and treats persons with speech, voice, hearing, communication, and swallowing disorders	Master's degree in speech/language pathology, 1 year supervised work experience, and national examination

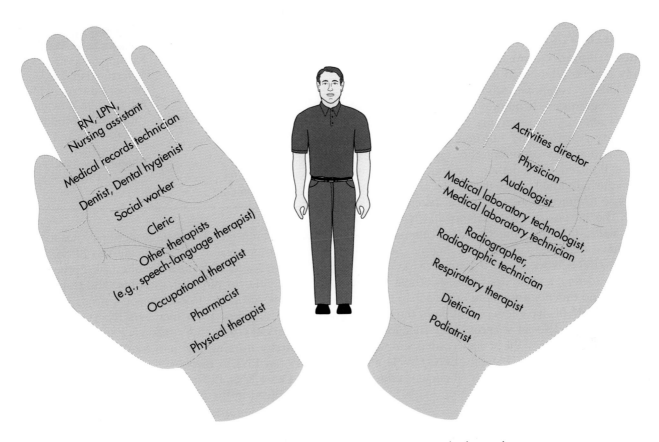

Fig. 1-4 Members the of the health team, with the person as the focus of care.

nursing assistants. Staff RNs report to the head nurse or nurse manager. LPNs/LVNs report to staff RNs or to the head nurses or nurse managers. You report to the RN or LPN/LVN supervising your work.

A nursing education department is also part of nursing service. Nursing education staff plan and present educational programs to nursing personnel so that current and safe care is given. This department also educates and trains nursing assistants. It also conducts new employee orientation programs.

THE NURSING TEAM

The nursing team involves RNs, LPNs/LVNs, and nursing assistants. Each has different roles and responsibilities. All are concerned with the physical, social, emotional, and spiritual needs of patients and residents and their families.

REGISTERED NURSES

A **registered nurse (RN)** studies for 2 years at a community college, 2 or 3 years in a hospital-based diploma program, or 4 years at a college or university. Nursing and the biological, social, and physical sciences are studied. The graduate nurse takes a licensing examination offered by a state board of nursing. The nurse must pass the examination to become *registered* and receive a license to practice. RNs must be licensed by the state in which they practice.

RNs assess, make nursing diagnoses, plan, implement, and evaluate nursing care. An RN identifies a person's nursing problems and develops a care plan. The RN carries out the plan. The RN also delegates nursing care to LPNs/LVNs and nursing tasks to nursing assistants. The RN then evaluates the effect of the care plan and nursing care on the person. The person is helped to become independent and is taught ways to stay or become healthy. Family teaching is provided.

The RN is responsible for carrying out the doctor's orders. The RN may carry out the orders or delegate them to LPNs/LVNs or nursing assistants. RNs do not diagnose diseases or illnesses or prescribe treatments or medications. However, RNs can study to become clinical nurse specialists or nurse practitioners. Special certification is required. These RNs are involved in diagnosing and prescribing.

RNs work as staff nurses, nurse managers, directors of nursing, and instructors. Their job opportunities depend on their education, professional abilities, and experience.

LICENSED PRACTICAL NURSES AND LICENSED VOCATIONAL NURSES

A **licensed practical nurse (LPN)** completes 1 year of study in a hospital-based nursing program, community college, vocational school, or technical school. Some programs are 18 months long. Some public high schools offer 2-year programs. Students study nursing, body structure and function, basic psychology, mathematics, and communication skills. Graduates take a licensing examination for practical nursing. When the individual passes the test, he or she receives a license to practice and the title of *licensed practical nurse.* The title *licensed vocational nurse (LVN)* is used in some states. Like RNs, practical or vocational nurses must have a license to practice nursing.

LPNs/LVNs work under the supervision of RNs, licensed doctors, and licensed dentists. Their responsibilities and functions are more limited than those of RNs. LPNs/LVNs have less education in the biological, physical, and social sciences. They function with little supervision when the person's care is simple and the person's condition is stable. LPNs/LVNs assist RNs in providing care to acutely ill persons and with complex procedures.

NURSING ASSISTANTS

Nursing assistants give basic nursing care under the supervision of RNs. Some states allow LPNs/LVNs to supervise nursing assistants. There are many titles for nursing assistants. The title depends on the setting and the nursing assistant's role and functions. **Assistive personnel** is a broad term that applies to nursing staff who assist nurses in giving care (Box 1-2). The term includes nursing assistants. Hospitals, long-term care centers, community colleges, technical schools, and high school vocational programs offer courses for assistive personnel. Assistive personnel are discussed in greater detail in Chapter 2.

NURSING CARE PATTERNS

Safe and effective nursing care is provided in different ways. The nursing care pattern depends on how many persons need care, the available staff, and the cost.

Functional nursing focuses on tasks and jobs. Each nursing team member has certain functions or tasks to do. For example, one RN gives all drugs. Another RN changes all dressings and gives all treatments. LPNs give baths, take vital signs, and weigh all patients. Nursing assistants make beds, serve meal trays, and feed patients or residents.

Team nursing involves a team of nursing staff led by an RN. The RN decides the amount and kind of care

Box 1-2	Titles for Assistive Personnel
Certified Nursing Assistant	Nursing Support Technician
Clinical Technician	Patient Care Assistant
Health Care Assistant	Patient Care Attendant
Health Care Technician	Patient Care Monitor
Licensed Nursing Assistant	Patient Care Technician
Nurse's Aide	Patient Care Worker
Nurse Extender	Support Partner
Nurse Technician	

each person needs. The team leader delegates the care of certain persons to other RNs and to LPNs/LVNs. The team leader delegates nursing tasks, procedures, and activities to nursing assistants. The team leader delegates according to the person's needs and team member abilities. Team members report to the team leader about observations made and the care given.

Primary nursing involves total care. The primary nurse (an RN) is responsible for the person's total care. Other RNs, LPNs/LVNs, and nursing assistants are involved in the person's care as needed. The RN gives bedside nursing care and teaches and counsels the person and family. The RN also plans the person's discharge. If necessary, home care or long-term care is arranged.

Case management is like primary nursing. A case manager (an RN) coordinates the person's care from admission through discharge and into the home setting. The case manager communicates with the person's doctor and with community agencies involved in the person's care. Some case managers work with the patients and residents of certain doctors. Others work only with persons having certain health problems. For example, one case manager works only with heart patients. Another works only with cancer patients.

Patient-focused care moves hospital services from departments to the bedside. Nurses and assistive personnel are cross-trained to perform basic skills performed by other health team members (see Chapter 2). The number of people caring for each person is reduced, which also reduces care costs.

PAYING FOR HEALTH CARE

Health care is costly. Even after the person leaves the hospital or nursing center, bills often continue for doctor visits, drugs, medical supplies, and home care. Most people cannot afford large medical bills. Some avoid medical care because they cannot pay. Others pay doctor bills even if it means going without food or medicine. Worry, fear, and emotional upset occur about paying for health care. If the person has insurance, part of or all health care costs are covered.

Health care is a major focus in today's society. The goals are to provide health care to everyone and to reduce the high cost of care. Government leaders have proposed many changes. Efforts to reduce health care costs include managed care and prospective payment systems. More changes are likely. Before managed care and prospective payment are presented, a general discussion of insurance programs is necessary.

- *Private insurance plans* are purchased by individuals and families. Depending on the plan, the insurance company pays for some or all health care costs.
- *Group insurance plans* cover individuals belonging to a group. Many employers provide health insurance for employees under group coverage.
- *Medicaid* is a health insurance program sponsored by federal and state governments. Benefits, rules, and eligibility requirements vary from state to state. Older, blind, and disabled people are usually eligible. So are those with low incomes. There is no insurance premium to pay.
- *Medicare* is a health insurance plan administered by the Social Security Administration of the federal government. Benefits are for older persons. Younger persons with a disability may be eligible. Medicare has two parts. Part A is for hospital costs. Part B helps pay for doctors' services, ambulance service, laboratory fees, and equipment and supplies. Part B is voluntary. That is, a person can choose to enroll in Part B and pay the required premium.

MANAGED CARE

Managed care deals with the delivery and payment of health care. Insurance companies contract with doctors and hospitals for reduced rates or discounts. The insured person uses those doctors and agencies providing the lower rates. If others are used, the care may be covered in part or not at all. The person pays for costs not covered by insurance.

Types of Managed Care.
Managed care limits the person's choice of where to go for health care and the services covered. It also places limits on which doctors provide the care. Health maintenance organizations and preferred provider organizations (Box 1-3) are common managed care arrangements. Managed care generally involves private and group insurance plans. However, many states require managed care for Medicaid and Medicare participants.

Managed Care as Preapproval for Services.
Many insurance companies must approve the need

Box 1-3   Types of Managed Care

Health Maintenance Organization (HMO)—provides health care services for a prepaid fee. For the fee, persons receive all needed services offered by the organization. Some need only an annual physical examination, but others require hospital care. Whatever services are used, the cost is covered by the prepaid fee. HMOs emphasize preventing disease and maintaining health. Keeping someone healthy costs far less than treating illness.

Preferred Provider Organization (PPO)—is a group of doctors and hospitals that provides health care at reduced rates. Usually the arrangement is made between the PPO and an employer or an insurance company. Employees or those insured are given reduced rates for the services used. The person can choose any doctor or hospital in the PPO.

---

for health care services. If the need is approved, the insurance company pays for the services. If pre-approval or precertification is not obtained, the person pays for the health care. This preapproval process and the monitoring of care is also called *managed care*. The purpose of managed care in this sense is to reduce unneeded medical and surgical services and procedures. The insurance company decides what to pay. With HMO or PPO contracts, the insurance company may decide where the person goes for the services.

Insurance companies have RNs who handle the preapproval process. The process varies depending on the insurance plan.

PROSPECTIVE PAYMENT SYSTEMS

Prospective payment systems limit the amounts paid by insurance companies, Medicare, and Medicaid. Prospective relates to *before* care. The amount paid for services is determined before the person enters the hospital.

Diagnosis-related groups (DRGs) help reduce Medicare and Medicaid costs. Under the DRG system, Medicare and Medicaid payments are determined *before* the person receives hospital care.

Each DRG has certain diagnoses. Length of stay and treatment costs are determined for each diagnosis. The hospital is paid the preset amount for persons covered by Medicare and Medicaid. If the hospital's treatment costs are less than the DRG amount, the hospital keeps the extra money. If costs are greater, the hospital takes the loss.

Long hospital stays are costly. Therefore early discharges are common. Patients often are still quite ill. Home care, subacute care, or long-term care often is required.

REVIEW

Circle the BEST answer.

1. Helping a person return to the best possible physical and psychological functioning is known as
   A. Detection and treatment of disease
   B. Promotion of health
   C. Rehabilitation
   D. Disease prevention

2. The governing body of a health care agency is called the
   A. Director of nursing
   B. Health team
   C. Board of trustees
   D. Nursing team

3. Who is responsible for the entire nursing staff and the activities involved in providing safe nursing care?
   A. The case manager
   B. The director of nursing
   C. The nursing supervisor
   D. A registered nurse

4. You are a member of
   A. The health team and nursing team
   B. The health team and the medical team
   C. The nursing team and the medical team
   D. An HMO and a PPO

5. The nursing team includes the following *except*
   A. Registered nurses
   B. Doctors
   C. Nursing assistants
   D. LVNs/LPNs

6. Who does *not* supervise LPNs/LVNs?
   A. Doctors
   B. RNs
   C. Dentists
   D. Assistive personnel

7. Nursing team members perform certain functions and tasks for all persons. This is
   A. Functional nursing
   B. Primary nursing
   C. Team nursing
   D. Case management

8. These statements are about insurance programs. Which is *false*?
   A. Preferred provider organizations provide health care at reduced rates.
   B. Health maintenance organizations provide health care for a prepaid fee.
   C. Medicare and Medicaid are government programs for anyone in need.
   D. Diagnosis-related groups affect Medicare payments.

Answers to these questions are on p. 833.

CHAPTER

2

THE NURSING
ASSISTANT

Define the key terms listed in this chapter

Explain the history and current trends affecting nursing assistants

Describe nurse practice acts and how they affect nursing assistants

Describe the Omnibus Budget Reconciliation Act of 1987

Explain the functions, roles, responsibilities, and role limits of nursing assistants

Explain why a job description is important

Describe the educational requirements for nursing assistants

Describe the delegation process and the "five rights of delegation"

Explain how you will use the "five rights of delegation"

Explain your responsibilities when accepting or not accepting a delegated task

Explain how to prevent negligent acts

Give examples of false imprisonment, defamation, assault, battery, and fraud

Describe how to protect the right to privacy

Explain the purpose of informed consent

Explain your role in preparing and signing wills

Describe child, elderly, and domestic abuse

KEY TERMS

accountable Being responsible for one's actions and the actions of others who perform delegated tasks; answering questions about and explaining one's actions and the actions of others

assault Intentionally attempting or threatening to touch a person's body without the person's consent

battery Unauthorized touching of a person's body without the person's consent

civil law Laws concerned with relationships between people; private law

crime An act that violates a criminal law

criminal law Laws concerned with offenses against the public and society in general; public law

defamation Injuring a person's name and reputation by making false statements to a third person

delegate Authorizing another person to perform a task

ethics Knowledge of what is right conduct and wrong conduct

false imprisonment Unlawful restraint or restriction of a person's movement

fraud Saying or doing something to trick, fool, or deceive another person

invasion of privacy Violating a person's right not to have his or her name, photograph, or private affairs exposed or made public without giving consent

law A rule of conduct made by a government body

libel Defamation through written statements

malpractice Negligence by a professional person

negligence An unintentional wrong in which a person fails to act in a reasonable and careful manner and causes harm to a person or to the person's property

preceptor A staff member who guides and teaches

responsibility The duty or obligation to perform some act or function

slander Defamation through oral statements

task A function, procedure, activity, or work that does not require an RN's professional knowledge or judgment

tort A wrong committed against a person or the person's property

will A legal statement of how a person's property is to be distributed after the person's death

Federal and state laws and agency policies combine to define the roles and functions of each health team member. All health care personnel must protect patients and residents from harm. To protect them from harm, you must understand your roles and responsibilities. You need to know what you can and cannot do, what is right conduct and wrong conduct, and your legal limits. Supervised by nurses, you perform selected nursing tasks. Laws, job descriptions, and the person's condition influence how you function. So does the amount of supervision you need.

Protecting patients and residents from harm also involves a complex set of rules and standards of conduct. These rules and standards form the legal and ethical aspects of care.

HISTORY AND CURRENT TRENDS

Nursing practice has a long history involving assistive personnel. For decades they assisted nurses in giving care. Commonly called *nurse's aides* or *nursing assistants*, assistive personnel gave basic bedside nursing care. Bathing and feeding patients and residents were common tasks. So were making beds, repositioning, and assisting with elimination. Their work was similar in hospitals and nursing homes throughout the United States. Until the 1980s, no training or experience was required by law. RNs gave on-the-job training. Some hospitals, nursing homes, and schools offered nursing assistant courses.

Before the 1980s, team nursing was a common nursing care pattern. Team members included RNs, LPNs/LVNs, and nursing assistants. An RN was the team leader. The RN made team member assignments according to each person's needs and condition. The education and experiences of each staff member also influenced assignments. Team members communicated with the team leader about the person's care and observations.

Primary nursing became popular in the 1980s. RNs planned and gave care. With this nursing care pattern, hospitals eliminated many LPN/LVN and nursing assistant positions. Often only RNs were hired to give care.

Meanwhile, nursing centers relied on nursing assistants for resident care. To improve the quality of life of nursing center residents, the U.S. Congress passed the Omnibus Budget Reconciliation Act of 1987 (OBRA). This law sets minimum training and competency evaluation requirements for nursing assistants working in nursing centers. Each state must have rules for nursing assistant training and evaluation. A state's requirements must be met before a person can work as a nursing assistant in a nursing center in that state.

Home care also increased during the 1980s. Prospective payment systems greatly affected this trend.

Prospective payment systems limit how much insurance companies, Medicare, and Medicaid pay for health care. To reduce care costs, hospitals limit how long patients stay in the hospital. Therefore early patient discharges are common. These persons are often still quite ill. Home care often is required.

The rising costs of health care became a major political issue in the early 1990s. The goal was to control and reduce these costs and to provide all persons with health care. Insurance companies, Medicare, and Medicaid further reduced payments for treating certain illnesses. Meanwhile, health care costs kept on increasing.

Efforts to reduce health care costs included:

- *Hospital closings*—Many hospitals closed for financial reasons. The amount of money coming into the hospital was not enough to meet expenses.
- *Hospital mergers*—Hospitals merged to share resources and to avoid offering the same costly services. For example, instead of two hospitals offering cardiac surgery services, only one does. The other hospital may offer maternity and pediatric services.
- *Health care systems*—A health care system involves health care agencies joining together as one provider of care (see Chapter 1). For example, a hospital patient needs long-term care. The system's ambulance service is used to transfer the person from the hospital to the system-owned nursing center. When the person is ready for discharge from the nursing center, home care is arranged with the system's home care agency. The person's care is kept within the system. There is full use of the system's resources.
- *Managed care*—Many insurance companies have contracts with doctors, hospitals, and health care systems (see Chapter 1). The contracts involve reduced rates or discounts. The insured person uses the doctors and agencies offering the lower rates. If others are used, the care is covered only in part or not at all. The person pays for costs not covered by insurance.
- *Return to a nursing staff mix*—Instead of hiring only RNs, hospitals began hiring assistive personnel. Today more and more hospitals are hiring assistive personnel. Some hospitals provide needed training. Others require completion of a state-approved nursing assistant training and competency evaluation program. More training is given for those nursing tasks not included in the training program but that are part of the person's job description.
- *Patient-focused care and cross-training*—This moves services from departments to the bedside. Staff members are cross-trained to perform basic skills performed by other health team members. Nurses and assistive personnel are often cross-trained to collect blood specimens (phlebotomy) and take

electrocardiograms (ECGs, EKGs). For example, a doctor orders a blood test for Ms. Tyler. The nurse tells the unit secretary, who then calls the laboratory. The laboratory secretary tells a medical laboratory technician. The technician sends a staff member to Ms. Tyler's room to draw the blood sample. Five people are involved so far. With patient-focused care and cross-training, Ms. Tyler's blood is drawn by a nurse or assistive person when the order is given. Ms. Tyler does not wait for laboratory staff to be notified and arrive. She is served faster and with fewer staff members. Care costs are reduced when fewer staff members are involved.

STATE AND FEDERAL LAWS

The tasks performed by assistive personnel vary from state to state and among agencies. They can also vary within agencies. For example, assistive personnel in the emergency room may perform different tasks from those performed by assistive personnel on a surgical nursing unit. The tasks may differ for assistive personnel working in the hospital's home care department.

Unlike long-term care, the work of assistive personnel in hospitals currently is not well defined. Concerns about assistive personnel training and job descriptions are prompting states to study the issue. Many states are regulating the training and practice of assistive personnel working in hospitals. State nurse practice acts and OBRA provide some direction.

NURSE PRACTICE ACTS

Each state has a nurse practice act. Intended to protect the public's welfare and safety, the law regulates nursing practice in that state. Definitions are given for RNs and LPNs/LVNs. Their scope of practice is described. So are education and license requirements. The law protects the public from persons practicing nursing without a license. That is, it prevents persons who do not meet the state's education and licensing requirements from performing nursing functions.

Under the law, a nurse's license may be revoked or suspended. The reasons for such action include:

- Being convicted of a crime in any state
- Selling or distributing drugs
- Using the patient's or resident's drugs for oneself
- Placing patients or residents in danger from the excessive use of alcohol or drugs
- Demonstrating grossly negligent nursing practice
- Being convicted of abusing or neglecting children or elderly persons
- Violating the act and its rules and regulations
- Demonstrating incompetent behaviors

- Aiding or assisting another person to violate the act and its rules and regulations
- Making medical diagnoses or prescribing drugs and treatments

A state's nurse practice act is used to determine the nursing tasks that assistive personnel can perform. Legal and advisory opinions about assistive personnel are based on the act. So are any state laws that regulate assistive personnel. If you perform a task beyond the legal limits of your role, you could be practicing nursing without a license. This creates serious legal problems for you and the nurse supervising your work.

THE OMNIBUS BUDGET RECONCILIATION ACT OF 1987

In 1987 the U.S. Congress passed the Omnibus Budget Reconciliation Act (OBRA). This law applies to all 50 states. The law addresses training for nursing assistants working in long-term care. It requires each state to have a nursing assistant training and competency evaluation program. Assistive personnel working in nursing centers and hospital long-term care units must meet federal and state training and competency requirements.

The Training Program. State requirements vary. However, OBRA requires at least 75 hours of instruction. Sixteen of those hours involve supervised practical training. Such training occurs in a laboratory or clinical setting (Fig. 2-1). The student actually performs nursing care and procedures on another person. An RN or LPN/LVN supervises this practical training (clinical practicum or clinical experience).

The training program includes the knowledge and skills needed to give basic nursing care. Areas of study include:

- Communication
- Infection control
- Safety and emergency procedures
- Residents' rights
- Basic nursing skills
- Personal care skills
- Feeding techniques
- Elimination procedures
- Skin care
- Transferring, positioning, and turning techniques
- Dressing
- Ambulating residents
- Range-of-motion exercises
- Signs and symptoms of common diseases and conditions
- How to care for cognitively impaired residents (those who have problems with thinking and memory)

Fig. 2-1 Nursing assistant training program. **A,** Students study in a classroom setting. **B,** Students practice nursing skills in a laboratory setting.

Competency Evaluation. The competency evaluation program includes a written test and a skills test. (See Appendix, p. 841.) The skills test involves demonstrating nursing skills learned in the training program.

The written and skills tests are taken after completing your training program. Your instructor tells you where the tests are given and helps you complete the application form. The required fee is sent with your application.

Preparation for the competency evaluation began the first day of your training program. If you listen, study hard, and practice safe care, you should do well on both the written and skills tests. If the first attempt was not successful, you can retest. OBRA allows 3 opportunities to successfully complete the evaluation.

Nursing Assistant Registry. OBRA requires that each state have a nursing assistant registry. The registry is an official record or listing of persons who have successfully completed a state-approved nursing assistant training and competency evaluation program. The registry contains the following information about each nursing assistant:

- Full name, including maiden name and any married names
- Last known home address
- Registration number and its expiration date
- Date of birth
- Last known employer, date hired, and date employment ended
- Date the competency evaluation was passed
- Information about findings of abuse, neglect, or dishonest use of property. Such information includes the nature of the offense and evidence supporting the finding. If a hearing was held, the date and its outcome are included. The individual has the right to include a statement disputing the finding. All of this information remains in the registry for at least 5 years.

Registry information is requested by any agency needing the information. The nursing assistant also receives a copy of all information in the registry relating to him or her. The copy is provided when first included in the registry and when information is changed or added. The nursing assistant can correct wrong information.

Other OBRA Requirements. OBRA also requires retraining and a new competency evaluation program for nursing assistants who have not worked for 2 consecutive years (24 months). (OBRA allows states to only require a new competency evaluation.) For example, Linda Ames completed a training and competency evaluation. After working as a nursing assistant, she quit her job to go back to school. Three years later she decides to work as a nursing assistant again. According to OBRA, she has to take another training and competency evaluation program. This is to ensure that she has current knowledge and skills to give safe care. It does not matter how long she worked as a nursing assistant. What matters is how long she did *not* work.

Regular in-service education and performance reviews are other OBRA requirements. Nursing centers must regularly provide educational programs to nursing assistants. The work of each nursing assistant must also be regularly evaluated. These requirements help ensure that nursing assistants have the knowledge and skills to give safe, effective care. (*See Focus on Home Care box on p. 16.*)

Focus On... HOME CARE

Many states have training and competency requirements for home health care assistants (home health
aides). If a home care agency receives Medicare
funds, assistive personnel must meet OBRA's training and competency evaluation requirements.

ROLES AND RESPONSIBILITIES

Nurse practice acts, OBRA, state laws, and legal and
advisory opinions give direction to what you can do.
To protect patients and residents from harm, you must
understand what you can do, what you cannot do,
and the legal limits of your role. In some states this is
called *scope of practice*.

You work under the supervision of RNs. Some
states allow LPNs/LVNs to supervise you. You assist
RNs and LPNs/LVNs in giving care. You also perform
nursing procedures and tasks involved in the person's
care. Often you function without a nurse in the room.
At other times you help nurses give bedside care. In
some agencies you assist doctors with diagnostic procedures. The rules listed in Box 2-1 will help you understand your role.

Nursing assistant functions and responsibilities
vary among states and agencies. The procedures in
this textbook are performed by nursing assistants. Before you perform a procedure make sure that:

- Your state allows nursing assistants to perform the
  procedure
- The procedure is in your job description
- You have the necessary training and education
- A nurse is available to answer questions and to su-
  pervise you

Generally, you assist nurses in meeting the hygiene, safety, nutrition, exercise, elimination, and oxygen needs of patients and residents. Related functions include lifting and moving patients and residents,
observing them, and helping promote physical comfort. You also assist with admissions and discharges
and measure temperatures, pulses, respirations, and
blood pressures. *(See Focus on Home Care box at right.)*

Box 2-2 describes the limits of your role. These are
the procedures and tasks that you never perform. Remember, you must understand what you *cannot* do.

You must remember that state laws and legal and
advisory opinions differ. Therefore you must know
what you can do in the state in which you are working. For example, if you live in Utah and move to New
Hampshire, you must become familiar with the laws

Box 2-1   Rules for Assistive Personnel

- You are an assistant to the nurse.
- A nurse determines and supervises your work.
- You do not decide what should or should not be
  done for a person.
- Review directions or instructions with the nurse
  before going to the person.
- Perform no function or task that you have not
  been prepared to do. Also, perform no function
  or task that you do not feel comfortable performing without a nurse's supervision.
- Perform only those functions and tasks that are
  allowed by your state and that are in your job
  description.

Focus On... HOME CARE

Home health care assistants provide personal care
and home services. Home services depend on the
needs of the person and family. They may include:
- Doing light housekeeping so rooms are clean and
  neat.
- Doing laundry. Clothing and linens are washed,
  ironed, and mended as needed. Family laundry
  may also be done.
- Shopping for groceries and household items as
  needed and directed.
- Preparing and serving nutritious meals. This includes planning menus, following special diets,
  and feeding the person if necessary.
Home health care assistants do not do heavy housekeeping. This includes moving heavy furniture,
waxing floors, shampooing carpets, washing windows, cleaning rugs or drapes, and carrying fire-
wood, coal, or ash containers.

---

and rules in New Hampshire. Sometimes nursing assistants work in two states. For example, you work
part-time at a nursing center in Illinois and part-time
at a nursing center in Iowa. What you can do in Illinois may be different from what you do in Iowa. You
must know the laws and rules of each state.

Some assistive personnel are also emergency medical technicians (EMTs). EMTs are trained to give
emergency care outside of health care settings. These
settings are called "in the field." EMTs work under the
direction of doctors in hospital emergency rooms.
Each state has laws and rules that apply to EMTs.
These laws and rules are different from those for assistive personnel. What EMTs do "in the field" is very
different from the work of assistive personnel. For example, Joan Woods is an EMT for a fire department.

Box 2-2   Role Limits for Nursing Assistants

- **Never give medications.** This includes drugs given orally, rectally, by injection, by application to the skin, or directly into the bloodstream through an intravenous line. Licensed nurses are responsible for giving drugs. They cannot delegate this responsibility to nursing assistants. (Some states allow assistive personnel to give medications under certain conditions. One condition is completing a state-required education and training program about giving medications. Other conditions include having the function in your job description and having the necessary supervision.)

- **Never insert tubes or objects into body openings or remove them from the body unless allowed by your state and job description.** You must not insert tubes into a person's bladder, esophagus, trachea, nose, ears, bloodstream, or surgically created body openings. Exceptions to this rule are procedures in this textbook that you will study and practice with your instructor's supervision. Giving enemas and inserting rectal tubes are examples. (Some states allow assistive personnel to insert catheters [tubes] into the urinary bladder, suction the upper airway, and collect blood specimens. Other states do not. If such advanced procedures are allowed, additional education, training, and supervision are required.)

- **Never take oral or telephone orders from doctors.** Politely give your name and title, ask the doctor to wait, and promptly find a nurse to speak with the doctor.

- **Never perform procedures that require sterile technique.** With sterile technique, all objects in contact with the person's body must be free of all microorganisms. Sterile technique and procedures require skills, knowledge, and judgment beyond the training you will receive. You may assist a nurse during a sterile procedure. However, you will not perform the procedure yourself. (In some states, assistive personnel are allowed to perform certain sterile procedures. They must receive additional education, training, and supervision.)

- **Never tell the patient, resident, or family the person's diagnosis or medical or surgical treatment plans.** The doctor is responsible for informing the person and family about the diagnosis and treatment. Nurses may further clarify what the doctor said.

- **Never diagnose or prescribe treatments or drugs for anyone.** Only doctors can diagnose and prescribe.

- **Never supervise other nursing assistants or assistive personnel.** RNs are legally responsible for supervising the work of other nursing assistants or assistive personnel. You will not be trained or paid to supervise the work of others. Supervising others can have serious legal consequences.

- **Never ignore an order or request to do something that you cannot do or that is beyond your legal limits.** Promptly explain to the nurse why you cannot carry out the order or request. The nurse assumes you are doing what you were told to do unless you explain otherwise. Patient and resident care cannot be neglected.

When off duty, she works as a nursing assistant at St. John's Hospital. Her state allows EMTs to start intravenous infusions (IVs) in the field. However, assistive personnel do not start IVs. Despite knowing how to start an IV, Joan cannot start IVs when working at the hospital as a nursing assistant.

The situation is similar for persons who served as medics or corpsmen in military service. Medics or corpsmen may suture wounds. Assistive personnel cannot do so. When employed in the assistive role, medics and corpsmen must follow the laws and rules that apply to assistive personnel in that state. As with EMTs, the ability to perform a task does not give a person the right to perform that task in all settings.

Nursing assistant functions are limited by state laws and rules. Job descriptions for nursing assistants reflect those laws and rules.

JOB DESCRIPTION

The job description lists the responsibilities and functions the agency expects you to perform (Box 2-3, pp. 18-23). Always request a written job description when you apply for a job. Ask questions about the job de-

scription during your job interview. Before accepting a job, tell the employer about any functions you do not know how to do. Also advise the employer of functions you are opposed to doing for moral or religious reasons. Have a clear understanding of what is expected of you before taking a job. Do not take a job that requires you to:

- Act beyond the legal limits of your role
- Function beyond your educational limits
- Perform acts that are against your moral or religious principles

No one can force you to perform a function, task, or procedure that is beyond the legal limits of your role. Jobs may be threatened for refusing to follow a nurse's orders. Often staff members obey out of fear. That is why you must understand the roles and responsibilities of nursing assistants. You also need to know the functions you can safely perform, the things you should never do, and your job description. Understanding the ethical and legal aspects of your role is equally important.

Text continued on p. 23

Box 2-3 **Sample Job Description**

OSF ST. JOSEPH MEDICAL CENTER
BLOOMINGTON, ILLINOIS
JOB DESCRIPTION/PERFORMANCE APPRAISAL

JOB TITLE: Nursing Assistant

DEPARTMENT: Medical/Surgical Services

GENERAL SUMMARY
The nursing assistant:
- Performs any combination of the following duties in giving patient care, under direction of a Registered Nurse
- Reports to the RN
- According to department policies, provides appropriate basic nursing care to patients based on the ages of the patients served on the unit
- Observes patients for physical/emotional changes
- Records pertinent information in medical record
- Communicates with other patient care providers to ensure continuity of care

The following are general characteristics of this job, although duties may vary by assigned shift. Provides care for patients and family/significant others across the life span based on physical, psychosocial, educational, safety, and related criteria appropriate to the age of patients served in assigned service area. May work nursing departments of Medical, Surgical, Pediatrics, SNF, PICU, Post-Partum, and Nursery.

	Medical	**Surgical**	**Skilled**
Age range	12-96	12-96	53-94
Average age	62	52	76
% Male	50	60	64
% Female	50	40	36
Average LOS	4.68	3.67	10.09

CORPORATE PHILOSOPHY:
It is the obligation of each employee of OSF St. Joseph Medical Center to abide by and promote the Philosophy, Values, Mission, and Vision of the Sisters of the Third Order of Saint Francis.

COMMENTS:
_____

_____

SKILLS OR SPECIALIZATION REQUIRED:
A. *Education:* Certification by the State of Illinois for nursing assistant and additional unit-specific and on-the-job training to learn procedures and develop proficiencies for specific nursing procedures.
B. *Work Experience:* Prior experience within the hospital environment in the previous 2 years is preferred but not mandatory.
C. *Job Knowledge:* Knowledge of the nursing process thereby enabling him/her to provide care in conjunction with an RN. Must possess current comprehensive cognitive knowledge and technical skills in nursing and health care. Must understand and practice patient confidentiality; displays problem identification and conflict resolution.
D. *Skills and abilities:*
   CPR skill validation
   MIS experience preferred
   Good telephone skills
   Ability to monitor various types of equipment ranging from but not limited non-invasive blood pressure monitors and other equipment involved in the care of the patient.
   Demonstrates Standard Precautions and Transmission-Based Precautions.
   Collects accurate patient data and completes documentation

PRINCIPAL DUTIES AND RESPONSIBILITIES:
The following statements are intended to describe the essential elements, functions, and requirements of the position as defined by the ADA, except for those that begin with the word "May." The list should not be taken as an exhaustive list of all responsibilities, duties, and skills required of individual assigned to this job. In accordance with the philosophy, objectives, and values of OSF St. Joseph Medical Center and the Sisters of the Third Order of St. Francis, the nursing assistant assumes the following duties and responsibilities:he/she demonstrates through his/her care that returning patients to expected state of health and maintaining their safety, security, and dignity are paramount.

Modified from OSF St. Joseph Medical Center, Bloomington, Ill.
Note that the job description is also a performance appraisal tool.

Box 2-3 **Sample Job Description—cont'd**

RATING GUIDE (1-5)
1 – Performance fails to meet job requirements.
2 – Performance results show inconsistent achievement.
3 – Performance consistently meets job requirements.
4 – Performance consistently meets all job requirements and often exceeds them.
5 – Performance consistently above job requirements.

A. PATIENT CARE:

1. Assists RN with admission, room orientation, data collection (e.g., vital signs, weights, heights).	
2. Assists patients with activities of daily living, including personal hygiene and grooming, bathing, eating.	
3. Performs basic nursing care procedures (e.g., sitz baths, enemas, daily weights, applying and changing non-sterile dressing and pads, applying warm or cold compresses, simple NG care, blood glucose testing, occupied bed making, care for patient in traction, CPM assists).	
4. Collects patient specimen (e.g., urine, stool, sputum), labels and sends to laboratory for analysis, and communicates to the RN.	
5. Monitors, collects, and documents data on a 24-hour flowsheet: hygiene, diet, percentage taken, stools, voidings, enema, empty ostomy equipment, patient activity, graphics, and I&Os.	
6. Has knowledge of patient's plan of care and interventions under the direction of the RN.	
7. Reinforces patient/significant other as indicated on the plan of care. Documents reinforcement of patient/significant other and his/her response.	
8. Provides care according to physician's orders and in conformance with the Standards of Practice and Care, Nursing Service policies and procedures, the Illinois Nurse Practice Act, and the guidelines of OSF Values.	
9. Responds to emergency situations in accordance with established policies and procedure.	
10. Maintains accurate record within the chart: graphics, I&Os, 24-hour UA.	
11. Assists physicians as indicated.	
12. Utilizes positive communication and interpersonal skills in performance of duties.	

B. PERSONNEL RESPONSIBILITIES

1. May assist in orientation of personnel as instructed by unit director.	
2. Promotes an atmosphere conducive to learning for personnel and nursing students.	
3. Shows concern and respect for the physical, spiritual, emotional, and economical well-being of co-workers.	
4. May be required to change patient assignments based on changing patient acuity and patient needs.	

C. MATERIALS MANAGEMENT

1. Ensures accurate charging for all patient care items.	
2. Cooperates in identification and application of cost-containment measures.	
3. Assists in maintaining equipment and department in optimal function order. Completes or ensures that work orders are completed to ensure all equipment is in proper working order and available when needed.	
4. Assists in ensuring adequate availability of supplies for oncoming shift.	
5. Ensures that charges are entered for all equipment.	
6. Ensures that a record is kept of all equipment and/or supplies borrowed by or from another department, if applicable.	

Continued

Box 2-3 **Sample Job Description—cont'd**

D. COMMUNICATION

1 Provides complete documentation of any incident or unusual happenings that occur.	
2. Reports any unusual occurrences in a nonjudgmental manner.	
3. Keeps resource RN, supervisor, and/or director of the unit informed of patient condition changes or immediate problems within the department.	
4. Listens carefully and is empathetic to expressed needs of patients and staff.	
5. Accepts constructive criticism with a positive, agreeable attitude.	
6. Fosters a harmonious working relationship.	

E. PROFESSIONAL DEVELOPMENT

1. Makes improvements in the quality of patient care via participation in and utilization of Quality Improvement monitors. Embraces and demonstrates the principles of Total Quality Management.	
2. Participates in continuing educational programs to maintain competence and gain additional skills.	
3. Maintains documentation of attendance at inservices and continuing education programs.	
4. Seeks and/or identifies need for opportunities for growth.	
5. Attends mandatory inservices.	
6. Completes quarterly one touch quality control.	
7. Work attendance reflects dependability.	
8. Appears neat and clean and follows dress code.	
9. Attends and contributes at departmental staff meetings.	
10. Supports, when possible, community organizations that seek to promote health needs of others.	

F. AGE-SPECIFIC CRITERIA-BASED

Demonstrates the minimum knowledge, skills, and abilities for the following patient groups:	Infancy (Birth-1 yr)	Pediatric (1-12 yrs)	Adolescence (12-18 yrs)	Adult (18-65 yrs)	Late Adulthood (65+ yrs)
PHYSICAL CARE					
1. Meets patient's physical care needs based on normal growth and development as directed.					
2. Assists in planning age-appropriate physical or therapeutic patient care.					
3. Implements age-appropriate physical or therapeutic care procedures as directed.					
4. Assists in evaluating effectiveness of identified age-specific interventions.					
PSYCHOSOCIAL CARE					
1. Meets age-appropriate psychosocial needs of patient as directed.					
2. Assists in planning age-appropriate psychosocial interventions.					
3. Implements appropriate psychosocial interventions as directed.					
4. Assists in evaluating effectiveness of age-specific psychosocial interventions.					

Box 2-3 **Sample Job Description—cont'd**

F. AGE-SPECIFIC CRITERIA-BASED—cont'd

Demonstrates the minimum knowledge, skills, and abilities for the following patient groups:	Infancy (Birth-1 yr)	Pediatric (1-12 yrs)	Adolescence (12-18 yrs)	Adult (18-65 yrs)	Late Adulthood (65+ yrs)
EDUCATIONAL CARE					
1. Meets age-specific learning needs of patient, family or significant other as directed.					
2. Assists in planning age-appropriate education.					
3. Assists in evaluating patient, family, and significant other's understanding of age-appropriate education.					
SAFETY: Identifies and applies age-specific safety needs of patients when performing own job duties in the following circumstances.					
1. Disasters/evacuation					
2. Transfer of patients					
3. Minimizing security risks					
4. Restraints/immobilization devices					
5. Use of equipment					

PSYCHOLOGICAL CONSIDERATIONS

Some stress is experienced because of changing patient acuity, census fluctuations, and spontaneous reaction to situations as they arise. The dynamics of working closely with physicians, other members of the health care team, and the public facilitates the stressful environment. Must display social sensitivity, acting suitable in all situations and adjusting behavior to fit the occasion and interpret how others are feeling. Behaviors must be flexible in response to changing situations to remain motivated with accuracy to reach a goal.

COMMENTS:

_____
_____
_____
_____
_____
_____
_____
_____

COGNITIVE SKILLS REQUIRED:

1. Ability to read and follow written English protocols as necessary.
2. Ability to follow verbal communications.
3. Ability to understand written and spoken English; to remember and to understand the written and spoken word.
4. Organize and express thoughts in spoken English words to others, so they will understand.
5. Ability to problem solve with a variety of variables, interpret instructions.
6. Problem sensitivity: ability to interpret assessments to tell when something is wrong or likely to go wrong; identify the whole problem.
7. Must be able to communicate with all educational levels and display good human relations.
8. Must be able to perform duties in an atmosphere of constant interruptions.
9. Ability to learn technical material and equipment.
10. Ability to enter and obtain information from a computer.
11. Ability to read and follow established hospital policy, nursing service policies and procedures, unit-specific policies and procedures, and standards of practice and care.
12. Memorization: must be able to remember words, numbers, procedures, and pieces of information.
13. Information ordering: follow rules correctly; arrange action in a certain order.
14. Must be able to organize and maintain flexible scheduling to coordinate all job responsibilities.
15. Must be able to perform duties in an atmosphere of frequent interruptions.

Continued

Box 2-3   Sample Job Description—cont'd

COMMENTS:

_____

_____

PHYSICAL REQUIREMENTS:
1. Must be able to sit for a portion of the work day, up to 50%.
2. Must be able to read a CRT to complete order entry, order verification, or to obtain results.
3. Must have visual acuity that enables the individual to monitor patient and to complete documentation—Frequency: hourly.
4. Must perform major visual functions, including acuity, depth perception, field of vision, accommodation, and color perception—Frequency: hourly.
5. Must be able to walk in order to provide patient care, transport objects and equipment and patients to various parts of the hospital and within the department. This includes heavy but not mobile equipment—Frequency: hourly. The equipment may weigh 100 pounds or more and may be transported by pushing or pulling using a wheeled cart—Frequency: seldom.
6. Must be able to stand for prolonged periods of time when assisting with procedures and/or providing patient care—Frequency: hourly.
7. Must be capable of maintaining equilibrium to prevent falling when walking or standing—Frequency: hourly.
8. Must be capable of stooping, bending, reaching, and squatting during patient care activities—Frequency: hourly.
9. Must be capable of carrying up to 50 pounds for transporting equipment and supplies—Frequency: hourly.
10. Must be capable of a wide range of hand, wrist, and finger motions including pinching, grasping, and fingering required for tasks such as writing, answering phones and call lights, adjusting dials and switches, order entry, carrying equipment and supplies, and caring for and positioning patients—Frequency: hourly.
11. Must have eye, hand, and foot coordination to perform technical aspects of job—Frequency: hourly.

COMMENTS:

_____

_____

MEASUREMENTS FOR EQUIPMENT AND/OR SUPPLIES:
Height: May range from floor level to 7 foot
Weight: May range from several ounces to 150 plus pounds
Bed: 27" to 6 feet
IV poles: 72" high, 2 lbs. to force move
Reach to floor and up to 3 feet above or from body

PHYSIOLOGICAL CONSIDERATIONS:
There is a potential for exposure to blood and body fluids, contagious and infectious diseases, including hepatitis and the HIV virus. There is also the potential for exposure to chemicals such as cleaning solutions and medications. There may be noxious odors present. Personal protective equipment and supplies are readily available within the work environment, and the employee is expected to follow established hospital policy regarding use of protective equipment and supplies.

COMMENTS:

_____

_____

ENVIRONMENTAL CONSIDERATIONS:
The normal work day is inside, protected from the elements; however, it may be necessary to exit the building to discharge patients or accompany patients to other facilities. Temperature changes may be experienced within the work environment.

COMMENTS:

_____

_____

REPORTING RELATIONSHIPS:
Reports to the director of Medical/Surgical Services or immediate supervisor (RN).

Box 2-3	**Sample Job Description—cont'd**

TOTAL RATINGS, ACTUAL, ALL STANDARDS ——

TOTAL RATINGS, POSSIBLE, ALL STANDARDS ——

APPROVALS

Department Director/Manager   Date

Assistant Administrator   Date

Asst Administrator–Human Resources   Date

The above is intended to describe the general content of and requirements for the performance of this job. It is not to be construed as an exhaustive statement of duties, responsibilities, or requirements.

Employee/Applicant Signature   Date

EDUCATIONAL REQUIREMENTS

Each agency has its own educational requirements for nursing assistants. These requirements are based on state laws or recommendations that limit what assistive personnel can do.

When employed, you will complete the agency's orientation program. Agency policies and procedures are explained and your skills checked. That is, the agency has you perform nursing procedures and tasks to make sure you can do them safely and correctly. Also, you are shown how to use the agency's supplies and equipment.

Some agencies have clinical preceptor programs. A **preceptor** is a staff member who guides and teaches. In a clinical preceptor program, nurses teach and train assistive personnel in the clinical area (Fig. 2-2). For example, you complete a training program for nursing assistants. A nurse preceptor works with you and supervises your work for a period of time. The nurse helps you adjust to your role, shows you how to use equipment and supplies, answers your questions, and makes sure that you give safe care. Depending on the agency, the preceptor program can last from 6 weeks to 3 months. It is designed to help you succeed in your new role and to ensure quality and safe care.

DELEGATION

Nurse practice acts give RNs and LPNs/LVNs certain responsibilities and the authority to perform nursing tasks. A **responsibility** is the duty or obligation to perform some act or function. For example, RNs are re-

Fig. 2-2 A nurse preceptor shows a new nursing assistant where to find supplies.

sponsible for supervising LPNs/LVNs and assistive personnel. Only RNs can carry out this responsibility.

In nursing, a **task** is a function, procedure, activity, or work that does not require an RN's professional knowledge or judgment. **Delegate** means to authorize another person to perform a task. The person must be competent to perform the task in a given situation. For example, you know how to give a complete bed bath. However, Mr. Jones has multiple injuries from an auto accident. He has neck injuries and is at risk for paralysis. His left leg is fractured in three places, and he has a full leg cast. His right lung was punctured, and he has chest tubes. He has two IVs, a retention catheter, a nasogastric tube, and a tracheostomy. In this situation, giving a bed bath to Mr. Jones is complicated. The RN gives the bath and asks you to assist.

WHO CAN DELEGATE

Nurse practice acts allow RNs to delegate tasks to LPNs/LVNs and assistive personnel. Some states allow LPNs/LVNs to delegate tasks to assistive personnel. RNs and LPNs/LVNs can delegate only tasks within their scope of practice.

When making delegation decisions, nurses must protect the person's health and safety. The delegating nurse remains **accountable** for the delegated task. To be accountable means to be responsible for one's actions and the actions of others who perform delegated tasks. It also involves answering questions about and explaining one's actions and the actions of others.

The delegating nurse must make sure that the task was completed safely and correctly. If the RN delegates, the RN is responsible for the delegated task. If the LPN/LVN delegates, the LPN/LVN is responsible for the delegated task. Remember, the RN is also responsible for supervising the practice of LPNs/LVNs. Therefore the RN also is accountable for the tasks that LPNs/LVNs delegate to assistive personnel. The RN is accountable for all patient and resident care. *(See Focus on Long-Term Care box.)*

Assistive personnel cannot delegate. You cannot delegate any task to other nursing assistants or assistive personnel. You can ask another assistive person to help you. However, you cannot ask or tell another person to do your work.

DELEGATION PROCESS

Delegated tasks must be within the legal limits of what assistive personnel can do. Before delegating tasks to you, the nurse must know:

- What tasks your state allows assistive personnel to perform
- The tasks included in your job description
- What you were taught in your training program
- What skills you learned and how they were evaluated
- About your work experiences

The nurse uses this information to make delegation decisions. The nurse is likely to discuss this information with you. This is so the nurse can get to know

---

Box 2-4 — Factors Affecting Delegation Decisions

- What is the person's condition? Is it stable or likely to change?
- What are the person's basic needs at this time?
- What is the person's mental function at this time?
- What are the person's emotional and spiritual needs at this time?
- Can the person assist with his or her care? Does the person depend on others for care?
- Is the task something the nurse can delegate?
- For this person, does the task require the knowledge, judgment, and skill of an RN or LPN/LVN?
- How often will the nurse have to assess the person?
- Can the task harm the person? If yes, how?
- What effect will the task have on the person?
- Is it safe for the person if the task is delegated to you?
- Do you have the training and experience to perform the task, given the person's current status? Is your training documented? How were your training and skills evaluated?
- How often have you performed the task?
- What other tasks were delegated to you?
- Do you have the time to perform the task safely?
- Is a nurse available to supervise you?
- How much supervision will you need?
- Will you need more directions as you perform the task?
- Is a nurse available to help or take over if the person's condition changes or problems arise?

---

you, your abilities, and your concerns. Whenever your work with a new nurse, you should meet to discuss your training and work experience. You may be a new employee or new to the nursing unit. Or the nurse may be someone new. In any case, it is wise for the nurse to get to know you and for you to get to know the nurse.

Agency policies, guidelines, and your job description state what tasks nurses can delegate to you. These documents must be in line with state laws, rules, and legal opinions about the roles and functions of assistive personnel. However, even if a task is in your job description, a nurse does not have to delegate it to you. The nurse must consider the circumstances when delegating.

The nurse makes delegation decisions after considering the questions in Box 2-4. The patient's or resident's needs, the task, and the person performing the task must fit. The nurse can decide to delegate the task to you. Or the nurse can decide not to delegate the task. If the person's needs and the task require the knowledge, judgment, and skill of an RN or LPN/LVN, the nurse completes the task. You may be asked to assist.

Focus On... LONG-TERM CARE

Some states allow LPNs/LVNs to have supervisory roles in long-term care settings. The LPN/LVN delegates tasks to assistive personnel. The LPN/LVN follows the delegation process and the "five rights of delegation."

Do not get offended or angry if you are not allowed to perform a task that is part of your job description and that is usually delegated to you. The nurse makes a decision that is best for the person at the time. That decision is also best for you at that time. You do not want to perform a task that requires a nurse's judgment and critical thinking skills. For example, you often care for Mrs. Mills. You give personal care and assist with walking. She visits her son during the weekend. When she returns to the nursing center, she has bruises on her face and arms. She reports falling down the stairs. The RN suspects abuse. Instead of asking you to bathe Mrs. Mills, the RN does so. The RN wants to assess Mrs. Mills for other signs of abuse and to talk with her. Although you are able to give Mrs. Mills a bath, at this time she needs the RN's knowledge and judgment.

The person's circumstances are central factors in making delegation decisions. Delegation decisions should always result in the best care for the person. A nurse places a person's health and safety at risk with poor delegation decisions. Also, the nurse may face serious legal problems. If you perform a task that places the person at risk, you can also face serious legal problems.

The Five Rights of Delegation. The National Council of State Boards of Nursing's five rights of delegation summarize the delegation process:

- *The right task*—Can the task be delegated? Does the nurse practice act allow the RN or LPN/LVN to delegate the task? Is the task in your job description?
- *The right circumstances*—What are the person's physical, mental, emotional, and spiritual needs at this time?
- *The right person*—Do you have the training and experience to safely perform the task for this person?
- *The right directions and communication*—The nurse must give clear directions. The nurse tells you what to do, when to do it, what observations to make, and when to report back. The nurse allows questions and helps you set priorities.
- *The right supervision*—The nurse guides, directs, and evaluates the care you give. The nurse demonstrates tasks as necessary and is available to answer questions. The less experience you have performing a task, the more supervision you need. Complex tasks require greater supervision than basic tasks. Also, the person's circumstances affect how much supervision you need. The nurse assesses how the task affected the person and how well you performed the task. To help you learn and give better care, the nurse tells you what you did well and what you can do to improve your work.

Box 2-5 — The Five Rights of Delegation for Assistive Personnel

THE RIGHT TASK
- Does your state allow you to perform the task?
- Were you trained to do the task?
- Do you have experience performing the task?
- Is the task in your job description?

THE RIGHT CIRCUMSTANCES
- Do you have experience performing the task, given the person's condition and needs?
- Do you understand the purpose of the task for the person?
- Can you perform the task safely under the current circumstances?
- Do you have the equipment and supplies to safely complete the task?
- Do you know how to use the equipment and supplies?

THE RIGHT PERSON
- Are you comfortable performing the task?
- Do you have concerns about performing the task?

THE RIGHT DIRECTIONS AND COMMUNICATION
- Did the nurse give clear directions and instructions?
- Did you review the task with the nurse?
- Do you understand what the nurse expects?

THE RIGHT SUPERVISION
- Is a nurse available to answer questions?
- Is a nurse available if the person's condition changes or if problems occur?

Modified from the National Council of State Boards of Nursing, Inc.

YOUR ROLE IN DELEGATION

You must remember that you perform delegated tasks for or on *a person*. You must perform the task safely to protect the person from harm.

You have two choices when a nurse delegates a task to you. You either *agree* or *refuse* to do the task. You should use the "five rights of delegation" to make your choice. Before accepting a delegated task, you need to answer the questions in Box 2-5.

Accepting a Task. When you agree to perform a task, you are responsible for your own actions. Remember, what you do or fail to do can harm the person. *You must complete the task safely.* You must ask for help when you are unsure or have questions about a task. You must communicate with the nurse by reporting what you did and your observations.

Refusing a Task. You have the right to say "no." Sometimes refusing to follow the nurse's directions is your right and duty. You should refuse to perform a task when:

- The task is beyond the legal limits of your role.
- The task is not in your job description.
- You were not prepared to perform the task safely.
- The task could harm the person.
- The person's condition has changed.
- You do not know how to use the supplies or equipment.
- The nurse's directions are unethical, illegal, or against agency policies.
- The nurse's directions are unclear or incomplete.
- A nurse is not available for supervision.

Protect patients, residents, and yourself by using common sense. Ask yourself if what you are doing is safe for the person.

As explained in Box 2-2, you must never ignore an order or request to do something. You must communicate your concerns to the nurse. If the task is within the legal limits of your role and in your job description, the nurse can help you feel more comfortable with the tasks. The nurse can answer your questions, demonstrate the task, and show you how to use supplies and equipment. The nurse can help you as needed, observe you performing the task, and check on you often. The nurse also can arrange for needed training.

With good communication, you and the nurse should be able to work out the problem. If not, try talking to the nurse's supervisor. When work problems continue, talk to someone whom you trust and can confide in. For example, your instructor or another professional can help you sort out work problems.

You must not refuse a delegated task simply because you do not like or want to do the task. You must have sound reasons for your refusal. Otherwise, you could place the person at risk for harm. You also risk losing your job.

ETHICAL ASPECTS

Ethics is concerned with what is right conduct and wrong conduct. It involves morals and making choices or judgments about what should or should not be done. An ethical person behaves and acts in the right way and does not bring harm to the person.

Ethical behavior also involves not being *prejudiced* or *biased*. A person who is prejudiced or biased makes judgments and has opinions before knowing the facts. Judgments and opinions usually are based on a person's own values and standards. Such values are derived from the person's culture, religion, education, and life experiences. The person's situation may be very different from your own. For example:

- Children decide that their elderly mother needs nursing home care after leaving the hospital. In your culture, children take care of elderly parents at home.
- A person has multiple tattoos and body piercings. You do not believe in tattooing or body piercing.
- An 80-year-old man has a living will that says he should not be resuscitated. You believe that everything possible should be done to save life.

You must not judge the person by your own values or standards. You must not avoid persons whose standards and values are different from your own.

Ethical dilemmas involve making choices. You must decide what is the right thing to do. For example:

- A co-worker was late for work 3 days this week. You find her in an empty room drinking from a thermos. You also smell alcohol on her breath. She asks you not to tell anyone.
- An older person has bruises all over her body. She told the RN that they are from a fall. Later she tells you that her son is very mean to her. She asks you not to tell anyone.

Professional groups have codes of ethics. The code involves rules, or standards of conduct, for group members to follow. The American Nurses Association (ANA) has a code of ethics for RNs. The National Federation of Licensed Practical Nurses (NFLPN) has one for LPNs/LVNs. No formal code of ethics exists for nursing assistants. However, the rules of conduct in Box 2-6 can guide your thinking and behavior. See Chapter 3 for ethical behavior in the workplace.

Box 2-6	Rules of Conduct for Nursing Assistants

- Respect each person as an individual.
- Perform no act that is not within the legal limits of your role.
- Perform no act for which you have not been adequately prepared.
- Take no drug without the prescription and supervision of a doctor.
- Carry out the directions and instructions of the nurse to your best possible ability.
- Complete each task safely.
- Be loyal to your employer and co-workers.
- Act as a responsible citizen at all times.
- Recognize the limits of your role and knowledge.
- Keep patient and resident information confidential.
- Consider the person's needs to be more important than your own.

LEGAL ASPECTS

Whereas ethics is concerned with what you *should or should not do*, laws tell you what you *can and cannot do*. A **law** is a rule of conduct made by a government body such as the U.S. Congress or a state legislature. Laws protect the public welfare and are enforced by the government.

Criminal laws are concerned with offenses against the public and against society in general. A violation of a criminal law is called a **crime**. A person found guilty of a crime is fined or sent to prison. Murder, robbery, rape, abuse, and kidnapping are examples of crimes.

Civil laws deal with the relationships between people. Examples of civil laws are those that involve contracts and nursing practice. A person found guilty of breaking a civil law usually has to pay a sum of money to the injured person.

TORTS

Tort comes from a French word meaning *wrong*. Torts are part of civil law. A tort is committed by an individual against another person or the person's property. Torts may be intentional or unintentional.

Unintentional Torts.

Negligence is an unintentional wrong. The person did not mean or intend to cause harm. The negligent person failed to act in a reasonable and careful manner and thereby caused harm to the person or property of another. The person at fault failed to do what a reasonable and careful person would have done. Or the individual did what a reasonable and careful person would not have done. The negligent individual may have to pay damages (a sum of money) to the injured person.

Malpractice is negligence by professionals. A person has professional status because of training, education, and the service provided. Nurses, doctors, dentists, lawyers, and pharmacists are examples of professional people.

Box 2-7 gives some common examples of negligent acts committed by nursing assistants. You are legally responsible *(liable)* for your own actions. What you do or do not do can lead to a lawsuit if harm results to the person or property of another. A nurse may direct you to do something beyond the legal limits of your role. Or you may be asked to do something beyond your education. Giving drugs is an example. You may be told not to worry—that the nurse is responsible if anything happens. The nurse is liable as your supervisor. However, you are not relieved of personal liability. *You are responsible for your own actions.* Remember, sometimes refusing to follow the nurse's directions is your right and duty.

Box 2-7   Common Negligent Acts of Nursing Assistants

- The nursing assistant leaves the bed in the raised positions. The resident falls out of bed and breaks a hip.
- A nursing assistant applied a warm water bottle that was too hot. The patient is burned.
- A nursing assistant drops a patient's dentures. The dentures break.
- A resident complains to the nursing assistant of chest pain and difficulty breathing. The complaints are not reported to the nurse. The person has a heart attack and dies.
- A resident puts on the signal light. The nursing assistant goes past the room several times but does not answer the signal light. The resident goes into shock because of sudden, severe bleeding.

Intentional Torts.

Intentional torts are acts meant to be harmful. Defamation (libel and slander), assault and battery, false imprisonment, invasion of privacy, and fraud are intentional torts.

Defamation is injuring the name and reputation of a person by making false statements to a third person. **Libel** is making false statements in print, writing, or through pictures or drawings. **Slander** is making false statements orally. Protect yourself from defamation by never making false statements about a patient, resident, co-worker, or any other person. Examples of defamation include:

- Implying or suggesting that a person has a sexually transmitted disease
- Saying that a person is insane or mentally ill
- Implying or suggesting that a person is corrupt or dishonest

Assault and battery may result in both civil and criminal charges. **Assault** is intentionally attempting or threatening to touch a person's body without the person's consent. The person fears bodily harm. Threatening to "tie down" an uncooperative patient is an example of assault. **Battery** is the actual touching of a person's body without the person's consent. Consent is the important factor in assault and battery. The person must consent to any procedure, treatment, or other act that involves touching the body. The person has the right to withdraw consent at any time.

Consent is more than a person's verbal okay or signature on a form. For consent to be valid, it must be *informed* consent. Protect yourself from assault and battery by explaining to the person what is to be done and getting the person's consent. Consent may be verbal ("yes" or "okay") or a gesture (a nod, turning over for a back rub, or holding out an arm for a blood pressure measurement).

False imprisonment is the unlawful restraint or restriction of a person's freedom of movement. Threat of restraint or actual physical restraint is false imprisonment. Preventing a person from leaving the agency also is false imprisonment.

Every person has the right not to have his or her name, photograph, or private affairs exposed or made public without having given consent. Violating this right is an **invasion of privacy.** You must treat patients and residents with respect and ensure their privacy. Only staff members who are involved in the person's care should see, handle, or examine the person's body. The precautions listed in Box 2-8 help ensure the right to privacy.

Box 2-8	**Protecting the Person's Right to Privacy**

- Keep all patient or resident information confidential.
- Make sure the person is covered when being moved in corridors.
- Screen the person as in Figure 2-3, and close the door when giving care. Also close drapes and window shades.
- Expose only the body part involved in a treatment or procedure.
- Do not discuss the person or the person's treatment with anyone except the nurse supervising your work. "Shop talk" is a common cause of invasion of privacy.
- Ask visitors to leave the room when care is given.
- Do not open the person's mail.
- Allow the person to visit with others and to use the telephone in private.

Fig. 2-3 Pulling the curtain around the bed helps protect the person's privacy.

Fraud is saying or doing something to trick, fool, or deceive another person. The act is fraud if it does or could cause harm to a person or the person's property. Telling a person or family that you are an RN is fraud. So is giving incomplete or inaccurate information on a job application.

INFORMED CONSENT

Informed consent recognizes a person's right to decide what will be done to his or her body and who can touch his or her body. The doctor is responsible for informing the person about all aspects of treatment. Consent is informed when the person clearly understands:

- The reason for a treatment
- What will be done
- How it will be done
- Who will do it
- The expected outcomes
- Other treatment options
- The effects of not having the treatment

Often consent is needed for persons under legal age (usually 18 years of age). A parent or legal guardian gives consent. Mentally incompetent persons also cannot give legal consent. Persons who are unconscious, sedated, or confused are not mentally competent to give legal consent. Persons with certain mental health disorders also are incompetent to give consent. Consent is given by a responsible party—a husband, wife, daughter, son, or legal representative. As with consent given by the person, consent by a responsible party must be informed consent.

Consent is given when the person enters the agency. A form is signed giving general consent to treatment. Special consent forms are required for surgery and other complex and invasive procedures. The doctor is responsible for informing the person about all aspects of the surgery or procedure. The RN may be given this responsibility. *You are never responsible for obtaining written consent.* However, you can witness the signing of a consent. When you are a witness, you must be present when the person signs the consent.

WILLS

A **will** is a legal statement of how a person wants property distributed after his or her death. A person may ask you to help prepare a will. You must politely refuse such a request. Explain that you do not have the knowledge or legal ability to prepare a will. Ask a nurse to speak to the person about contacting a lawyer.

Legally, you can witness the signing of a will. However, many agencies have policies about staff members witnessing wills. Make sure you know the policy of your agency. Do not witness a person's will if you are named in the will. To do so prevents you from receiving what was left to you. If you are a witness, you must be prepared to testify that the person was of sound mind when the will was signed. Also, be prepared to testify that the person stated that the document being signed was the person's last will. Be sure to tell your supervisor that you were a witness to a person's will.

REPORTING ABUSE

Abuse is a crime. Abuse has one or more of the following elements:

- Willful causing of injury
- Unreasonable confinement
- Intimidation (to make afraid with threats of force or violence)
- Punishment
- Deprivation of goods or services needed for physical, mental, or psychosocial well-being

With abuse, one or more of these elements result in physical harm, pain, or mental anguish. Protection against abuse extends to persons in a coma. With child and elderly abuse, the abuser is usually a family member or a caregiver. All states require the reporting of child abuse and elderly abuse. In domestic abuse (domestic violence), the abuser is a partner. The victim is responsible for reporting the abuse and filing criminal charges.

ELDERLY ABUSE

There are different forms of elderly abuse:

- *Physical abuse* involves hitting, slapping, kicking, pinching, and beating. It also includes corporal punishment—punishment inflicted directly on the body, such as beatings, lashings, or whippings. Neglect is also physical abuse. It involves depriving the person of needed medical services or treatment. Neglect is also failure to provide food, clothing, hygiene, and other basic needs. In health care, neglect includes but is not limited to leaving persons lying or sitting in urine or feces, isolating persons in their rooms or other locations, and failing to answer signal lights.
- *Verbal abuse* is the use of oral or written words or statements that speak badly of, sneer at, criticize, or condemn the person. Verbal abuse includes unkind gestures.
- *Involuntary seclusion* is confining the person to a certain area. Older people have been locked in closets, basements, attics, and other spaces.
- *Financial abuse* is when the elderly person's money is used by another person.

- *Mental abuse* includes humiliation, harassment, and threats of being punished or deprived of needs such as food, clothing, care, a home, or a place to sleep.
- *Sexual abuse* is when the person is harassed about sex or is attacked sexually. The person may be forced to perform sexual acts out of fear of punishment or physical harm.

There are many signs of elderly abuse. The abused person may show only some of the signs listed in Box 2-9.

Federal and state laws require the reporting of elderly abuse. If abuse is suspected, it must be reported. Where and how to report suspected abuse vary in each state. You may suspect that a person is being abused. If so, discuss the situation and your observations with the RN. Give as much information as possible. The RN then contacts the appropriate members of the health team. Community agencies that investigate elderly abuse also are contacted. They act immediately if there is a life-threatening situation. Sometimes the help of police or the courts is necessary.

Helping abused elderly persons is not always easy or possible. The abuse may never be reported or recognized, or the investigating agency may be unable to gain access to the person. Sometimes elderly persons are abused by their children. A victim may want to

---

Box 2-9   Signs of Elderly Abuse

- Living conditions are unsafe, unclean, or inadequate.
- Personal hygiene is lacking. The person is unclean, and clothes are dirty.
- Weight loss—there are signs of poor nutrition and inadequate fluid intake.
- Frequent injuries—circumstances behind the injuries are strange or seem impossible.
- Old bruises and new bruises are seen.
- The person seems very quiet or withdrawn.
- The person seems fearful, anxious, or agitated.
- The person does not seem to want to talk or answer questions.
- The person is restrained or locked in a certain area for long periods. Toilet facilities, food and water, and other necessary items cannot be reached.
- Private conversations are not allowed. The caregiver is present during all conversations.
- The person seems anxious to please the caregiver.
- Medications are not taken properly. Drugs are not purchased, or too much or too little medicine is taken.
- Visits to the emergency room may be frequent.
- The person may go from one doctor to another. Some people do not have a doctor.

protect the child. Some victims are embarrassed or believe the abuse is deserved. A victim may be afraid of what will happen. He or she may think that the present situation is better than no care at all. Some people fear not being believed if they report the abuse themselves. *(See Focus on Long-Term Care box.)*

CHILD ABUSE

Child abuse occurs at every social level. It occurs in low-, middle-, and high-income families. The abuser may have little education or be highly educated. The abuser is usually a household member (parent, a parent's partner, brother or sister, nanny) or someone known to the family. Risk factors for child abuse include the following:

- Stress
- Family crisis (divorce, unemployment, relocation, poverty, crowded living conditions)
- Drug or alcohol abuse
- Abuser history of being abused as a child
- Discipline beliefs that include physical punishment
- Lack of emotional attachment to the child
- A child with birth defects or chronic illness

- A child with a personality or behaviors that the abuser considers "different" or unacceptable
- Unrealistic expectations for the child's behavior or performance
- Families that move frequently and do not have family or friends nearby

Types of Child Abuse. Abuse differs from neglect. *Physical neglect* involves depriving the child of food, clothing, shelter, and medical care. *Emotional neglect* involves not meeting the child's need for affection and attention.

Physical abuse is intentionally injuring the child. Death can occur from physical abuse. *Sexual abuse* is using, persuading, or forcing a child to engage in sexual conduct. It may take several forms:

- *Rape*—forced sexual intercourse without the child's consent.
- *Molestation*—sexual advances toward a child. Molesting includes kissing, touching, or fondling sexual areas. The abuser may kiss, touch, or fondle the child. Or the child is forced to kiss, touch, or fondle the abuser.
- *Incest*—sexual activity between family members. The abuser may be a parent, stepparent, brother or sister, stepbrother or stepsister, aunt or uncle, cousin, or grandparent.
- *Child pornography*—photographing or videotaping a child involved in sexual acts.
- *Child prostitution*—forcing a child to engage in sexual activity for money. Usually the child is forced to have many sexual partners.

Box 2-10 lists the signs of physical and sexual abuse in children. Behaviors of the child and parents may arouse suspicion that something is wrong. The child may be quiet and withdrawn and fear adults. Sometimes children are afraid to go home. Sudden behavior changes are common in sexual abuse. Bedwetting, thumb-sucking, loss of appetite, poor grades, and running away from home are some examples.

Parents give different stories about what happened. Injuries are blamed on play accidents or other children. Frequent emergency room visits are common.

Child abuse is a complex syndrome. Many more behaviors, signs, and symptoms are present than discussed here. Health care professionals must be alert for signs and symptoms of child abuse. State laws require the reporting of suspected child abuse. However, it is important not to falsely accuse someone. If you suspect child abuse, share your concerns with the RN. As with elderly abuse, give as much information as you can. The RN will contact appropriate members of the health team and child protection agencies.

Focus On... LONG-TERM CARE

OBRA requires that nursing centers not employ persons who were convicted of abuse, neglect, or mistreatment of persons in a nursing center, hospital, home agency, or other health care agency. Before hiring a person, the center must thoroughly check the applicant's past work history. All references must be checked and efforts made to find out about any criminal prosecutions. For nursing assistant job applicants, the employer also checks the nursing assistant registry for any findings about abuse, neglect, or mistreatment of residents or misappropriation (misuse, stealing) of their property. For nurses or other staff, the appropriate licensing authority is contacted.

The center must take certain actions if abuse is suspected within the center:
- The incident must be reported immediately to the administrator and to other officials as required by federal and state laws.
- All claims of abuse must be thoroughly investigated.
- The center must prevent further potential for abuse while the investigation is in progress.
- Investigation results must be reported to the center administrator and to other officials as required by federal and state laws within 5 days of the incident.
- Corrective action must be taken if the claim is found to be true.

Box 2-10	**Signs and Symptoms of Child Abuse**

PHYSICAL ABUSE

- Bruises on the face (lips, mouth, cheeks), back, buttocks, abdomen, chest, and inner thighs
- Welts on the face (lips, mouth, cheeks), back, buttocks, abdomen, chest, and inner thighs
  - The shape of the object causing the welt may be seen. The shape may be of a belt, belt buckle, wooden spoon, chain, clothes hanger, rope, or other object.
- Burns and scalds on the feet, hands, back, or buttocks
  - Intentional burns leave a pattern from the item causing the burn: cigarettes, irons, curling irons, ropes, stove burners, and radiators.
  - In scalds, the area immersed in the hot liquid is clearly marked. For example, with a scald to the hand, the hand looks like a glove. A scald to a foot looks like a sock.
- Fractures of the nose, skull, arms, or legs
- Bite marks

SEXUAL ABUSE

- Bleeding, cuts, and bruises of the genitalia, anus, or mouth
- Stains or blood on underclothing
- Painful urination
- Vaginal discharge
- Genital odor
- Difficulty walking or sitting
- Pregnancy

DOMESTIC ABUSE

Domestic abuse occurs in relationships. One partner has power and control over the other. Such power and control occurs through abuse. Fear and harm occur. Types of abuse include physical, sexual, verbal, economic, or social. Usually more than one type of abuse is present in the relationship:

- *Physical abuse* is unwanted punching, slapping, biting, pulling hair, or kicking. Other forms of violence include burns and the use of weapons. Physical injuries occur. Death is a constant threat.
- *Sexual abuse* is unwanted sexual contact.
- *Verbal abuse* involves unkind and hurtful remarks. The remarks leave the person feeling unwhole, unattractive, and with little value.
- *Economic abuse* involves controlling money. Having or not having a job, paychecks, money gifts from family and friends, and money for household expenses (food, clothing) are controlled by the abuser.
- *Social abuse* is controlling friendships and other relationships. The abuser controls phone calls, use of the car, leaving the home, and visits with family and friends.

Like child and elderly abuse, domestic abuse is complex. The victim often hides the abuse and protects the abusive partner, However, unlike child and elderly abuse, all states do not require that health professionals report suspected domestic abuse. However, health professionals have an ethical responsibility to provide emotional support and to give information about safety and community resources. If you suspect that a person is a victim of domestic abuse, share your concerns with the RN. The RN will gather additional information as necessary to help the person.

Circle the BEST answer.

1. Which health care trend moves services from departments to the bedside?
   A. Managed care
   B. Health care systems
   C. Staffing mix
   D. Patient-focused care

2. Nursing practice is regulated by
   A. The Omnibus Budget Reconciliation Act of 1987
   B. Medicare and Medicaid
   C. Nurse practice acts
   D. Codes of ethics

3. What state law affects what assistive personnel can do?
   A. The state's nurse practice act
   B. The Omnibus Budget Reconciliation Act of 1987
   C. Medicare
   D. Medicaid

4. You perform a nursing task not allowed by your state. Which is *true*?
   A. If an RN delegated the task, there is no legal problem.
   B. You could be found guilty of practicing nursing without a license.
   C. Performing the task is allowed if it is in your job description.
   D. If you complete the task safely, there is no legal problem.

5. An RN asks you to start an IV. Which is *true*?
   A. Nursing assistants do not start IVs.
   B. The RN must supervise your work.
   C. You must be trained to start IVs.
   D. You must know how the IV affects the person.

6. These statements are about delegation. Which is *false*?
   A. RNs can delegate their responsibilities to you.
   B. A delegated task must be safe for the person.
   C. The delegated task must be in your job description.
   D. The delegating nurse is responsible for the safe completion of the task.

7. A task is in your job description. Which is *false*?
   A. The RN must always delegate the task to you.
   B. The RN delegates the task to you if the person's circumstances are right.
   C. The RN must make sure you have the necessary education and training.
   D. You must have clear directions before you perform the task.

8. An RN delegates a task to you. You must
   A. Complete the task
   B. Decide if you can accept the task or if you must say "no"
   C. Delegate the task to someone else if you are too busy to complete the task
   D. Ignore the request if you do not know how to perform the task

9. You are responsible for
   A. Completing delegated tasks safely
   B. Delegation
   C. The "five rights of delegation"
   D. Delegating tasks to other assistive personnel

10. You can refuse to perform a task for the following reasons *except*
    A. The task is beyond the legal limits of your role
    B. The task is not in your job description
    C. You do not like the task
    D. A nurse is not available to supervise you

11. You decide to refuse to perform a task. Your first action is to
    A. Delegate the task to someone else
    B. Communicate your concerns to the nurse
    C. Ignore the request
    D. Talk to the nurse's supervisor

12. Ethical standards
    A. Are federal laws
    B. Are state laws
    C. Are about right conduct and wrong conduct
    D. Are rules stating what you can and cannot do

13. The doctor orders several laboratory tests for a person. The person wants to know why. Who is responsible for telling the person?
    A. The doctor
    B. You
    C. The RN
    D. Any health team member

14. Which is *not* a crime?
    A. Negligence
    B. Murder
    C. Robbery
    D. Rape

15. These statements are about negligence. Which is *false*?
    A. It is an unintentional tort.
    B. The negligent person did not act in a reasonable manner.
    C. Harm was caused to a person or a person's property.
    D. A prison term is likely.

16. The intentional attempt or threat to touch a person's body without the person's consent is
    A. Assault
    B. Battery
    C. Defamation
    D. False imprisonment

17. The illegal restraint of another person's movement is
    A. Assault
    B. Battery
    C. Defamation
    D. False imprisonment

18. Mr. Blue's photograph is made public without his consent. This is
    A. Battery
    B. Fraud
    C. Invasion of privacy
    D. Malpractice

19. Which will *not* protect the person's right to privacy?
    A. Getting the person's consent for treatment
    B. Screening the person when giving care
    C. Exposing only the body part involved in the treatment or procedure
    D. Asking visitors to leave the room when care is given

20. A family member asks if you are a nurse. You answer "yes." This is
    A. Negligence
    B. Fraud
    C. Libel
    D. Slander

21. Who is responsible for obtaining the person's informed consent?
    A. The doctor
    B. The RN
    C. The LPN
    D. The nursing assistant

22. Which is *not* a sign of elderly abuse?
    A. Stiff joints and joint pain
    B. Old bruises and new bruises
    C. Poor personal hygiene
    D. Frequent injuries

23. A child is deprived of food and clothing. This is
    A. Physical neglect
    B. Physical abuse
    C. Emotional neglect
    D. Sexual abuse

24. These statements are about domestic abuse. Which is *true*?
    A. Suspected abuse must be reported to the police.
    B. Domestic abuse always involves violence.
    C. One partner has control over the other partner.
    D. Only one type of abuse is usually present.

25. You suspect a person was abused. What should you do?
    A. Tell the family.
    B. Call a state agency.
    C. Tell an RN.
    D. Ask the person if he or she was abused.

Answers to these questions are on p. 833.

CHAPTER

3

WORK ETHICS

Define the key terms listed in this chapter

Identify good health and personal hygiene practices

Describe the practices for professional appearance

Describe the qualities and characteristics of a successful nursing assistant

Explain what you should do to get a job

Prepare for work by planning for childcare and transportation

Describe ethical behavior on the job

Explain what is meant by harassment and sexual harassment

Explain how to resign from a job

Identify the common reasons for losing a job

KEY TERMS

confidentiality To trust others with personal and private information

courtesy A polite, considerate, or helpful comment or act

gossip To spread rumors or talk about the private matters of others

harassment To trouble, torment, offend, or worry a person by one's behavior or comments

work ethics Behavior in the workplace

As explained in Chapter 2, ethics deals with right conduct and wrong conduct. It involves making choices and judgments about what or what not to do. An ethical person does the right thing. In the workplace, certain behaviors (conduct), choices, and judgments are expected. Therefore **work ethics** deals with behavior in the workplace. Your conduct reflects your choices and judgments. Work ethics involves how you look, what you say, how you behave, and how you treat and work with others. To get and keep a job, you must conduct yourself in the right way.

PERSONAL HEALTH, HYGIENE, AND APPEARANCE

The health team sets an example for others. Patients, residents, and families expect the team to look and act healthy. A person has reason to question health team members who smoke, especially when the person is told to stop smoking. If you look unclean or unhealthy, the person and family wonder if you give good care. You are a member of the health team. Therefore your personal health, appearance, and hygiene deserve careful attention.

YOUR HEALTH

Patients, residents, and employers trust you. They believe you will give careful and effective care. To deserve this trust you must be physically and mentally healthy. Otherwise you cannot function at your best.

- *Diet*—Good nutrition involves eating a balanced diet from the Food Guide Pyramid (see Chapter 18). Start your day with a good breakfast. To maintain your weight, the number of calories taken in must equal your energy needs. To lose weight, take in fewer calories than your energy needs. Avoid foods from the fats, oils, and sweets group, salty foods, and crash diets.
- *Sleep and rest*—Sleep and rest are needed to stay healthy and to do your job well. Most adults need about 7 hours of sleep daily. Fatigue, lack of energy, and irritability mean you need more rest and sleep.
- *Body mechanics*—You will bend, carry heavy objects, and lift, move, and turn patients and residents. These activities place stress and strain on your body. You need to use your muscles in the right way (see Chapter 11).
- *Exercise*—Exercise is needed for muscle tone, circulation, and weight control. Walking, running, swimming, and biking are good forms of exercise.

You will feel better physically and mentally with regular exercise. Consult your doctor before starting a vigorous exercise program.

- *Your eyes*—Good vision is needed in your work. You will read instructions and measure blood pressures and temperatures. These involve fine measurements. Wrong readings can place patients and residents in danger. Have your eyes checked, and wear needed glasses or contact lenses. Make sure you have enough light when reading or doing fine work.
- *Smoking*—Smoking causes lung cancer, lung diseases, and many heart and circulatory disorders. Cigarette, cigar, and pipe smoke can offend others. Smoke odors stay on a person's breath, hands, clothing, and hair. Therefore handwashing and good personal hygiene are essential.
- *Drugs*—Some drugs affect thinking, feeling, behavior, and function. They affect a person's ability to work effectively. A person who works under the influence of drugs places patients and residents in danger. Take only those drugs ordered by a doctor and only in the way prescribed.
- *Alcohol*—Alcohol is a drug that depresses the brain. It affects thinking, balance, coordination, and mental alertness. Never report to work under the influence of alcohol or drink alcohol while working. Alcohol presents safety risks to patients and residents, co-workers, and you.

YOUR HYGIENE

You must pay careful attention to your personal cleanliness. Prevent offensive body odors by bathing daily and using a deodorant or antiperspirant. Brush your teeth after meals and use a mouthwash to prevent breath odors. Shampoo often, and style your hair in an attractive and simple way. Keep fingernails clean, short, and neatly shaped.

Special hygiene measures are needed during menstrual periods. Change tampons or sanitary napkins often, especially if flow is heavy. Wash your genital area with soap and water at least twice a day. Wash your hands after going to the bathroom, changing tampons or sanitary napkins, and washing the genital area.

YOUR APPEARANCE

Good health and personal hygiene practices help you look and feel well. Box 3-1 describes practices and suggestions to help you look neat, clean, and professional (Fig. 3-1).

GETTING A JOB

You may know where you want to work. If not, there are some simple ways to find out about job openings. One place is the *classified ad* sections of newspapers. The local *state employment service* is also a source. You may hear about jobs from *people you know*. You can also directly *contact the agencies* where you would like to work. Phone book yellow pages list health care agencies.

The agency for your student clinical experience is another place to look. The staff always looks at students as future employees. They watch how students treat patients or residents and co-workers. They look

---

Box 3-1 **Practices for a Professional Appearance**

- Uniforms fit well and are modest in length and style.
- Uniforms are clean, pressed, and mended. Wear a clean uniform daily.
- Wear your name badge or photo ID at all times when on duty.
- Underclothes are clean and fit properly. They are changed daily and are an appropriate color. Colored undergarments can be seen through white and light-colored uniforms.
- Cover tatooes. They may offend patients, residents, families, and co-workers.
- Jewelry is not worn. This includes adornments in body piercings. Most agencies let employees wear wedding rings; some allow engagement rings. Large rings and bracelets can scratch patients and residents. Confused or combative persons can easily pull off necklaces, bracelets, and earrings. Young children also like to pull on jewelry.

- Stockings and socks are clean, well-fitting, and changed daily.
- Shoes are comfortable, give needed support, and fit properly.
- Clean and polish shoes often. Wash laces, and replace them as necessary.
- Fingernails are clean, short, and neatly shaped. Long nails can scratch patients and residents.
- Nail polish is not worn. Chipped nail polish provides a place for microorganisms to grow and multiply.
- Hairstyles are simple and attractive. Hair is off your collar and away from your face. Use simple pins, combs, barrettes, and bands to keep long hair up and in place.
- Makeup is modest in amount and moderate in color. Avoid a painted and severe look.
- Perfume, cologne, and after-shave lotions are not worn. They may offend, nauseate, or cause breathing problems in patients and residents.

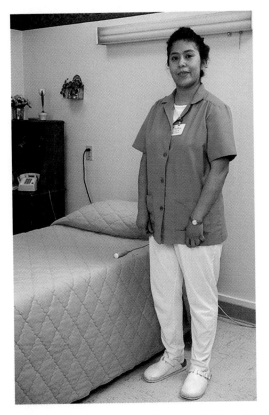

Fig. 3-1 The assistive person is well-groomed. Her uniform and shoes are clean. Her hair has a simple style and is out of her face and off of her collar. No jewelry is worn.

for the qualities and characteristics described in Box 3-2. So you are really being considered for a job while still a student. This is one more reason to always display good work ethics. If that agency is not hiring, the staff may advise you where to apply.

WHAT EMPLOYERS LOOK FOR

Before applying for a job or interviewing, think about what employers want in those they hire. If you had your own business, whom would you want to hire? Answering that question helps you better understand the employer's point of view.

Employers want employees who:

- Are well groomed
- Are dependable
- Have the skills and training needed to do the job
- Have the values and attitudes that fit with the agency

Caring about others is a common trait of health team members. You must care enough to want to make the life of a person happier, easier, or less painful. Good work ethics involves certain traits, attitudes, and manners. These qualities and characteristics are described in Box 3-2. They are necessary for you to function effectively in your role (Fig. 3-2, p. 38). *(See Focus on Home Care box on p. 38.)*

Box 3-2   Qualities and Characteristics for Good Work Ethics

Caring   Have concern for the person. Help make the person's life happier, easier, or less painful.

Dependability   Report to work on time and when scheduled. Perform delegated tasks and keep obligations and promises.

Consideration   Respect the person's physical and emotional feelings. Be gentle and kind toward patients, residents, families, and co-workers.

Cheerfulness   Greet and talk to people in a pleasant manner. Do not be moody, bad tempered, or unhappy while at work.

Empathy   Empathy is seeing things from the person's point of view—to put yourself in the person's position. Always ask yourself how you would feel if you had the person's problem?

Trustworthiness   Patients, residents, and staff members have confidence in you. They believe you will keep the person's information confidential. They trust you not to gossip about patients, residents, doctors, or the health team.

Respectfulness   Patients and residents have rights, values, beliefs, and feelings. If they differ from yours, do not criticize or condemn the person. Treat the person with respect and dignity at all times. Also show respect for supervisors and co-workers.

Courtesy   Be polite and courteous to patients, residents, families, visitors, and co-workers. Address people by title and name ("Mr. Tyler," "Ms. Crane," "Dr. Gilson"). Other courtesies include explaining to the person what you are going to do, saying "please" and "thank you," and not interrupting others.

Conscientiousness   Be careful, alert, and exact in following instructions. Give thorough care with knowledge and skill. Always give your best possible effort.

Honesty   Truthfully and accurately report the amount and kind of care given, your observations, and any errors.

Cooperation   Willingly help and work with others. Also take that "extra step" during busy and stressful times.

Enthusiasm   Be eager, interested, and excited about your work. What you are doing is important.

Self-Awareness   Know your own feelings, strengths, and weaknesses. You need to understand yourself before you can understand your patients and residents.

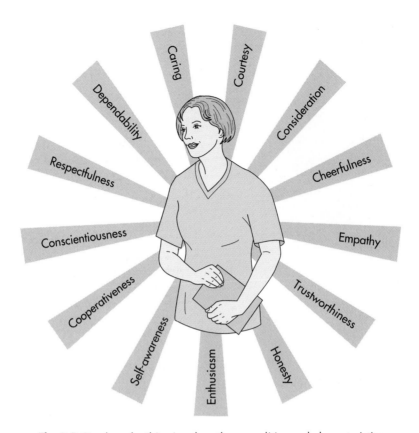

Fig. 3-2 Good work ethics involves these qualities and characteristics.

Focus On... HOME CARE

Home health care assistants also must be able to work alone and have self-discipline. You work alone in the home. An RN can be reached by phone. The RN makes some home visits. However, an RN is not immediately available to you at the bedside if problems occur. You must be able to perform procedures skillfully and safely.

Self-discipline also is essential. You must arrive at homes on time. Organize activities so personal care needs and housekeeping tasks are fulfilled. Avoid temptations. This includes watching TV, talking on the telephone, visiting, and stopping for an extra cup of coffee.

Honesty is very important. You may be asked to shop. You must be honest and thrifty with the person's money. Accurately report to the person or family the items purchased, their cost with receipts, total amount spent, and amount of money returned.

Respecting the person's property also is important. Assistive personnel handle valuables and personal property in health care settings. However, access to the person's property is greater in the home. Home furnishings, appliances, linens, and household items are used for personal care and housekeeping. Treat personal and family property with respect. Prevent damage. Read the manufacturer's instructions before using any appliance. Clean the appliance after use.

Applicants who look good communicate many things to the employer. You have only one chance to make a good first impression. A well-groomed person is likely to get the job over someone who is sloppy, has wrinkled or dirty clothes, and has body or breath odors. Proper dress for an interview is discussed later in this section.

Being dependable is very important. Health care agencies provide services to people. Staff must be at work on time and when scheduled. Undependable people cause everyone problems. Other staff members take on extra work. Fewer people give care. Quality of care can easily suffer. Supervisors spend time trying to find out if the person is coming to work. They also have to find someone else to cover for the absent employee. If you had your own business, you would want people to be at work when expected. Otherwise your business would be less efficient and productive.

Employers need to know that you can perform required job skills. The employer requests proof of required training. A certificate of course completion or a high school, college, or technical school transcript documents your training. Some employers accept a copy of an official grade report (report card).

Give the employer only a *copy* of your certificate, transcript, or grade report. Never give the original to the employer. Keep the original for future use. The employer may want the transcript sent directly from the school or college. *(See Focus on Long-Term Care box and Focus on Home Care box.)*

JOB APPLICATIONS

The agency asks you to complete a job application (Fig. 3-3, pp. 40-43). You get the application from the *personnel office* or *human resources office*. You may be asked to complete the application in that office. Some agencies have you take the application home and return it by mail or in person. Make sure you are well groomed and behave pleasantly when seeking or returning a job application. It may be your first chance to make a good impression.

Refer to the guidelines in Box 3-3 on p. 44 when completing a job application. How you fill it out may mean the difference between getting or not getting the job. Often the application is your first chance to impress the employer. A neat, legible, and complete application gives a better image than one that is sloppy or incomplete. Remember, employers use applications to screen out unqualified applicants.

THE JOB INTERVIEW

A job interview is the employer's chance to get to know and evaluate you. It also lets you find out more about the agency. Remember, employers hire well-groomed, dependable, and skilled people.

The interview may be when you complete the job application. Some employers review the application first to see if you are qualified. Box 3-4 on p. 44 lists common interview questions. Prepare your answers to these questions before the interview. Also prepare a typed list of your skills to give to the interviewer.

Your appearance is important. You must make a good impression. You need to be neat, clean, and well groomed (Fig. 3-4). The way you dress is also important. Box 3-5 on p. 45 gives guidelines on how to dress for an interview.

You must be on time. It shows you are dependable. If you have not been to the agency or do not know where it is, a *dry run* is useful. Go to the agency some day before your interview. Note how long it takes to get there and where to park. Also ask where to find the personnel office. A dry run gives you an idea of the time it takes to get from your home to the personnel office.

When you arrive for the interview, tell the receptionist your name and why you are there. Also give the interviewer's name. Then take a seat in the waiting area. Sit quietly in a professional manner. Do not smoke or chew gum. Use the time to review your answers to the common interview questions. Remember, waiting may be part of the interview. The interviewer may ask the receptionist about you—how you presented yourself when you arrived and what you did

---

Focus On... LONG-TERM CARE

OBRA requires that long-term care centers hire nursing assistants who have completed a state-approved training and competency evaluation program. The employer requests proof of training and also checks your record in the state nursing assistant registry.

Focus On... HOME CARE

Home care agencies receiving Medicare funds must meet OBRA requirements. Assistive personnel must meet the training and competency evaluation requirements outlined in OBRA. Some states have additional training requirements for assistive personnel employed by home care agencies.

---

while waiting. You must be polite and friendly at all times. Remember to smile.

Greet the interviewer in a polite, courteous manner. A firm handshake is correct for both men and women. Address the interviewer as Mr., Mrs., Ms., Miss, or Doctor. Then remain standing until asked to take a seat. When sitting, use good posture and sit in a professional manner (see Fig. 3-4). If the interviewer offers you a beverage, it is correct to accept. Remember to thank the person.

Good eye contact with the interviewer is important. Look directly at the interviewer when answering or asking questions. Poor eye contact can communicate negative information. This negative information includes being shy, insecure, dishonest, or lacking interest. Also watch your body language (see Chapter 5). Body language relates to facial expressions, gestures, postures, and body movements. What you say is important. However, how you use and move your body also communicates a great deal. Avoid distracting habits such as biting your nails, playing with jewelry or clothing, crossing your arms, and swinging your legs back and forth. Keep your mind on the interview. Do not touch or read things on the interviewer's desk.

The interview lasts 15 to 45 minutes. Answer honestly and to the best of your ability. Speak clearly and with confidence. Avoid short and long answers. "Yes" and "no" answers give little information. You generally want to give a brief explanation of "yes" and "no" responses.

The interviewer is likely to ask about your skills. Give him or her your skill list. The employer may ask about a skill not on your list. Explain that you are willing to learn the skill if your state allows assistive personnel to perform the task.

Text continued on p. 45

OSF℠ HEALTHCARE
A commitment to life.

OSF St. Francis Hospital
3401 Ludington Street, Escanaba, MI 49829

OSF Saint Joseph Hospital
1005 Julien Street, Belvidere, IL 61008

OSF Saint Anthony Medical Center
5666 E State Street, Rockford, IL 61108

OSF Saint James Hospital
610 E Water Street, Pontiac, IL 61764

OSF St. Joseph Medical Center
2200 E Washington Street, Bloomington, IL 61701

OSF Saint Francis Medical Center
530 NE Glen Oak Avenue, Peoria, IL 61637

OSF St. Mary Medical Center
3333 N Seminary, Galesburg, IL 61401

**OSF St. Francis Continuation Care and
Nursing Home Center**
210 S Fifth Street, Burlington, IA 52601

OSF St. Anthony's Continuing Care Center
767 30th Street, Rock Island, IL 61201

OSF HEALTHPLANS, INC.
300 SW Jefferson Street, Peoria, IL 61602

OSF SAINT FRANCIS, INC.
4541 N Prospect, Peoria, IL 61614

OSF HEALTHCARE SYSTEM
800 NE Glen Oak Avenue, Peoria, IL 61603

APPLICATION FOR EMPLOYMENT

OSF HealthCare is an equal opportunity employer and does not discriminate because of age, sex, race, creed, color, religion, national origin, marital status, disability, or other protected status.

NAME — LAST — FIRST — MIDDLE INITIAL — POSITION DESIRED — DATE

PLEASE PRINT

LAST NAME	FIRST NAME	MIDDLE INITIAL	SOCIAL SECURITY NO.

STREET ADDRESS, CITY, STATE, ZIP	HOME PHONE ( )
	ALTERNATE PHONE ( )

POSITION(S) DESIRED	DATE AVAILABLE	PAYRATE DESIRED

HAVE YOU EVER APPLIED AT OSF HEALTHCARE BEFORE? ☐ YES ☐ NO	WHEN?	WHERE?	WHAT POSITION?

WERE YOU EVER EMPLOYED BY OSF HEALTHCARE BEFORE? ☐ YES ☐ NO	IF YES, WHEN? — UNDER WHAT LAST NAME?	WHAT FACILITY?	WHAT CAPACITY?

IF UNDER AGE 18, GIVE BIRTHDATE.	ARE YOU A U.S. CITIZEN OR AN ALIEN LEGALLY AUTHORIZED TO WORK IN THE U.S.A.? ☐ YES ☐ NO

DO YOU HAVE ANY RELATIVES WORKING AT THIS FACILITY? ☐ YES ☐ NO	IF YES, PLEASE LIST NAMES AND RELATIONSHIP

Have you ever pled guilty to or been convicted of any criminal offense (other than minor traffic violations)? ☐ Yes ☐ No
If "yes," please explain. Note: A criminal conviction is not an automatic bar to employment.

_____

_____

EMPLOYMENT DATA

WHAT SHIFT(S) ARE YOU WILLING TO WORK? 1ST 2ND 3RD OTHER: _____	CIRCLE DAYS YOU CAN WORK MON. TUES. WED. THURS. FRI. SAT. SUN. ARE YOU WILLING TO WORK OT IF REQUIRED? ☐ YES ☐ NO	ARE YOU WILLING TO WORK WEEKENDS? ☐ YES ☐ NO HOLIDAYS? ☐ YES ☐ NO	STATUS DESIRED ☐ FULL-TIME ☐ PART-TIME

WHAT PROMPTED YOUR APPLICATION? (PLEASE BE SPECIFIC)

☐ EMPLOYEE REFERRAL _____

☐ NEWSPAPER _____

☐ OWN ACCORD _____

☐ JOB LINE _____

☐ OTHER _____

☐ PRN

☐ TEMPORARY

IF APPLYING FOR PART-TIME, HOW MANY HOURS PER WEEK ARE YOU ABLE TO WORK? _____

Form No. Z8020 (Rev. 10/96) **MFI**

Fig. 3-3 A sample job application. *(Courtesy OSF St. Joseph Medical Center, Bloomington, Ill.)*

EDUCATION

	NAME & ADDRESS OF SCHOOL	COURSE OF STUDY	CIRCLE LAST YEAR COMPLETED	DID YOU GRADUATE	LIST DEGREE OR DIPLOMA
HIGH SCHOOL			1 2 3 4	☐ YES ☐ NO	
COLLEGE			1 2 3 4	☐ YES ☐ NO	
POST GRADUATE			1 2 3 4	☐ YES ☐ NO	
OTHER					

IF NOW ATTENDING SCHOOL, PLEASE GIVE ANTICIPATED GRADUATION DATE.

EMPLOYMENT HISTORY

PRESENT OR MOST RECENT EMPLOYER

NAME OF EMPLOYER	STREET ADDRESS, CITY, STATE, ZIP	PHONE NUMBER ( )
YOUR LAST NAME AT THAT TIME?	JOB TITLE	DATE OF EMPLOYMENT FROM: TO:
REASON FOR LEAVING?	SUPERVISOR'S NAME	ENDING SALARY
CONTACT FOR REFERENCE? IF NO WHY? ☐ YES ☐ NO	DUTIES, SKILLS. EQUIPMENT USED:	

PREVIOUS EMPLOYERS LIST MOST RECENT FIRST

NAME OF EMPLOYER	STREET ADDRESS, CITY, STATE, ZIP	PHONE NUMBER ( )
YOUR LAST NAME AT THAT TIME?	JOB TITLE	DATE OF EMPLOYMENT FROM: TO:
REASON FOR LEAVING?	SUPERVISOR'S NAME	ENDING SALARY
CONTACT FOR REFERENCE? IF NO, WHY? ☐ YES ☐ NO	DUTIES, SKILLS, EQUIPMENT USED:	

NAME OF EMPLOYER	STREET ADDRESS, CITY, STATE, ZIP	PHONE NUMBER ( )
YOUR LAST NAME AT THAT TIME?	JOB TITLE	DATE OF EMPLOYMENT FROM: TO:
REASON FOR LEAVING?	SUPERVISOR'S NAME	ENDING SALARY
CONTACT FOR REFERENCE? IF NO, WHY? ☐ YES ☐ NO	DUTIES, SKILLS, EQUIPMENT USED:	

NAME OF EMPLOYER	STREET ADDRESS, CITY, STATE, ZIP	PHONE NUMBER
YOUR LAST NAME AT THAT TIME?	JOB TITLE	DATE OF EMPLOYMENT FROM: TO:
REASON FOR LEAVING?	SUPERVISOR'S NAME	ENDING SALARY
CONTACT FOR REFERENCE? IF NO, WHY? ☐ YES ☐ NO	DUTIES, SKILLS, EQUIPMENT USED:	

I HEREBY GIVE PERMISSION TO OSF HEALTHCARE TO CONTACT THE EMPLOYERS LISTED ABOVE TO OBTAIN ANY INFORMATION DEEMED RELEVANT. I COMPLETELY RELEASE OSF HEALTHCARE AND THE PROVIDERS OF THE INFORMATION FROM ANY AND ALL LIABILITY ARISING OUT OF INQUIRIES MADE OR INFORMATION PROVIDED RELATIVE TO MY APPLICATION FOR EMPLOYMENT EVEN IF SUCH INFORMATION IS NEGATIVE AND/OR ADVERSELY AFFECTS MY APPLICATION FOR EMPLOYMENT.

_____   _____
DATE   APPLICANT SIGNATURE

Fig. 3-3, cont'd For legend see opposite page.

Continued

PROFESSIONAL LICENSES, REGISTRATIONS, AND/OR CERTIFICATIONS

ARE YOU CURRENTLY: ☐ REGISTERED   ☐ LICENSED   ☐ CERTIFIED

TYPE	STATE ISSUED	DATE	NO.
TYPE	STATE ISSUED	DATE	NO.
TYPE	STATE ISSUED	DATE	NO.

HAVE YOU EVER HAD YOUR LICENSES, REGISTRATION OR CERTIFICATION REVOKED, SUSPENDED OR PUT ON PROBATION?   ☐ YES ☐ NO
IF YES, PLEASE EXPLAIN.

IF THE JOB YOU ARE APPLYING FOR REQUIRES THE DRIVING OF A MOTOR VEHICLE WHILE ON DUTY, PLEASE PROVIDE THE FOLLOWING INFORMATION:

DRIVER'S LICENSE NO. _____ STATE _____

ADDITIONAL SKILLS

PLEASE CHECK ANY SKILLS BELOW IN WHICH YOU ARE PROFICIENT:

☐ TYPING _____ WPM

☐ SHORTHAND OR SPEEDWRITING

☐ MACHINE TRANSCRIPTION

☐ MEDICAL TERMINOLOGY

☐ FOREIGN LANGUAGE _____

☐ OTHER: _____

COMPUTER SKILLS: (SPECIFY SOFTWARE)

☐ WINDOWS

☐ WORD PROCESSING

☐ SPREADSHEET

☐ DATABASES

☐ GRAPHICS

☐ ALPHANUMERIC DATA ENTRY _____ SPH

PLEASE NOTE ANY ADDITIONAL SKILLS, EXPERIENCE, OR TRAINING THAT YOU FEEL IS IMPORTANT. PLEASE INCLUDE EQUIPMENT OR COMPUTER SOFTWARE USED.

I UNDERSTAND THAT IF I MAKE ANY FALSE STATEMENTS, MISREPRESENTATIONS, OR OMISSIONS ON THIS APPLICATION OR DURING THE HIRING PROCESS, I MAY BE REFUSED EMPLOYMENT OR, IF EMPLOYED, I MAY BE TERMINATED, REGARDLESS OF WHEN DISCOVERED. IN CONSIDERATION OF MY EMPLOYMENT, I AGREE TO CONFORM TO THE RULES, REGULATIONS AND PHILOSOPHY AND VALUES OF OSF HEALTHCARE. I UNDERSTAND THIS APPLICATION IS NOT INTENDED TO BE A CONTRACT OF EMPLOYMENT. I UNDERSTAND THAT MY EMPLOYMENT CAN BE TERMINATED AT ANY TIME AND FOR ANY REASON, AT THE OPTION OF EITHER OSF HEALTHCARE OR MYSELF. I UNDERSTAND THAT NO ONE OTHER THAN AN ADMINISTRATOR HAS ANY AUTHORITY TO ENTER INTO ANY AGREEMENT FOR EMPLOYMENT FOR ANY SPECIFIED PERIOD OF TIME OR TO MAKE ANY AGREEMENT CONTRARY TO THE FOREGOING AND THAT ANY SUCH AGREEMENT MUST BE IN WRITING, SIGNED BY AN ADMINISTRATOR, AND NOTARIZED. I ALSO UNDERSTAND THAT I WILL BE REQUIRED TO COMPLETE A MEDICAL EXAMINATION WHICH MAY INCLUDE A DRUG SCREEN AND A CRIMINAL BACKGROUND CHECK BEFORE BEGINNING EMPLOYMENT. I UNDERSTAND THIS APPLICATION AND ANY INFORMATION IN IT MAY BE SHARED WITH ANY OSF HEALTHCARE ENTITY.

_____   _____
APPLICANT SIGNATURE   DATE

Fig. 3-3 A sample job application. (*Courtesy OSF St. Joseph Medical Center, Bloomington, Ill.*)

APPLICANT DO NOT WRITE IN THIS SPACE - FOR OFFICE USE ONLY

HR / INTERVIEWER / MANAGER COMMENTS: (INCLUDE DATES)

EXTEND APPLICANT A CONDITIONAL OFFER OF EMPLOYMENT AT THE STARTING RATE OF $_____

_____ AND FOR _____ HOURS PER PAY PERIOD ON THE _____ SHIFT AS A

❏ REGULAR   ❏ TEMPORARY EMPLOYEE.   DESIRED START DATE: _____

DO NOT OFFER EMPLOYMENT.   EXPLAIN: _____

SIGNATURE: _____   DATE: _____

COPIES SENT TO: (INCLUDE DATES) _____

INTERVIEWED WITH: (INCLUDE DATES) _____

TO BE COMPLETED BY HUMAN RESOURCES

ID #:	NEW HIRE:	REHIRE:	TRANSFER:	FACILITY #:
BIRTH DATE	FACILITY DATE	SYSTEM DATE	BENEFIT DATE	PENSION DATE
PAY FREQUENCY	REGULAR / TEMP / PRN	HOURS PER PAY PERIOD	SHIFT	PHYSICAL DATE
TIME CARD STATUS	EXEMPT / NONEXEMPT	ANNUAL SALARY	HOURLY RATE	TABLE / GRADE / STEP
DEPARTMENT #	COST CENTER	JOB TITLE		JOB CODE
MALE / FEMALE	MARITAL STATUS	EEOC	CITIZENSHIP	
BACKGROUND SENT	BACKGROUND ID #	HR AUTHORIZATION		DATE

Fig. 3-3, cont'd For legend see opposite page.

Box 3-3   Guidelines for Completing a Job Application

- Read the directions first and then follow them. The directions may ask you to use black ink and to print. Following directions is important on the job. Employers look at job applications to see if you can follow directions.
- Write neatly. Your writing must be legible. A messy application gives a bad image. Legible writing lets the employer have the correct information. You will not be contacted if the employer cannot read your telephone number. You may miss getting the job.
- Complete the entire application. If something does not apply to you, write "N/A" for nonapplicable or draw a line through the space. This tells the employer that you read the section and that you did not skip the item on purpose.
- Report any felony arrests or convictions as directed. Write "no" or "none" as appropriate. Some states require criminal background checks.
- Provide information about employment gaps. If you did not work for a time, the employer wonders why. Provide this information to give the employer a good impression about your honesty. Some reasons include going to school, staying home to raise children, caring for an ill family member, or your own illness.
- Tell why you left a job, if asked. Be brief but honest. People leave jobs for one that pays better or for career advancement. Other reasons include those given above for employment gaps. If you were fired from a job, give an honest but positive response. However, do not talk badly about a former employer.
- Provide references as requested. Be prepared to give the names, titles, addresses, and telephone numbers of at least three references. You should have this information written down before completing an application. (Always ask references if an employer can contact them.) You may get the job faster or over another applicant if the employer can quickly check references. If reference information is missing or incomplete, the employer waits for all of the information. This wastes your time and the employer's time. Also, the employer wonders if you are hiding something with incomplete reference information.
- Be honest in all your responses. Lying on an application is fraud. It is grounds for being fired.

Box 3-4   Common Interview Questions

- Tell me about yourself.
- Please tell me about your career goals.
- What are you doing currently to achieve these goals?
- Describe what you consider to be *professional* behavior.
- Tell me about your last job.
- What did you like the most about your last job? What did you like the least?
- Why did you leave your last job?
- What would your supervisor and co-workers tell me about your dependability? Your skills? Your ability to adapt?
- Of all your functions, which presented the most difficulty for you?
- How did you handle this difficulty?
- How do you set priorities?
- In what ways have your past experiences prepared you for this position?
- If there is one thing that you could change about your last job, what would it be?
- How do you handle problems with patients, residents, and co-workers?
- Why do you want to work here?
- Why should this agency hire you?

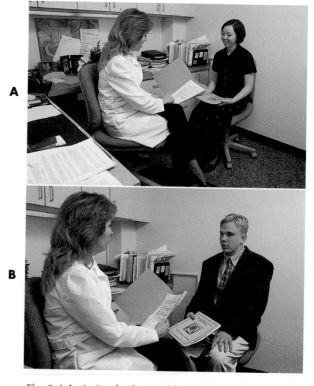

Fig. 3-4 A, A simple skirt and blouse are worn for a job interview. Note that the applicant sits with her back straight and legs together. **B,** This man is wearing light slacks, a shirt and tie, and a jacket for his interview.

Box 3-5	Grooming and Dressing for an Interview

- Take a bath, brush your teeth, and wash your hair.
- Use a deodorant or antiperspirant.
- Make sure your hands and fingernails are clean.
- Apply makeup in a simple, attractive manner.
- Style your hair so that it is neat and attractive. You may want to wear it as you would for work.
- Do not wear jeans, shorts, tank tops, halter tops, or other casual clothing.
- Wear a simple dress, skirt and blouse, or suit (women). Men should wear a suit or dark slacks, shirt and tie, and a jacket. A long-sleeved white or light-blue shirt is best.
- Make sure clothing is pressed and in good repair. Sew on loose buttons and mend garments as needed.
- Wear socks (men and women) or hose (women). Hose should be free of runs and snags.
- Make sure shoes are polished and in good repair.
- Avoid heavy perfumes, colognes, and after-shaves. A lightly scented fragrance is acceptable.
- Wear only simple jewelry that complements your clothes. Avoid adornments in body piercings. If you have multiple ear piercings, wear only one set of earrings.
- Stop in the restroom when you arrive at the interview location. Check to make sure that your hair, makeup, and clothes are in place.

Box 3-6	Questions to Ask the Interviewer

- Which of the job functions do you think are the most important?
- What employee qualities and characteristics are most important to you?
- What nursing care pattern is used here? (See Chapter 1).
- Who will I be working with?
- When are performance evaluations done? Who does them? How are they done?
- What performance factors are evaluated?
- How does the supervisor handle problems?
- What are the most common reasons that nursing assistants quit their jobs here?
- What are the most common reasons that nursing assistants lose their jobs here?
- How do you see this job in the next year? In the next 5 years?
- What is the greatest reward from this job?
- What is the greatest challenge of this job?
- What do you like the most about nursing assistants who work here?
- What do you like the least about nursing assistants who work here?
- Why should I work here rather than in another agency?
- Why are you interested in hiring me?
- May I have a tour of the agency and the unit I will be working on? Will you introduce me to the nurse manager and unit staff?
- Can I have a few minutes to talk with my nurse manager?

Whenever you look for employment, you want to find the right job for you. A right match is important. You do not want a job that is not right for you. Nor does the employer want to hire someone who will not be happy in the job or at the agency. At the end of the interview, you will have the chance to ask questions. Box 3-6 lists some questions to ask during your interview. The interviewer's answer will help you decide if the job is right for you.

You should also review the job description with the interviewer. If you have any questions, ask them at this time. Also advise the interviewer of any functions you cannot perform because of training, legal, ethical, or religious reasons. An honest talk with the interviewer prevents problems later.

Also ask questions about starting salary, work hours, your job description, uniform requirements, and the agency's new-employee orientation program. Remember to ask about benefits such as health and disability insurance, vacation, and continuing education.

The interviewer signals when the interview is over. You will be thanked for coming for the interview. You may be offered a job at this time. Or the interviewer tells you when to expect a call. Follow-up is acceptable. Ask the interviewer when you can check on your application. Before leaving, thank the interviewer and tell the person that you look forward to hearing from him or her.

A written thank-you note is advised (Fig. 3-5, p. 46). Write this the day of or the day after the interview. Your writing must be neat and legible. Use a computer or typewriter if your writing is hard to read. The thank-you note should include:

- The date
- The interviewer's formal name using Mr., Mrs., Ms., Miss, or Dr.
- A statement thanking the person for the interview
- Comments about the interview, the agency, and your eagerness to hear about the job
- Your signature using your first and last names

ACCEPTING A JOB

Accept the job that is best for you. You can apply at several places and have many interviews. Take time to think about any offers before accepting one. If you have more questions about the agency, ask them before accepting the job. Discussing the offer with a relative, friend, co-worker, or your instructor may help you with your decision.

December 12

Dear Ms. Miller,

Thank you for the interview yesterday. I enjoyed meeting you and learning more about the nursing center. I was impressed by the friendliness of the staff and would enjoy working in that environment.

Again, thank you. I look forward to hearing from you soon.

Sincerely,

Jane M. Doe

Fig. 3-5 Sample thank-you note written after a job interview.

When you accept a job, agree on a starting date and time. Find out where to report on your first day. Ask for the employee handbook and other agency information. Read all materials before you start working.

PREPARING FOR WORK

Having a job is a privilege. It is not a right or something due to you. You earned the job by getting the required education and training. You succeeded in a job interview. Now you must function well and work well with others to keep your job.

You must work when scheduled. This means getting to work on time and staying the entire shift. Absences and tardiness (being late) are among the most common reasons for losing a job. Childcare and transportation issues often interfere with getting to work and getting to work on time. You need to plan for childcare and transportation. Do not wait until it is time to leave for work.

CHILDCARE

Someone needs to care for your children when you leave for work, while you are at work, and before you get home from work. Also plan for the following emergencies:

- Your childcare provider is ill or cannot care for your children that day
- A child becomes ill while you are at work
- You will be late getting home from work

TRANSPORTATION

Plan for how you get to and from work. If you drive your own car, keep the car in good working order. Keep plenty of gas in the car, or leave early enough to get gas.

Car pooling is another option. Car pool members have responsibilities to each other. If the driver is late leaving or picking one person up, everyone is late for work. If one person is not ready when the driver arrives, everyone in the car pool is late for work. Car pool with persons you trust to be ready and on time. When you drive, make sure you leave and pick others up on time. When you are a passenger, be ready when the driver arrives.

Public transportation (buses and trains) is common in large cities. Know your bus or train schedule. Know what other bus or train you can take if delays occur. Always make sure you have enough money for your fares to and from work.

Always have a back-up transportation plan. Your car may not start, the car pool driver may not go to work, or public transportation may not operate. If you have a back-up plan, you can get to work on time.

ON THE JOB

You will have contact with patients, residents, visitors, and co-workers. How you look, how you behave, and what you say affect everyone in the agency. Working when scheduled, being cheerful and friendly, performing delegated tasks, helping others, and being kind in what you do and say are part of good work ethics. The *Employee Handbook* of OSF Saint Francis Medical Center (Peoria, Ill.) says it best:

You are what people see when they arrive here; yours are the eyes they look into when they're frightened and lonely. Yours are the voices people hear when they ride the elevators, when they try to sleep, and when they try to forget their problems. You are what they hear on their way to appointments which could affect their destinies, and what they hear after they leave those appointments. Yours are the comments people hear when you think they can't.

Yours is the intelligence and caring that people hope they'll find here. If you're noisy, so is the medical center. If you're rude, so is the medical center. And if you're wonderful, so is the medical center.

ATTENDANCE

You must report to work when scheduled and on time. The entire unit is affected when just one person is late. You must call your supervisor if you will be late or cannot go to work. Agency attendance policies are explained in its employee handbook. You must follow these policies. Poor attendance can cause you to lose your job.

Being on time does not mean arriving at the agency when your shift begins. It means being *ready to work* when your shift starts. Remember you need to store your coat, purse, backpack, and other personal items. You might need to use the restroom when you arrive at the agency. Plan to arrive on your nursing unit a few minutes early. This gives you time to greet others and settle yourself.

Attendance is more than getting to work when scheduled and on time. You must stay the entire shift. Preparing for childcare emergencies is important. Watching the clock so that you can leave as soon as the shift ends gives a bad image. Working overtime is sometimes necessary. You need to prepare to stay longer if necessary. (*See Focus on Home Care box.*)

YOUR ATTITUDE

You need to show a good attitude about your job. Show that you are happy to be at the agency and that you enjoy your work. Listen to others and be willing to learn. Stay busy and use your time well. You must demonstrate the qualities and characteristics described in Box 3-2.

The work you do is very important. Nurses, patients, residents, and families rely on you to give good care. You need to believe that you and your work are valuable to the agency.

Always think before you speak. The following statements signal a bad attitude:

- "I can't. I'm too busy."
- "I didn't do it."
- "It's not my fault."
- "Don't blame me."
- "It's not my turn. I did it yesterday."
- "Nobody told me."
- "I can't come to work today. I have a headache."
- "That's not my job."
- "You didn't tell me that you needed it right away."
- "I work harder than anyone else."
- "No one appreciates what I do."

GOSSIP

To **gossip** means to spread rumors or talk about the private matters of others. Gossiping is unprofessional.

Focus On... HOME CARE

Home care assignments must be completed. You must never leave in the middle of an assignment. Nor should you leave before someone from the next shift arrives. Unfortunately, conflicts or problems may occur. Make every effort to finish the assignment. Explain the problem to your supervisor. The supervisor will try to make any needed changes. You must not walk out on the person. That would leave the person in an unsafe situation. Walking out is a most unethical behavior.

It can hurt others. The following guidelines will help you to avoid being a part of gossip:

- Remove yourself from a group or situation where gossip is occurring.
- Do not make or repeat any comment that can hurt a person, family member, co-worker, or the agency.
- Do not make or repeat any comment that you do not know to be true. Remember, making or writing false statements about another person is defamation (see Chapter 2).
- Do not talk about patients, residents, visitors, family members, co-workers, or the agency at home or in social settings.

CONFIDENTIALITY

The person's information is private and personal. **Confidentiality** means to trust others with personal and private information. Patient or resident information is shared only among health team members involved in the person's care. The person has the right to privacy and confidentiality (see Chapter 2). Agency and co-worker information also is confidential.

Avoid talking about patients, residents, the agency, or co-workers where others are present. Only share information with the nurse supervising your work. Avoid talking about patients, residents, the agency, or co-workers in hallways, elevators, dining areas, or outside the agency. Others not involved in the situation may overhear you. Patients, residents, and visitors are very alert to what is said. Those persons overhearing you may think you are talking about them or their loved ones. This leads to misinformation and the wrong impressions about the person's condition. You can easily upset the person or family. Therefore you must be very careful about what you say, how you say it, when you say it, and where you say it.

Avoid eavesdropping. To eavesdrop means to listen in or overhear the conversations of others. When you eavesdrop, you invade another person's privacy.

Intercom systems require special considerations (see Chapter 4). Many agencies have intercom systems to allow communication between the bedside and the nurses' station. The person uses the intercom to signal when help is needed. The intercom is answered by a staff member at the nurses' station. The nursing team also uses the intercom to communicate with other team members. Be careful what you say over the intercom. It is like a loudspeaker. Others nearby can hear what you are saying.

PERSONAL HYGIENE AND APPEARANCE

How you look affects the way people think about you and the agency. If staff are clean and neat, people think the agency is clean and neat. They think the agency is unclean if staff are messy and unkempt. People also wonder about the quality of care given.

Attire accepted in home and social settings is often improper in the work setting. You cannot wear jeans, halter tops, tank tops, or short skirts. Clothing must not be tight, revealing, or sexual in nature. That is, females cannot show cleavage, the tops of breasts, or the upper thigh. Males must avoid tight pants and exposing their chests. Only the top shirt button is open.

Follow these guidelines for good personal hygiene and appearance in the work setting:

- Practice personal hygiene.
- Follow the guideline for professional appearance listed in Box 3-1.
- Follow the agency's dress code.
- Tend to grooming needs in private. Use the restroom to brush hair, freshen make-up, apply lipstick, floss, or brush your teeth.
- Do not smoke or chew gum or tobacco while on duty.
- Cover tattoos. They may offend residents, visitors, and co-workers.

SPEECH AND LANGUAGE

Your speech and language must be professional. Accepted speech and language in home and social settings may be unacceptable at work. The words you use when talking to family and friends may offend patients, residents, visitors, and co-workers. Remember the following:

- Do not swear or use foul, vulgar, or abusive language.
- Do not use slang.
- Control the volume and tone of your voice. Speak softly and gently.
- Speak clearly. Persons with hearing problems may have difficulty hearing you (see Chapter 29).
- Do not shout or yell.
- Do not fight or argue with the person, family, or co-workers.

COURTESIES

A **courtesy** is a polite, considerate, or helpful comment or act. Courtesies are easy. They require little time or energy. And they mean so much to people. Even the smallest act of kindness can brighten someone's day.

- Address others by Miss, Mrs., Ms., Mr., or Doctor. Call a person by first name only if he or she asks you to do so.
- Say "please." Begin or end each request with "please."
- Say "thank you" whenever someone does something for you.
- Apologize to others. Say "I'm sorry" whenever you make a mistake or hurt someone. Even little things—like bumping into someone in the hallway—require an apology.
- Be thoughtful of others. Compliment others as appropriate. Wish others a happy birthday, a happy day or weekend off, or a happy holiday.
- Wish the person and family well when they leave the agency. "Stay well" or "stay healthy" are good phrases to use.
- Hold doors open for others. If you are at the door first, open the door and let others pass through. In business, males and females hold doors open for each other.
- Hold elevator doors open for others coming down the hallway.
- Help others willingly when asked.
- Praise others. If you see a co-worker do or say something that impresses you, tell that person. Also tell your co-workers.
- Do not take credit for another person's deed. Give the person credit for the action.

PERSONAL MATTERS

You are employed to do a job. Personal matters cannot interfere with the job. Otherwise care is neglected. You could lose your job for tending to personal matters while at work. Practice the following to keep personal matters out of the work place:

- Make personal phone calls only during breaks. Use public pay phones.
- Do not let family and friends visit you on the unit. If they must see you, arrange for them to meet you during a break.
- Arrange personal appointments (doctor, dentist, lawyer, beauty, and others) for times when you are not scheduled to work.
- Do not use agency computers, printers, fax machines, photocopiers, or other equipment for your personal use.
- Do not take agency supplies (pens, paper, and others) for your personal use.

- Do not discuss personal problems at work.
- Control your emotions. If you need to cry or express anger, do so in a private place. Get yourself together quickly and return to your work.
- Avoid borrowing money from or lending money to co-workers. This includes meal money and bus or train fares. Borrowing and lending can lead to problems with co-workers.
- Do not engage in selling or fund-raising activities at work. Do not sell your child's candy or raffle tickets to co-workers.
- Do not carry personal pagers or cellular phones while at work.

MEALS AND BREAKS

Meal breaks are usually 30 minutes long. Other breaks are usually for 15 minutes. Meals and breaks are scheduled so that some staff is always on the unit. Staff remaining on the unit cover for the staff on break.

Staff members are responsible to each other. Leave for and return from your meal or break on time. That way other staff can have their breaks. Do not take longer than you are allowed. Also remember to tell the nurse when you leave and return to the unit.

JOB SAFETY

Safety involves protecting patients, residents, visitors, co-workers, and yourself from harm. Every employee is responsible for job safety. Negligent behavior affects the safety of others (see Chapter 2). Safety practices are presented throughout this book. The following guidelines are important no matter what you are doing:

- Understand the roles, functions, and responsibilities in your job description.
- Be familiar with the contents and policies in personnel and procedure manuals.
- Know the difference between right and wrong.
- Know what you can and cannot do.
- Develop the desired qualities and characteristics of nursing assistants.
- Follow the nurse's directions and instructions.
- Question unclear instructions and things you do not understand.
- Help others willingly when asked.
- Follow agency rules and regulations.
- Ask for any training that you might need.
- Report measurements, observations, the care given, the person's complaints, and any errors accurately.
- Accept responsibility for your actions. Admit when you are wrong or make mistakes. Do not blame others. Do not make excuses for your actions. Learn what you did wrong and why. Always try to learn from your mistakes.

PLANNING AND ORGANIZING YOUR WORK

Working well with others includes working in an organized and efficient way. You will give nursing care to patients and residents. You also will perform routine tasks on the nursing unit. You must complete some assignments by a certain time. Other tasks or functions are done by the end of the shift. You must plan and organize your work to give safe, thorough care and to make good use of your time (Box 3-7).

HARASSMENT

Harassment means troubling, tormenting, offending, or worrying a person by one's behavior or comments. Harassment can be sexual. Or it can involve one's age, race, ethnic background, religion, or disability. What you say and do must be respectful of others. You must not offend others by your gestures, remarks, or use of touch. Nor can you offend others with jokes or pictures. Harassment is not legal in the work place.

Box 3-7	**Planning and Organizing Your Work**

- Discuss priorities with the nurse.
- Know the routine of your shift and nursing unit.
- List care or procedures that are on a schedule. Some persons are turned or offered the bedpan every 2 hours.
- Estimate how much time is needed for each person, procedure, and task.
- Identify which tasks and procedures can be done while patients or residents are eating, visiting, or involved in activities or therapies.
- Plan care around mealtimes, visiting hours, and therapies. If working in a nursing center, also consider daily recreation and social activities.
- Identify situations in which you will need help from a co-worker. Ask a co-worker to help you, and give the time when you will need help.
- Schedule any equipment or rooms if necessary. Some agencies have only one shower or bathtub to a nursing unit. You need to schedule the room for the person's use.
- Review the procedures and gather needed supplies beforehand.
- Do not waste time. Stay focused on your work.
- Do not leave a messy work area. Make sure rooms are neat and orderly. Also clean utility areas.
- Be a self-starter. That is, have initiative. Ask others if they need help, follow unit routines, stock supply areas, and clean utility rooms. Stay busy.

SEXUAL HARASSMENT

Sexual harassment involves unwanted sexual behaviors by another. The behavior may be a sexual advance or request for a sexual favor. Some comments or touch are sexual. The behavior interferes with the person's work and comfort. In extreme cases, the person's job is threatened if sexual favors are not granted.

Victims of sexual harassment may be men or women. Men harass women or men. Women harass men or women. If you feel that you are being harassed, you must report the situation to your supervisor and the human resource officer.

You must be careful about what you say or do. Even innocent remarks and behaviors can be viewed as harassment. Employee orientation programs include information about harassment. If you are not sure about your own or another person's remarks or behaviors, discuss the situation with the nurse. You cannot be too careful.

RESIGNING FROM A JOB

A new job closer to home, with better pay, or with new opportunities may prompt you to leave your current job. Going to school, childcare, and illness are other reasons. Or you may not like your job or the work setting. Whatever the reason, you need to inform your employer. Give a written notice. Prepare a letter of resignation or complete a form in the human resources office. Giving two weeks notice is a good practice. Include the following in your written notice:

- Your reason for leaving
- The last date you will work
- Comments thanking the employer for the opportunity to work in the agency

An exit interview is common practice. You and the employer talk before you leave the agency. Usually the employer asks what you liked about the agency and your job. Often employees are asked how the agency can improve.

LOSING A JOB

Remember, a job is a privilege. You must perform your job well and protect patients and residents from harm. No pay raise or losing your job result from poor performance. Failure to follow an agency policy is often grounds for termination. So is failure to get along with others. Box 3-8 lists the many reasons why you can lose your job. Protect your job by performing to the best of your ability. Always practice good work ethics.

Box 3-8	**Common Reasons for Losing a Job**

- Poor attendance—not showing up for work or excessive tardiness (being late)
- Abandonment—leaving the job during your shift
- Falsifying a record—application or a person's record
- Violent behavior in the workplace
- Possessing weapons in the work setting—guns, knives, explosives, or other dangerous items
- Possessing, using, or distributing alcohol in the work setting
- Possessing, using, or distributing drugs in the work setting (this excludes taking drugs ordered by a doctor)
- Taking a person's drug for your own use or distribution to others
- Harassment—see p. 49
- Using offensive speech and language
- Stealing the agency's or a person's property
- Destroying the agency's or a person's property
- Showing disrespect to patients, residents, visitors, co-workers, or supervisors
- Abusing or neglecting a person
- Invading a person's privacy
- Failing to maintain patient, resident, agency, or co-worker confidentiality (includes access to computer information)
- Using the employer's supplies and equipment for your own use
- Defamation—see Chapter 2 and Gossip, p. 47
- Abusing meal breaks and break periods
- Sleeping on the job
- Violating agency dress code
- Violating any agency policy
- Tending to personal matters while on duty

REVIEW

Circle the **BEST** answer.

1. To perform your job well you need the following *except*
   A. Adequate sleep and rest
   B. To exercise regularly
   C. To use drugs and alcohol
   D. To have good nutrition

2. Good personal hygiene for work involves the following *except*
   A. Bathing daily
   B. Using a deodorant or antiperspirant
   C. Brushing teeth after meals
   D. Keeping fingernails long and polished

3. You are getting ready for work. You should do the following *except*
   A. Press and mend your uniform
   B. Wear your name badge or photo ID
   C. Wear jewelry
   D. Style your hair so it is up and off the collar

4. When should you ask questions about your job description?
   A. After completing the application
   B. Before completing the application
   C. When your interview is scheduled
   D. During the interview

5. Lying on an employment application is
   A. Negligence
   B. Fraud
   C. Libel
   D. Slander

6. When completing a job application you should do the following *except*
   A. Write neatly and clearly
   B. Provide references
   C. Give information about employment gaps
   D. Leave spaces blank that do not apply to you

7. Which of these qualities and characteristics do employers look for the most?
   A. Cooperation
   B. Courtesy
   C. Dependability
   D. Empathy

8. Empathy is
   A. Feeling sorry for patients and residents
   B. Seeing things from the other person's point of view
   C. Being polite to others
   D. All of the above

9. What should you wear to a job interview?
   A. A uniform
   B. Party clothes
   C. A simple dress or suit
   D. What is most comfortable

10. Which behavior is inappropriate during a job interview?
    A. Good eye contact with the interviewer
    B. Shaking hands with the interviewer
    C. Asking the interviewer questions
    D. Crossing your arms and legs

11. Which response to an interview question is best?
    A. "Yes" or "no"
    B. Long answers
    C. Brief explanations
    D. A written response

12. Which statement reflects a positive work attitude?
    A. "It's not my fault."
    B. "Please show me how this works."
    C. "That's not my job."
    D. "I did it yesterday. It's her turn."

13. A co-worker tells you that a doctor and nurse are dating. This is
    A. Gossip
    B. Eavesdropping
    C. Confidential information
    D. Sexual harassment

14. Which is professional speech and language?
    A. Speaking clearly
    B. Using vulgar and abusive words
    C. Shouting
    D. Arguing

15. Which is *not* a courteous act?
    A. Saying "please" and "thank you"
    B. Expecting others to open doors for you
    C. Saying "I'm sorry"
    D. Complimenting others

16. You are on your meal break. Which is *false?*
    A. You can make personal phone calls.
    B. Family members can meet you.
    C. You can take a few extra minutes if necessary.
    D. The RN needs to know that you are off the unit.

17. You are organizing your work. You should do the following *except*
    A. Discuss priorities with the nurse
    B. Ask others if they need help
    C. Stay busy
    D. Plan care so that you can watch the person's TV

18. Which is not harassment?
    A. Using touch to comfort a person
    B. Joking about a person's religious practices
    C. Asking for a sexual favor
    D. Imitating a person's disability

19. A letter of resignation should include the following *except*
    A. Your reason for leaving
    B. The last day you will work
    C. A thank you to the employer
    D. What problems you had during your work

20. You can lose your job for the following reasons *except*
    A. Sharing the person's information with others
    B. Arriving at the agency after your shift begins
    C. Following the agency's dress code
    D. Using the agency's computer for your own use

Answers to these questions are on p. 833.

COMMUNICATING WITH THE HEALTH TEAM

OBJECTIVES

Define the key terms listed in this chapter

Explain why health team members need to communicate

Describe the rules for effective communication

Explain the purpose, parts, and information found in the medical record

Describe the legal and ethical aspects of medical records

Describe the purpose of the Kardex

Explain your role in the nursing process

Identify information to collect about a person using sight, hearing, touch, and smell

List the information to include when reporting to the nurse

List the basic rules for recording

Use the 24-hour clock

Explain how computers are used in health care

Explain how to protect the person's right to privacy when using computers

Describe the rules for answering the telephone

Explain how to deal with conflict

KEY TERMS

assessment Collecting information about the person; a step in the nursing process

chart Another term for the medical record

communication The exchange of information—a message sent is received and interpreted by the intended person

conflict A clash between opposing interests or ideas

evaluation To measure if goals are met or if progress is made; a step in the nursing process

goal That which is desired in or by the person as a result of nursing care

implementation To perform or carry out; a step in the nursing process

Kardex A type of card file that summarizes information found in the medical record; includes drugs and treatments, diagnosis, routine care measures, and special equipment used by the person

medical diagnosis The identification of a disease or condition by a doctor

medical record A written account of a person's illness and response to the treatment and care given by the health team; chart

minimum data set (MDS) A form used by nurses in nursing centers to assess a resident's mental, physical, and psychosocial functioning

nursing care plan A written guide giving direction about the nursing care a person should receive

nursing diagnosis A statement describing a health problem that is treated by nursing measures; a step in the nursing process

nursing intervention An action or measure taken by the nursing team to help the person reach a goal

nursing process The method used by RNs to plan and deliver nursing care; its five steps are assessment, nursing diagnosis, planning, implementation, and evaluation

objective data Information that is seen, heard, felt, or smelled by another person; signs

observation Using the senses of sight, hearing, touch, and smell to collect information about a person

KEY TERMS *continued*

planning Setting priorities and goals; a step in the nursing process

recording Writing or charting patient or resident care and observations

reporting A verbal account of patient or resident care and observations

resident assessment protocol (RAP) Triggers and guidelines used in developing the comprehensive care plan

signs Objective data

subjective data That which is reported by a person and is not observed by others using the senses; symptoms

symptoms Subjective data

triggers Clues that direct the caregiver to the appropriate resident assessment protocol (RAP)

Health team members must communicate with each other to give coordinated and effective care to the person. Information is shared about what was done and what needs to be done for the person. Information about the person's response to treatment also is shared.

Consider this example of communication among the health team. Dr. Hart orders a blood test for Mrs. Kemp. For the test, Mrs. Kemp must fast from midnight until after the blood is drawn. Therefore Mrs. Kemp cannot have breakfast at the usual time. A nurse tells the dietary department not to send the breakfast tray until notified. A technician draws the blood and then tells the nurse that Mrs. Kemp may have breakfast. The nurse orders the meal. A dietary department aide brings the tray to the nursing unit. You take Mrs. Kemp's tray to her. When she is done eating, you remove the tray and observe what she ate. You report your observations to the nurse, who then records the information in Mrs. Kemp's record. Because health team members communicated with one another, Mrs. Kemp had coordinated and effective care.

You need to understand the basic elements and rules of communication. Then you can learn how to communicate information to the nursing and health teams.

COMMUNICATION

Communication is the exchange of information—a message sent is received and interpreted by the intended person. Words must have the same meaning for both the sender and the receiver of the message. The words "small," "moderate," and "large" mean different things to different people. Is small the size of a dime or the size of a half dollar? In health care, different meanings can cause serious problems. Try to avoid words with more than one meaning.

Use familiar words when communicating. You will learn medical terminology as you study and gain experience in health care. If someone uses an unfamiliar term, ask for an explanation. If you do not understand the message sent to you, communication did not occur. Likewise, do not use terms that are unfamiliar to the person and family.

Try to be brief and concise when communicating. Do not add unrelated or unneeded information. You must stay on the subject, avoid wandering in thought, and not get wordy. Being brief and concise reduces the possibility of omitting important details.

Give information in a logical and orderly manner. Organize your thoughts so you can present them logically and in sequence. Think about what happened step by step. Present information to the nurse in that way.

Present facts and be specific when giving information. Give the receiver a clear picture of what you are communicating. Asking for clarification or for more information should not be necessary. Telling the nurse that a person's temperature is 100.2° F is more specific, factual, and descriptive than saying the "temperature is up."

The rules for communication are summarized in Box 4-1 on p. 56.

THE MEDICAL RECORD

The **medical record (chart)** is a written account of a person's illness and response to treatment and care. It provides a way for the health team to communicate information about the person. The record is permanent and can be retrieved years later if the person's health history is needed. The record is a legal document. It can be used in court as evidence of the person's problems, treatment, and care.

The record has many forms organized into sections for easy use. Each page is stamped with the person's name, room number, and other identifying information. This helps prevent errors and improper placement of records. The record includes the person's:

Box 4-1   Rules for Communication

- Try to avoid words with more than one meaning.
- Use familiar words.
- Ask for an explanation of an unfamiliar term.
- Be brief and concise.
- Do not add unrelated or unneeded information.
- Stay on the subject.
- Avoid wandering in thought.
- Do not get wordy.
- Organize your thoughts so you can present them logically and in sequence.
- Give information in a logical and orderly manner.
- Present facts and be specific when giving information.

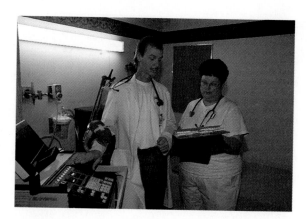

Fig. 4-1 The nurse and respiratory therapist review a resident's chart.

- History
- Physical examination results
- Doctor's orders
- Doctor's progress notes
- Graphic sheet
- X-ray examination reports
- IV therapy record
- Respiratory therapy record
- Consultation reports
- Surgery and anesthesia reports
- Admission sheet
- Other reports (e.g., physical therapy, occupational therapy, speech therapy)
- Special consents

Health team members record information on the forms for their department and service. The information is read by other health team members who need to know the care provided and the person's response (Fig. 4-1).

Each agency has policies about the contents of medical records and who has access to them. Policies state how often to make recordings and who records on the specific forms. Policies address acceptable abbreviations, how to correct errors, the color of ink to use, and how to sign entries. You need to know your agency's policies.

All professional staff involved in the person's care have access to the medical record. Those not directly involved usually cannot review the person's record. Cooks, laundry and housekeeping staff, and office clerks do not need to see medical records.

If you have access to medical records, you must keep the information confidential. This is an ethical and legal responsibility. Only health team members involved in the person's care need to read the chart. If you know someone in the agency and you are not involved in that person's care, you have no right to review that person's chart. To do so is an invasion of privacy.

Many agencies let patients and residents see their records if they so request. Know your employer's policy about patients and residents seeing their charts. If a person asks you for the chart, report the request to the RN. The RN is responsible for dealing with the person's request.

The following parts of the medical record relate to your work.

THE ADMISSION SHEET

The admission sheet is completed when the person is admitted to the agency. It has identifying information about the person:

- Legal name
- Birth date
- Age
- Gender (male or female)
- Current address
- Marital status (single, married, divorced, widowed)
- Social Security number
- Known allergies
- Religion
- Church
- Occupation
- Employer
- Insurance coverage
- Person's nearest relative or legal representative
- Name and number of the person to notify in an emergency
- Diagnosis
- Date and time of admission
- Doctor's name
- Identification (ID) number (given when admitted to the agency)
- Advance directives (living will or other instructions about life support measures—see Chapter 37)

The admission sheet is useful for filling out other forms that require some of the same information. That way the person does not have to answer the same question several times.

NURSING HISTORY

A nurse completes the nursing history when the person is admitted (Fig. 4-2, pp. 58-59). The nurse interviews the person. The nurse asks about why the person sought health care, signs and symptoms, drugs, and prior illnesses. You can use the form to learn about the person's background and health history.

THE GRAPHIC SHEET

The graphic sheet is used to record measurements and observations that are made every shift or 3 to 4 times per day (Fig. 4-3, p. 61). Information may include the person's blood pressure, temperature, pulse, respirations, height, and weight. Some graphic sheets have places to chart the intake and output, routine care, bowel movements, and doctor's visits.

Text continued on p. 61

BARNES HOSPITAL ST. LOUIS, MISSOURI		
Person to Contact:	Emergency Phone:	

Why you came to the hospital?

Allergies (food, drugs, latex, environment)?

Items brought in from home?
☐ Medications ☐ Dentures
☐ Contacts ☐ Glasses
☐ Hearing Aid

Did you bring:
☐ Money ☐ Jewelry ☐ Credit Cards ☐ Checkbook/Checks ☐ Other _____
(These need to be locked up with security or sent home. Hospital will not be responsible for valuables left in room)

MEDICINE NAMES	Dose & How Often Taken	Reason You Take Medicine	Time of Last Dose
Prescribed by a Doctor			
Non-Prescription			

Do you have any problems with your medicines?

Do you smoke? ☐ Yes ☐ No	Do you use "street" drugs? ☐ Yes ☐ No	How much caffeine do you drink or eat?
Do you chew tobacco? ☐ Yes ☐ No	How much alcohol do you drink?_____	

Medical History:
☐ Epilepsy   ☐ Cancer   ☐ Chicken Pox/Shingles   ☐ Menstrual Disease
☐ Heart Disease   ☐ Stroke   ☐ Hepatitis   ☐ Fainting/Dizzy Spells ☐ Circulation Problems
☐ Lung Disease   ☐ Diabetes   ☐ High Blood Pressure   ☐ Stomach Problems   ☐ Swelling
☐ Liver Disease   ☐ TB   ☐ Rheumatic Disease   ☐ Bladder Problems   ☐ Bleeding
☐ Immune Disorders   ☐ Sexually Transmitted Disease: _____
☐ Other _____

HISTORY COMMENTS:

Could you be pregnant?   ☐ Yes   ☐ No   When was your last Period?_____

What surgeries or procedures have you had? (Date)

Family Health History: ☐ Hypertension ☐ Diabetes ☐ Heart Disease ☐ Stroke ☐ Cancer ☐ Other _____

Which of the following have you had in the past 12 months?
☐ Self Breast Exam   ☐ Prostate Check   ☐ Glaucoma Check   ☐ Rectal Check (over 40)   ☐ Dental Exam
☐ Mammogram (over 40)   ☐ Testicular Check   ☐ Pelvic Exam   ☐ Hearing Check   ☐ Vision Check

Are your immunizations current?   ☐ Yes   ☐ No   ☐ Unknown
(Call ID Specialist)

Fig. 4-2 Nursing history. *(Courtesy Barnes-Jewish Hospital, St Louis.)*

Are you on a special diet?	How is your appetite?
Any foods you can't eat, and why?	Any difficulty eating or swallowing?
Nutritional supplements/or diet substitutions (e.g., vitamins, artificial sweeteners, salt, substitutes)	Weight loss/gain (amount) in the last 12 months?

How often do you have a BM?
Do you have any difficulty having a bowel movement?
☐ use laxatives   ☐ hemorrhoids
☐ use stool softeners   ☐ black/tarry stools

Do you tire easily?   ☐ Yes   ☐ No

Have you fallen recently?   ☐ Yes   ☐ No

Do you have any difficulty urinating?

☐ burning   ☐ blood   ☐ leaking   ☐ frequency

Do you get regular exercise?   ☐ Yes   ☐ No
What kind?_____   How often? _____

What activities do you need help with?
☐ Feeding/eating   ☐ Meal preparation
☐ Dressing   ☐ Transportation
☐ Grooming/bathing   ☐ Housework
☐ Taking medications ☐ Handling finances
☐ Toileting   ☐ Grocery shopping
☐ Moving/positioning

☐ Walking on level surfaces
☐ Walking on stairs
☐ Paying for Medicines

(RN consider appropriate consults)

Aides used at home:
☐ Eye glasses   ☐ Contact lenses
☐ Hearing aid   ☐ Cane
☐ Walker   ☐ Wheelchair
☐ Prosthesis: _____
DENTURES: ☐ Upper ☐ Lower
PARTIALS: ☐ Upper ☐ Lower

Is it difficult for you to carry out prescribed health care regimens (Diet, Activity, Medications)?   ☐ Yes   ☐ No
If YES, explain:

How much sleep do you normally get?

What helps you fall asleep?

Who do you live with?   ☐ Alone   ☐ Spouse only   ☐ Family   ☐ Friends   ☐ Nursing Home

Who helps you at home?   ☐ Spouse   ☐ Family   ☐ Friends   ☐ Home Health   ☐ Visiting Nurse

Do you have concerns about your family while you are in the hospital?

What major changes have you had in your life in the past 12 months?

Do you feel you deal successfully with stress? ☐ Yes ☐ No	Would you like additional resources? ☐ Yes ☐ No

Do you have concerns that your illness/hospitalization will affect:
☐ appearance   ☐ job   ☐ male/female roles   ☐ how you feel about yourself

Is religion important in your life? ☐ Yes ☐ No	Will this illness/hospitalization interfere with any religious beliefs/practices? ☐ Yes ☐ No

What do you expect from us while in the hospital?

Do you have a Living Will?   ☐ Yes   ☐ No   Do you have a Power of Attorney?   ☐ Yes   ☐ No
Do you have a copy with you?   ☐ Yes   ☐ No

Patient/Significant Other Signature: Relationship:	Date	Staff Signature Title:	Date

☐ REVIEWED BY REGISTERED NURSE   SIGNATURE: DATE:

TO BE COMPLETED BY STAFF ONLY

Patient provided: ☐ Admit kit   ☐ ID band   ☐ Sensitivity/Allergy band on patient   ☐ Allergy sticker on chart
Patient instructed: ☐ Valuables policy   ☐ Waiver signed   ☐ Smoking   ☐ Visitation
                      ☐ Nursing call/Emergency   ☐ TV/phone   ☐ Fall precautions/band on wrist
                      ☐ Patient's Rights/responsibilities   ☐ Received copy of Personal Directions for My Healthcare

Time patient arrived on Division:_____   SIGNATURE: _____

Fig. 4-2, cont'd For legend see opposite page.

Med-Forms, Inc.
FORM #MF37079 (Rev 9/95)

OSF
ST. JOSEPH MEDICAL CENTER
Bloomington, Illinois 61701

DAILY SUMMARY AND GRAPHIC

TEMPERATURE
Write in 105¹ or over

	2400	0400	0800	1200	1600	2000	2400	0400	0800	1200	1600	2000	2400	0400	0800	1200	1600	2000	2400	0400	0800	1200	1600	2000
DATE																								
HOSPITAL DAY																								
POST OP DAY																								
HOUR	2400	0400	0800	1200	1600	2000	2400	0400	0800	1200	1600	2000	2400	0400	0800	1200	1600	2000	2400	0400	0800	1200	1600	2000
B/P																								

TEMPERATURE

104   40
102.2   39
100.4   38
98.6   37
96.6   36

PULSE																								
RESPIRATION																								
WEIGHT																								
DR. VISIT																								

INTAKE	2300-0700	0700-1500	1500-2300	TOTAL	2300-0700	0700-1500	1500-2300	TOTAL	2300-0700	0700-1500	1500-2300	TOTAL	2300-0700	0700-1500	1500-2300	TOTAL
Oral																
IV																
Tube Feedings																
PPN/TPN/Lipids																
Blood/Blood Products																
IV Meds																
Chemotherapy																
Unreturned irr. sol.																
TOTAL INTAKE																
OUTPUT	2300-0700	0700-1500	1500-2300	TOTAL	2300-0700	0700-1500	1500-2300	TOTAL	2300-0700	0700-1500	1500-2300	TOTAL	2300-0700	0700-1500	1500-2300	TOTAL
Urine																
GI																
Emesis																
Drains																
TOTAL OUTPUT																
Feces																

Fig. 4-3 Graphic sheet. *(Courtesy OSF St. Joseph Medical Center, Bloomington, Ill.)*

Progress Notes

Progress notes are a written description of nursing care given, the person's response to care, and any observations about the person's condition (Fig. 4-4, p. 62). They are used to record information about special treatments and drugs. Teaching, counseling, and procedures performed by the doctor and visits by health team members also are recorded in the progress notes. *(See Focus on Long-Term Care box below.)*

Flow Sheets

A flow sheet is used to record measurements or observations that are made often. For example, a person's blood pressure, pulse, and respirations may be taken every 15 minutes or more often. The graphic sheet does not have enough room for frequent measurements. A flow sheet designed for this purpose does. The intake and output record kept at the bedside is another type of flow sheet (see Chapter 18). *(See Focus on Long-Term Care and Focus on Home Care boxes below.)*

Text continued on p. 67

 Focus On ... LONG-TERM CARE

Interdisciplinary progress notes are used in long-term care. They contain information similar to that found in nurses' notes. Nurses chart about a change in the resident's condition, unusual events, or problems. Summaries of care are written about the person's progress toward goals and response to care.

Daily recordings are not necessary. Center policies state how often recordings are made. However, OBRA requires that a summary be written every 3 months.

Focus On ... LONG-TERM CARE

An activities-of-daily-living flow sheet is common in long-term care (Fig. 4-5, pp. 63-67). The form contains information about hygiene, food and fluids, elimination, rest and sleep, activity, and social interactions.

Focus On ... HOME CARE

A weekly client care record is used in home care. The form has boxes for each day of the week and for care activities. The form includes boxes for temperature, pulse, respirations, blood pressure, and weight. The home health care assistant checks the box for the day care was given or records the measurement on the day it was done.

ST. JOSEPH MEDICAL CENTER

Bloomington, Illinois 61701

PATIENT CARE
PROGRESS NOTES

DATE TIME	DEPT. CODE	FOCUS	PROGRESS NOTES

DEPARTMENT CODES:

FORM # MF9087 (Rev. 5/96)

Med-Forms, Inc. ™

1. All Physicians	5. Rehab. Services	9. Endoscopy	13. Pastoral Care
2. Nursing	6. Pharmacy	10. Home Care	14. Social Services
3. Medical Imaging	7. Cardiology Services	11. Hospice	15. Laboratory
4. Respiratory	8. Neurology	12. Nutrition	16. Other

Fig. 4-4 Progress notes. Note that other members of the health team also record on the notes. *(Courtesy OSF St. Joseph Medical Center, Bloomington, Ill.)*

WC# _____   Walker# _____

199__   JAN FEB MAR APR MAY JUN JUL AUG SEP OCT NOV DEC
(days 1 – 31)

DATE	ORDER/INSTRUCTION	TIME
	Bath & Shampoos every ___ & ___ on ___ shift / Tub, Shower, Bedbath	11-7
		7-3
		3-11
	Oral Care / Own/Dentures/None / I = Independent A = Assist / SU = Setup	11-7
		7-3
		3-11
	Dressing / I = Independent A = Assist / SU = Setup T = Total Care	11-7
		7-3
		3-11
	Grooming: Washing, Face, Hands, Combing Hair / I = Independent A = Assist / SU = Setup T = Total Care	11-7
		7-3
		3-11
	Trim nails weekly	11-7
		7-3
		3-11
	Lotion arms and legs twice daily	11-7
		7-3
		3-11
	Shave men daily	11-7
		7-3
		3-11
	Initials	11-7
		7-3
		3-11

SIGNATURE	INITIALS	SIGNATURE	INITIALS	SIGNATURE	INITIALS

DIAGNOSIS   ALLERGIES   SPECIAL INSTRUCTIONS:

PATIENT STICKER

(revised 2/97)

Fig. 4-5 Activities-of-daily-living flow sheet. *(Courtesy Bonell Good Samaritan Center, Greeley, Colo.)*   *Continued*

WC#	Walker#	199__	JAN									FEB	MAR			APR				MAY					JUN			JUL				AUG				SEP	OCT					NOV		DEC			
DATE	ORDER/INSTRUCTION	TIME	1	2	3	4	5	6	7	8	9	10	11	12	13	14	15	16	17	18	19	20	21	22	23	24	25	26	27	28	29	30	31													
	Bowel Movements L = Large M = Medium S = Small I = Incontinent	11-7																																													
		7-3																																														
		3-11																																														
	Weight Bearing Status TT = Toe Touch AT = As tol P = Partial F = Full NWB = Not wt bearing	11-7																																														
		7-3																																														
		3-11																																														
	Transfer Status ML = Medilift SBA = Stand By Assist; Assist of 1 or 2	11-7																																														
		7-3																																														
		3-11																																														
	Activity A = Ambulate GC = Gerichair T = Turn every 2 hrs W/C = Wheelchair	11-7																																														
		7-3																																														
		3-11																																														
	Safety LT = Lap Tray SR = Siderails BA = Bed Alarm SB = Seat Belt	11-7																																														
		7-3																																														
		3-11																																														
	Feeding Status I = Independen S = Set up/cue F = Staff feed SP = Swallow Precautions; TL = Thickened Liquids	Breakfast																																														
		Lunch																																														
		Supper																																														
	Amount of Food Taken in %	Breakfast																																														
		Lunch																																														
		Supper																																														
	Initials	11-7																																														
		7-3																																														
		3-11																																														

INITIALS	SIGNATURE	INITIALS	SIGNATURE	INITIALS	SIGNATURE	INITIALS	SIGNATURE

PATIENT STICKER DIAGNOSIS ALLERGIES SPECIAL INSTRUCTIONS:

Fig. 4-5 Activities-of-daily-living flow sheet. (*Courtesy Bonell Good Samaritan Center, Greeley, Colo.*)

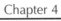

The table below represents the grid/chart shown.

WC# _____ Walker# _____	199_ JAN	FEB	MAR	APR	MAY	JUN	JUL	AUG	SEP	OCT	NOV	DEC	
DATE	ORDER/INSTRUCTION	TIME	1 2 3 4 5 6 7 8 9 10 11 12 13 14 15 16 17 18 19 20 21 22 23 24 25 26 27 28 29 30 31											
	Amount of Snacks Taken in %	AM												
		PM												
		HS												
	Vital Signs Every _____	11-7												
		7-3												
		3-11												
	Weight Every _____													
	Intake and Output	11-7												
		7-3												
		3-11												
	Initials	11-7												
		7-3												
		3-11												

INITIALS   SIGNATURE   INITIALS   SIGNATURE   INITIALS   SIGNATURE

DIAGNOSIS   ALLERGIES   SPECIAL INSTRUCTIONS:

PATIENT STICKER

Fig. 4-5, cont'd *For legend see opposite page.*

Continued

Fig. 4-5 Activities-of-daily-living flow sheet. *(Courtesy Bonell Good Samaritan Center, Greeley, Colo.)*

THE KARDEX

The **Kardex** is a type of card file. For each person there is a card that contains some of the information found in the medical record. The Kardex is a summary of the current drugs and treatments ordered by the doctor, the person's current diagnosis, routine care measures, and special equipment needs. The nursing care plan (see pp. 80-81) also may be found in the Kardex. The Kardex is a quick, easy source of information about the person (Fig. 4-6).

Fig. 4-6 A sample Kardex. *(From Potter PA, Perry AG:* Fundamentals of nursing: concepts, process, and practice, *ed 4 St Louis, 1997, Mosby.)*

NURSING PROCESS

Nurses must communicate with each other about the person's problems, needs, and care. Information is communicated through the nursing process. The **nursing process** is the method used by nurses to plan and deliver nursing care. It has five steps: assessment, nursing diagnosis, planning, implementation, and evaluation. The purpose of the nursing process is to meet the person's nursing needs. It requires good communication between the person and the nursing team.

Each step is important. If done in order with good communication, the nursing process help the person reach desired goals. Nursing care is organized and has purpose. All members of the nursing team do the same things for the person and have the same goals. The person feels safe and secure with consistent care.

The nursing process is used by nurses in all health care settings. It is used for all age-groups. The nursing process is ongoing. That is, it constantly changes as new information is gathered and as the persons' needs change. You will see the continuous nature of the nursing process as each step is explained.

ASSESSMENT

Assessment involves collecting information about the person. Nurses gather information from many sources. A nursing history is taken about current and past health problems. The family's health history also is important. Many diseases are genetic. That is, the risk for certain diseases is inherited from parents. For example, if a mother had breast cancer, her daughters are at risk. The nurse reviews the information collected by the doctor. If available, past medical records are reviewed. The nurse also reviews laboratory and other test reports.

The RN performs a physical assessment. Information is collected about each body system. The RN also assesses the person's mental status. Information is gathered by observing the person. You play an important role in the assessment step. You make many observations as you give care and talk to the person.

Observation is using the senses of sight, hearing, touch, and smell to collect information. You *see* the way the person lies, sits, or walks. You see flushed or pale skin and reddened or swollen body areas. You *listen* to the person breathe, talk, and cough. You use a stethoscope to listen to the heartbeat and to measure blood pressure. When *touching* the person, you collect information about skin temperature and if the skin is moist or dry. You also use touch to take the person's pulse. *Smell* is used to detect body, wound, and breath odors and unusual odors from urine and bowel movements.

Information observed about a person is called objective data. **Objective data (signs)** are seen, heard, felt, or smelled. You can feel a pulse, and you can see urine. However, you cannot feel or see the person's pain, fear, or nausea. **Subjective data (symptoms)** are things a person tells you about that you cannot observe through your senses.

Box 4-2 lists the basic observations you need to make and report to the nurse. Make notes of your observations. They help later when you report to the nurse. They also help when recording observations. Carry a note pad and pen in your pocket to note observations as you make them.

The assessment step never ends. The nursing team collects new information with every patient or resident contact. New observations are made, and the person shares more information. The family often adds more information. *(See Focus on Long-Term Care box.)*

Text continued on p. 78

Focus On... LONG-TERM CARE

OBRA requires the use of the **minimum data set (MDS)** for residents in nursing centers (Fig. 4-7, pp. 70-77). The MDS is an assessment and screening tool. The form is completed when the resident is admitted to the center. It provides extensive information about the person. Examples include the person's memory, communication, hearing and vision, physical function, and activities. The form is updated before each care conference. A new MDS is completed once a year and whenever the person's condition changes.

Box 4-2 Basic Observations

ABILITY TO RESPOND
- Is the person easy or difficult to arouse?
- Can the person give his or her name, the time, and location when asked?
- Does the person identify others accurately?
- Does the person answer questions correctly?
- Does the person speak clearly?
- Are instructions followed correctly?
- Is the person calm, restless, or excited?
- Is the person conversing, quiet, or talking a lot?

MOVEMENT
- Can the person squeeze your fingers with each hand?
- Can the person move arms and legs?
- Are the person's movements shaky or jerky?
- Does the person complain of stiff or painful joints?

PAIN OR DISCOMFORT
- Where is the pain located? (Ask the person to point to the pain.)
- Does the pain go anywhere else?
- When did the pain begin?
- What was the person doing when the pain began?
- How long does the pain last?
- How does the person describe the pain?
  - Sharp
  - Severe
  - Knifelike
  - Dull
  - Burning
  - Aching
  - Comes and goes
  - Depends on position
- Was medication given?
- Did medication help relieve the pain? Is pain still present?
- Is the person able to sleep and rest?
- What is the position of comfort?

SKIN
- Is the skin pale or flushed?
- Is the skin cool, warm, or hot?
- Is the skin moist or dry?
- What color are the lips and nails?
- Is the skin intact? Are there broken areas? If so, where?
- Are sores or reddened areas present?
- Are bruises present? Where are they located?
- Does the person complain of itching?

EYES, EARS, NOSE, AND MOUTH
- Is there drainage from the eyes? What color is the drainage?
- Are the eyelids closed?
- Are the eyes reddened?
- Does the person complain of spots, flashes, or blurring?
- Is the person sensitive to bright lights?
- Is there drainage from the ears?
- Can the person hear? Is repeating necessary? Are questions answered appropriately?
- Is there drainage from the nose? What color is the drainage?
- Can the person breathe through the nose?
- Is there breath odor?
- Does the person complain of a bad taste in the mouth?

RESPIRATIONS
- Do both sides of the person's chest rise and fall with respirations?
- Is breathing noisy?
- Does the person complain of difficulty breathing?
- What is the amount and color of sputum?
- What is the frequency of the person's cough? Is it dry or productive?

BOWELS AND BLADDER
- Is the abdomen firm or soft?
- Does the person complain of gas?
- What is the amount, color, and consistency of bowel movements?
- Does the person have pain or difficulty urinating?
- What is the amount of urine?
- Is the person able to control the passage of urine?
- What is the frequency of urination?
- What is the frequency of bowel movements?
- Is the person able to control bowel movements?

APPETITE
- Does the person like the diet?
- How much of the food on the tray is eaten?
- What are the person's food preferences?
- Is the person able to chew food?
- How much liquid was taken?
- What are the person's liquid preferences?
- How often does the person drink liquids?
- Is the person able to swallow food and liquids?
- Is the person experiencing nausea?
- What is the amount and color of material vomited?
- Does the person have hiccups?
- Is the person belching?

ACTIVITIES OF DAILY LIVING
- Can the person perform personal care without help?
  - Bathing
  - Brushing teeth
  - Combing and brushing hair
  - Shaving
- Does the person use the toilet, commode, bedpan, or urinal?
- Is the person able to feed self?
- Is the person able to walk?
- What amount and kind of assistance is needed?

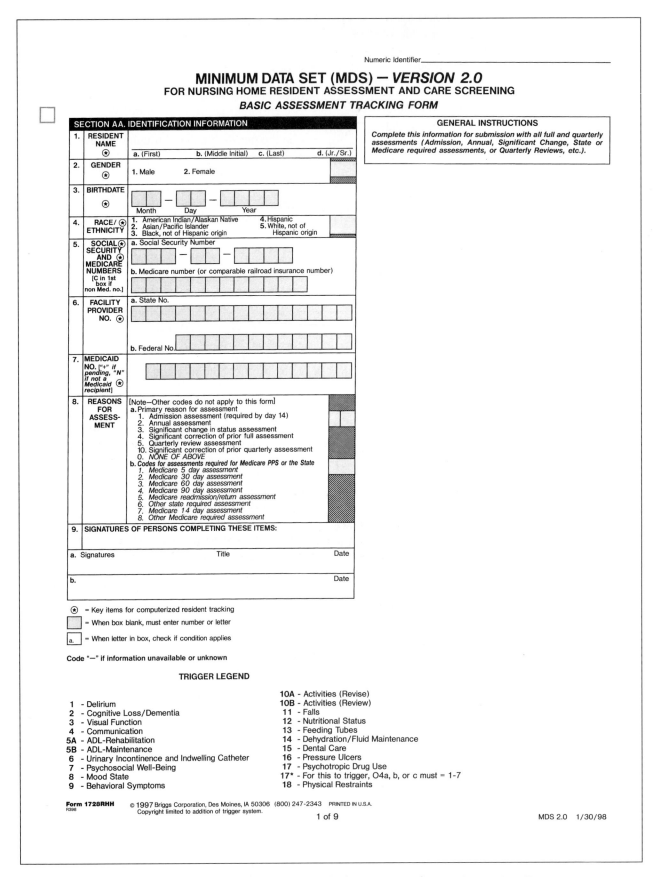

Fig. 4-7 Minimum data set (MDS). *(Reprinted with permission of Briggs Corporation, Des Moines, Iowa.)*

Resident _____ Numeric Identifier _____

MINIMUM DATA SET (MDS) — *VERSION 2.0*
FOR NURSING HOME RESIDENT ASSESSMENT AND CARE SCREENING
BACKGROUND (FACE SHEET) INFORMATION AT ADMISSION

SECTION AB. DEMOGRAPHIC INFORMATION

1. DATE OF ENTRY
Date the stay began. Note — Does not include readmission if record was closed at time of temporary discharge to hospital, etc. In such cases, use prior admission date.

☐☐ — ☐☐ — ☐☐☐☐
Month   Day   Year

2. ADMITTED FROM (AT ENTRY)
1. Private home/apt. with no home health services
2. Private home/apt. with home health services
3. Board and care/assisted living/group home
4. Nursing home
5. Acute care hospital
6. Psychiatric hospital, MR/DD facility
7. Rehabilitation hospital
8. Other

3. LIVED ALONE (PRIOR TO ENTRY)
0. No   1. Yes   2. In other facility

4. ZIP CODE OF PRIOR PRIMARY RESIDENCE
☐☐☐☐☐

5. RESIDEN-TIAL HISTORY 5 YEARS PRIOR TO ENTRY
(Check all settings resident lived in during 5 years prior to date of entry given in item AB1 above.)
Prior stay at this nursing home ... a.
Stay in other nursing home ... b.
Other residential facility — board and care home, assisted living, group home ... c.
MH/psychiatric setting ... d.
MR/DD setting ... e.
NONE OF ABOVE ... f.

6. LIFETIME OCCUPA-TION(S) *(Put "/" between two occupations)*

7. EDUCATION *(Highest level completed)*
1. No schooling   5. Technical or trade school
2. 8th grade/less   6. Some college
3. 9-11 grades   7. Bachelor's degree
4. High school   8. Graduate degree

8. LANGUAGE *(Code for correct response)*
a. Primary Language
0. English   1. Spanish   2. French   3. Other
b. If other, specify ☐☐☐☐☐☐☐☐☐☐

9. MENTAL HEALTH HISTORY
Does resident's RECORD indicate any history of mental retardation, mental illness, or developmental disability problem?
0. No   1. Yes

10. CONDITIONS RELATED TO MR/DD STATUS
(Check all conditions that are related to MR/DD status that were manifested before age 22, and are likely to continue indefinitely)
Not applicable — no MR/DD (Skip to AB11) ... a.
MR/DD with organic condition
  Down's syndrome ... b.
  Autism ... c.
  Epilepsy ... d.
  Other organic condition related to MR/DD ... e.
MR/DD with no organic condition ... f.

11. DATE BACK-GROUND INFORMA-TION COMPLETED
☐☐ — ☐☐ — ☐☐☐☐
Month   Day   Year

☐ = When box blank, must enter number or letter
a. = When letter in box, check if condition applies
Code "—" if information unavailable or unknown

NOTE: Normally, the MDS Face Sheet is completed once, when an individual first enters the facility. However, the face sheet is also required if the person is reentering this facility after a discharge where return had not previously been expected. It is not completed following temporary discharges to hospitals or after therapeutic leaves/home visits.

SECTION AC. CUSTOMARY ROUTINE

1. CUSTOMARY ROUTINE
(In year prior to DATE OF ENTRY to this nursing home, or year last in community if now being admitted from another nursing home)

(Check all that apply. If all information UNKNOWN, check last box only)

CYCLE OF DAILY EVENTS
Stays up late at night (e.g., after 9 pm) ... a.
Naps regularly during day (at least 1 hour) ... b.
Goes out 1+ days a week ... c.
Stays busy with hobbies, reading, or fixed daily routine ... d.
Spends most of time alone or watching TV ... e.
Moves independently indoors (with appliances, if used) ... f.
Use of tobacco products at least daily ... g.
NONE OF ABOVE ... h.

EATING PATTERNS
Distinct food preferences ... i.
Eats between meals all or most days ... j.
Use of alcoholic beverage(s) at least weekly ... k.
NONE OF ABOVE ... l.

ADL PATTERNS
In bedclothes much of day ... m.
Wakens to toilet all or most nights ... n.
Has irregular bowel movement pattern ... o.
Showers for bathing ... p.
Bathing in PM ... q.
NONE OF ABOVE ... r.

INVOLVEMENT PATTERNS
Daily contact with relatives/close friends ... s.
Usually attends church, temple, synagogue (etc.) ... t.
Finds strength in faith ... u.
Daily animal companion/presence ... v.
Involved in group activities ... w.
NONE OF ABOVE ... x.
UNKNOWN — Resident/family unable to provide information ... y.

END

SECTION AD. FACE SHEET SIGNATURES

SIGNATURES OF PERSONS COMPLETING FACE SHEET:

a. Signature of RN Assessment Coordinator .... Date

b. Signatures .... Title .... Sections .... Date

c. .... Date

d. .... Date

e. .... Date

f. .... Date

g. .... Date

Form 1728RHH   © 1997 Briggs Corporation, Des Moines, IA 50306 (800) 247-2343   PRINTED IN U.S.A.
Copyright limited to addition of trigger system.
2 of 9   MDS 2.0 1/30/98

Fig. 4-7, cont'd For legend see opposite page.

Continued

Resident _____ Numeric Identifier _____

MINIMUM DATA SET (MDS) — *VERSION 2.0*
FOR NURSING HOME RESIDENT ASSESSMENT AND CARE SCREENING
FULL ASSESSMENT FORM
(Status in last 7 days, unless other time frame indicated)

SECTION A. IDENTIFICATION AND BACKGROUND INFORMATION

1. RESIDENT NAME
a. (First) b. (Middle Initial) c. (Last) d. (Jr./Sr.)

2. ROOM NUMBER

3. ASSESSMENT REFERENCE DATE
a. Last day of MDS observation period
Month — Day — Year
b. Original (0) or corrected copy of form (enter number of correction)

4a. DATE OF REENTRY
Date of reentry from most recent temporary discharge to a hospital in last 90 days (or since last assessment or admission if less than 90 days)
Month — Day — Year

5. MARITAL STATUS
1. Never married 3. Widowed 5. Divorced
2. Married 4. Separated

6. MEDICAL RECORD NO.

7. CURRENT PAYMENT SOURCES FOR N.H. STAY
(Billing Office to indicate; check all that apply in last 30 days)
Medicaid per diem — a.
Medicare per diem — b.
Medicare ancillary part A — c.
Medicare ancillary part B — d.
CHAMPUS per diem — e.
VA per diem — f.
Self or family pays for full per diem — g.
Medicaid resident liability or Medicare co-payment — h.
Private insurance per diem (including co-payment) — i.
Other per diem — j.

8. REASONS FOR ASSESSMENT
[Note—If this is a discharge or reentry assessment, only a limited subset of MDS items need be completed]
a. Primary reason for assessment
1. Admission assessment (required by day 14)
2. Annual assessment
3. Significant change in status assessment
4. Significant correction of prior full assessment
5. Quarterly review assessment
6. Discharged—return not anticipated
7. Discharged—return anticipated
8. Discharged prior to completing initial assessment
9. Reentry
10. Significant correction of prior quarterly assessment
0. NONE OF ABOVE
b. Codes for assessments required for Medicare PPS or the State
1. Medicare 5 day assessment
2. Medicare 30 day assessment
3. Medicare 60 day assessment
4. Medicare 90 day assessment
5. Medicare readmission/return assessment
6. Other state required assessment
7. Medicare 14 day assessment
8. Other Medicare required assessment

9. RESPONSIBILITY/ LEGAL GUARDIAN
(Check all that apply)
Legal guardian — a.
Other legal oversight — b.
Durable power of attorney/health care — c.
Durable power of attorney/financial — d.
Family member responsible — e.
Patient responsible for self — f.
NONE OF ABOVE — g.

10. ADVANCED DIRECTIVES
(For those items with supporting documentation in the medical record, check all that apply)
Living will — a.
Do not resuscitate — b.
Do not hospitalize — c.
Organ donation — d.
Autopsy request — e.
Feeding restrictions — f.
Medication restrictions — g.
Other treatment restrictions — h.
NONE OF ABOVE — i.

SECTION B. COGNITIVE PATTERNS

1. COMATOSE (Persistent vegetative state/no discernible consciousness)
0. No 1. Yes (If yes, skip to Section G)

2. MEMORY (Recall of what was learned or known)
a. Short-term memory OK—seems/appears to recall after 5 minutes
0. Memory OK 1. Memory problem 2
b. Long-term memory OK—seems/appears to recall long past
0. Memory OK 1. Memory problem 2

☐ = When box blank, must enter number or letter.
a. = When letter in box, check if condition applies
Code "—" if information unavailable or unknown

3. MEMORY/ RECALL ABILITY (Check all that resident was *normally able to recall during last 7 days*)
Current season — a.
Location of own room — b.
Staff names/faces — c.
That he/she is in a nursing home — d.
NONE OF ABOVE are recalled — e.

4. COGNITIVE SKILLS FOR DAILY DECISION-MAKING (Made decisions regarding tasks of daily life)
0. INDEPENDENT—decisions consistent/reasonable
1. MODIFIED INDEPENDENCE—some difficulty in new situations only 2
2. MODERATELY IMPAIRED—decisions poor; cues/ supervision required 2
3. SEVERELY IMPAIRED—never/rarely made decisions 2, 5B

5. INDICATORS OF DELIRIUM— PERIODIC DISORDERED THINKING/ AWARENESS (Code for behavior in the last 7 days.) [Note: Accurate assessment requires conversations with staff and family who have direct knowledge of resident's behavior over this time.]
0. Behavior not present
1. Behavior present, not of recent onset
2. Behavior present, over last 7 days appears different from resident's usual functioning (e.g., new onset or worsening)
a. EASILY DISTRACTED—(e.g., difficulty paying attention; gets sidetracked) 2 = 1, 17*
b. PERIODS OF ALTERED PERCEPTION OR AWARENESS OF SURROUNDINGS—(e.g., moves lips or talks to someone not present; believes he/she is somewhere else; confuses night and day) 2 = 1, 17*
c. EPISODES OF DISORGANIZED SPEECH—(e.g., speech is incoherent, nonsensical, irrelevant, or rambling from subject to subject; loses train of thought) 2 = 1, 17*
d. PERIODS OF RESTLESSNESS—(e.g., fidgeting or picking at skin, clothing, napkins, etc.; frequent position changes; repetitive physical movements or calling out) 2 = 1, 17*
e. PERIODS OF LETHARGY—(e.g., sluggishness; staring into space; difficult to arouse; little body movement) 2 = 1, 17*
f. MENTAL FUNCTION VARIES OVER THE COURSE OF THE DAY—(e.g., sometimes better, sometimes worse; behaviors sometimes present, sometimes not) 2 = 1, 17*

6. CHANGE IN COGNITIVE STATUS Resident's cognitive status, skills, or abilities have changed as compared to status of 90 days ago (or since assessment if less than 90 days)
0. No change 1. Improved 2. Deteriorated 1, 17*

SECTION C. COMMUNICATION/HEARING PATTERNS

1. HEARING (With hearing appliance, if used)
0. HEARS ADEQUATELY—normal talk, TV, phone
1. MINIMAL DIFFICULTY when not in quiet setting 4
2. HEARS IN SPECIAL SITUATIONS ONLY—speaker has to adjust tonal quality and speak distinctly 4
3. HIGHLY IMPAIRED/absence of useful hearing 4

2. COMMUNICATION DEVICES/ TECHNIQUES (Check all that apply in last 7 days)
Hearing aid, present and used — a.
Hearing aid, present and not used regularly — b.
Other receptive comm. techniques used (e.g., lip reading) — c.
NONE OF ABOVE — d.

3. MODES OF EXPRESSION (Check all used by resident to make needs known)
Speech — a.
Writing messages to express or clarify needs — b.
American sign language or Braille — c.
Signs/gestures/sounds — d.
Communication board — e.
Other — f.
NONE OF ABOVE — g.

4. MAKING SELF UNDERSTOOD (Expressing information content—however able)
0. UNDERSTOOD
1. USUALLY UNDERSTOOD—difficulty finding words or finishing thoughts 4
2. SOMETIMES UNDERSTOOD—ability is limited to making concrete requests 4
3. RARELY/NEVER UNDERSTOOD 4

5. SPEECH CLARITY (Code for speech in the last 7 days)
0. CLEAR SPEECH—distinct, intelligible words
1. UNCLEAR SPEECH—slurred, mumbled words
2. NO SPEECH—absence of spoken words

6. ABILITY TO UNDERSTAND OTHERS (Understanding verbal information content—however able)
0. UNDERSTANDS
1. USUALLY UNDERSTANDS—may miss some part/ intent of message 2, 4
2. SOMETIMES UNDERSTANDS—responds adequately to simple, direct communication 2, 4
3. RARELY/NEVER UNDERSTANDS 2, 4

7. CHANGE IN COMMUNICATION/ HEARING Resident's ability to express, understand, or hear information has changed as compared to status of 90 days ago (or since last assessment if less than 90 days)
0. No change 1. Improved 2. Deteriorated 17*

TRIGGER LEGEND
1 - Delirium
2 - Cognitive Loss/Dementia
4 - Communication
5B - ADL Maintenance
17* - Psychotropic Drugs
(For this to trigger, O4a, b, or c must = 1-7)

Form 1728RHH © 1997 Briggs Corporation, Des Moines, IA 50306 (800) 247-2343 PRINTED IN U.S.A.
Copyright limited to addition of trigger system.
3 of 9
MDS 2.0 1/30/98

Fig. 4-7 Minimum data set (MDS). *(Reprinted with permission of Briggs Corporation, Des Moines, Iowa.)*

Fig. 4-7, cont'd For legend see opposite page.

Continued

Resident _____ Numeric Identifier _____

| 2. | BATHING | How resident takes full-body bath/shower, sponge bath, and transfers in/out of tub/shower (EXCLUDE washing of back and hair). *Code for most dependent in self-performance and support. A = 1, 2, 3 or 4 =5A* (A) BATHING SELF-PERFORMANCE codes appear below.
 0. Independent—No help provided (A) (B)
 1. Supervision—Oversight help only
 2. Physical help limited to transfer only
 3. Physical help in part of bathing activity
 4. Total dependence
 8. Activity itself did not occur during entire 7 days
 (Bathing support codes are as defined in Item 1, code B above) |

| 3. | TEST FOR BALANCE (See training manual) | *(Code for ability during test in the last 7 days)*
 0. Maintained position as required in test
 1. Unsteady, but able to rebalance self without physical support
 2. Partial physical support during test; or stands (sits) but does not follow directions for test
 3. Not able to attempt test without physical help
 a. Balance while standing
 b. Balance while sitting—position, trunk control 1, 2, or 3 = **17*** |

| 4. | FUNCTIONAL LIMITATION IN RANGE OF MOTION (see training manual) | *(Code for limitations during last 7 days that interfered with daily functions or placed resident at risk of injury)*
 (A) RANGE OF MOTION (B) VOLUNTARY MOVEMENT
 0. No limitation 0. No loss
 1. Limitation on one side 1. Partial loss
 2. Limitation on both sides 2. Full loss (A) (B)
 a. Neck
 b. Arm—Including shoulder or elbow
 c. Hand—Including wrist or fingers
 d. Leg—Including hip or knee
 e. Foot—Including ankle or toes
 f. Other limitation or loss |

| 5. | MODES OF LOCOMOTION | *(Check all that apply during last 7 days)*
 Cane/walker/crutch a. Wheelchair primary mode of locomotion d.
 Wheeled self b.
 Other person wheeled c. NONE OF ABOVE e. |

| 6. | MODES OF TRANSFER | *(Check all that apply during last 7 days)*
 Bedfast all or most of time **16** a. Lifted mechanically d.
 Bed rails used for bed mobility or transfer b. Transfer aid (e.g., slide board, trapeze, cane, walker, brace) e.
 Lifted manually c. NONE OF ABOVE f. |

| 7. | TASK SEGMENTATION | Some or all of ADL activities were broken into subtasks during **last 7 days** so that resident could perform them
 0. No 1. Yes |

| 8. | ADL FUNCTIONAL REHABILITATION POTENTIAL | Resident believes he/she is capable of increased independence in at least some ADLs **5A** a.
 Direct care staff believe resident is capable of increased independence in at least some ADLs **5A** b.
 Resident able to perform tasks/activity but is very slow c.
 Difference in ADL Self-Performance or ADL Support, comparing mornings to evenings d.
 NONE OF ABOVE e. |

| 9. | CHANGE IN ADL FUNCTION | Resident's ADL self-performance status has changed as compared to status of **90 days ago** (or since last assessment if less than 90 days)
 0. No change 1. Improved 2. Deteriorated |

SECTION H. CONTINENCE IN LAST 14 DAYS

1.	CONTINENCE SELF-CONTROL CATEGORIES *(Code for resident's PERFORMANCE OVER ALL SHIFTS)* 0. CONTINENT—Complete control (includes use of indwelling urinary catheter or ostomy device that does not leak urine or stool) 1. USUALLY CONTINENT—BLADDER, incontinent episodes once a week or less; BOWEL, less than weekly 2. OCCASIONALLY INCONTINENT—BLADDER, 2 or more times a week but not daily; BOWEL, once a week 3. FREQUENTLY INCONTINENT—BLADDER, tended to be incontinent daily, but some control present (e.g., on day shift); BOWEL, 2-3 times a week 4. INCONTINENT—Had inadequate control. BLADDER, multiple daily episodes; BOWEL, all (or almost all) of the time
a.	BOWEL CONTINENCE	Control of bowel movement, with appliance or bowel continence programs, if employed 1, 2, 3 or 4 = **16**
b.	BLADDER CONTINENCE	Control of urinary bladder function (if dribbles, volume insufficient to soak through underpants), with appliances (e.g., foley) or continence programs, if employed 2, 3 or 4 = **6**
2.	BOWEL ELIMINATION PATTERN	Bowel elimination pattern regular—at least one movement every three days a. Constipation **17*** b. Diarrhea c. Fecal impaction **17*** d. NONE OF ABOVE e.

| 3. | APPLIANCES AND PROGRAMS | Any scheduled toileting plan a. Did not use toilet room/commode/urinal f.
 Bladder retraining program b. Pads/briefs used **6** g.
 External (condom) catheter **6** c. Enemas/irrigation h.
 Indwelling catheter **6** d. Ostomy present i.
 Intermittent catheter **6** e. NONE OF ABOVE j. |

| 4. | CHANGE IN URINARY CONTINENCE | Resident's urinary continence has changed as compared to status of **90 days ago** (or since last assessment if less than 90 days)
 0. No change 1. Improved 2. Deteriorated |

SECTION I. DISEASE DIAGNOSES

Check only *those diseases that have a relationship* to current ADL status, cognitive status, mood and behavior status, medical treatments, nursing monitoring, or risk of death. (Do not list inactive diagnoses)

1.	DISEASES	*(If none apply, CHECK the NONE OF ABOVE box)*
	ENDOCRINE/METABOLIC/NUTRITIONAL		Hemiplegia/Hemiparesis	v.
	Diabetes mellitus	a.	Multiple sclerosis	w.
	Hyperthyroidism	b.	Paraplegia	x.
	Hypothyroidism	c.	Parkinson's disease	y.
	HEART/CIRCULATION		Quadriplegia	z.
	Arteriosclerotic heart disease (ASHD)	d.	Seizure disorder	aa.
	Cardiac dysrhythmias	e.	Transient ischemic attack (TIA)	bb.
	Congestive heart failure	f.	Traumatic brain injury	cc.
	Deep vein thrombosis	g.	PSYCHIATRIC/MOOD	
	Hypertension	h.	Anxiety disorder	dd.
	Hypotension **17***	i.	Depression **17***	ee.
	Peripheral vascular disease **16**	j.	Manic depression (bipolar disease)	ff.
	Other cardiovascular disease	k.	Schizophrenia	gg.
	MUSCULOSKELETAL		PULMONARY	
	Arthritis	l.	Asthma	hh.
	Hip fracture	m.	Emphysema/COPD	ii.
	Missing limb (e.g., amputation)	n.	SENSORY	
	Osteoporosis	o.	Cataracts **3**	jj.
	Pathological bone fracture	p.	Diabetic retinopathy	kk.
	NEUROLOGICAL		Glaucoma **3**	ll.
	Alzheimer's disease	q.	Macular degeneration	mm.
	Aphasia	r.	OTHER	
	Cerebral palsy	s.	Allergies	nn.
	Cerebrovascular accident (stroke)	t.	Anemia	oo.
	Dementia other than Alzheimer's disease	u.	Cancer	pp.
			Renal failure	qq.
			NONE OF ABOVE	rr.

2.	INFECTIONS	*(If none apply, CHECK the NONE OF ABOVE box)*
	Antibiotic resistant infection (e.g., Methicillin resistant staph)	a.	Septicemia	g.
	Clostridium difficile (c. diff.)	b.	Sexually transmitted diseases	h.
	Conjunctivitis	c.	Tuberculosis	i.
	HIV infection	d.	Urinary tract infection in last 30 days **14**	j.
	Pneumonia	e.	Viral hepatitis	k.
	Respiratory infection	f.	Wound infection	l.
			NONE OF ABOVE	m.

| 3. | OTHER CURRENT OR MORE DETAILED DIAGNOSES AND ICD-9 CODES | Dehydration 276.5 = **14** a. •
 b. •
 c. •
 d. •
 e. • |

SECTION J. HEALTH CONDITIONS

1.	PROBLEM CONDITIONS	*(Check all problems present in last 7 days unless other time frame is indicated)*
	INDICATORS OF FLUID STATUS		Dizziness/Vertigo **11, 17***	f.
	Weight gain or loss of 3 or more pounds within a 7 day period **14**	a.	Edema	g.
	Inability to lie flat due to shortness of breath	b.	Fever **14**	h.
	Dehydrated; output exceeds input **14**	c.	Hallucinations **17***	i.
	Insufficient fluid; did NOT consume all/almost all liquids provided during last 3 days **14**	d.	Internal bleeding **14**	j.
			Recurrent lung aspirations in last 90 days **17***	k.
	OTHER		Shortness of breath	l.
	Delusions	e.	Syncope (fainting) **17***	m.
			Unsteady gait **17***	n.
			Vomiting	o.
			NONE OF ABOVE	p.

TRIGGER LEGEND
3 - Visual Function
5A - ADL Rehabilitation
6 - Urinary Incontinence/Indwelling Catheter
11 - Falls
14 - Dehydration/Fluid Maintenance
16 - Pressure Ulcers
17* - Psychotropic Drugs
(*For this to trigger, O4a, b, or c must = 1-7)

Form 1728RHH © 1997 Briggs Corporation, Des Moines, IA 50306 (800) 247-2343 PRINTED IN U.S.A.
 Copyright limited to addition of trigger system. MDS 2.0 1/30/98

5 of 9

Fig. 4-7 Minimum data set (MDS). *(Reprinted with permission of Briggs Corporation, Des Moines, Iowa.)*

Resident _____   Numeric Identifier _____

2.	PAIN SYMPTOMS	*(Code the **highest level of pain** present in the **last 7 days**)* **a. FREQUENCY** with which resident complains or shows evidence of pain 0. No pain *(skip to J4)* 1. Pain less than daily 2. Pain daily **b. INTENSITY** of pain 1. Mild pain 2. Moderate pain 3. Times when pain is horrible or excruciating
3.	PAIN SITE	*(If pain present, **check all sites** that apply in **last 7 days**)* Back pain — a. Incisional pain — f. Bone pain — b. Joint pain (other than hip) — g. Chest pain while doing usual activities — c. Soft tissue pain (e.g., lesion, muscle) — h. Headache — d. Stomach pain — i. Hip pain — e. Other — j.
4.	ACCIDENTS	*(Check all that apply)* Fell in past 30 days **11, 17*** — a. Fell in past 31-180 days **11, 17*** — b. Hip fracture in last 180 days **17*** — c. Other fracture in last 180 days — d. NONE OF ABOVE — e.
5.	STABILITY OF CONDITIONS	Conditions/diseases make resident's cognitive, ADL, mood or behavior patterns unstable—(fluctuating, precarious, or deteriorating) — a. Resident experiencing an acute episode or a flare-up of a recurrent or chronic problem — b. End-stage disease, 6 or fewer months to live — c. NONE OF ABOVE — d.

SECTION K. ORAL/NUTRITIONAL STATUS

1.	ORAL PROBLEMS	Chewing problem — a. Swallowing problem **17*** — b. Mouth pain **15** — c. NONE OF ABOVE — d.
2.	HEIGHT AND WEIGHT	*Record (a.) height in inches and (b.) weight in pounds. Base weight on most recent measure in last 30 days; measure weight consistently in accord with standard facility practice—e.g., in a.m. after voiding, before meal, with shoes off, and in nightclothes.* **a. HT (in.)** **b. WT (lb.)**
3.	WEIGHT CHANGE	**a. Weight loss**—5% or more in **last 30 days**; or 10% or more in **last 180 days** 0. No 1. Yes **12** **b. Weight gain**—5% or more in **last 30 days**; or 10% or more in **last 180 days** 0. No 1. Yes
4.	NUTRI- TIONAL PROBLEMS	Complains about the taste of many foods **12** — a. Leaves 25% or more of food uneaten at most meals **12** — c. Regular or repetitive complaints of hunger — b. NONE OF ABOVE — d.
5.	NUTRI- TIONAL APPROACH- ES	*(Check all that apply in **last 7 days**)* Parenteral/IV **12, 14** — a. Feeding tube **13, 14** — b. Mechanically altered diet **12** — c. Syringe (oral feeding) **12** — d. Therapeutic diet **12** — e. Dietary supplement between meals — f. Plate guard, stabilized built-up utensil, etc. — g. On a planned weight change program — h. NONE OF ABOVE — i.
6.	PARENTERAL OR ENTERAL INTAKE	*(Skip to Section L if neither 5a nor 5b is checked)* **a.** Code the proportion of **total calories** the resident received through parenteral or tube feedings in the **last 7 days** 0. None 3. 51% to 75% 1. 1% to 25% 4. 76% to 100% 2. 26% to 50% **b.** Code the average **fluid intake** per day by IV or tube in **last 7 days** 0. None 3. 1001 to 1500 cc/day 1. 1 to 500 cc/day 4. 1501 to 2000 cc/day 2. 501 to 1000 cc/day 5. 2001 or more cc/day

SECTION L. ORAL/DENTAL STATUS

1.	ORAL STATUS AND DISEASE PREVEN- TION	Debris (soft, easily movable substances) present in mouth prior to going to bed at night **15** — a. Has dentures or removable bridge — b. Some/all natural teeth lost—does not have or does not use dentures (or partial plates) **15** — c. Broken, loose, or carious teeth **15** — d. Inflamed gums (gingiva); swollen or bleeding gums; oral abscesses; ulcers or rashes **15** — e. Daily cleaning of teeth/dentures or daily mouth care—by resident or staff Not ✓ = **15** — f. NONE OF ABOVE — g.

SECTION M. SKIN CONDITION

			Number at Stage
1.	ULCERS (Due to any cause)	*(Record the number of ulcers at each ulcer stage—regardless of cause. If none present at a stage, record "0" (zero). Code all that apply during **last 7 days**. Code 9 = 9 or more.)* **[Requires full body exam.]** **a. Stage 1.** A persistent area of skin redness (without a break in the skin) that does not disappear when pressure is relieved. **b. Stage 2.** A partial thickness loss of skin layers that presents clinically as an abrasion, blister, or shallow crater. **c. Stage 3.** A full thickness of skin is lost, exposing the subcutaneous tissues—presents as a deep crater with or without undermining adjacent tissue. **d. Stage 4.** A full thickness of skin and subcutaneous tissue is lost, exposing muscle or bone.	
2.	TYPE OF ULCER	*(For each type of ulcer, **code for the highest stage** in the last 7 days using scale in item M1—i.e., 0=none; stages 1, 2, 3, 4)* **a.** Pressure ulcer—any lesion caused by pressure resulting in damage of underlying tissue 1 = **16**; 2, 3 or 4 = **12, 16** **b.** Stasis ulcer—open lesion caused by poor circulation in the lower extremities	
3.	HISTORY OF RESOLVED ULCERS	Resident had an ulcer that was resolved or cured in **LAST 90 DAYS** 0. No 1. Yes **16**	
4.	OTHER SKIN PROBLEMS OR LESIONS PRESENT	*(Check all that apply during **last 7 days**)* Abrasions, bruises — a. Burns (second or third degree) — b. Open lesions other than ulcers, rashes, cuts (e.g., cancer lesions) — c. Rashes—e.g., intertrigo, eczema, drug rash, heat rash, herpes zoster — d. Skin desensitized to pain or pressure **16** — e. Skin tears or cuts (other than surgery) — f. Surgical wounds — g. NONE OF ABOVE — h.	
5.	SKIN TREAT- MENTS	*(Check all that apply during **last 7 days**)* Pressure relieving device(s) for chair — a. Pressure relieving device(s) for bed — b. Turning/repositioning program — c. Nutrition or hydration intervention to manage skin problems — d. Ulcer care — e. Surgical wound care — f. Application of dressings (with or without topical medications) other than to feet — g. Application of ointments/medications (other than to feet) — h. Other preventative or protective skin care (other than to feet) — i. NONE OF ABOVE — j.	
6.	FOOT PROBLEMS AND CARE	*(Check all that apply during **last 7 days**)* Resident has one or more foot problems—e.g., corns, calluses, bunions, hammer toes, overlapping toes, pain, structural problems — a. Infection of the foot—e.g., cellulitis, purulent drainage — b. Open lesions on the foot — c. Nails/calluses trimmed during **last 90 days** — d. Received preventative or protective foot care (e.g., used special shoes, inserts, pads, toe separators) — e. Application of dressings (with or without topical medications) — f. NONE OF ABOVE — g.	

SECTION N. ACTIVITY PURSUIT PATTERNS

1.	TIME AWAKE	*(Check appropriate time periods over **last 7 days**)* Resident awake all or most of time (i.e., naps no more than one hour per time period) in the: **10B** only if BOTH N1a = ✓ and N2 = 0 Morning **10B** — a. Evening — c. Afternoon — b. NONE OF ABOVE — d.
		(IF RESIDENT IS COMATOSE, SKIP TO SECTION O)
2.	AVERAGE TIME INVOLVED IN ACTIVITIES	*(When awake and not receiving treatments or ADL care)* 0. Most—more than 2/3 of time **10B** 2. Little—less than 1/3 of time **10A** 1. Some—from 1/3 to 2/3 of time 3. None **10A**
3.	PREFERRED ACTIVITY SETTINGS	*(Check all settings in which activities are **preferred**)* Own room — a. Day/activity room — b. Outside facility — d. Inside NH/off unit — c. NONE OF ABOVE — e.
4.	GENERAL ACTIVITY PREFER- ENCES (Adapted to resident's current abilities)	*(Check all PREFERENCES whether or not activity is currently available to resident)* Cards/other games — a. Trips/shopping — g. Crafts/arts — b. Walking/wheeling outdoors — h. Exercise/sports — c. Watching TV — i. Music — d. Gardening or plants — j. Reading/writing — e. Talking or conversing — k. Spiritual/religious activities — f. Helping others — l. NONE OF ABOVE — m.

TRIGGER LEGEND

10A - Activities (Revise)   13 - Feeding Tubes   17* - Psychotropic Drugs
10B - Activities (Review)   14 - Dehydration/Fluid Maintenance   (*For this to trigger, O4a, b, or c must = 1-7)
11 - Falls   15 - Dental Care
12 - Nutritional Status   16 - Pressure Ulcers

Form 1728RHH   © 1997 Briggs Corporation, Des Moines, IA 50306 (800) 247-2343   PRINTED IN U.S.A.
 Copyright limited to addition of trigger system.   6 of 9   MDS 2.0   1/30/98

Fig. 4-7, cont'd For legend see opposite page.

Continued

Resident _____   Numeric Identifier _____

5.	PREFERS CHANGE IN DAILY ROUTINE	Code for resident preferences in daily routines 0. No change 1. Slight change 2. Major change	
		a. Type of activities in which resident is currently involved 1 or 2 = **10A**	
		b. Extent of resident involvement in activities 1 or 2 = **10A**	

SECTION O. MEDICATIONS

1.	NUMBER OF MEDICATIONS	*(Record the number of different medications used in the last 7 days; enter "0" if none used)*	
2.	NEW MEDICA-TIONS	*(Resident currently receiving medications that were initiated during the last 90 days)* 0. No 1. Yes	
3.	INJECTIONS	*(Record the number of DAYS injections of any type received during the last 7 days; enter "0" if none used)*	
4.	DAYS RECEIVED THE FOLLOWING MEDICATION	*(Record the number of DAYS during last 7 days; enter "0" if not used. Note—enter "1" for long-acting meds used less than weekly)* (NOTE: For **17** to actually be triggered, O4a, b, or c MUST = 1-7 AND at least one additional item marked **17*** must be indicated. See sections B, C, E, G, H, I, J, and K.)	

a. Antipsychotic 1-7 = **17**   d. Hypnotic

b. Antianxiety 1-7 = **11, 17**   e. Diuretic 1-7 = **14**

c. Antidepressant 1-7 = **11, 17**

SECTION P. SPECIAL TREATMENTS AND PROCEDURES

1.	SPECIAL TREAT-MENTS, PROCE-DURES, AND PROGRAMS	**a. SPECIAL CARE**—*Check treatments or programs received during the last 14 days*

TREATMENTS
- Chemotherapy   a.
- Dialysis   b.
- IV medication   c.
- Intake/output   d.
- Monitoring acute medical condition   e.
- Ostomy care   f.
- Oxygen therapy   g.
- Radiation   h.
- Suctioning   i.
- Tracheostomy care   j.
- Transfusions   k.

PROGRAMS
- Ventilator or respirator   l.
- Alcohol/drug treatment program   m.
- Alzheimer's/dementia special care unit   n.
- Hospice care   o.
- Pediatric unit   p.
- Respite care   q.
- Training in skills required to return to the community (e.g., taking medications, house work, shopping, transportation, ADLs)   r.
- *NONE OF ABOVE*   s.

b. THERAPIES—*Record the number of days and total minutes each of the following therapies was administered (for at least 15 minutes a day) in the last 7 calendar days (Enter 0 if none or less than 15 min. daily) [Note—count only post admission therapies]*

(A) = # of days administered for **15 minutes or more**

(B) = total # of minutes provided in **last 7 days**

	DAYS (A)	MIN (B)
a. Speech-language pathology and audiology services		
b. Occupational therapy		
c. Physical therapy		
d. Respiratory therapy		
e. Psychological therapy (by any licensed mental health professional)		

2.	INTERVEN-TION PROGRAMS FOR MOOD, BEHAVIOR, COGNITIVE LOSS	(Check all interventions or strategies used in **last 7 days**—no matter where received)
		Special behavior symptom evaluation program a.
		Evaluation by a licensed mental health specialist in **last 90 days** b.
		Group therapy c.
		Resident-specific deliberate changes in the environment to address mood/behavior patterns—e.g., providing bureau in which to rummage d.
		Reorientation—e.g., cueing e.
		NONE OF ABOVE f.

3.	NURSING REHABILI-TATION/ RESTOR-ATIVE CARE	Record the NUMBER OF DAYS each of the following rehabilitation or restorative techniques or practices was **provided to the resident for more than or equal to 15 minutes** per day in the **last 7 days** *(Enter 0 if none or less than 15 min. daily.)*

- a. Range of motion (passive)
- b. Range of motion (active)
- c. Splint or brace assistance

TRAINING AND SKILL PRACTICE IN:
- d. Bed mobility
- e. Transfer
- f. Walking
- g. Dressing or grooming
- h. Eating or swallowing
- i. Amputation/prosthesis care
- j. Communication
- k. Other

4.	DEVICES AND RESTRAINTS	*(Use the following codes for last 7 days:)* 0. Not used 1. Used less than daily 2. Used daily	
		Bed rails	
		a. —Full bed rails on all open sides of bed	
		b. —Other types of side rails used (e.g., half rail, one side)	
		c. Trunk restraint 1 = **11, 18**; 2 = **11, 16, 18**	
		d. Limb restraint 1 or 2 = **18**	
		e. Chair prevents rising 1 or 2 = **18**	
5.	HOSPITAL STAY(S)	Record number of times resident was admitted to hospital with an overnight stay in **last 90 days** (or since last assessment if less than 90 days). *(Enter 0 if no hospital admissions)*	
6.	EMERGENCY ROOM (ER) VISIT(S)	Record number of times resident visited ER without an overnight stay in **last 90 days** (or since last assessment if less than 90 days). *(Enter 0 if no ER visits)*	
7.	PHYSICIAN VISITS	In the **LAST 14 DAYS** (or since admission if less than 14 days in facility) how many days has the physician (or authorized assistant or practitioner) examined the resident? *(Enter 0 if none)*	
8.	PHYSICIAN ORDERS	In the **LAST 14 DAYS** (or since admission if less than 14 days in facility) how many days has the physician (or authorized assistant or practitioner) changed the resident's orders? *Do not include order renewals without change.* (Enter 0 if none)	
9.	ABNORMAL LAB VALUES	Has the resident had any abnormal lab values during the **last 90 days** (or since admission)? 0. No 1. Yes	

SECTION Q. DISCHARGE POTENTIAL AND OVERALL STATUS

1.	DISCHARGE POTENTIAL	a. Resident expresses/indicates preference to return to the community 0. No 1. Yes	
		b. Resident has a support person who is positive toward discharge 0. No 1. Yes	
		c. Stay projected to be of a short duration—discharge projected **within 90 days** (do not include expected discharge due to death) 0. No 2. Within 31-90 days 1. Within 30 days 3. Discharge status uncertain	
2.	OVERALL CHANGE IN CARE NEEDS	Resident's overall self sufficiency has changed significantly as compared to status of **90 days ago** (or since last assessment if less than 90 days) 0. No change 1. Improved—receives fewer supports, needs less restrictive level of care 2. Deteriorated—receives more support	

SECTION R. ASSESSMENT INFORMATION

1.	PARTICI-PATION IN ASSESSMENT	a. Resident: 0. No 1. Yes	
		b. Family: 0. No 1. Yes 2. No family	
		c. Significant other: 0. No 1. Yes 2. None	

2. SIGNATURES OF PERSONS COMPLETING THE ASSESSMENT:

a. Signature of RN Assessment Coordinator (sign on above line)

b. Date RN Assessment Coordinator signed as complete

Month	Day	Year

c. Other Signatures	Title	Sections	Date
d.			Date
e.			Date
f.			Date
g.			Date
h.			Date

TRIGGER LEGEND

10A - Activities (Revise)

11 - Falls

14 - Dehydration/Fluid Maintenance

16 - Pressure Ulcers

17 - Psychotropic Drugs

17* - For this to trigger, O4a, b, or c must = 1-7

18 - Physical Restraints

7 of 9   MDS 2.0   1/30/98

Fig. 4-7 Minimum data set (MDS). *(Reprinted with permission of Briggs Corporation, Des Moines, Iowa.)*

Resident _____   Numeric Identifier _____

SECTION T. THERAPY SUPPLEMENT FOR MEDICARE PPS		
1.	**SPECIAL TREAT-MENTS AND PROCE-DURES**	**a. RECREATION THERAPY**—*Enter number of days and total minutes of recreation therapy administered* **(for at least 15 minutes a day)** *in the* **last 7 days** *(Enter 0 if none)* (A) = **# of days** administered for 15 minutes or more (B) = **total # of minutes** provided in last 7 days

	DAYS	MIN
	(A)	(B)

Skip unless this is a Medicare 5 day or Medicare readmission/return assessment.

b. ORDERED THERAPIES—*Has physician ordered any of following therapies to begin in FIRST 14 days of stay—physical therapy, occupational therapy, or speech pathology service?*

0. No   1. Yes

If not ordered, skip to item 2

c. Through day 15, provide an estimate of the number of days when at least 1 therapy service can be expected to have been delivered.

d. Through day 15, provide an estimate of the number of therapy minutes (across the therapies) than can be expected to be delivered.

| **2.** | **WALKING WHEN MOST SELF SUFFICIENT** | *Complete item 2 if ADL self-performance score for TRANSFER (G.1.b.A) is 0, 1, 2, or 3 AND at least one of the following are present:*
• Resident received physical therapy involving gait training (P.1.b.c)
• Physical therapy was ordered for the resident involving gait training (T.1.b)
• Resident received nursing rehabilitation for walking (P.3.f)
• Physical therapy involving walking has been discontinued within the past 180 days
Skip to item 3 if resident did not walk in last 7 days
FOR FOLLOWING FIVE ITEMS, BASE CODING ON THE EPISODE WHEN THE RESIDENT WALKED THE FARTHEST WITHOUT SITTING DOWN. INCLUDE WALKING DURING RE-HABILITATION SESSIONS.) |

a. Furthest distance walked without sitting down during this episode.
0. 150+ feet   3. 10-25 feet
1. 51-149 feet   4. Less than 10 feet
2. 26-50 feet

b. Time walked without sitting down during this episode.
0. 1-2 minutes   3. 11-15 minutes
1. 3-4 minutes   4. 16-30 minutes
2. 5-10 minutes   5. 31+ minutes

c. Self-Performance in walking during this episode.
0. *INDEPENDENT*—No help or oversight
1. *SUPERVISION*—Oversight, encouragement or cueing provided
2. *LIMITED ASSISTANCE*—Resident highly involved in walking; received physical help in guided maneuvering of limbs or other nonweight bearing assistance
3. *EXTENSIVE ASSISTANCE*—Resident received weight bearing assistance while walking

d. Walking support provided associated with this episode (code regardless of resident's self-performance classification).
0. No setup or physical help from staff
1. Setup help only
2. One person physical assist
3. Two+ persons physical assist

e. Parallel bars used by resident in association with this episode.
0. No   1. Yes

| **3.** | **CASE MIX GROUP** | Medicare [ ][ ][ ][ ][ ]   State [ ][ ][ ][ ][ ] |

Form 1728RHH   © 1997 Briggs Corporation, Des Moines, IA 50306 (800) 247-2343   PRINTED IN U.S.A.
Copyright limited to addition of trigger system.   MDS 2.0   1/30/98

Fig. 4-7, cont'd For legend see opposite page.

NURSING DIAGNOSIS

The RN uses information from the assessment to make a nursing diagnosis. A **nursing diagnosis** is a statement describing a health problem that is treated by nursing measures. The health problem may exist or may develop. Nursing diagnoses and medical diagnoses are different. A **medical diagnosis** is the identification of a disease or condition by a doctor. Medical diagnoses include cancer, pneumonia, chickenpox, stroke, heart attack, infection, AIDS, and diabetes. Drugs, therapies, and surgery are ordered by doctors to cure or heal.

A person may have more than one nursing diagnosis. Remember, nursing deals with the total person. Therefore nursing diagnoses involve the person's physical, emotional, social, and spiritual needs. Box 4-3 lists the nursing diagnoses approved by the North American Nursing Diagnosis Association (NANDA).

Text continued on p. 80

Box 4-3	Nursing Diagnoses Approved by the North American Nursing Diagnosis Association (Nanda)

- Activity Intolerance
- Activity Intolerance, Risk for
- Adaptive Capacity: Intracranial, Decreased
- Adjustment, Impaired
- Airway Clearance, Ineffective
- Anxiety
- Aspiration, Risk for
- Body Image Disturbance
- Body Temperature, Risk for Altered
- Breastfeeding, Effective
- Breastfeeding, Ineffective
- Breastfeeding, Interrupted
- Breathing Pattern, Ineffective
- Cardiac Output, Decreased
- Caregiver Role Strain
- Caregiver Role Strain, Risk for
- Communication, Impaired Verbal
- Community Coping, Ineffective
- Community Coping, Potential for Enhanced
- Confusion, Acute
- Confusion, Chronic
- Constipation
- Constipation, Colonic
- Constipation, Perceived
- Decisional Conflict (Specify)
- Defensive Coping
- Denial, Ineffective
- Diarrhea
- Disorganized Infant Behavior
- Disorganized Infant Behavior, Risk for
- Disuse Syndrome, Risk for
- Diversional Activity Deficit
- Dysfunctional Ventilatory Weaning Response
- Dysreflexia
- Energy Field Disturbance
- Environmental Interpretation Syndrome, Impaired

- Family Coping: Compromised, Ineffective
- Family Coping: Disabling, Ineffective
- Family Coping: Potential for Growth
- Family Processes; Alcoholism, Altered
- Family Processes, Altered
- Fatigue
- Fear
- Fluid Volume, Deficit
- Fluid Volume, Risk for Deficit
- Fluid Volume, Excess
- Gas Exchange, Impaired
- Grieving, Anticipatory
- Grieving, Dysfunctional
- Growth and Development, Altered
- Health Maintenance, Altered
- Health-Seeking Behaviors (Specify)
- Home Maintenance Management, Impaired
- Hopelessness
- Hyperthermia
- Hypothermia
- Incontinence, Bowel
- Incontinence, Functional
- Incontinence, Reflex
- Incontinence, Stress
- Incontinence, Total
- Incontinence, Urge
- Individual Coping, Ineffective
- Infant Feeding Pattern, Ineffective
- Infection, Risk for
- Injury, Risk for
- Knowledge Deficit (Specify)
- Loneliness, Risk for
- Management of Therapeutic Regimen: Community, Ineffective
- Management of Therapeutic Regimen: Families, Ineffective

From North American Nursing Diagnosis Association: *NANDA nursing diagnoses: definitions and classification 1999-2000,* Philadelphia, 1999, The Association.

Box 4-3	Nursing Diagnoses Approved by the North American Nursing Diagnosis Association (Nanda)—cont'd

- Management of Therapeutic Regimen: Individual, Effective
- Management of Therapeutic Regimen (Individuals), Ineffective
- Management of Therapeutic Regimen, Noncompliance (Specify)
- Memory, Impaired
- Nutrition, Altered: Less Than Body Requirements
- Nutrition, Altered: More Than Body Requirements
- Nutrition: Potential for More Than Body Requirements
- Oral Mucous Membrane: Altered
- Organized Infant Behavior, Potential for Enhanced
- Pain
- Pain, Chronic
- Parent/Infant/Child Attachment, Risk for Altered
- Parental Role Conflict
- Parenting, Altered
- Parenting, Risk for Altered
- Perioperative Positioning Injury, Risk for
- Peripheral Neurovascular Dysfunction, Risk for
- Personal Identity Disturbance
- Physical Mobility, Impaired
- Poisoning, Risk for
- Post-Trauma Response
- Powerlessness
- Protection, Altered
- Rape-Trauma Syndrome
- Rape-Trauma Syndrome: Compound Reaction
- Rape-Trauma Syndrome: Silent Reaction
- Relocation Stress Syndrome
- Role Performance, Altered

- Self-Care Deficit
  - Bathing/Hygiene
  - Feeding
  - Dressing/Grooming
  - Toileting
- Self-Esteem, Chronic Low
- Self-Esteem Disturbance
- Self-Esteem, Situational Low
- Self-Mutilation, Risk for
- Sensory/Perceptual Alterations (Specify visual, auditory, kinesthetic, gustatory, tactile, olfactory)
- Sexual Dysfunction
- Sexuality Patterns, Altered
- Skin Integrity, Impaired
- Skin Integrity, Risk for Impaired
- Sleep Pattern Disturbance
- Social Interaction, Impaired
- Social Isolation
- Spiritual Distress
- Spiritual Well-Being, Potential for Enhanced
- Suffocation, Risk for
- Swallowing, Impaired
- Thermoregulation, Ineffective
- Thought Process, Altered
- Tissue Integrity, Impaired
- Tissue Perfusion, Altered (Specify renal, cerebral, cardiopulmonary, gastrointestinal, or peripheral)
- Trauma, Risk for
- Unilateral Neglect
- Urinary Elimination, Altered
- Urinary Retention
- Ventilatory Weaning Response, Dysfunctional (DVWR)
- Violence, Risk for Self-Directed or Directed at Others

Nursing diagnosis	Goal	Intervention
Constipation related to lack of privacy.	Patient will have regular bowel movements by 6/30.	Ask patient to use call light when urge to have bowel movement is felt. Answer call light promptly. Assist patient to bathroom. Close bathroom door for privacy. Leave the room if the patient can be alone; tell the patient you are leaving and that you will return when he turns on the call light.
Sleep pattern disturbance related to noisy environment.	Patient will report a restful sleep by 6/29.	Perform any necessary care measures before bedtime. Close the door to the patient's room. Turn off television or radio or keep volume low if patient prefers. Ask staff to avoid unnecessary talking outside the patient's room. Ask staff to speak in low voices. Turn off unneeded equipment.

Fig. 4-8 Nursing care plan. Each nursing diagnosis has a goal. There are nursing measures for each goal.

PLANNING

Planning involves setting priorities and goals. Nursing measures or actions are chosen to help the person meet the goals (Fig. 4-8). The person, family, and nursing team all help the RN plan. Other health workers may be involved.

Priorities relate to what is most important for the person. Maslow's theory of basic needs is useful for setting priorities (see Chapter 5). Maslow describes the needs that all humans have. The needs are arranged in order of importance. Some needs are re-

quired for life and survival, such as oxygen, water, and food. The needs necessary for life and survival must be met before all other needs. They have priority and must be met first.

Goals are then set. A **goal** is that which is desired in or by a person as a result of nursing care. Goals are aimed at the person's highest level of well-being and functioning: physical, emotional, social, spiritual. Goals promote health and prevent health problems. They also promote the person's rehabilitation.

The nursing interventions are chosen. An intervention is an action or measure. A **nursing intervention** is an action or measure taken by the nursing team to help the person reach a goal. In this book, nursing intervention, nursing action, and nursing measure mean the same thing. A nursing intervention does not need a doctor's order. However, some nursing measures come from a doctor's order. For example, a doctor orders that Mrs. Kemp walk 50 yards two times a day. The RN includes this order in the care plan.

The **nursing care plan** is a written guide about the care a person should receive. The plan has the person's nursing diagnoses and goals. It also has the measures or actions for each goal. The nursing care plan is a communication tool. Nursing staff use the care plan to see what care to give. The plan helps ensure that the nursing team gives the same care. The written care plan is found in the medical record, Kardex, or on computer (see Fig. 4-6).

The RN may conduct a care conference to share information and ideas about the person's care. The purpose is to develop or revise a person's nursing care plan for effective care. Assistive personnel are usually included in the conference. You are encouraged to share your suggestions and observations.

The plan must be carried out. The plan may change if the person's nursing diagnoses change. Remember, nursing diagnoses may change as new information is gained during assessment. *(See Focus on Long-Term Care box.)*

IMPLEMENTATION

Implementation means to perform or carry out. The **implementation** step is performing or carrying out nursing measures in the nursing care plan. Care is given in this step.

Nursing measures range from simple to complex. The nurse delegates measures to you that are within the legal limits of your role and job description. Nurses often ask you to assist with complex measures.

You report to the nurse the care given. Some agencies allow you to record the care given. Reporting and recording are done after giving care, not before. Also remember to report or record your observations. Observing is part of assessment. New observations may change the nursing diagnoses, causing changes in the nursing care plan. You need to know about any changes in the nursing care plan so you can give the correct care.

Focus On... LONG-TERM CARE

OBRA requires the use of **resident assessment protocols (RAPs)** for developing care plans. The problems identified on the MDS (minimum data set) give **triggers** (clues) for the resident assessment protocols. RAPs are triggers and guidelines that help the team develop the resident's care plan (Fig. 4-9, p. 82). For example, the MDS shows that Mrs. Reece cannot do her activities of daily living (ADL). This triggers the RAPs, which provide guidelines for actions to solve the problems. The goal is for Mrs. Reece to be independent in all ADL. The actions to help Mrs. Reece reach the goal are as follows:

- Occupational therapy to work with the resident on ADL
- Physical therapy to work with the resident on strengthening exercises daily
- A nursing staff member to walk the resident 50 feet twice daily

OBRA also requires regular interdisciplinary care planning (IDCP) conferences for each resident. It is attended by health team members (called the *interdisciplinary health team* by OBRA) involved in the person's care.

EVALUATION

Evaluation means to measure. The **evaluation** step involves measuring if the goals in the planning step were met. The RN evaluates the progress made. Goals may be met totally, in part, or not at all. Information from assessment is used for evaluation. Changes in nursing diagnoses, goals, and the care plan may result from evaluation.

The nursing process never ends. Nurses constantly collect information about the person. As the person's needs change, the nursing process changes. Nursing diagnoses, goals, and the care plan may change. You play an important part in the nursing process. You make and report observations. The nurse uses the information for nursing diagnoses, goals, and the care plan. You may help develop the care plan. In the implementation step, you perform nursing actions and measures written in the care plan. Your observations are used for the evaluation step.

SECTION V. RESIDENT ASSESSMENT PROTOCOL SUMMARY   Numeric Identifier_____

Resident's Name:	Medical Record No.:

1. Check if RAP is triggered.
2. For each triggered RAP, use the RAP guidelines to identify areas needing further assessment. Document relevant assessment information regarding the resident's status.

- Describe:
  - Nature of the condition (may include presence or lack of objective data and subjective complaints).
  - Complications and risk factors that affect your decision to proceed to care planning.
  - Factors that must be considered in developing individualized care plan interventions.
  - Need for referrals/further evaluation by appropriate health professionals.
- Documentation should support your decision-making regarding whether to proceed with a care plan for a triggered RAP and the type(s) of care plan interventions that are appropriate for a particular resident.
- Documentation may appear anywhere in the clinical record (e.g., progress notes, consults, flowsheets, etc.).

3. Indicate under the <u>Location of RAP Assessment Documentation</u> column where information related to the RAP assessment can be found.
4. For each triggered RAP, indicate whether a new care plan, care plan revision, or continuation of current care plan is necessary to address the problem(s) identified in your assessment. The Care Planning Decision column must be completed within 7 days of completing the RAI (MDS and RAPs).

A. RAP Problem Area	(a) Check if Triggered	Location and Date of RAP Assessment Documentation	(b) Care Planning Decision—check if addressed in care plan
1. DELIRIUM			
2. COGNITIVE LOSS			
3. VISUAL FUNCTION			
4. COMMUNICATION			
5. ADL FUNCTIONAL/ REHABILITATION POTENTIAL			
6. URINARY INCONTINENCE AND INDWELLING CATHETER			
7. PSYCHOSOCIAL WELL-BEING			
8. MOOD STATE			
9. BEHAVIORAL SYMPTOMS			
10. ACTIVITIES			
11. FALLS			
12. NUTRITIONAL STATUS			
13. FEEDING TUBES			
14. DEHYDRATION/FLUID MAINTENANCE			
15. ORAL/DENTAL CARE			
16. PRESSURE ULCERS			
17. PSYCHOTROPIC DRUG USE			
18. PHYSICAL RESTRAINTS			

B. _____   2. ☐☐ – ☐☐ – ☐☐☐☐
1. Signature of RN Coordinator for RAP Assessment Process   Month   Day   Year

_____   4. ☐☐ – ☐☐ – ☐☐☐☐
3. Signature of Person Completing Care Planning Decision   Month   Day   Year

Form 1728RHH   © 1997 Briggs Corporation, Des Moines, IA 50306 (800) 247-2343   PRINTED IN U.S.A.
Copyright limited to addition of trigger system.
9 of 9   MDS 2.0   1/30/98

Fig. 4-9 Resident assessment protocols (RAPs). *(Reprinted with permission of Briggs Corporation, Des Moines, Iowa.)*

REPORTING AND RECORDING

Reporting and recording promote communication among health team members. Both are accounts of what was done for and observed about the person. **Reporting** is the verbal account of care and observations. **Recording** (or *charting*) is the written account of observations and care.

REPORTING

You report to the nurse patient or resident care and observations. Reports must be prompt, thorough, and accurate. Always tell the nurse the person's name, room and bed number, and the time your observations were made or the care was given. Report only those things that you observed or did yourself. Give reports as often as the person's condition requires or as often as requested by the nurse. Immediately report any changes from normal or changes in the person's condition. Use your written notes to give a specific, concise, and descriptive report (Fig. 4-10).

The nurse gives a report at the end of the shift to the nursing team of the oncoming shift (called the *end-of-shift report*). Information is shared about the care given and the care that must be given to patients or residents. Information about the person's condition also is included. Some agencies have all nursing team members hear the end-of-shift report as they come on duty. Others have nursing assistants perform routine tasks while RNs and LPNs hear the report.

RECORDING

When recording on the person's chart, you must communicate clearly and thoroughly. You must follow the rules in Box 4-4. Anyone who reads your charting should know:

- What you observed
- What you did
- The person's response

Fig. 4-10 The nursing assistant uses notes when reporting.

Box 4-4   Rules for Recording

- Always use ink. Follow agency policy for the color of ink to use.
- Include the date and the time whenever a recording is made. Use conventional time (AM or PM) or 24-hour clock time according to agency policy (see p. 84).
- Make sure writing is legible and neat.
- Use only agency approved abbreviations (see p. 84).
- Use correct spelling, grammar, and punctuation.
- Never erase or use correction fluid if you make an error. Cross out the incorrect part, write "error" or "mistaken entry" over it, and rewrite the part. Follow agency policy for correcting errors.
- Sign all entries with your name and title as required by agency policy.
- Do not skip lines. Draw a line through the blank space of a partially completed line or to the end of a page. This prevents others from recording in a space with your signature.
- Make sure each form is stamped with the person's name and other identifying information.
- Record only what you observed and did yourself.
- Never chart a procedure or treatment until after its completion.
- Be accurate, concise, and factual. Do not record judgments or interpretations.
- Record in a logical and sequential manner.
- Be descriptive. Avoid terms with more than one meaning.
- Use the person's exact words whenever possible. Use quotation marks to show that the statement is a direct quote.
- Chart any changes from normal or changes in the person's condition. Also chart that you informed the nurse and the time you made the report.
- Do not omit information.
- Record safety measures such as raising bed rails, assisting a person when up, or reminding someone not to get out of bed. This will help protect you if the person falls.

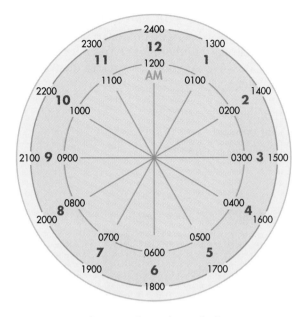

Fig. 4-11 The 24-hour clock.

Box 4-5	24-Hour Clock	
CONVENTIONAL TIME		**24-HOUR CLOCK**
1:00 AM		0100
2:00 AM		0200
3:00 AM		0300
4:00 AM		0400
5:00 AM		0500
6:00 AM		0600
7:00 AM		0700
8:00 AM		0800
9:00 AM		0900
10:00 AM		1000
11:00 AM		1100
12:00 NOON		1200
1:00 PM		1300
2:00 PM		1400
3:00 PM		1500
4:00 PM		1600
5:00 PM		1700
6:00 PM		1800
7:00 PM		1900
8:00 PM		2000
9:00 PM		2100
10:00 PM		2200
11:00 PM		2300
12:00 MIDNIGHT		2400 or 0000

Recording Time. The 24-hour clock (military time or international time) involves using a four-digit number for time (Fig. 4-11). The first two digits are for the hour: 0100 = 1:00 AM; 1300 = 1:00 PM. The last two digits are for minutes: 0110 = 1:10 AM. The AM and PM abbreviations are not used.

As Box 4-5 shows, morning hours are the same but AM is not used. For PM times, add 12 to the clock time. If it is 2:00 PM, add 12 plus 2 for 1400. For 8:35 PM, add 12 and 835 for 2035.

Communication is better when using the 24-hour clock. The AM and PM abbreviations must be used with conventional clock time. Someone may forget to use AM or PM, or writing may be unclear. If this happens, the correct time is not communicated. Harm to the person could result if time is not accurately recorded.

MEDICAL TERMINOLOGY AND ABBREVIATIONS

Medical terminology and abbreviations are used to communicate in health care (see Chapter 38). They are presented throughout this book. If a word or phrase is used that you do not understand, ask a nurse to explain its meaning. Otherwise, communication does not occur. You also may want to buy a medical dictionary so you can learn new words.

COMPUTERS IN HEALTH CARE

Computer information systems collect, send, record, and store information. Information is retrieved when needed. Medical records and care plans are on computer in many agencies. Instead of recording on the person's chart, information is entered into the computer (Fig. 4-12). Using a computer is easier, faster, and more efficient than writing on the chart. Recordings are more accurate, legible, and reliable.

Agency departments communicate with the nursing unit by computer. Instead of sending a typed report by messenger for the chart, the information is entered into the computer. The information is accessed at the computer in the nurses' station or at the bedside. These computer communication links reduce clerical work and telephone calls. Information is communicated with greater speed and accuracy.

Fig. 4-12 The nurse enters information into the computer.

The computer is used for many other functions. For example, computers are used to monitor certain measurements such as blood pressures, temperatures, heart rates, and heart function. The computer recognizes normal and abnormal measurements. When the abnormal is sensed, an alarm alerts the nursing staff. Computer monitoring is accurate and promotes early detection of life-threatening events.

Doctors can use computers when diagnosing. Signs and symptoms are entered into the computer. The computer asks questions, and the doctor responds. Eventually the computer offers possible diagnoses. The doctor can also use the computer also to prescribe medicines. The person's diagnosis is entered along with any requested information. The computer analyzes the information and suggests medicines and dosages.

Computers save time. Quality care and safety are increased. Fewer recording errors occur. Records are more complete and staff more efficient.

Computer information is easy to access. Therefore the person's right to privacy must be protected. Only certain staff are allowed to use the computer. They have their own codes (passwords) to access computer files. If allowed access, you will learn how to use the agency's system. You must follow the ethical and legal considerations relating to privacy, confidentiality, and defamation (see Chapter 2). Also follow the rules in Box 4-6.

Box 4-6   Rules to Protect Privacy When Using the Computer

- Do not tell anyone your password. If someone has your password, that person can access the computer under your name. It will be hard to prove that someone else made the entries.
- Change your password on a regular basis.
- Follow the rules for recording listed in Box 4-4 (see p. 83).
- Enter information carefully. Double-check your entries.
- Prevent others from seeing what is on the screen. Do not leave the computer unattended. Log off after making an entry.
- Position equipment so that the screen cannot be seen in the hallway.
- Do not leave printouts where others can read them or pick them up.
- Destroy or shred any computer-printed worksheets.
- Use e-mail wisely.
  - Send e-mail only to the people who need the information.
  - Do not use e-mail for information that requires immediate reporting. Tell the individual in person. (The recipient may not read e-mail in a timely manner.)
  - Do not use e-mail to report confidential information. The e-mail system may not be secure.

TELEPHONE COMMUNICATIONS

Often it is necessary to answer phones at the nurses' station or in the person's room. Good telephone communication skills are needed. The caller cannot see you. But you give much information by your tone of voice, how clearly you speak, and your attitude. When answering the phone, behave as if you are speaking to someone face-to-face.

Agencies have policies about answering telephones. You must be professional and courteous. Good work ethics apply when on the phone. Follow the guidelines in Box 4-7 on p. 86. *(See Focus on Home Care box on p. 86.)*

Box 4-7	Guidelines for Answering Telephones

- Answer the call after the first ring if possible. Business manners call for the phone to be answered by the fourth ring.
- Do not answer the phone in a rushed or hasty manner.
- Give a courteous greeting, identify the area, and give your name and title. For example: "Good morning. Three center. John Hayne, nursing assistant."
- Write the following information when taking a message: the caller's name and telephone number (include area code and extension number), the date and time, and the message.
- Repeat the message and telephone number back to the caller.
- Ask the caller to "Please hold" if necessary. However, find out who is calling first; then ask if the caller can hold. Do not put callers with an emergency on hold.
- Do not lay the phone down or cover the receiver with your hand when not speaking to the caller. The caller may overhear confidential conversations.
- Return to a caller on hold within 30 seconds. Ask if the caller can wait longer or if the call can be returned.
- Do not give confidential information to any caller. Remember, information about patients, residents and employees is confidential. Refer such calls to a RN.
- Transfer the call if appropriate. Tell the caller that you are going to transfer the call. Give the name of the department if appropriate. Give the caller the phone number in case the call gets disconnected or the line is busy.
- End the conversation politely. Thank the person for calling, and say good-bye.
- Give the message to the appropriate person.

Focus On... HOME CARE

When answering phones in patient homes, simply answer with "hello." This is for everyone's safety—the patient's, the family's, and your own. The caller has too much information when you give the patient's name ("Price residence") or your own name and title. People call homes for many reasons. They call to sell things or to obtain donations for charity. Others call with criminal intent. They want to know who is in the home. By saying that you are a home health assistant, you tell the caller that an ill, older, or disabled person is in the home. These people have difficulty defending themselves and are easy prey for criminals. Do not give your name or the patient's name until you know who is calling and why that person is calling. Give the information only when it is someone you are sure that you want to talk to—the patient's family or friend, your supervisor, or a caller expected by the patient.

DEALING WITH CONFLICT

People bring their own values, attitudes, opinions, experiences, and expectations to the work setting. Differences often lead to conflict. **Conflict** is described as a clash between opposing interests and ideas. Disagreements, misunderstandings, arguments, and unrest occur.

Conflicts arise over issues or events. Work schedules, absences, and the amount and quality of work performed are examples. The problems must be worked out. Otherwise, unkind words or actions may occur. The work environment becomes unpleasant, and care is affected.

Communication and good work ethics are essential for preventing and resolving conflicts. Identify and solve problems before they become major issues. The following guidelines can help you deal with conflict:

- Ask your supervisor for some time to talk privately. Explain the situation, and ask for advice in solving the problem. Give facts and specific examples.
- Approach the person with whom you have a conflict. Ask to talk privately. Be polite and professional in your approach.
- Agree on a time and place to talk.
- Talk in a private setting. Others should not see or hear you and your co-worker.
- Explain the problem and what is bothering you. Give facts and specific behaviors. Focus on the problem, not on the person.
- Listen to the person's response. Do not interrupt the person.
- Identify ways to solve the problem. Offer your own thoughts, and ask for the co-worker's ideas.
- Schedule a date and time to review the situation.
- Thank the person for meeting with you.
- Implement the solutions.
- Review the situation as scheduled.

CROSS-TRAINING OPPORTUNITIES

Receptionists and unit secretaries (ward clerks) use much of what you learned in this chapter. A receptionist answers the telephone and greets visitors. Information is also given about where to find patient or resident rooms and the various departments. A unit secretary or ward clerk works on a nursing unit. The person maintains the medical record, writes information on the Kardex, orders supplies, and communicates with the health team. Answering the phone, taking messages, and working with the computer are other duties.

You may be asked to cross-train for one or both of these roles. Should you choose to do so, your job opportunities will be greater. You will also learn more about what these workers do. That will help you better understand and appreciate their roles and functions.

Circle the BEST answer.

1. When communicating, you should do all of the following *except*
   A. Use terms that have more than one meaning
   B. Be brief and concise
   C. Present information logically and in sequence
   D. Give facts and be specific

2. Mrs. Kemp is discharged from the agency. Her medical record is
   A. Destroyed to protect her right to privacy
   B. Sent home with her
   C. Permanent
   D. On computer

3. These statements are about medical records. Which is *false?*
   A. The record is used to communicate information about the person.
   B. The record is a written account of the person's illness and response to treatment.
   C. The record can be used in a court of law.
   D. Anyone working in the agency can read the medical record.

4. A person is weighed daily. The measurement is recorded on the
   A. Admission sheet
   B. Graphic sheet
   C. Flow sheet
   D. Nurses' notes

5. Where does the RN describe the nursing care given?
   A. Nursing care plan
   B. Progress notes
   C. Graphic sheet
   D. Kardex

6. Which is a symptom?
   A. Redness
   B. Vomiting
   C. Pain
   D. Pulse rate of 78

7. Measures in the nursing care plan are carried out. What step of the nursing process is this?
   A. Nursing diagnosis
   B. Planning
   C. Implementation
   D. Evaluation

8. Which statement is *true?*
   A. The nursing process is done without the person's involvement.
   B. Nursing assistants are responsible for the nursing process.
   C. The nursing process is used to communicate the person's care.
   D. All of the above

9. The nursing care plan
   A. Is written by the doctor
   B. Consists of actions the nursing team takes to help a person
   C. Is the same for all persons
   D. Is also called the Kardex

10. When recording information, you should do the following, *except*
    A. Use ink
    B. Include the date and time
    C. Erase if you make an error
    D. Sign all entries with your name and title

11. These statements are about recording. Which is *false?*
    A. Use the person's exact words when possible.
    B. Record only what you observed and did yourself.
    C. Do not skip lines.
    D. To save time, chart a procedure before it is completed.

12. In the evening you note that the clock says 9:26. In 24-hour clock time you record this as
    A. 9:26 PM
    B. 926
    C. 0926
    D. 2126

13. These statements are about computers in health care. Which is *false?*
    A. Computers are used to collect, send, record, and store information.
    B. The person's privacy must be protected.
    C. All employees have the same password.
    D. Computers link one department to another.

14. You answer a person's phone in the agency. How should you answer?
    A. "Good morning. Mrs. Kemp's room."
    B. "Good morning. Third floor."
    C. "Hello."
    D. "Good morning. Mrs. Kemp's room. Joan Bates, nursing assistant, speaking."

15. A co-worker is often late for work. You have extra work in her absence. In resolving the conflict you should do the following *except*
    A. Explain the problem to your supervisor
    B. Discuss the matter during the end-of-shift report
    C. Give facts and specific instances
    D. Suggest ideas to solve the problem

Answers to these questions are on p. 833.

UNDERSTANDING THE PERSON

OBJECTIVES

Define the key terms listed in this chapter

Identify the parts that make up the whole person

Describe the basic needs identified by Abraham Maslow

Explain how culture and religion influence health and illness

Identify the psychological and social effects of illness

Describe persons cared for in health care agencies

Explain the American Hospital Association's *A Bill of Rights*

Identify the elements needed for effective communication

Describe how verbal and nonverbal communication are used

Explain the techniques and barriers to effective communication

Explain why family and visitors are important to patients and residents

Identify the courtesies you should give to patients, residents, and visitors

Explain how to deal with the angry person

KEY TERMS

body language Facial expressions, gestures, posture, and body movements that send messages to others

culture The language, values, beliefs, habits, likes, dislikes, customs, and characteristics of a group that are passed from one generation to the next

esteem The worth, value, or opinion one has of a person

geriatrics The branch of medicine concerned with the problems and diseases of old age and older persons

holism A concept that considers the whole person; the whole person has physical, social, psychological, and spiritual parts that are woven together and cannot be separated

need That which is necessary or desirable for maintaining life and mental well-being

nonverbal communication Communication that does not involve words

obstetrics The branch of medicine concerned with the care of women during pregnancy, labor, and childbirth and for the 6 to 8 weeks after birth

paraphrasing Restating the person's message in your own words

pediatrics The branch of medicine concerned with the growth, development, and care of children ranging in age from the newborn to the adolescent

psychiatry The branch of medicine concerned with the diagnosis and treatment of people with mental health problems

religion Spiritual beliefs, needs, and practices

self-actualization Experiencing one's potential

self-esteem Thinking well of yourself and being thought well of by others

verbal communication Communication that uses the written or spoken word

The patient or resident is the most important person in the agency. Age, religion, nationality, culture, education, occupation, and life-style are some factors that make each person unique. The person is treated as a human being with value. The person is important and special. You must treat the person as someone who thinks, acts, and makes decisions.

Each person has fears, needs, and rights. This chapter focuses on understanding the persons you serve and help.

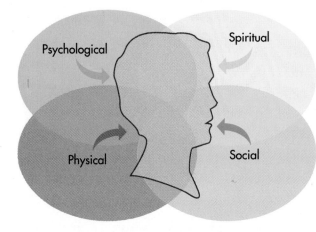

Fig. 5-1 A person is a physical, psychological, social, and spiritual being. The parts overlap and cannot be separated.

CARING FOR THE PERSON

The person is someone who lives, works, loves, and has fun. When the person is ill or disabled, things are done to and for him or her. The person is told when to eat, sleep, bathe, have visitors, sit in a chair, walk, and use the bathroom. It is easy to forget that the person once did these things without help. No wonder patients and residents often complain that they are treated as things, not as people.

Too often the person is treated as a physical disease or problem: "the heart attack in 310" rather than "John Porter in 310." Most patients and residents have physical problems. However, to provide good care, you must be aware of the whole person.

Holism means *whole*. With **holism,** the whole person has physical, social, psychological, and spiritual parts. The parts are woven together and cannot be separated (Fig. 5-1). Each part relates to and depends on the others. As a social being, a person speaks and communicates with others. Physically, the brain, mouth, tongue, lips, and throat structures must function for speech. Communication is also highly psychological. It involves the thinking and reasoning abilities of the mind. Considering only the physical part is ignoring the person's ability to think, make decisions, and interact with others. It also ignores the person's experiences, joys, sorrows, and needs.

BASIC NEEDS

A **need** is that which is necessary or desirable for maintaining life and mental well-being. According to Abraham Maslow, a famous psychologist, certain basic needs must be met for a person to survive and

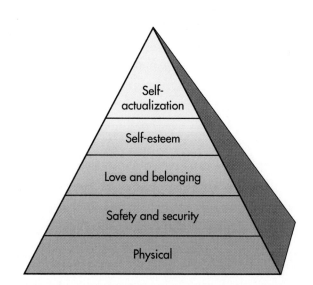

Fig. 5-2 Basic needs for life as described by Maslow. These needs, from the lowest to the highest level, are physical needs, the need for safety and security, the need for love and belonging, the need for self-esteem, and the need for self-actualization. *(From Maslow, Abraham H., Motivation and personality, © 1954, 1987. © 1970 by Abraham H. Maslow. Adapted by permission of Prentice-Hall, Inc., Upper Saddle River, NJ.)*

function. These needs are arranged in order of importance (Fig. 5-2). Lower-level needs must be met before the higher-level needs. These basic needs are, from the lowest level to the highest level:

- Physical needs
- The need for safety and security
- The need for love and belonging
- The need for self-esteem
- The need for self-actualization

People normally meet their own needs every day. When they cannot, it is usually because of illness or injury. When ill, they usually seek health care.

PHYSICAL NEEDS

Oxygen, food, water, elimination, rest, and shelter are required for life. These needs are the most important for survival. They must be met before higher-level needs. A person dies within minutes without oxygen. Without food or water, a person feels weak and ill within a few hours. The kidneys and intestines must function normally. Otherwise poisonous wastes build up in the blood. If the problem is not corrected, the person dies. Without enough rest and sleep, a person becomes exhausted.

THE NEED FOR SAFETY AND SECURITY

Safety and security needs relate to protection from harm, danger, and fear. Many people are afraid of health care. Many procedures involve frightening equipment, require entering the body, and cause pain or discomfort. People feel safer and more secure if they understand the procedure. Even for a simple bed bath, they should know:

- Why a procedure is to be done
- Who will do it
- How it will be performed
- What sensations or feelings to expect

THE NEED FOR LOVE AND BELONGING

The need for love and belonging relates to love, closeness, affection, belonging, and meaningful relationships with others. There are many cases in which people were slow to recover or died because of lack of love and belonging. This is particularly true of children and older persons. The need for love and belonging can be met by family, friends, and health workers.

THE NEED FOR SELF-ESTEEM

Esteem is the worth, value, or opinion one has of a person. **Self-esteem** relates to thinking well of yourself and of being thought well of by others. People often lack self-esteem when ill or injured. Think about the following:

- How does a father feel when he cannot work and support his family because of an illness?
- Does a woman feel whole and pretty after having a breast removed?
- Does a person with a leg amputation feel complete and attractive?

THE NEED FOR SELF-ACTUALIZATION

Self-actualization means experiencing one's potential. It involves learning, understanding, and creating to the limit of a person's capacity. This is the highest need. Rarely, if ever, is it totally met. Most people constantly try to learn and understand more. The need for self-actualization can be postponed, and life will continue.

CULTURE AND RELIGION

Culture is the characteristics of a group of people—the language, values, beliefs, habits, likes, dislikes, and customs—passed from one generation to the next. The person's culture influences health beliefs and practices. Culture also influences behavior during illness.

You will care for people from different cultural backgrounds. Besides Americans of various nationalities, you may care for people from other countries. These people have family practices, food preferences, hygiene habits, and clothing styles different from

> ### Caring About Culture
>
> #### HEALTH CARE BELIEFS
> Some cultures believe that health involves a balance between hot and cold. In *Mexico* and the *Dominican Republic*, hot and cold imbalances are thought to cause disease. "Hot" conditions include fever, infections, diarrhea, constipation, and ulcers. "Cold" conditions include cancer, earaches, menstrual periods, headaches, colds, and paralysis.
>
> In *Vietnam*, foods and medicine are given to restore the hot-cold balance. Hot foods and medicines are given for "cold" illnesses. Cold foods and medicines are given for "hot" illnesses.
>
> *Remember, individuals may not follow every belief and practice of their culture and religion. Each person is unique. Do not judge the person by your own standards.*

Modified from Giger JN, Davidhizar RE: *Transcultural nursing: assessment and interventions,* ed 2, St Louis, 1995, Mosby.

yours. The person may speak and understand another language. Some cultural groups have beliefs about the causes and cures of illnesses. *(See Caring About Culture [Health Care Beliefs] box.)* They may perform certain rituals aimed at ridding the body of disease. Many have beliefs and rituals about dying and death. Culture also is a factor in communication.

Religion relates to spiritual beliefs, needs, and practices. Like culture, a person's religion influences health and illness practices. Religions may have beliefs and practices relating to daily living habits, behaviors, relationships with others, diet, healing, days of worship, birth and birth control, medicine, and death.

Many people rely on religion for support and comfort during illness. They may want to pray and observe certain religious practices. A visit from their spiritual leader or adviser may be helpful. If a person asks to see a member of the clergy, promptly report the request to the nurse. Make sure the person's room is neat and orderly, and place a chair by the bed. Ensure privacy during the visit.

The nursing process reflects the person's culture and religion. The RN and the person plan measures that include the person's cultural and religious practices. You must show respect and accept the person's culture and religion. When you meet people from other cultures or religions, take time to learn about their beliefs and practices. This will help you to understand the person and give better care.

Individuals may not follow every belief and practice of their culture or religion. Remember, each person is unique. Do not judge the person by your own standards. (See Focus on Home Care box on p. 94.)

Focus On... HOME CARE

Culture is reflected in the home. Homes vary in size, cleanliness, and furnishings. Some homes are expensive. Others reflect poverty. Whether rich or poor, treat each person and family with respect, kindness, and dignity. Do not judge the person's life-style, habits, religion, or culture.

BEING SICK

People cannot choose between health or illness. Illness and injury do occur. Besides physical effects, illness has some psychological and social effects.

Normal activities—such as working, going to school, preparing meals, doing house or yard work, and taking part in sports or hobbies—may seem difficult or impossible. Daily activities bring personal satisfaction, worth, and contact with others. Most people are frustrated and angry when unable to perform them. These feelings may become even greater if others must perform routine functions for the person.

Sick people have many fears and anxieties. They fear death, disability, chronic illness, and loss of function. Some explain why they are afraid. Others keep their feelings to themselves. They fear being laughed at for being afraid. A person with a broken leg may fear having a limp or not walking again. Persons having surgery often fear cancer. These fears and anxieties are normal and expected. You need to understand how people are affected by illness. Think about how you would feel and react if you had the person's illness and problems.

Sick people are expected to behave in a certain way. They need to see a doctor, stay in bed, and rely on others for care and comfort. These behaviors are accepted so the person can get well. When recovery is delayed or does not occur, the normal psychological and social effects of illness become greater.

Culture and religion are also factors in how people think and behave when ill. (See Caring About Culture [Sick Care Practices] box.)

PERSONS YOU WILL CARE FOR

Patients and residents are grouped in health care agencies by their problems, needs, and age. Doctors and nurses have special knowledge and skills to care for certain people.

- *Mothers and newborns*—**Obstetrics** is the branch of medicine concerned with the care of women during pregnancy, labor, and childbirth and during the

Caring About Culture

SICK CARE PRACTICES

Folk practices are common in the *Vietnamese* culture. Such practices include *cao gio*—rubbing the skin with a coin. This is done to treat the common cold. Skin pinching *(bat gio)* is used for headaches and sore throats. Herbal teas and soups are common remedies for many different signs and symptoms.

Russian folk practices also include herbs. Herbs are taken through drinks or enemas. For headaches, an ointment is placed behind the ears and temples. It is also placed at the back of the neck. There are different treatments for backache. One involves making a dough of dark rye flour and honey. The dough is placed on the spinal column.

Folk healers are seen in *Mexico* and among some *Mexican Americans*. Folk healers include a family member skilled in healing practices passed down from one generation to another. Folk healers are sometimes sought outside the family. A *jerbero* uses herbs and spices to prevent or cure disease. A *curandero* (*curandera* if female) deals with serious physical and mental illnesses. Witches use magic. A male witch is a called a *brujos;* a female witch is called a *brujas.*

Remember, individuals may not follow every belief and practice of their culture and religion. Each person is unique. Do not judge the person by your own standards.

Modified from Giger JN, Davidhizar RE: *Transcultural nursing: assessment and interventions,* ed 2, St Louis, 1995, Mosby.

6 to 8 weeks after birth. Patients are seen in clinics or doctors' offices during pregnancy. When labor begins, these women usually are admitted to the obstetrical (maternity) department. Pregnancy, labor, and childbirth are normal and natural events. However, complications can occur at any time during pregnancy through the 6 to 8 weeks after childbirth.

- *Children*—**Pediatrics** is the branch of medicine concerned with the growth, development, and care of children ranging in age from the newborn to the adolescent. When hospital care is needed, children are admitted to a pediatric unit. The unit is designed and equipped to meet the needs of children and parents. The nursing staff is concerned with the child's physical, safety, and emotional needs (Fig. 5-3). (See Focus on Children boxes throughout this book.)
- *Adults with medical problems*—Medical problems are illnesses, diseases, or injuries that do not need surgery. People may have acute, chronic, or terminal illnesses. Examples are infections, strokes, or heart attacks.

Fig. 5-3 The nursing assistant gives care to a sick child.

- *Persons having surgery*—Surgical patients are those being prepared for or who have had surgery. Surgeries range from simple to very complex. An appendectomy (removal of the appendix) is a simple surgery. Open-heart and brain surgeries are complex. Preoperative care involves preparing the person for what to expect after surgery. The person's fears and anxieties are also dealt with. Needs after surgery relate to relieving pain and discomfort, preventing complications, and adjusting to body changes.
- *Persons with mental health problems*—**Psychiatry** is the branch of medicine concerned with the diagnosis and treatment of people with mental health problems. Problems vary from mild to severe mental and emotional disorders. Some persons function normally but need help making decisions or coping with life stresses. Others are severely disturbed. They cannot do simple things such as eating, bathing, or dressing. Special precautions and treatments are necessary for persons who are dangerous to themselves or others.
- *Older persons*—**Geriatrics** is the branch of medicine concerned with the problems and diseases of old age and older persons. Aging is a normal process. It is not an illness or disease. Many older people enjoy good health. Others suffer from acute or chronic illnesses. Some have degenerative diseases common in older persons. Body changes normally occur with the aging process. Social and psychological changes also occur. (See Chapter 8). Sometimes the changes are so severe that the person requires long-term care (Fig. 5-4). *(See Focus on Older Persons boxes throughout this book.)*
- *Persons in special care areas*—Some people have special problems or are seriously ill. They need special care and equipment. Special care units are designed and equipped to treat and prevent life-threatening problems and complications. These special care areas include intensive care units, coronary care units (Fig. 5-5), kidney dialysis units, burn units, and emergency rooms.

Fig. 5-4 This older persons lives in a nursing center.

Fig. 5-5 A room in an intensive care unit.

- *Persons requiring rehabilitation*—As described in Chapter 1, rehabilitation is the process of restoring the disabled person to the highest level of functioning possible. The person may need to regain functions lost from surgery, illness, or accidents. Persons with birth defects need to learn skills using existing abilities.
- *Persons requiring subacute care*—Subacute care has a strong rehabilitation focus. Persons needing subacute care have a longer recovery period than persons with acute illnesses. However, long-term care or lengthy rehabilitation is not needed. Persons may need subacute care after joint replacement surgery. Persons with some lung and nervous system disorders may have longer recovery periods and need rehabilitation.

THE PERSON'S RIGHTS

Patients' rights came about when people demanded more information about their health problems and treatment. They also demanded better care at lower costs and greater involvement in treatment decisions. Patients were not willing to be helpless and to accept the doctor's advice without question.

A Patient's Bill of Rights was issued by the American Hospital Association (AHA). It has an ethical and legal basis. The right to privacy and informed consent are involved. Although the relationship between the doctor and the patient is stressed, there are important messages for the health team. The basic points of *A Patient's Bill of Rights* are presented in Box 5-1. (*See Focus on Long-Term Care box.*)

Focus On... LONG-TERM CARE

Residents have rights as citizens of the United States. They also have rights under OBRA (see Chapter 8). These rights relate to their everyday lives and care in the nursing center. The center must protect and promote resident rights. Residents must be free to exercise their rights without center interference. Some residents are incompetent (not able) and cannot exercise their rights. Legal representatives exercise rights for them.

Nursing centers must inform residents of their rights. They must be informed orally and in writing. Such information is given before or during admission to the center. It must be given in the language used and understood by the resident.

Box 5-1 Patient Rights

The right to CONSIDERATION AND RESPECT
- The patient is treated as a person and given kind and thoughtful care.
- Personal values, beliefs, cultural practices, and personality are considered when planning and providing care.

The right to INFORMATION
- The patient receives information from the doctor about the diagnosis, treatment, and prognosis in terms the patient can understand.
- Unfamiliar medical terminology is avoided.
- An interpreter is needed if the patient does not understand or speak English.
- The nearest relative or legal representative is informed of the patient's diagnosis, treatment, and prognosis if it is unwise to tell the patient.

The right to INFORMED CONSENT
- The patient receives information and explanations about any treatments or procedures.
- The doctor provides information about a treatment's purpose, risks, alternatives, and the probable length of recovery.
- The patient is told who will perform the treatment or procedure.

The right to REFUSE TREATMENT
- The person can refuse treatment.
- The patient does not have to consent to each treatment or procedure recommended by the doctor.
- The doctor must inform the patient of the risks to life and health involved in refusing the treatment.

The right to PRIVACY
- The patient's body, record, care, and personal affairs are kept private.
- The right to privacy is still protected after death.

The right to CONFIDENTIALITY
- Information is shared with other health workers in a wise and careful manner.
- All health workers must recognize the confidential nature of patient information.

The right to HOSPITAL SERVICES
- The patient has the right to expect that the hospital can provide needed services.
- After immediate needs are met, the patient may be transferred to another agency better equipped to handle the patient's problems and needs.
- The patient is informed of the reason for the transfer and of other alternatives.

The right to INFORMATION ABOUT THE HOSPITAL'S RELATIONSHIP TO OTHER AGENCIES
- The patient is informed of any relationships with schools and other health care agencies.
- Patients have the right to know about these relationships and to know the names of students or other persons providing or involved in their care.

The right to INFORMATION ON RESEARCH AND HUMAN EXPERIMENTATION
- The patient receives information and explanations about research for making an informed decision about participating.
- The patient's consent is obtained before involvement in human experimentation or research.
- The patient may refuse to participate.

The right to CONTINUING CARE
- The patient is informed of the care needed after discharge.
- The patient is given written information about the times and locations of appointments with doctors.

The right to THE PATIENT'S BILL
- The patient has the right to examine bills and receive an explanation of the items in the bill.
- This right exists even if the bill is to be paid by an insurance company or the government.

The right to KNOW HOSPITAL RULES AND REGULATIONS
- The patient is informed of any rules and regulations applying to his or her conduct as a patient.
- The patient and family are given pamphlets that explain the rules and regulations.

Reprinted with permission of the American Hospital Association, copyright 1992.

COMMUNICATING WITH THE PERSON

Several elements are necessary for effective communication between you and the person:

- You must understand and respect the patient or resident as a person.
- You must view the person as more than a disease or an illness. The person is a physical, psychological, social, and spiritual human being.
- You must appreciate the person's problems and frustrations from being sick.
- You need to recognize and respect the person's rights.
- You must accept and respect the person's religion and culture.

The rules for communication discussed in Chapter 4 apply when you communicate with patients and residents:

- Use words that have the same meaning to both you and the person.
- Avoid using medical terminology and other words that are unfamiliar to the person.
- Communicate in a logical and orderly manner. Do not wander in thought.
- Give specific and factual information.
- Be brief and concise.

Verbal and nonverbal communication are used when relating to patients and residents. You must use both methods effectively.

VERBAL COMMUNICATION

Words are used in **verbal communication.** The words are spoken or written. Verbal communication is used to talk with patients or residents, to find out how they are feeling, and to share information with them.

Most verbal communication involves the spoken word. Shouting, whispering, and mumbling cause ineffective communication. You need to:

- Control the loudness and tone of your voice
- Speak clearly, slowly, and distinctly
- Avoid using slang or vulgar words
- Repeat information as needed
- Ask one question at a time, and wait for the answer. Do not ask several questions at once

The written word is used when persons cannot speak or hear. If a person cannot speak, provide a way for the person to send messages. A Magic Slate, paper and pencil, electronic talking aid, picture board, or communication board can be used (Fig. 5-6). Write messages to communicate with deaf persons or those with severe

Fig. 5-6 **A,** Magic Slate, **B,** Electronic talking aid. **C,** Communication board. (**B,** *Courtesy Mayer-Johnson Co., Solana Beach, Calif.*)

hearing problems (Fig. 5-7, p. 98). Deaf persons may use sign language to communicate (see Chapter 29).

Communication between you and the person should be on a professional level. You should not become personally involved with the patient or resident.

NONVERBAL COMMUNICATION

Nonverbal communication does not involve words. Gestures, facial expressions, posture, body movements, touch, and smell are ways of sending messages without words. Nonverbal messages more accurately reflect a person's feelings. They are usually involuntary and hard to control. A person may say one thing but act in a different way. Therefore you need to watch the person's eyes, hand movements, gestures, posture, and other actions.

Fig. 5-7 The nursing assistant writes a note to a person who is hearing impaired.

Touch. Touch is a very important form of nonverbal communication. It conveys comfort, caring, love, affection, interest, trust, concern, and reassurance. Touch means different things to different people. The meaning depends on the person's age, gender (male or female), life experiences, and culture. *(See Caring About Culture [Touch Practices] box.)* All cultural groups have rules or practices about touch. They relate to who can touch, when touch can occur, and where the body can be touched.

Some people do not like being touched. However, do not be afraid to use touch to convey caring and warmth. Patients and residents often are comforted by stroking or having their hands held. Touch should be gentle, not hurried or rough. Touch should not be sexual in nature.

Body Language. People send messages through their **body language.** Body language includes:

- Posture
- Gait
- Facial expressions *(See Caring About Culture [Facial Expressions in Americans] box and Caring About Culture [Facial Expressions in Other Cultures] box.)*
- Eye contact
- Hand movements
- Gestures
- Body movements
- Appearance (dress, hygiene, and adornments such as jewelry, perfume, and cosmetics)

Slumped posture may mean the person is not happy or feeling well. A person may deny pain but protects the affected body part by standing, lying, or sitting in a certain way. People send many other messages with body language.

Caring About Culture

TOUCH PRACTICES
Touch practices vary widely among cultural groups. Touch is used often in *Mexico.* Some people believe that using touch while complimenting a person is important. It is thought to neutralize the power of the evil eye *(mal ojo).*

Persons from the *United Kingdom* tend not to use touch. However, it is important in nonverbal communication among the people of Russia. They commonly kiss three times on the cheek for greetings and farewells. Hugging and kissing on the cheek is also common in *Poland.*

In *India,* men shake hands with other men. Men do not shake hands with women. Similar practices occur in the *Vietnamese* culture.

People from *China* do not like being touched by strangers. A nod or slight bow is given during introductions.

Remember, individuals may not follow every belief and practice of their culture and religion. Each person is unique. Do not judge the person by your own standards.

From Geissler EM: *Pocket guide to cultural assessment,* ed 2, St Louis, 1998, Mosby.

Caring About Culture

FACIAL EXPRESSIONS IN AMERICANS
- Coldness—constant stare; face muscles do not move
- Fear—eyes wide open; eyebrows raised; mouth tense with the lips drawn back
- Anger—eyes fixed in a hard stare; upper lids lowered; eyebrows drawn down; lips tightly compressed
- Tiredness—eyes rolled upward
- Disapproval—eyes rolled upward
- Disgust—eyes narrowed; upper lip curled; nose moving
- Embarrassment—eyes turned away or down; face flushed; pretend smile; rub eyes, nose, or face; twitch hair, beard, or mustache
- Surprise—direct gaze with raised eyebrows
  Remember, individuals may not follow every belief and practice of their culture and religion. Each person is unique. Do not judge the person by your own standards.

Modified from Giger JN, Davidhizar RE: *Transcultural nursing: assessment and intervention,* ed 2, St Louis, 1995, Mosby.

Caring About Culture

FACIAL EXPRESSIONS OF OTHER CULTURES

Italian, Jewish, African-American, and Spanish-speaking persons smile readily. They also use many facial expressions and gestures to communicate happiness, pain, or displeasure. *Irish, English, and Northern European* persons tend to have less facial expression.

In some cultures, facial expressions mean the opposite of what the person is feeling. For example, *Asians* may conceal negative emotions with a smile.

Remember, individuals may not follow every belief and practice of their culture and religion. Each person is unique. Do not judge the person by your own standards.

Modified from Giger JN, Davidhizar RE: *Transcultural nursing: assessment and intervention*, ed 2, St Louis, 1995, Mosby.

Caring About Culture

EYE CONTACT

In the *American* culture, eye contact is a sign of a good self-concept, openness, interest in others, attention, and honesty. Eye contact also communicates warmth. Lack of eye contact can communicate:

- Shyness
- Lack of interest
- Subordination
- Humility
- Guilt
- Embarrassment
- Low self-esteem
- Rudeness
- Dishonesty

Many cultures are uncomfortable with eye contact. For some *Asian* and *Native American* cultures, eye contact is impolite and an invasion of privacy. In certain *Indian* cultures, eye contact is avoided with persons of higher or lower socioeconomic class. It is also given a special sexual meaning.

Direct eye contact is practiced among the people of *Poland* and *Russia*. However, direct eye contact is rude in *Mexican* and *Vietnamese* cultures. In the *United Kingdom,* staring is a part of good listening.

Blinking also has meaning. In the *Vietnamese* culture, blinking means that a message is received. It indicates understanding in the *United Kingdom.*

Remember, individuals may not follow every belief and practice of their culture and religion. Each person is unique. Do not judge the person by your own standards.

Modified from Giger JN, Davidhizar RE: *Transcultural nursing: assessment and intervention*, ed 2, St Louis, 1995, Mosby; Geissler EM: *Pocket guide to cultural assessment*, ed 2, St Louis, 1998, Mosby.

You also send messages by the way you act and move. Your facial expressions and how you stand, sit, walk, and look at a person all send messages. Your body language should show interest and enthusiasm about your work. It should also show caring and respect for the person. You need to control your body language in many instances. For example, do not react to odors from excretions or the person's body. Many odors are beyond the person's control. The person's embarrassment and humiliation increase if you react to the odor.

TECHNIQUES FOR EFFECTIVE COMMUNICATION

Certain techniques help you communicate with patients, residents, and families. The techniques result in a better relationship with these persons. You also gain more information for the nursing process. Such information is used for the assessment and evaluation steps of the nursing process. As you communicate with the person, you also find out about the person's likes and dislikes. These are useful when the nurse plans care.

Listening. Listening means being attentive to the person's verbal and nonverbal communication. You use the senses of sight, hearing, touch, and smell. You must concentrate on what the person is saying. You also must observe nonverbal clues. The person's nonverbal communication can support what the person says. Or it can show other feelings. For example, Mr. Hart says, "I want to go to a nursing home. That way my daughter does not have to stay home to care

for me." However, you see tears in his eyes and he looks away from you. His verbal says happy, but his nonverbal shows sadness.

Listening requires that you care and have interest. The following guidelines are important:

- Face the person.
- Have good eye contact with the person. *(See Caring About Culture [Eye Contact] box.)*
- Lean toward the person (Fig. 5-8, p. 100). Do not sit back with your arms crossed.
- Respond to the person. Nod your head. Say "uh huh," "mmm," and "I see." Repeat what the person says, and ask questions.
- Avoid the communication barriers (see p. 100).

Fig. 5-8 Listen by facing the person, having good eye contact, and leaning toward the person.

Paraphrasing. **Paraphrasing** is restating the person's message in your own words. You use fewer words than the person did to send the message. Paraphrasing serves three purposes:

- It shows you are listening.
- It lets the person see if you understand the message sent.
- It promotes further communication.

The person generally responds to your statement. For example:

Mr. Hart: My wife left here crying after she spoke with the doctor. I don't know what he said to her.
You: You don't know why your wife was crying.
Mr. Hart: He must have told her that I have a tumor.

Direct Questions. Direct questions focus on specific information. You ask the person something you need to know. Some direct questions have "yes" or "no" answers. Others require that the person give more information. For example:

You: Mr. Hart, do you want to shave this morning?
Mr. Hart: Yes.
You: When would you like to shave and have your bath?
Mr. Hart: Could we start in about 15 minutes? I'd like to call my son first.
You: Yes, we can start in 15 minutes. Did you have a bowel movement today, Mr. Hart?
Mr. Hart: No.
You: You said you didn't eat well this morning. Can you tell me what you ate?
Mr. Hart: I only had toast and coffee. I just don't feel like eating this morning.

Open-Ended Questions. Open-ended questions lead or invite the person to share thoughts, feelings, or ideas. The person chooses what to talk about. Answers require more than a "yes" or "no." However, the person controls what is talked about and the information given. Consider these examples:

- "What do you like about living with your daughter?"
- "Tell me about your grandson."
- "What was your wife like?"
- "What do you like about being retired?"

The person chooses how to answer the question. Responses to open-ended questions are longer and give more information than direct questions.

Clarifying. Clarifying lets you make sure that you understand the message. You can ask the person to repeat the message, say you do not understand, or restate the message. For example:

- "Could you say that again?"
- "I'm sorry, Mr. Hart. I don't understand what you mean."
- "Are you saying that you want to go home?"

Focusing. Focusing is dealing with a certain topic. It is useful when a person rambles or wanders in thought. For example, Mr. Hart talks at length about his favorite foods and places to eat. You need to know why he did not feel like eating breakfast. You focus the conversation on breakfast by saying: "Let's talk about today's breakfast. You said you didn't feel like eating."

Silence. Silence is a very powerful way to communicate. Sometimes, especially during sad times, you do not need to say anything. Just being there shows you care. At other times, silence gives you or the person time to think, organize thoughts, or choose words. Silence is useful when making difficult decisions. It is useful also when the person is upset and needs time to regain control. Silence on your part shows caring and respect for the person's situation and feelings.

Sometimes pauses or long silences are uncomfortable. Do not think you need to talk when the person is silent. The person may need silence. Dealing with silence gets easier as you gain experience in your role. *(See Caring About Culture [Meaning of Silence] box.)*

COMMUNICATION BARRIERS

Communication barriers prevent sending and receiving messages. Communication fails. You must avoid the following barriers:

Caring About Culture

THE MEANING OF SILENCE

In the *English* and *Arabic* cultures, silence is used for privacy. Among *Russian, French, and Spanish* cultures, silence means agreement between parties. In some *Asian* cultures, silence is a sign of respect, particularly to an older person.

Remember, individuals may not follow every belief and practice of their culture and religion. Each person is unique. Do not judge the person by your own standards.

Modified from Giger JN, Davidhizar RE: *Transcultural nursing: assessment and interventions,* ed 2, St Louis, 1995, Mosby.

- *Using unfamiliar language.* You and the person must use and understand the same language. If not, messages are not accurately interpreted.
- *Cultural differences.* The person may attach different meanings to verbal and nonverbal communication. *(See Caring About Culture [Communicating With Persons From Other Cultures] box.)*
- *Changing the subject.* Either you or the person changes the subject when the topic is uncomfortable. Avoid changing the subject whenever possible.
- *Giving your opinion.* This tells the person that you are judging his or her values, behavior, or feelings. Let others express their feelings and concerns without adding your opinion, making a judgment, or jumping to conclusions.
- *Talking a lot when others are silent.* Excessive talking is usually because of nervousness and discomfort with silence. Silences have meaning. They convey acceptance, rejection, fear, or the need for quiet and time to think.
- *Failing to listen.* Communication is blocked if you fail to listen with interest and sincerity. Do not pretend to listen. This causes inappropriate responses and conveys a lack of interest and caring. You can miss important complaints of pain, discomfort, or other abnormal sensations that must be reported to the nurse.
- *Giving pat answers.* "Don't worry," "Everything will be okay," and "Your doctor knows best" block communication. These make patients and residents feel that you are ridiculing their concerns, feelings, and fears. They think you do not care about what they think or feel.
- *Illness.* Some central nervous system disorders affect speech and body movements. The person may be unable to speak. Disorders that affect movement interfere with nonverbal communication.

Caring About Culture

COMMUNICATING WITH PERSONS FROM OTHER CULTURES

- Ask the nurse about the beliefs and values of the person's culture. Learn as much as you can about the person's culture.
- Do not judge the person by your own attitudes, values, beliefs, and ideas.
- Follow the person's care plan. The nurse plans care that includes the person's cultural beliefs and customs.
- Do the following when communicating with foreign-speaking persons:
  - Convey comfort by your tone of voice and body language.
  - Do not speak loudly or shout. It will not help the person understand English.
  - Speak slowly and distinctly.
  - Keep messages short and simple.
  - Be alert for words the person seems to understand.
  - Use gestures and pictures.
  - Repeat the message in different ways.
  - Avoid using medical terms and abbreviations.
  - Be alert for signs that the person is pretending to understand. Nodding and answering "yes" to all questions are signs that the person does not understand what you are saying.

Modified from Geissler EM: *Pocket guide to cultural assessment,* ed 2, St Louis, 1998, Mosby.

THE FAMILY AND VISITORS

Family, relatives, and friends help meet the person's needs for safety and security, love and belonging, and self-esteem. They offer support and comfort and lessen loneliness. Some also help with the person's care—meals, bathing, brushing and combing hair, and other care. The presence or absence of significant family members or friends can affect recovery. *(See Caring About Culture [Family Roles in Sick Care] box.)*

The person should visit with family and friends in private and without unnecessary interruptions (Fig. 5-9, p. 102). Sometimes care must be given when visitors are present. Politely ask them to leave the room, and show them a comfortable waiting area. Do not expose the person's body in front of visitors. Promptly tell visitors when they may return to the room.

Family and visitors are treated with courtesy and respect. They have concerns and fears about the person's condition. They need support and understanding

Caring About Culture

FAMILY ROLES IN SICK CARE

In *Vietnam,* all family members are involved in the person's care. A similar practice is common in Russia and in *China.* Family members bathe, feed, and comfort the person. However, women in *Mexico* cannot give care at home if it involves touching the genitals of adult men.

Remember, individuals may not follow every belief and practice of their culture and religion. Each person is unique. Do not judge the person by your own standards.

Modified from Geissler EM: *Pocket guide to cultural assessment,* ed 2, St Louis, 1998, Mosby.

Fig. 5-9 This man has a private visit with his son.

Focus On... OLDER PERSONS

Sometimes older brothers, sisters, and cousins live together. They provide companionship and share living expenses. They care for each other during illness or disability. One may be the caregiver if the other is ill or disabled.

Some older people live with their adult children. The older parent may be healthy, need some supervision, or be ill or disabled. The older parent (or parents) moves in with the child, or the child moves into the parent's home. Living with a child can help the older person feel safe and secure. Often the adult child is a caregiver for an ill or disabled parent.

Adult children often need to work even though the older parent cannot be left alone. Adult day care centers provide meals, supervision, and activities for older persons. Activities include cards, board games, movies, crafts, dancing, walks, and lectures. Some provide bowling and swimming. All activities are supervised. Assistance is given as needed. Some provide transportation from home to the center.

Living with an adult child is a social change. The parent, adult child, and the child's family all need to adjust. The adult child's family still needs time alone. Other brothers, sisters, and family members may help give care. Respite care provides a break for the family. The older person enters a nursing center for a few days or weeks. This gives caregivers a vacation, rest, or simply a break from the stress of giving care. Community and church groups often have volunteers who can help give care.

from the nursing team. However, do not discuss the person's condition with them. Refer their questions to the nurse.

Visitors often have questions about visiting rules. The number of visitors allowed and the visiting hours vary among agencies. Often they depend on the person's age or condition. A child's parents usually can visit as often and as long as they want. Only short visits are allowed in special care units. Dying persons usually can have family members present constantly. Know your agency's visiting policies and the special needs of each person. Visitors may also have questions about where to find the chapel, gift shop, business office, lounge, or dining room. You must know the location, special rules, and hours of these facilities.

Sometimes a visitor can upset or tire a person. Report your observations to the nurse. The nurse will speak with the visitor about the person's needs.

(See Focus on Older Persons box and Focus on Home Care box.)

THE ANGRY PERSON

Anger is a common emotion seen in patients, residents, and families. The many causes of anger include fear, pain, and death and dying. Loss of body function and losing control of one's health and life also cause anger. So do long waits for treatment or to see the doctor.

Anger also is a symptom of diseases that affect thinking and behavior. Persons who abuse alcohol and drugs are likely to show anger. Also, some people are generally angry. Few things please or make them happy.

Anger is communicated verbally and nonverbally. Verbal outbursts, shouting, raised voices, and rapid speech are common. The person tells you what to do or threatens you or the agency. Some people are silent when angry. Others are uncooperative and may refuse to answer questions. Nonverbal signs of anger include rapid movements, pacing, clenched fists, and a reddened face. Glaring and getting close to you when speaking are other signs. Violent behaviors can occur.

Good communication is important to prevent and deal with anger. Follow the guidelines in Box 5-2.

Box 5-2 Dealing With the Angry Person

- Recognize frustrating and frightening situations. Put yourself in the person's situation. How would you feel? How would you want to be treated?
- Treat the person with dignity and respect.
- Answer the person's questions clearly and thoroughly. Ask the nurse to answer questions you cannot answer.
- Keep the person informed. Tell the person what you are going to do and when.
- Do not keep the person waiting for long periods. Answer signal lights promptly. If you tell the person that you will do something for him or her, do it promptly.
- Explain the reason for long waits. Ask if there is something you can get or do for the person to increase his or her comfort.
- Stay calm and professional if the person directs anger and hostility toward you. Often the person is not angry at you, but at another person or situation.
- Do not argue with the person.
- Listen and use silence. The person may feel better if able to express angry feelings.
- Protect yourself from violent behaviors (see Chapter 9).
- Report the person's behavior to the nurse. Discuss how you should deal with the person.

Circle the BEST answer.

1. Sally Jones had surgery to remove her gallbladder. You must be concerned
   A. Only with what is on her nursing care plan
   B. With her physical, safety and security, and esteem needs
   C. With her as a physical, psychological, social, and spiritual person
   D. Only with her cultural and religious needs

2. Which basic need is the most essential?
   A. Self-actualization
   B. Self-esteem
   C. Love and belonging
   D. Safety and security

3. Based on Maslow's theory of basic needs, which person's needs must be met first?
   A. Mr. Hart, who wants another blanket
   B. Miss Parks, who asks you to read her mail to her
   C. Ms. Street, who asks for more water
   D. Mr. Hill, who is crying

4. Sally Jones says, "I don't know what they are going to do to me." What basic need is not being met?
   A. Physical needs
   B. The need for safety and security
   C. The need for love and belonging
   D. Self-esteem needs

5. Mr. Hart is a nursing center resident. He wants a little vegetable garden out behind the center's garage. What need does this relate to?
   A. Self-actualization
   B. Self-esteem needs
   C. Love and belonging
   D. Safety and security

6. Which is *false?*
   A. A person's culture influences health and illness practices.
   B. Culture and religion influence food practices.
   C. A person's religious and cultural practices are not allowed in the health care agency.
   D. A person may not follow all of the beliefs and practices of his or her religion or culture.

7. Which is *true?*
   A. An obstetrical patient is one who is pregnant, in labor, or giving birth or who has given birth during the previous 6 to 8 weeks.
   B. Pediatrics is concerned only with sick children.
   C. Geriatric persons suffer from a disease commonly known as aging.
   D. All of the above

8. As a patient, Sally Jones has the right to
   A. Considerate and respectful care *
   B. Information about her diagnosis, treatment, and prognosis
   C. Refuse treatment
   D. All of the above

9. The right to privacy is protected after death.
   A. True
   B. False

10. Which is *false?*
    A. Verbal communication involves the written or spoken word.
    B. Verbal communication is the truest reflection of a person's feelings.
    C. Messages can be sent by facial expressions, gestures, posture, body movements, appearance, and eye contact.
    D. Touch means different things to different people.

11. To communicate with Sam Long you should
    A. Use medical words and phrases
    B. Change the subject often to show you care about his interests and concerns
    C. Give your opinion when he is sharing fears and concerns
    D. Be quiet when he is silent

12. You and Sam Long are talking. You do the following. Which might mean that you are not listening?
    A. You sit facing him.
    B. You have good eye contact with him.
    C. You sit with your arms crossed.
    D. You ask him questions.

13. You and Sally Jones are talking about her surgery. Which is a direct question?
    A. "Do you feel better now?"
    B. "Tell me what your plans are for home."
    C. "What will you do when you get home?"
    D. "You said that you will be off work for awhile."

14. Sally Jones wants to take a shower. You say, "You would like a shower." This is
    A. Focusing
    B. Clarifying
    C. Paraphrasing
    D. An open-ended question

15. Focusing is a useful communication tool when
    A. A person is rambling
    B. You want to make sure you understand the message
    C. You want the person to share thoughts and feelings
    D. You need certain information

16. Which will promote communication?
    A. "Don't worry."
    B. "Everything will be just fine."
    C. "This is a good hospital."
    D. "Why are you crying?"

17. A person is angry. Which is *true?*
    A. The person probably has a disease that affects thinking and behavior.
    B. Drug or alcohol abuse is likely.
    C. You can tell the person to calm down and that everything will be fine.
    D. Listening and the use of silence are important.

18. Sally Jones has many visitors. Which is *false?*
    A. Family and friends can help meet her basic needs.
    B. Privacy should be allowed.
    C. Visitors should be politely asked to leave the room when care must be given.
    D. Questions about gift shop and lounge hours are directed to the nurse.

Answers to these questions on are on p. 833.

CHAPTER 6

BODY STRUCTURE AND FUNCTION

Define the key terms listed in this chapter

Identify the basic structures of the cell, and explain how cells divide

Describe four types of tissue

Identify the structures of each body system

Describe the functions of each body system

KEY TERMS

artery A blood vessel that carries blood away from the heart

capillary A tiny blood vessel; food, oxygen, and other substances pass from the capillaries to the cells

cell The basic unit of body structure

digestion The process of physically and chemically breaking down food so that it can be absorbed for use by the cells

hemoglobin The substance in red blood cells that carries oxygen and gives blood its color

hormone A chemical substance secreted by the glands into the bloodstream

immunity Protection against a disease or condition; the person will not get or be affected by the disease

menstruation The process in which the lining of the uterus breaks up and is discharged from the body through the vagina

metabolism The burning of food for heat and energy by the cells

organ Groups of tissues with the same function

peristalsis Involuntary muscle contractions in the digestive system that move food through the alimentary canal

respiration The process of supplying the cells with oxygen and removing carbon dioxide from them

system Organs that work together to perform special functions

tissue A group of cells with similar function

vein A blood vessel that carries blood back to the heart

NOTE: Students are responsible for only those terms mentioned in the text. Additional terms used in labeling figures throughout this chapter are for illustrative purposes only.

You will help patients and residents meet their basic needs. Their bodies do not work at peak efficiency because of illness, disease, or injury. You will provide care and perform procedures to promote comfort, healing, and recovery. A basic knowledge of the body's normal structure and function will help you understand certain signs and symptoms, reasons for care, and purposes of procedures. This knowledge should result in safer and more efficient patient and resident care.

CELLS, TISSUES, AND ORGANS

The basic unit of body structure is the **cell.** Each cell has the same basic structure. However, the function, size, and shape of cells may be different. Cells are so small that a microscope is needed to see them. Cells need food, water, and oxygen to live and perform their functions.

The cell and its basic structures are shown in Figure 6-1, p. 108. The *cell membrane* is the outer covering that encloses the cell and helps it hold its shape. The *nucleus* is the control center of the cell; it directs the cell's activities. The nucleus is in the center of the cell. The *cytoplasm* is the portion of the cell that surrounds the

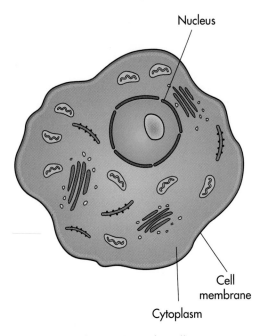

Fig. 6-1 Parts of a cell.

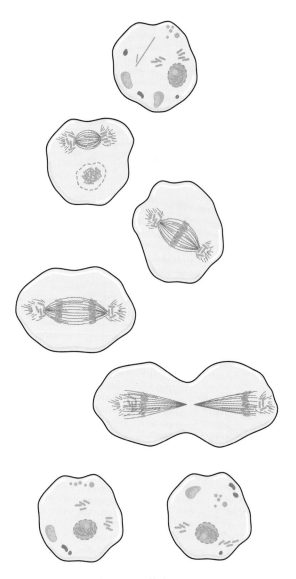

Fig. 6-2 Cell division.

nucleus. Cytoplasm contains many smaller structures that perform cell functions. The *protoplasm,* which means "living substance," refers to all of the structures, substances, and water within the cell. Protoplasm is a semiliquid substance much like an egg white.

Chromosomes are threadlike structures within the nucleus. Each cell has 46 chromosomes. Chromosomes contain *genes.* Genes control the physical and chemical traits inherited by children from their parents. Inherited traits include height, eye color, and skin color.

Besides controlling cell activities, the nucleus is responsible for cell reproduction. Cells reproduce by dividing in half. The process of cell division is called *mitosis.* Cell division is needed for growth and repair of body tissues. During mitosis, the 46 chromosomes arrange themselves in 23 pairs. As the cell divides, the 23 pairs of chromosomes are pulled in half. The two new cells are identical, and each contains 46 chromosomes (Fig. 6-2).

The cells are the body's building blocks. Groups of cells with similar functions combine to form **tissues.** The body has four basic types of tissue:

- *Epithelial tissue* covers internal and external body surfaces. Tissue that lines the nose, mouth, respiratory tract, stomach, and intestines is epithelial tissue. So are the skin, hair, nails, and glands.

- *Connective tissue* anchors, connects, and supports other body tissues. Connective tissue is found in every part of the body. Bones, tendons, ligaments, and cartilage are connective tissue. Blood is a form of connective tissue.
- *Muscle tissue* allows the body to move by stretching and contracting. There are three types of muscle tissue, p. 111.
- *Nerve tissue* receives and carries impulses to the brain and back to body parts.

Groups of tissues form **organs.** An organ performs one or more functions. Examples of organs are the heart, brain, liver, lungs, and kidneys. **Systems** are formed by organs that work together to perform special functions (Fig. 6-3).

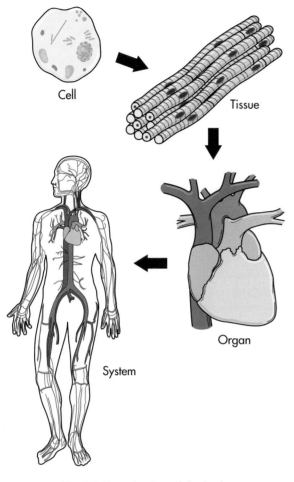

Fig. 6-3 Organization of the body.

THE INTEGUMENTARY SYSTEM

The *integumentary system,* or skin, is the largest system of the body. *Integument* means covering. The skin is the body's natural covering. Skin is made up of epithelial, connective, and nerve tissue, as well as oil and sweat glands. There are two skin layers: the epidermis and the dermis (Fig. 6-4). The *epidermis* is the outer layer; it contains living and dead cells. The dead cells were once deeper in the epidermis and were pushed upward as other cells divided. Dead cells constantly flake off and are replaced by living cells. Living cells also die and flake off. Living cells of the epidermis contain *pigment.* Pigment gives skin its color. The epidermis has no blood vessels and few nerve endings. The *dermis* is the inner layer of the skin and is made up of connective tissue. Blood vessels, nerves, sweat and oil glands, and hair roots are found in the dermis.

Oil and *sweat glands, hair,* and *nails* are skin appendages. The entire body, except the palms of the hands and soles of the feet, is covered with hair. Hair in the nose, eyes, and ears protects these organs from dust, insects, and other foreign objects. Nails protect the tips of fingers and toes. Nails help fingers pick up and handle small objects. Sweat glands help the body regulate temperature. Sweat consists of water, salt, and a small amount of wastes. Sweat is secreted through pores in the skin. The body is cooled as sweat evaporates. Oil glands lie near hair shafts. They secrete an oily substance into the space near the hair shaft. Oil travels to the skin surface, helping to keep the hair and skin soft and shiny.

Fig. 6-4 Layers of the skin.

The skin has many important functions. It is the protective covering of the body. Bacteria and other substances are prevented from entering the body. The skin prevents excessive amounts of water from leaving the body and protects organs from injury. Nerve endings in the skin sense both pleasant and unpleasant stimulation. There are nerve endings over the entire body. The body is protected because cold, pain, touch, and pressure are sensed. The skin helps regulate body temperature. Blood vessels dilate (widen) when temperature outside the body is high. More blood is brought to the body surface for cooling during evaporation. When blood vessels constrict (narrow), the body retains heat because less blood reaches the skin.

THE MUSCULOSKELETAL SYSTEM

The musculoskeletal system provides the framework for the body and allows the body to move. This system also protects and gives the body shape. Besides bones and muscles, the system has ligaments, tendons, and cartilage.

BONES

The human body has 206 bones (Fig. 6-5). There are four types of bones:

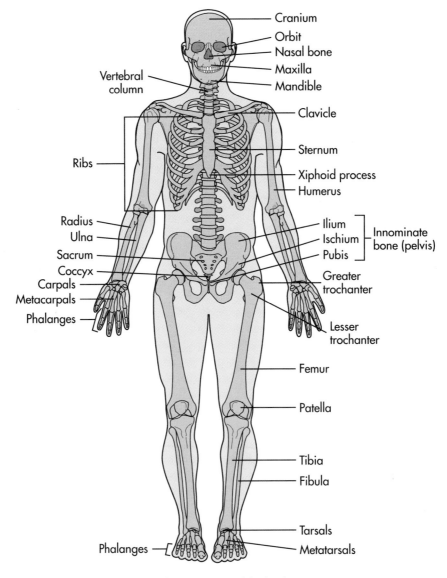

Fig. 6-5 Bones of the body.

- *Long bones* bear the weight of the body. Leg bones are long bones.
- *Short bones* allow skill and ease in movement. Bones in the wrists, fingers, ankles, and toes are short bones.
- *Flat bones* protect the organs. Such bones include the ribs, skull, pelvic bones, and shoulder blades.
- *Irregular bones* are the vertebrae in the spinal column. They allow various degrees of movement and flexibility.

Bones are hard, rigid structures that are made up of living cells. They are covered by a membrane called *periosteum*. Periosteum contains blood vessels that supply bone cells with oxygen and food. Inside the hollow centers of the bones is a substance called *bone marrow*. Blood cells are manufactured in the bone marrow.

JOINTS

A *joint* is the point at which two or more bones meet. Joints allow movement (see Chapter 20). *Cartilage* is the connective tissue at the end of long bones. Cartilage cushions the joint so that bone ends do not rub together. The *synovial membrane* lines the joints. The membrane secretes *synovial fluid*. Synovial fluid acts as a lubricant so the joint can move smoothly. Bones are held together at the joint by strong bands of connective tissue called *ligaments*.

There are three types of joints (Fig. 6-6):

- *Ball-and-socket joint* allows movement in all directions. It is made up of the rounded end of one bone and the hollow end of another bone. The rounded end of one fits into the hollow end of the other. The joints of the hips and shoulders are ball-and-socket joints.
- *Hinge joint* allows movement in one direction. The elbow is a hinge joint.
- *Pivot joint* allows turning from side to side. The skull is connected to the spine by a pivot joint.

MUSCLES

There are more than 500 muscles in the human body (Figs. 6-7 and 6-8, pp. 112-113). Some are voluntary, and others are involuntary. *Voluntary* muscles can be consciously controlled. Muscles attached to bones *(skeletal muscles)* are voluntary. Arm muscles do not work unless you move your arm; likewise for leg muscles. Skeletal muscles are *striated;* that is, they look striped or streaked. *Involuntary muscles* work automatically and cannot be consciously controlled. Involuntary muscles control the action of the stomach, intestines, blood vessels, and other body organs. In-

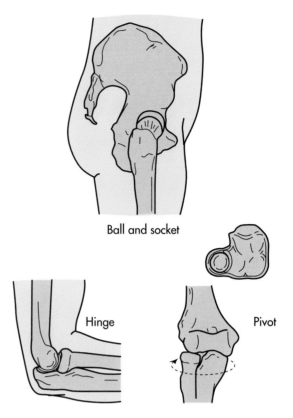

Fig. 6-6 Types of joints.

Ball and socket

Hinge

Pivot

voluntary muscles are also called *smooth muscles.* They look smooth—not streaked or striped. *Cardiac muscle* is in the heart. Although it is an involuntary muscle, it appears striated like skeletal muscle.

Muscles perform three important body functions:

- Movement of body parts
- Maintenance of posture
- Production of body heat

Strong, tough connective tissues called *tendons* connect muscles to bones. When muscles contract (shorten), tendons at each end of the muscle cause the bone to move. The body has many tendons; the Achilles tendon is shown in Figure 6-8. Some muscles constantly contract to maintain the body's posture. When muscles contract, they burn food for energy, resulting in the production of heat. The greater the muscular activity, the greater the amount of heat produced in the body. Shivering is a way the body produces heat when exposed to cold. The shivering sensation is from rapid, general muscle contractions.

Text continued on p. 114

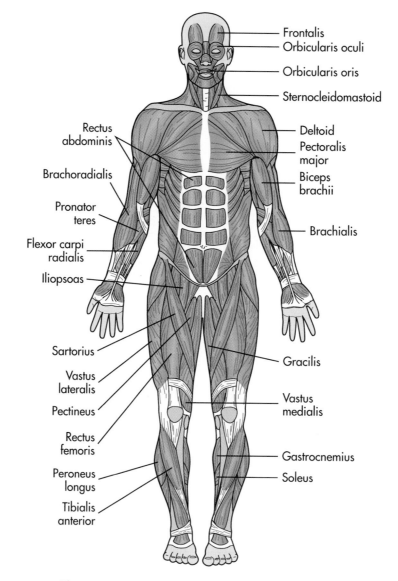

Fig. 6-7 Anterior (front) view of the muscles of the body.

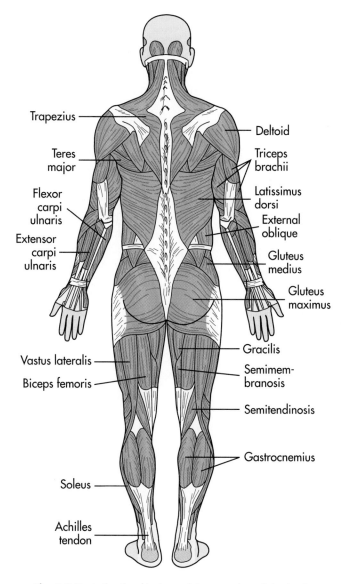

Trapezius

Deltoid

Teres
major

Triceps
brachii

Flexor
carpi
ulnaris

Latissimus
dorsi

External
oblique

Extensor
carpi
ulnaris

Gluteus
medius

Gluteus
maximus

Gracilis

Vastus lateralis

Semimem-
branosis

Biceps femoris

Semitendinosis

Gastrocnemius

Soleus

Achilles
tendon

Fig. 6-8 Posterior (back) view of the muscles of the body.

THE NERVOUS SYSTEM

The nervous system controls, directs, and coordinates body functions. The two main divisions of the nervous system are the *central nervous system* (CNS) and the *peripheral nervous system*. The central nervous system consists of the *brain* and *spinal cord* (Fig. 6-9). The peripheral nervous system involves the *nerves* throughout the body (Fig. 6-10). Nerves carry messages or impulses to and from the brain. Nerves are connected to the spinal cord.

Nerves are easily damaged and take a long time to heal. Some nerve fibers have a protective covering called a *myelin sheath*. The myelin sheath also insulates the nerve fiber. Nerve fibers covered with myelin can conduct impulses faster than those fibers without the protective covering.

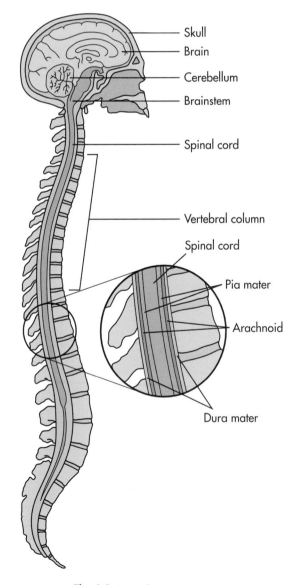

Fig. 6-9 Central nervous system.

Skull
Brain
Cerebellum
Brainstem
Spinal cord
Vertebral column
Spinal cord
Pia mater
Arachnoid
Dura mater

THE CENTRAL NERVOUS SYSTEM

The central nervous system consists of the brain and spinal cord. The brain is covered by the skull. The three main parts of the brain are the *cerebrum*, the *cerebellum*, and the *brain stem* (Fig. 6-11).

The cerebrum is the largest part of the brain. It is the center of thought and intelligence. The cerebrum is divided into two halves called the right and left *hemispheres*. The right hemisphere controls movement and activities on the body's left side. The left hemisphere controls the right side. The outside of the cerebrum is called the *cerebral cortex*. The cerebral cortex controls the highest functions of the brain. These include reasoning, memory, consciousness, speech, voluntary muscle movement, vision, hearing, sensation, and other activities.

The cerebellum regulates and coordinates body movements. The smooth movements of voluntary muscles and balance are possible because of control by the cerebellum. Injury to the cerebellum results in jerky movements, loss of coordination, and muscle weakness.

The brain stem connects the cerebrum to the spinal cord. Important structures within the brain stem are the *midbrain, pons,* and *medulla*. The midbrain and pons relay messages between the medulla and the cerebrum. The medulla is directly below the pons. Heart rate, breathing, blood vessel size, swallowing, coughing, and vomiting are some functions controlled by the medulla. The brain is connected to the spinal cord at the lower end of the medulla.

The spinal cord lies within the spinal column. The cord is about 18 inches long. Pathways that conduct messages to and from the brain are contained within the cord.

The brain and spinal cord are covered and protected by three layers of connective tissue called *meninges*. The outer layer lies next to the skull. It is a tough covering called the *dura mater*. The middle layer is called the *arachnoid*. The inner layer is the *pia mater*. The space between the middle and inner layers is the *arachnoid space*. The space is filled with fluid called *cerebrospinal fluid*. It circulates around the brain and spinal cord. Cerebrospinal fluid protects the central nervous system. It cushions shocks that could easily injure structures of the brain and spinal cord.

THE PERIPHERAL NERVOUS SYSTEM

The peripheral nervous system has 12 pairs of *cranial nerves* and 31 pairs of *spinal nerves*. Cranial nerves conduct impulses between the brain and the head, neck, chest, and abdomen. They conduct impulses for smell, vision, hearing, pain, touch, temperature, pressure, and voluntary and involuntary muscle control. Spinal nerves carry impulses from the skin, extremities, and the internal body structures not supplied by cranial nerves.

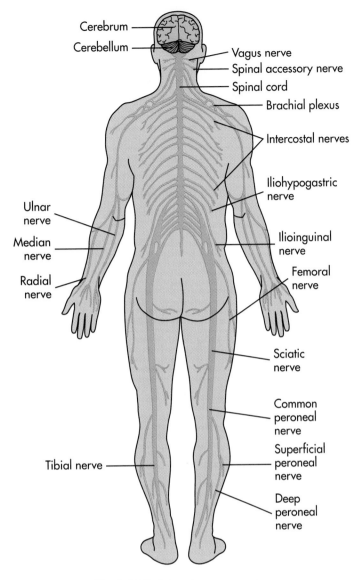

Cerebrum

Cerebellum

Vagus nerve

Spinal accessory nerve

Spinal cord

Brachial plexus

Intercostal nerves

Iliohypogastric nerve

Ilioinguinal nerve

Femoral nerve

Ulnar nerve

Median nerve

Radial nerve

Sciatic nerve

Common peroneal nerve

Superficial peroneal nerve

Tibial nerve

Deep peroneal nerve

Fig. 6-10 Peripheral nervous system.

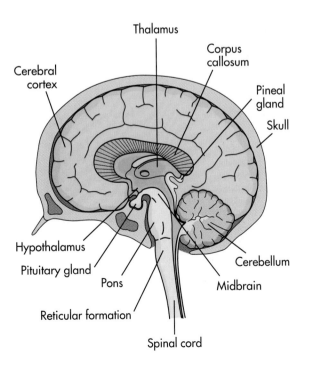

Thalamus

Corpus callosum

Cerebral cortex

Pineal gland

Skull

Fig. 6-11 The brain.

Hypothalamus

Pituitary gland

Pons

Reticular formation

Cerebellum

Midbrain

Spinal cord

Some peripheral nerves with special functions form the *autonomic nervous system.* This system controls involuntary muscles and certain body functions. The functions include the heartbeat, blood pressure, intestinal contractions, and glandular secretions. These functions occur automatically. The autonomic nervous system is divided into the *sympathetic nervous system* and the *parasympathetic nervous system.* These divisions balance one another. The sympathetic nervous system tends to speed up functions. The parasympathetic nervous system slows them down. When you are angry, frightened, excited, or exercising, the sympathetic nervous system is stimulated. The parasympathetic system is activated when you relax or when the sympathetic system is under stimulation for too long.

THE SENSE ORGANS

The five major senses are sight, hearing, taste, smell, and touch. Receptors for taste are in the tongue and are called *taste buds.* Receptors for smell are in the nose. Touch receptors are found in the dermis, especially in the toes and fingertips.

The Eye. Receptors for vision are in the eyes. The eye is a delicate organ that can be easily injured. Bones of the skull, eyelids and eyelashes, and tears protect the eyes from injury. Eye structures are shown in Figure 6-12. The eye has three layers:

- The *sclera,* the white of the eye, is the outer layer. It is made of tough connective tissue.
- The *choroid* is the second layer. Blood vessels, the *ciliary muscle,* and the *iris* make up the choroid. The iris gives the eye its color. The opening in the middle of the iris is the *pupil.* Pupil size varies with the amount of light entering the eye. The pupil constricts (narrows) in bright light and dilates (widens) in dim or dark places.
- The *retina* is the inner layer of the eye. Receptors for vision and the nerve fibers of the optic nerve are contained in the retina.

Light enters the eye through the *cornea.* The cornea is the transparent part of the outer layer that lies over the eye. Light rays pass to the *lens,* which lies behind the pupil. The light is then reflected to the retina and carried to the brain by the optic nerve.

The *aqueous chamber* separates the cornea from the lens. The chamber is filled with a fluid called *aqueous humor.* The fluid helps the cornea keep its shape and position. The *vitreous body* is behind the lens. The vitreous body is a gelatin-like substance that supports the retina and maintains the eye's shape.

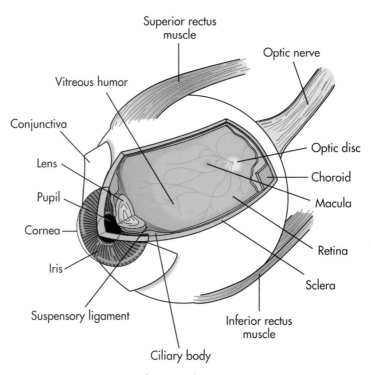

Fig. 6-12 The eye.

The Ear. The ear is a sense organ that functions in hearing and balance. It is divided into the *external ear, middle ear,* and *inner ear.* Ear structures are shown in Figure 6-13.

The external ear (outer part) is called the *pinna* or *auricle.* Sound waves are guided through the external ear into the *auditory canal.* Glands in the auditory canal secrete a waxy substance called *cerumen.* The auditory canal extends about 1 inch to the *eardrum.* The eardrum *(tympanic membrane)* separates the external ear and middle ear.

The middle ear is a small space that contains the *eustachian tube* and three small bones called *ossicles.* The eustachian tube connects the middle ear and the throat. Air enters the eustachian tube so that there is equal pressure on both sides of the eardrum. The ossicles amplify sound received from the eardrum and transmit the sound to the inner ear. The three ossicles are:

- The *malleus,* which looks like a hammer
- The *incus,* which resembles an anvil
- The *stapes,* which is shaped like a stirrup

The inner ear consists of the *semicircular canals* and the *cochlea.* The cochlea, which looks like a snail shell, contains fluid. The fluid carries sound waves received from the middle ear to the *auditory nerve.* The auditory nerve then carries the message to the brain.

The three semicircular canals are involved with balance. They sense the head's position and changes in position and send messages to the brain.

THE CIRCULATORY SYSTEM

The circulatory system is made up of the blood, heart, and blood vessels. The heart pumps blood through the blood vessels. The circulatory system has many important functions. Blood carries food, oxygen, and other substances to the cells. Blood also removes waste products from cells. Regulation of body temperature is aided by the blood and blood vessels. Heat from muscle activity is carried by the blood to other body parts. Blood vessels in the skin dilate if the body needs to be cooled. They constrict if heat should be kept in the body. The circulatory system also produces and carries cells that defend the body from disease-causing microorganisms.

THE BLOOD

The blood consists of blood cells and a liquid called *plasma.* Plasma is mostly water. It carries blood cells to other body cells. Plasma also carries other substances needed by cells for proper functioning. Food (proteins, fats, and carbohydrates), hormones, chemicals, and waste products are among the many substances carried in the plasma.

Red blood cells are called *erythrocytes.* They give the blood its red color because of a substance in the cell called **hemoglobin.** As red blood cells circulate through the lungs, hemoglobin picks up oxygen. The hemoglobin carries oxygen to the cells. When the blood is bright red, hemoglobin in the red blood cells is saturated (filled) with oxygen. As blood circulates through the

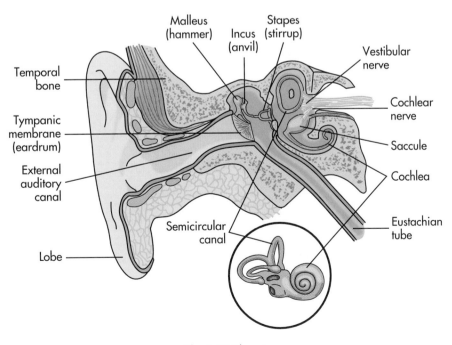

Fig. 6-13 The ear.

body, oxygen is given to the cells. The cells release carbon dioxide (a waste product), which is picked up by the hemoglobin. Red blood cells saturated with carbon dioxide make the blood look dark red.

There are about 25 trillion (25,000,000,000,000) red blood cells in the body. About $4\frac{1}{2}$ to 5 million cells are in a cubic millimeter of blood (the size of a tiny drop). These cells live for 3 or 4 months. They are destroyed by the liver and spleen as they wear out. Bone marrow produces new red blood cells. About 1 million new red blood cells are produced every second.

White blood cells, called *leukocytes*, are colorless. They protect the body against infection. There are 5,000 to 10,000 white blood cells in a cubic millimeter of blood. At the first sign of infection, white blood cells rush to the site of the infection and begin to multiply rapidly. The number of white blood cells increases when there is an infection in the body. White blood cells are also produced by the bone marrow. They live about 9 days.

Platelets (thrombocytes) are necessary for the clotting of blood. They are also produced by the bone marrow. There are about 200,000 to 400,000 platelets in a cubic millimeter of blood. A platelet lives about 4 days.

THE HEART

The heart is a muscle. It pumps blood through the blood vessels to the tissues and cells. The heart lies in the middle to lower part of the chest cavity toward the left side (Fig. 6-14). The heart is hollow and has three layers (Fig. 6-15):

- The *pericardium* is the outer layer. It is a thin sac covering the heart.
- The *myocardium* is the second layer. This layer is the thick, muscular portion of the heart.
- The *endocardium* is the inner layer. The endocardium is the membrane lining the inner surface of the heart.

The heart has four chambers (see Fig. 6-15). Upper chambers receive blood and are called the *atria*. The *right atrium* receives blood from body tissues. The *left atrium* receives blood from the lungs. Lower chambers are called *ventricles*. Ventricles pump blood. The *right ventricle* pumps blood to the lungs for oxygen. The *left ventricle* pumps blood to all parts of the body.

Valves are located between the atria and ventricles. The valves allow blood to flow in one direction. They prevent blood from flowing back into the atria from the ventricles. The *tricuspid valve* is between the right atrium and right ventricle. The *mitral valve (bicuspid valve)* is between the left atrium and left ventricle.

There are two phases of heart action. During *diastole*, the resting phase, heart chambers fill with blood. During *systole*, the working phase, the heart contracts. Blood is pumped through the blood vessels when the heart contracts.

Fig. 6-14 Location of the heart in the chest cavity.

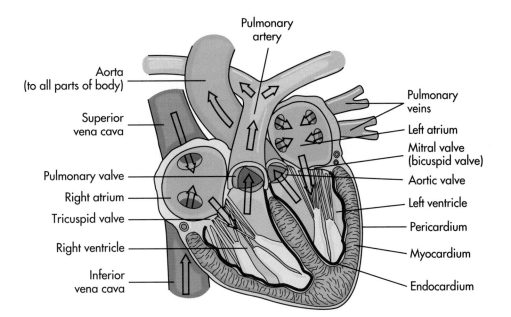

Fig. 6-15 Structures of the heart.

THE BLOOD VESSELS

Blood flows to body tissues and cells through the blood vessels. There are three groups of blood vessels: arteries, capillaries, and veins. **Arteries** carry blood away from the heart. Arterial blood is rich in oxygen. The *aorta* is the largest artery. The aorta receives blood directly from the left ventricle. The aorta branches into other arteries that carry blood to all parts of the body (Fig. 6-16). These arteries branch into smaller parts within the tissues. The smallest branch of an artery is an *arteriole.* Arterioles connect with blood vessels called **capillaries.** Capillaries are very tiny vessels. Food, oxygen, and other substances pass from capillaries into the cells. Waste products, including carbon dioxide, are picked up from cells by the capillaries. Waste products are carried back to the heart by the veins.

Veins return blood to the heart. They are connected to the capillaries by *venules.* Venules are small veins. Venules begin branching together to form veins. The many branches of veins also branch together as they near the heart to form two main veins (see Fig. 6-16). The two main veins are the *inferior vena cava* and the *superior vena cava.* Both empty into the right atrium. The inferior vena cava carries blood from the legs and trunk. The superior vena cava carries blood from the head and arms. Venous blood is dark red because it contains little oxygen and a lot of carbon dioxide.

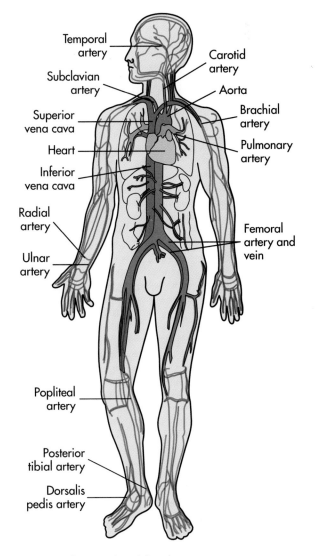

Fig. 6-16 Arterial and venous systems.

Blood flow through the circulatory system is diagrammed in Figure 6-15 and can be summarized as follows. Venous blood, poor in oxygen, empties into the right atrium. Blood flows through the tricuspid valve into the right ventricle. The right ventricle pumps blood into the lungs to pick up oxygen. Oxygen-rich blood from the lungs enters the left atrium. Blood from the left atrium passes through the mitral valve into the left ventricle. The left ventricle pumps the blood to the aorta, which branches off to form other arteries. The arterial blood is carried to the tissues by arterioles and to the cells by capillaries. The cells and capillaries exchange oxygen and nutrients for carbon dioxide and waste products. Capillaries connect with venules. Venules carry blood that contains carbon dioxide and waste products. The venules form veins. Veins return blood to the heart.

THE RESPIRATORY SYSTEM

Oxygen is needed for survival. Every cell needs oxygen. Air contains about 20% oxygen—enough to meet body needs under normal conditions. The respiratory system brings oxygen into the lungs and eliminates carbon dioxide. The process of supplying the cells with oxygen and removing carbon dioxide from them is called **respiration.** Respiration involves *inhalation* (breathing in) and *exhalation* (breathing out). The terms *inspiration* (breathing in) and *expiration* (breathing out) are also used. The respiratory system is shown in Figure 6-17.

Air enters the body through the *nose.* The air then passes into the *pharynx* (throat), a tube-shaped passageway for both air and food. Air passes from the pharynx into the *larynx* (the voice box). A piece of cartilage called the *epiglottis* acts like a lid over the larynx. The epiglottis prevents food from entering the airway during swallowing. During inhalation the epiglottis

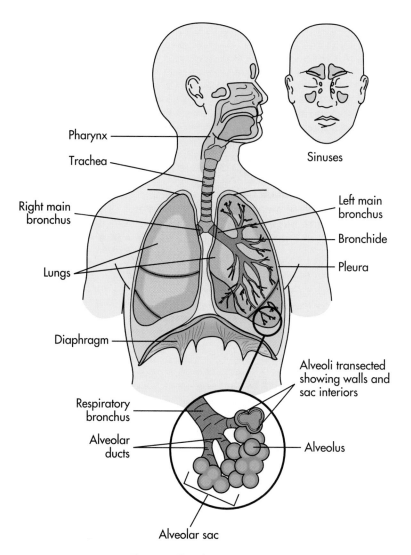

Fig. 6-17 Respiratory system.

lifts up to let air pass over the larynx. Air passes from the larynx into the *trachea* (the windpipe). The trachea divides at its lower end into the *right bronchus* and *left bronchus.* Each bronchus enters a lung. Upon entering the lungs, the bronchi further divide several times into smaller branches called *bronchioles.* Eventually the bronchioles subdivide and end in tiny one-celled air sacs called *alveoli.* Alveoli look like small clusters of grapes. They are supplied by capillaries. Oxygen and carbon dioxide are exchanged between the alveoli and capillaries. Blood in the capillaries picks up oxygen from the alveoli. Then the blood is returned to the left side of the heart and pumped to the rest of the body. Alveoli pick up carbon dioxide from the capillaries for exhalation.

The lungs are spongy tissues filled with alveoli, blood vessels, and nerves. Each lung is divided into lobes. The right lung has three lobes; the left lung has two. The lungs are separated from the abdominal cavity by a muscle called the *diaphragm.* Each lung is covered by a two-layered sac called the *pleura.* One layer is attached to the lung and the other to the chest wall.

The pleura secretes a very thin fluid that fills the space between the layers. The fluid prevents the layers from rubbing together during inhalation and exhalation. A bony framework consisting of the ribs, sternum, and vertebrae protects the lungs.

THE DIGESTIVE SYSTEM

The digestive system breaks down food physically and chemically so it can be absorbed for use by the cells. This process is called **digestion**. The digestive system is also called the *gastrointestinal system (GI system).* The system also eliminates solid wastes from the body. The digestive system consists of the *alimentary canal (GI tract)* and the accessory organs of digestion (Fig. 6-18). The alimentary canal is a long tube extending from the mouth to the anus. Its major parts are the mouth, pharynx, esophagus, stomach, small intestine, and large intestine. The accessory organs of digestion are the teeth, tongue, salivary glands, liver, gallbladder, and pancreas.

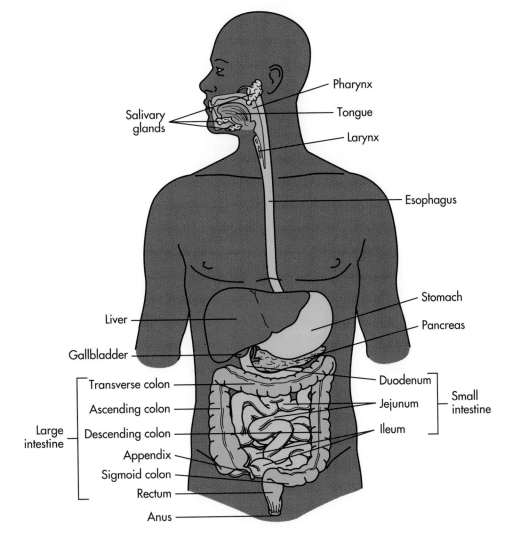

Fig. 6-18 Digestive system.

Digestion begins in the *mouth.* The mouth is also called the *oral cavity.* The oral cavity receives food and prepares it for digestion. Using chewing motions, the *teeth* cut, chop, and grind food into smaller particles for digestion and swallowing. The *tongue* aids in chewing and swallowing. *Taste buds* on the tongue's surface contain nerve endings. Taste buds allow sweet, sour, bitter, and salty tastes to be sensed. *Salivary glands* in the mouth secrete *saliva.* Saliva moistens food particles for easier swallowing and begins to digest food. During swallowing, the tongue pushes food into the pharynx.

The *pharynx* (throat) is a muscular tube. The act of swallowing is continued as the pharynx contracts. Contraction of the pharynx pushes food into the *esophagus.* The esophagus is a muscular tube about 10 inches long. It extends from the pharynx to the stomach. Involuntary muscle contractions called **peristalsis** move food down the esophagus into the stomach.

The *stomach* is a muscular, pouchlike sac in the upper left portion of the abdominal cavity. Strong stomach muscles stir and churn food to break it up into even smaller particles. The stomach is lined with a mucous membrane containing glands that secrete *gastric juices.* Food is mixed and churned with the gastric juices to form a semiliquid substance called *chyme.* Through peristalsis, the chyme is pushed from the stomach into the small intestine.

The *small intestine* is about 20 feet long and has three parts. The first part is the *duodenum.* In the duodenum, more digestive juices are added to the chyme. One is called *bile.* Bile is a greenish liquid produced by the *liver* and stored in the *gallbladder.* Juices from the *pancreas* and small intestine are also added to the chyme. The digestive juices chemically break down food so that it can be absorbed.

Peristalsis moves the chyme through the two remaining portions of the small intestine: the *jejunum* and the *ileum.* Tiny projections called *villi* line the small intestine. Villi absorb the digested food into the capillaries. Most of the absorption of food takes place in the jejunum and ileum.

Some chyme remains undigested. The undigested chyme passes from the small intestine into the *large intestine (large bowel* or *colon).* The colon absorbs most of the water from the chyme. The remaining semisolid material is called *feces.* Feces consist of a small amount of water, solid wastes, and some mucus and germs. These are the waste products of digestion. Feces pass through the colon into the *rectum* by peristalsis. Feces pass out of the body through the *anus.*

THE URINARY SYSTEM

Wastes are removed from the body through the respiratory system, the digestive system, and the skin. The digestive system rids the body of solid wastes. The lungs rid the body of carbon dioxide. Water and other substances are contained in sweat. There are other waste products in the blood as a result of body cells burning food for energy. The functions of the urinary system are to remove waste products from the blood and to maintain water balance within the body. The structures of the urinary system are shown in Figure 6-19.

The *kidneys* are two bean-shaped organs in the upper abdomen. They lie against the muscles of the back on each side of the spine. They are protected by the lower edge of the rib cage.

Each kidney has over a million tiny *nephrons* (Fig. 6-20). The nephron is the basic working unit of the kidney. Each nephron has a *convoluted tubule,* which is a tiny, coiled tubule. Each convoluted tubule has a *Bowman's capsule* at one end. The capsule partially surrounds a cluster of capillaries called a *glomerulus.* Blood passes through the glomerulus and is filtered by the capillaries. The fluid portion of the blood is squeezed into the Bowman's capsule. The fluid then passes into the tubule. Most of the water and other necessary substances are reabsorbed by the blood and recirculated in the body. The rest of the fluid and the waste products form *urine* in the tubule. Urine flows through the tubule to a *collecting tubule.* All of the collecting tubules within the millions of nephrons drain into the *renal pelvis* within the kidney.

A tube, called the *ureter,* is attached to the renal pelvis of the kidney. Each ureter is about 10 to 12 inches long. The ureters carry urine from the kidneys to the *bladder.* The bladder is a hollow, muscular sac situated toward the front in the lower part of the abdominal cavity. Urine is stored in the bladder until the desire to urinate is felt. The need to urinate usually occurs when there is about half a pint (250 ml) of urine in the bladder. Urine passes from the bladder through the *urethra.* The opening at the end of the urethra is the *meatus.* Urine passes from the body through the meatus. Urine is a clear, yellowish fluid.

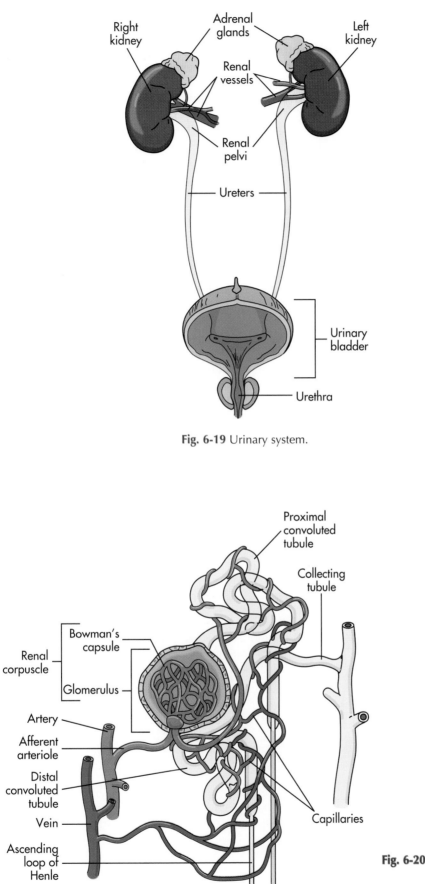

Fig. 6-19 Urinary system.

Fig. 6-20 A nephron.

THE REPRODUCTIVE SYSTEM

Human reproduction results from the union of a female sex cell and a male sex cell. Structures of the male reproductive system and female reproductive system are different. The differences allow for the process of reproduction.

THE MALE REPRODUCTIVE SYSTEM

The structures of the male reproductive system are shown in Figure 6-21. The *testes (testicles)* are the male sex glands. Sex glands are also called *gonads.* The two testes are oval or almond-shaped glands. Male sex cells are produced in the testes. Male sex cells are called *sperm* cells. *Testosterone,* the male hormone, is also produced in the testes. This hormone is needed for the functioning of the reproductive organs and for the development of the male's secondary sex characteristics (Chapter 7). The testes are suspended between the thighs in a sac called the *scrotum.* The scrotum is made of skin and muscle.

Sperm travel from the testis to the *epididymis.* The epididymis is a coiled tube on top and to the side of the testis. From the epididymis, sperm travel through a tube called the *vas deferens.* Eventually each vas deferens joins a *seminal vesicle.* The two seminal vesicles store sperm and produce *semen.* Semen is a fluid that carries sperm from the male reproductive tract. The ducts of the seminal vesicles unite to form the *ejaculatory duct.* The ejaculatory duct passes through the prostate gland.

The *prostate gland,* shaped like a doughnut, lies just below the bladder. The gland secretes fluid into the semen. As the ejaculatory ducts leave the prostate, they join the *urethra,* which also runs through the prostate. The urethra is the outlet for both urine and semen. The urethra is contained within the penis.

The *penis* is outside of the body and has *erectile* tissue. When a man becomes sexually excited, blood fills the erectile tissue. This causes the penis to become enlarged, hard, and erect. The erect penis can enter the vagina of the female reproductive tract. The semen, which contains sperm, is then released into the female vagina.

THE FEMALE REPRODUCTIVE SYSTEM

The structures of the female reproductive system are shown in Figure 6-22. The female gonads are two almond-shaped glands called *ovaries.* There is an ovary on each side of the uterus in the abdominal cavity. The ovaries contain *ova* or eggs. Ova are the female sex cells. One ovum (egg) is released monthly during the woman's reproductive years. Release of an ovum from an ovary is called *ovulation.* The ovaries also secrete the female hormones *estrogen* and *progesterone.* These hormones are needed for the functioning of the reproductive system and the development of secondary sex characteristics in the female (Chapter 7).

When an ovum is released from an ovary, it travels through a *fallopian tube.* There are two fallopian tubes, one on each side. The tubes are attached at one end to

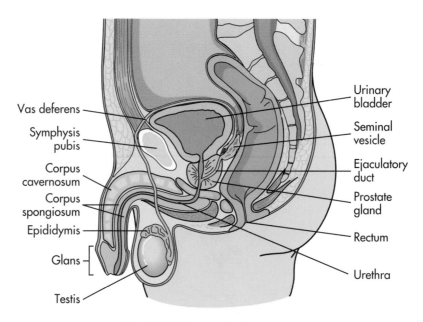

Fig. 6-21 Male reproductive system.

the uterus. The ovum travels through the fallopian tube to the *uterus*. The uterus is a hollow, muscular organ shaped like a pear. The uterus is in the center of the pelvic cavity behind the bladder and in front of the rectum. The main part of the uterus is the *fundus*. The neck or narrow section of the uterus is the *cervix*. Tissue lining the uterus is called the *endometrium*. There are many blood vessels in the endometrium. If sex cells from the male and female unite into one cell, that cell implants into the endometrium, where it grows into a baby. The uterus serves as a place for the unborn baby to grow and receive nourishment.

The cervix of the uterus projects into a muscular canal called the *vagina*. The vagina opens to the outside of the body and is located just behind the urethra. The vagina receives the penis during sexual intercourse and serves as part of the birth canal. Glands in the vaginal wall keep it moistened with secretions. In young girls, the external vaginal opening is partially closed by a membrane called the *hymen*. The hymen ruptures when the female has intercourse for the first time.

The external genitalia of the female are referred to as the *vulva* (Fig. 6-23). The *mons pubis* is a rounded, fatty pad over a bone called the *symphysis pubis.* The mons pubis is covered with hair in the adult female. The *labia majora* and *labia minora* are two folds of tissue on each side of the vaginal opening. The *clitoris* is a small organ composed of erectile tissue. The clitoris becomes hard when sexually stimulated.

The *mammary glands (breasts)* are considered organs of reproduction because they secrete milk after childbirth. The glands are located on the outside of the chest. They are made up of glandular tissue and fat (Fig. 6-24, p. 126). The milk drains into ducts that open onto the nipple.

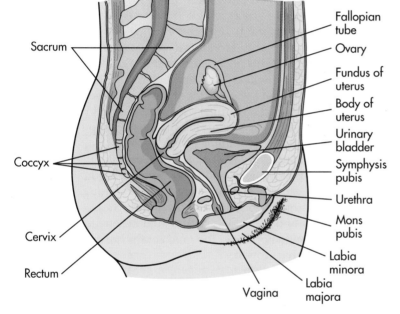

Fig. 6-22 Female reproductive system.

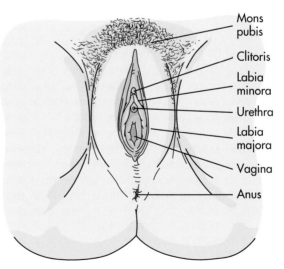

Fig. 6-23 External female genitalia.

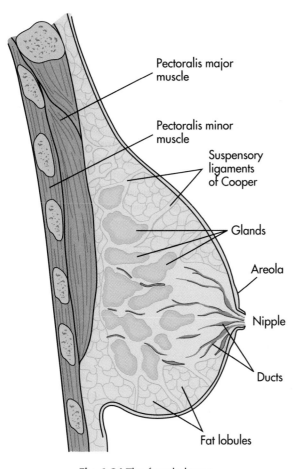

Fig. 6-24 The female breast.

Pectoralis major muscle

Pectoralis minor muscle

Suspensory ligaments of Cooper

Glands

Areola

Nipple

Ducts

Fat lobules

Menstruation. The endometrium is rich in blood to nourish the cell that grows into an unborn baby *(fetus).* If pregnancy does not occur, the endometrium breaks up and is discharged through the vagina to the outside of the body. This process is called **menstruation**. Menstruation occurs about every 28 days. Therefore it is also called the *menstrual cycle.*

The first day of the cycle begins with menstruation. Blood flows from the uterus through the vaginal opening. Menstrual flow usually lasts 3 to 7 days. Ovulation occurs during the next phase of the cycle. An ovum matures in an ovary and is released. Ovulation usually occurs on or about day 14 of the cycle. Meanwhile, estrogen and progesterone (the female hormones) are secreted by the ovaries. These hormones cause the endometrium to thicken for possible pregnancy. If pregnancy does not occur, the hormones decrease in amount. Blood supply to the endometrium decreases because of the decrease in hormones. The endometrium breaks up and is discharged through the vagina. Another menstrual cycle begins.

FERTILIZATION

For reproduction to occur, a male sex cell (sperm) must unite with a female sex cell (ovum). The uniting of the sperm and ovum into one cell is called *fertilization*. A sperm has 23 chromosomes, and an ovum has 23 chromosomes. When the two cells unite, the fertilized cell has 46 chromosomes.

During intercourse, millions of sperm are deposited in the vagina. Sperm travel up the cervix, through the uterus, and into the fallopian tubes. If a sperm and an ovum unite in a fallopian tube, fertilization occurs and results in pregnancy. The fertilized cell travels down the fallopian tube to the uterus. After a short time, the fertilized cell implants in the thick endometrium and grows during pregnancy.

THE ENDOCRINE SYSTEM

The endocrine system is made up of glands called the *endocrine glands* (Fig. 6-25). The endocrine glands secrete chemical substances called **hormones** into the bloodstream. Hormones regulate the activities of other organs and glands in the body.

The *pituitary gland* is called the *master gland.* About the size of a cherry, it is at the base of the brain behind the eyes. The pituitary gland is divided into the anterior pituitary lobe and the posterior pituitary lobe. The *anterior pituitary lobe* secretes important hormones. *Growth hormone* is needed for the growth of muscles, bones, and other organs. Adequate amounts of growth hormone are needed throughout life to maintain normal-size bones and muscles. Growth is stunted if a baby is born with deficient amounts of the growth hormone. Too much of the hormone causes excessive growth.

Thyroid-stimulating hormone (TSH) also is secreted by the anterior pituitary lobe. The thyroid gland requires thyroid-stimulating hormone for proper functioning. *Adrenocorticotropic hormone* (ACTH) is another hormone secreted by the anterior lobe. This hormone stimulates the adrenal gland. The anterior lobe also secretes hormones that regulate the growth, development, and function of the male and female reproductive systems.

The *posterior pituitary lobe* secretes *antidiuretic hormone* (ADH) and *oxytocin.* ADH prevents the kidneys from excreting excessive amounts of water. Oxytocin causes the uterine muscles to contract during childbirth.

The *thyroid gland*, shaped like a butterfly, is in the neck in front of the larynx. *Thyroid hormone* (TH) is secreted by the thyroid gland. Thyroxine is another term for thyroid hormone. Thyroid hormone regulates **metabolism**. Metabolism is the burning of food for heat and energy by the cells. Too little thyroid hormone results in slowed body processes, slowed movements, and weight gain. Too much of the hor-

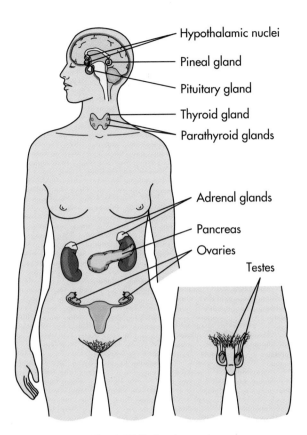

Fig. 6-25 Endocrine system.

mone causes increased metabolism, excess energy, and weight loss. If a baby is born with deficient amounts of thyroid hormone, physical and mental growth will be stunted.

The *parathyroid glands* secrete *parathormone*. There are four parathyroid glands. Two are located on each side of the thyroid gland. Parathormone regulates the body's use of calcium. Calcium is needed for the proper functioning of nerves and muscles. Insufficient amounts of calcium cause *tetany*. Tetany is a state of severe muscle contraction and spasm. If untreated, tetany can cause death.

There are two *adrenal glands*. An adrenal gland is on the top of each kidney. The adrenal gland has two parts: the *adrenal medulla* and the *adrenal cortex*. The adrenal medulla secretes *epinephrine* and *norepinephrine.* These hormones stimulate the body to quickly produce energy during emergencies. Heart rate, blood pressure, muscle power, and energy all increase. The adrenal cortex secretes three groups of hormones that are essential for life. The *glucocorticoids* regulate metabolism of carbohydrates. They also control the body's response to stress and inflammation. The *mineralocorticoids* regulate the amount of salt and water that is absorbed and lost by the kidneys. The adrenal cortex also secretes small amounts of male and female sex hormones.

The *pancreas* secretes *insulin.* Insulin regulates the amount of sugar in the blood available for use by the cells. Insulin is needed for sugar to enter the cells. If there is too little insulin, sugar cannot enter the cells. If sugar cannot enter the cells, excess amounts of sugar build up in the blood. This condition is called *diabetes mellitus.*

The *gonads* are the glands of human reproduction. Male sex glands (testes) secrete *testosterone.* Female sex glands (ovaries) secrete *estrogen* and *progesterone.*

THE IMMUNE SYSTEM

The immune system protects the body from disease and infection. Abnormal body cells can grow into tumors. Sometimes the body produces substances that cause the body to attack itself. Microorganisms (bacteria, viruses, and other germs) in the environment can lead to an infection. The immune system defends against threats inside and outside the body.

The immune system functions to provide the body with immunity. **Immunity** means that a person has protection against a disease or condition. The person will not get or be affected by the disease. *Specific immunity* is the body's reaction to a specific threat. *Nonspecific immunity* is the body's reaction to anything it does not recognize as a normal body substance.

Special cells and substances function to produce immunity:

- *Antibodies*—normal body substances that recognize abnormal or unwanted substances. They attack and destroy such substances.
- *Antigens*—abnormal or unwanted substances. An antigen causes the body to produce antibodies. The antibodies attack and destroy the antigens.
- *Phagocytes*—type of white blood cell that digests and destroys microorganisms and other unwanted substances.
- *Lymphocytes*—type of white blood cell that produces antibodies. Lymphocyte production increases as the body responds to an infection.
- *B lymphocytes (B cells)*—type of cell that causes the production of antibodies that circulate in the plasma. The antibodies react to specific antigens.
- *T lymphocytes (T cells)*—type of cell that destroys invading cells. *Killer T cells* produce poisonous substances near the invading cells. Some T cells attract other cells; these other cells destroy the invaders.

When the body senses an antigen (an unwanted substance), the immune system is activated. Phagocyte and lymphocyte production increases. Phagocytes destroy the invaders through digestion. The lymphocytes produce antibodies that attack and destroy the unwanted substances.

Circle the BEST answer.

1. The basic unit of body structure is the
   A. Cell
   B. Neuron
   C. Nephron
   D. Ovum

2. The outer layer of the skin is called the
   A. Dermis
   B. Epidermis
   C. Integument
   D. Myelin

3. Which is *not* a function of the skin?
   A. Providing the protective covering for the body
   B. Regulating body temperature
   C. Sensing cold, pain, touch, and pressure
   D. Providing the shape and framework for the body

4. Which parts allow movement?
   A. Bone marrow and periosteum
   B. Synovial membrane and tendons
   C. Joints
   D. Ligaments

5. Skeletal muscles
   A. Are under involuntary control
   B. Appear smooth
   C. Are under voluntary control
   D. Appear striped and smooth

6. The highest functions of the brain take place in the
   A. Cerebral cortex
   B. Medulla
   C. Brain stem
   D. Spinal nerves

7. Besides hearing, the ear is involved with
   A. Regulating body movements
   B. Balance
   C. Smoothness of body movements
   D. Controlling involuntary muscles

8. The liquid part of the blood is the
   A. Hemoglobin
   B. Red blood cell
   C. Plasma
   D. Alveolus

9. Which part of the heart pumps blood to the body?
   A. Right atrium
   B. Right ventricle
   C. Left atrium
   D. Left ventricle

10. Which carry blood away from the heart?
    A. Capillaries
    B. Veins
    C. Venules
    D. Arteries

11. Oxygen and carbon dioxide are exchanged
    A. In the bronchi
    B. Between the alveoli and capillaries
    C. Between the lungs and the pleura
    D. In the trachea

12. The process of digestion begins in the
    A. Mouth
    B. Stomach
    C. Small intestine
    D. Colon

13. Most food absorption takes place in the
    A. Stomach
    B. Small intestine
    C. Colon
    D. Large intestine

14. Urine is formed by the
    A. Jejunum
    B. Kidneys
    C. Bladder
    D. Liver

15. Urine passes from the body through
    A. The ureters
    B. The urethra
    C. The anus
    D. Nephrons

16. The male sex gland is called the
    A. Penis
    B. Semen
    C. Testis
    D. Scrotum

17. The male sex cell is the
    A. Semen
    B. Ovum
    C. Gonad
    D. Sperm

18. The female sex gland is the
    A. Ovary
    B. Fallopian tube
    C. Uterus
    D. Vagina

19. The discharge of the lining of the uterus is called
    A. The endometrium
    B. Ovulation
    C. Fertilization
    D. Menstruation

20. The endocrine glands secrete substances called
    A. Hormones
    B. Mucus
    C. Semen
    D. Insulin

21. The immune system protects the body from
    A. Low blood sugar
    B. Disease and infection
    C. Falling and loss of balance
    D. Stunted growth and loss of fluid

Answers to these questions are on p. 834.

GROWTH AND DEVELOPMENT

Define the key terms listed in this chapter

Understand the principles of growth and development

Identify the stages of growth and development and the normal age ranges for each stage

Identify the developmental tasks for each age-group

Describe the normal growth and development for each age-group

KEY TERMS

adolescence A time of rapid growth and psychological and social maturity

development Changes in a person's psychological and social functioning

developmental task That which the person must complete during a stage of development

ejaculation The release of semen

growth The physical changes that can be measured and that occur in a steady, orderly manner

menarche The time when menstruation first begins

menopause The time when menstruation stops

primary caregiver The person in the child's environment who is mainly responsible for providing or assisting with the child's basic needs

puberty The period when the reproductive organs begin to function and secondary sex characteristics appear

reflex An involuntary movement

You will care for people in different stages of development. A basic understanding of growth and development helps you give better care. The person's needs also are easier to understand. This chapter presents the basic changes that occur in normal, healthy persons from birth through old age.

Human growth and development are presented in nine stages. Age ranges and normal characteristics are given for each stage. Only basic descriptions are given. The stages overlap. This makes it hard to see clear-cut endings and beginnings of the stages. Also, the rate of growth and development varies with each person.

Growth and development theories generally involve the two-parent family. In our society, many households have only one parent. Often children are raised by a relative while the parent works or attends school. *Primary caregiver* is used in this chapter where *mother* or *father* would have been used. The **primary caregiver** is that person in the child's environment who is mainly responsible for providing or assisting with the child's basic needs. The primary caregiver may be a mother, father, grandparent, aunt, uncle, or court-appointed guardian. The words *parent* and *par-*

ents are used in this chapter. However, another primary caregiver may have the parent role.

PRINCIPLES

Growth is the physical changes that are measured and that occur in a steady and orderly manner. Growth is measured in height and weight. Changes in physical appearance and body functions also are measures of growth.

Development relates to changes in psychological and social functioning. A person behaves and thinks in certain ways in different stages of development. A 2-year-old thinks in simple terms and needs a primary caregiver for many basic needs. A 40-year-old thinks in complex ways and meets most basic needs without help from others.

Growth and development affect the entire person. Although each is defined, growth and development:

* Overlap
* Depend on each other
* Occur at the same time

For example, an infant cannot say simple syllables (development) until the physical structures needed for speech are strong enough (growth). The basic principles of growth and development are:

- Growth and development occur from the moment of fertilization until death.
- The process proceeds from the simple to the complex. A baby learns to sit before standing, to stand before walking, and to walk before running.
- Growth and development occur in certain directions:
  - From the head to the foot—babies learn to hold up their heads before they learn to sit. After learning to sit, they learn to stand.
  - From the center of the body outward—babies control shoulder movements before they control hand movements.
- Growth and development occur in a sequence, order, and pattern. Certain **developmental tasks** must be completed during each stage. A stage cannot be skipped. Each stage lays the foundation for the next stage.
- The rate of growth and development is uneven—not at a set pace. Growth is more rapid during infancy. Also, children have growth spurts. Some children develop rapidly; others develop slowly.
- Each stage of growth and development has its own characteristics and developmental tasks.

INFANCY (BIRTH TO 1 YEAR)

Infancy is the first year of life. Rapid physical, psychological, and social growth and development occur during this time. The developmental tasks of infancy are:

- Learning to walk
- Learning to eat solid foods
- Beginning to talk and communicate with others
- Beginning to have emotional relationships with primary caregivers, brothers, and sisters
- Developing stable sleep and feeding patterns

The *neonatal period* of infancy is the first 28 days after birth. A baby is called a *neonate* or a *newborn* during this time.

The average newborn is 19 to 21 inches long and weighs 7 to 8 pounds at birth. Birth weight usually doubles by the age of 5 to 6 months and triples by the first birthday. Babies are usually 20 to 30 inches long at the end of the first year.

The newborn's head is large compared with the rest of the body. The skin is wrinkled, and the baby appears red. Arms and legs seem short compared with

Fig. 7-1 A newborn.

the trunk. The abdomen is large and round. Eyes are a deep blue. The newborn has fat, pudgy cheeks, a flat nose, and a receding chin (Fig. 7-1).

The central nervous system is not well developed. Movements are uncoordinated and lack purpose. Babies can see at birth, although vision is not clear. They seem attracted to patterns. As babies develop, they prefer colors. Babies hear well. They are startled by loud noises and soothed by soft sounds. Babies respond better to female than to male voices. Infants react to touch, and the senses of smell and taste are developed.

Newborns have certain **reflexes** (involuntary movements). These reflexes decline and then disappear as the central nervous system develops.

- The *Moro reflex (startle reflex)* occurs when a baby is frightened by a loud noise or sudden movement. The arms are thrown apart, the legs extend, and the head is thrown back.
- The *rooting reflex* is stimulated when the infant's cheek is touched at or near the mouth. The baby's head turns toward the touch. The rooting reflex is necessary for feeding; it helps guide the baby's mouth to the nipple.
- The *sucking reflex* is produced by touching the cheeks or side of the lips.
- The *grasping reflex* occurs when the infant's palm is stimulated, causing the fingers to close around the object (Fig. 7-2). This reflex begins to decline around the second month and disappears by the third month.

Infants sleep most of the time during the first few weeks of life. They awaken when hungry and fall asleep right after eating. The time between feedings lengthens as infants grow and develop. They stay awake more and sleep less as growth and development occur.

Body movements are uncoordinated and without purpose. They are generally involuntary. As the cen-

Fig. 7-2 The grasping reflex.

A

B

Fig. 7-3 The 1-month-old infant can lift the head when lying on the stomach.

Fig. 7-4 A 2-month-old child. **A,** Child smiles. **B,** Child follows objects with the eyes.

tral nervous system and muscular system develop, infants develop specific, voluntary, and coordinated movements. Newborns cannot hold their heads up. At 1 month, infants can hold their heads up when held and can lift and turn their heads when lying on their stomachs (Fig. 7-3). At 2 months, they can smile and follow objects with their eyes (Fig. 7-4).

Three-month-old infants can raise their heads and shoulders when lying on their stomachs (Fig. 7-5, p. 134). They can sit for a short while when supported and can hold a rattle. Infants 4 months of age should be able to roll over. They can sit up if supported and may sleep all night. The Moro and rooting reflexes have disappeared. Tears are shed when crying. A rattle is held with both hands, objects are put in the mouth, and the infant babbles when spoken to. At 5 months, infants can grasp objects and play with their toes. Teeth start to come through (Fig. 7-6, p. 134).

Six-month-old infants usually have two lower front teeth and start to chew and bite finger foods. They can hold a bottle for feeding and can sit alone for a short time (Fig. 7-7, p. 134). At 7 months the upper teeth start to erupt. Babies respond to their names, can say "dada," and show a fear of strangers. At age 8 months, infants may be able to stand when holding onto something. They react to the word "no." Infants at this age do not like to be dressed or have diapers changed. Nine-month-old infants crawl (Fig. 7-8, p. 134), and more upper teeth appear.

At 10 months, most infants can walk around while holding on to furniture (Fig. 7-9, p. 135). They understand the words "bye-bye," "mama," and

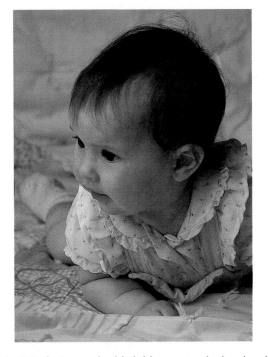

Fig. 7-5 The 3-month-old child can raise the head and shoulders.

Fig. 7-6 The 5-month-old child puts objects into the mouth as teeth begin to erupt.

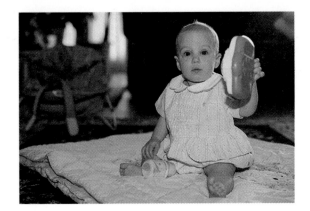

Fig. 7-7 A 6-month-old child can sit alone for a short time.

Fig. 7-8 A 9-month-old child is able to crawl.

Fig. 7-9 A 10-month-old child can walk while holding onto furniture.

Fig. 7-10 A toddler is able to use a spoon.

"dada." They smile when looking into a mirror. Infants at 11 months of age may begin to take steps and can hold a crayon. Many infants start to walk at 1 year of age. They can hold a cup for drinking. One-year-olds know more words, can say "no," and shake their heads for "no."

During the first 6 months, the infant's diet is mainly breast milk or formula. Solid foods (strained fruits and vegetables) are usually added at 5 to 6 months. Junior foods are added during the eighth and ninth months. A 1-year-old can eat table foods.

TODDLERHOOD (1 TO 3 YEARS)

Physical growth during the second year of life is not as rapid as during infancy. The developmental tasks during this period are:

- Tolerating separation from the primary caregiver
- Gaining control of bowel and bladder function
- Using words to communicate with others
- Becoming less dependent on the primary caregiver

Toddlers have the need to assert independence. Therefore the toddler years are known as the "terrible twos." The ability to move about and walk increases. So does the child's curiosity. Toddlers get into anything and everything. They touch, smell, and taste everything within reach. As toddlers become more coordinated, they start to climb. These new and increasing skills allow exploration of the environment. The child ventures farther away from the primary caregiver. The toddler also learns that some things can be done without the primary caregiver. By the age of 3 years, the toddler can run, jump, climb, ride a tricycle, and walk up and down stairs.

Increased hand coordination gives toddlers new skills. The need to feel, smell, and taste things is shown in their incr*easing ability to feed themselves. They progress from eating with fingers to using a spoon (Fig. 7-10). Toddlers can drink from cups. They can scribble, build towers with blocks, string beads, and turn book pages. Right- or left-handedness is seen during the second year.

Toilet training is a major developmental task for toddlers. Bowel and bladder control is related to central nervous system development. Children must be psychologically and physically ready for toilet training. The process starts with bowel control. Bowel control is easier because the frequency of bowel movements per day is less than urination. Bowel training usually is complete at about 2½ years of age. Bladder control during the day occurs before bladder control at night. Bladder training is complete usually at about 3 years of age.

Speech and language skills increase. Speech is clearer, and vocabulary increases. Words are learned by imitating others. Toddlers understand more words than they use. They are capable of 2- or 3-word sentences. By 3 years of age, children should be able to speak in short sentences.

Play ability increases. The child plays alongside other children but does not play with them. There is no sharing of toys with others. The toddler is very possessive and does not understand sharing. The word "mine" is often used.

Temper tantrums and saying "no" are common during this stage. When disciplined, the toddler often kicks and screams. The temper tantrum is the child's way of objecting to having independence challenged. The use of "no" can frustrate primary caregivers. Almost every request may be answered "no," even if the toddler is following the request.

Another developmental task is tolerating separation from the primary caregiver. As toddlers start to explore their environments, they tend to venture away from primary caregivers. When discomfort, frustration, or injury occur, they quickly return to primary caregivers or cry for their attention. If the primary caregiver is consistently present whenever needed, a child learns to feel secure. Thus toddlers learn to tolerate brief periods of separation.

PRESCHOOL (3 TO 6 YEARS)

The preschool years (early childhood) are from the ages of 3 to 6. Children grow taller but gain little weight. Preschoolers are thinner, more coordinated, and more graceful than toddlers. The developmental tasks of the preschool years include:

- Increasing the ability to communicate and understand others
- Performing self-care activities
- Learning the differences between the sexes and developing sexual modesty
- Learning right from wrong and good from bad
- Learning to play with others
- Developing family relationships

THE 3-YEAR-OLD

Three-year-olds become more coordinated. They can walk on tiptoe, balance on one foot for a few seconds, and run, jump, and climb with ease. Personal care skills increase. They can put on shoes, dress themselves, manage buttons, wash their hands, and brush their teeth (Fig. 7-11). They can feed themselves, pour from a bottle, and help set the table without breaking dishes. Hand skills also include drawing circles and crosses.

Most three-year-olds know about 1000 words, imitate new words, and talk and ask questions constantly. Sentences are brief—usually 3 or 4 words. Three-year-olds can name body parts, family members, friends, and animals. They like talking dolls and musical toys.

Play is important. Three-year-olds play in small groups with 2 or 3 other children and share toys. They play simple games and learn to follow simple rules. Imaginary playmates and imitating adults during play are common. They enjoy coloring books and crayons, scissors and paper, and playing "house" and "dress-up" (Fig. 7-12).

At 3 years old, children know that there are two sexes. They know that male and female bodies are different. They also know their own sex. Little girls may wonder how the penis works and why they do not have one. Little boys may wonder how girls can urinate without a penis.

Fig. 7-11 A 3-year-old has increased coordination.

Fig. 7-12 Three-year-olds enjoy cutting paper and using coloring books and crayons.

The concept of time develops. Children 3 years of age may speak of the past, present, and future. "Yesterday" and "tomorrow" are still confusing. Children may be afraid of the dark and need a night-light in the bedroom.

Three-year-olds are less fearful of strangers. They tolerate separation from primary caregivers for short periods. They are less jealous than toddlers of a new baby. Things are done to please primary caregivers at this age.

THE 4-YEAR-OLD

Four-year-olds can hop, skip, and throw and catch a ball. They can lace shoes, draw faces, copy a square, and try to print letters. They can bathe with some help and usually tend to toileting needs with help.

Vocabulary increases to about 1500 words. The child continues to ask many questions and tends to exaggerate when telling stories. The 4-year-old can sing simple songs, repeat four numbers, count to three, and name a few colors.

Fig. 7-13 Four-year-olds play "dress-up" and imitate adults.

Fig. 7-14 Five-year-olds enjoy doing things with the parent of the same sex.

Children 4 years of age may tend to attack others. They also tease, tattle, and tell fibs. They are more impatient and may blame an imaginary playmate when in trouble. Bragging, telling tales about family members, and showing off are common. They can play cooperatively with other children. Four-year-olds are proud of their accomplishments but have mood swings.

Children in this age-group enjoy playing "dress-up," wearing costumes, and telling and hearing stories. They like to draw and make things. Imagination, drama, and imitation of adults are seen during play (Fig. 7-13). They play in groups of two or three and tend to be bossy. Playing "doctor and nurse" is common as curiosity about the opposite sex continues.

Four-year-olds strongly prefer the primary caregiver of the other sex. Rivalries with brothers and sisters are seen, especially when younger children take the 4-year-old's possessions. Rivalries also occur when older children have more and different privileges. Family members are often the focus of the child's frustrations and aggressive behavior. Some 4-year-olds try to run away from home.

THE 5-YEAR-OLD

Coordination continues to develop. Five-year-olds can jump rope, skate, tie shoelaces, dress, and bathe. They can use a pencil well and copy diamond and triangle shapes. They can print a few letters and numbers and their first names. Drawings of people include the body, head, arms, legs, and feet.

Communication skills also increase. Vocabulary consists of about 14,000 words. Sentences have 6 to 8 words. They ask fewer questions than before, but questions have more meaning. They want definitions for unknown terms and take part in conversations. Four or more colors, coins, days of the week, and months can be named. They specify what they draw and give detailed descriptions of drawings.

Five-year-olds are more responsible and truthful, and they quarrel less than before. There is greater awareness of rules and an eagerness to do things the right way. They have manners, are independent, and can be trusted within limits. Five-year-olds have fewer fears but may have nightmares and dreams. They are also proud of their accomplishments.

Simple number and word games are enjoyed by 5-year-olds. Although they may cheat to win, they like rules and try to follow them. They imitate adults during play and have a greater interest in watching television. They also enjoy activities with the primary caregiver of the same sex (Fig. 7-14). Such activities include cooking, housecleaning, shopping, yard work, and sports.

These children tolerate brothers and sisters well. Although younger children are considered a nuisance, 5-year-olds usually protect them.

MIDDLE CHILDHOOD (6 TO 8 YEARS)

Preschoolers often have nursery school and kindergarten experiences. However, middle childhood is the time for school. Children enter the world of peer groups, games, and learning. The developmental tasks of middle childhood are:

- Developing the social and physical skills needed for playing games
- Learning to get along with other children of the same age and background (peers)
- Learning behaviors and attitudes appropriate to one's own sex
- Learning basic reading, writing, and arithmetic skills
- Developing a conscience and morals
- Developing a good feeling and attitude about oneself

Fig. 7-15 Six-year-olds begin to prefer playing with children of the same sex.

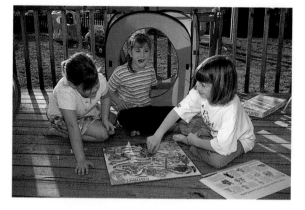

Fig. 7-16 Seven-year-olds enjoy board games.

THE 6-YEAR-OLD

The 6-year-old grows about 2 inches taller and gains 3 to 6 pounds. Baby teeth are lost, and replacement with permanent teeth begins. Children are very active and are skilled at running, jumping, skipping, hopping, and riding a bicycle. They seem to be constantly on the go. Sitting is tolerated for only a short time.

Six-year-olds enter the first grade and the world of school, activities, and other children. Children this age are often described as bossy, opinionated, charming, argumentative, and "know-it-alls." They have set ways of doing things and like to have their own way. They may have temper tantrums. Six-year-olds play well with children of both sexes. However, they begin to prefer playing with children of the same sex (Fig. 7-15). There is more sharing with others, and the child may have a "best friend." A child may cheat to win or leave a game before it is over to avoid losing. Tattling is common.

Six-year-olds have a vocabulary of about 16,500 words. They know the alphabet and begin to read and spell. They communicate thoughts and feelings better than before.

Play interests range from rough play to quiet activities such as playing with cards, paints, clay, and checkers. Collections are started of odds and ends rather than specific things like stamps, rocks, or butterflies. More active play includes tag, hide-and-seek, playing with balls, skating, and playing in mud or sand.

THE 7-YEAR-OLD

Seven-year-olds grow about 2 inches in height. The average 7-year-old weighs about 49 to 56 pounds and is 47 to 49 inches tall. Hand coordination increases. Children learn to write rather than print. They are quieter than 6-year-olds and spend much time alone. They are more serious, less stubborn, and more con-

cerned about being well liked. Seven-year-olds are more aware of themselves, their bodies, and the reactions of others. They do not like being teased or criticized and are sensitive about how others treat them. They like going to school, learning, and reading. There are concerns about grades and what the teacher thinks about them. Reading skills increase, and the child can tell time.

Play includes swimming, biking, collecting and trading objects, playing ball and games with rules, and working puzzles and magic tricks (Fig. 7-16). They play in groups. However, boys prefer to play with boys and girls prefer to play with girls. They may join scouting groups, such as the Cub Scouts or Brownies.

THE 8-YEAR-OLD

The 8-year-old enters the third grade. Growth in height and weight continues. More permanent teeth appear. Movements are faster and more graceful.

Peer group activities and opinions are important. Being accepted and included in peer groups are important for love and belonging and self-esteem (Fig. 7-17). Children this age get along with adults. However, they prefer peer group fads, opinions, and activities. Boys and girls play separately. Their interests relate to group games, collections, television, and movies.

Eight-year-olds are sometimes described as defensive, opinionated, practical, and outgoing. They give advice freely to others. However, they do not accept criticism well. They often do household tasks such as vacuuming, cooking, and yard work but expect to be paid. They expect more privileges than younger brothers and sisters.

Learning continues. They are curious about science, history, and other places and countries. School also provides social opportunities with peers. Eight-year-olds are daring in the classroom. They may pass notes or

Fig. 7-17 Belonging to a peer group is important to the 8-year-old.

Fig. 7-18 Movements are smooth and graceful in late childhood.

throw paper airplanes when they think the teacher is not looking. Despite this mischief, they are mannerly, relate well to adults, and take part in adult conversations. They are also friendly and affectionate.

LATE CHILDHOOD (9 TO 12 YEARS)

Late childhood (preadolescence) is between leaving childhood and dependency on others and entering adolescence. Developmental tasks are similar to those of middle childhood. However, a preadolescent is expected to show more refinement and maturity in achieving the following tasks:

- Becoming independent of adults and learning to depend on oneself
- Developing and keeping friendships with peers
- Understanding the physical, psychological, and social roles of one's sex
- Developing moral and ethical behavior
- Developing greater muscular strength, coordination, and balance
- Learning how to study

Boys grow about 1 inch per year. Girls grow about 2 inches per year. Boys gain about 3½ to 4 pounds each year. Girls gain between 4 and 5 pounds each year. Girls are usually taller than boys during late preadolescence. Many permanent teeth erupt.

Body movements are more graceful and coordinated (Fig. 7-18). Muscular strength and physical skills increase. Skill in team sports is important.

Body changes occur as the onset of puberty nears. In girls, the pelvis becomes broader, fat appears on the hips and chest, and the budding of breasts occurs. Boys show fewer signs of maturing sexually during this time. Genital organs begin to grow.

These children must have factual sex education. Information about sex that is shared among friends is often incomplete and inaccurate. Parents and children may be uncomfortable discussing sex with each other and may avoid the subject. When children do ask questions, honest and complete answers must be given in terms the children can understand.

Peer groups are the center of preadolescent activities. The group begins to affect the child's attitudes and behavior. Preference for companions of the same sex continues. Boys need to show their strength and toughness and may give each other nicknames. Arguments between boys and girls are common, and boys often tease girls.

Preadolescents are more aware of the mistakes and weaknesses of adults. They do not accept adult standards and rules without question. Rebellion against adults is common. Disagreements between parents and children increase, although the parents continue to be important for the child's development.

By the age of 12, the child uses about 7,000 words in conversation and understands about 50,000 words in reading. Dictionary, encyclopedia, and other references use increases. Interest in science, history, and geography continues. Girls often enjoy reading romantic books and stories. Boys usually prefer science fiction, mysteries, and adventure stories.

ADOLESCENCE (12 TO 18 YEARS)

Adolescence is a time of rapid growth and psychological and social maturity. The stage begins with puberty. **Puberty** is the period during which the reproductive organs begin to function and the secondary sex characteristics appear. Girls experience puberty between the ages of 10 and 14. Most boys reach puberty between the ages of 12 and 16.

Because the age of puberty varies, adolescence ranges from the ages of 12 and 18 years. The developmental tasks of adolescence include:

- Accepting changes in the body and appearance
- Developing appropriate relationships with males and females of the same age
- Accepting the male or female role appropriate for one's age
- Becoming independent from parents and adults
- Developing morals, attitudes, and values needed for functioning in society

Menarche, the beginning of menstruation, marks the onset of puberty in girls. Secondary sex characteristics appear. These include:

- Increase in breast size
- Appearance of pubic and axillary (underarm) hair
- Slight deepening of the voice
- Widening and rounding of the hips

During late childhood, male sex organs begin to increase in size. This growth continues during adolescence. **Ejaculation** (the release of semen) signals the onset of puberty in boys. *Nocturnal emissions* ("wet dreams") occur. During sleep *(nocturnal)*, the penis becomes erect and semen is released *(emission)*. Other secondary sex characteristics appear. These include:

- Appearance of facial hair and growth of a beard
- Pubic and axillary (underarm) hair
- Hair on the arms, chest, and legs
- Deepening of the voice
- Increases in neck and shoulder size

A growth spurt occurs. Boys grow about 4 to 16 inches and gain 15 to 60 pounds. They usually stop growing between the ages of 18 and 21. Some continue to grow until about age 25. Girls grow about 2 to 9 inches and gain between 15 and 50 pounds. They usually stop growing between the ages of 17 and 18. Some continue to grow until about age 21.

Adolescence is described as the awkward stage. Awkwardness and clumsiness are caused by the uneven growth of muscles and bones. Coordination and graceful body movements develop as muscle and bone growth even out.

Changes in appearance are often hard to accept. Some girls are embarrassed about breast development, especially very large or small breast size. Some are embarrassed about wearing a bra. Others wear tight sweaters so the breasts are noticed. Genital size may be a concern of boys. Height is a problem for both boys and girls. Being short limits play in some sports. Boys do not like being much shorter than their peers. Tall girls may feel embarrassed about being different and taller than other girls and boys.

Fig. 7-19 This teenager has a part-time job.

Emotional reactions vary from high to low. Adolescents can be happy one moment and sad the next. Predicting a reaction to a comment or event is difficult. Teenagers can control their emotions better later in this stage. Older adolescents (15- to 18-year-olds) can still become sad and depressed. However, they can better control the time and place of their emotional reactions.

Adolescents need to become independent of adults, especially their parents. They must learn to function, make decisions, and act in a responsible manner without adult supervision. Many teenagers work toward this independence with part-time jobs, babysitting, going to dances and parties, dating, taking part in school clubs and organizations, shopping without an adult, and staying home alone (Fig. 7-19).

Judgment and reasoning are not always sound. Guidance, discipline, and emotional and financial support are still needed from parents. Disagreements with parents are common, especially about behavior and activity restrictions and limits. Teenagers would rather be with peers than do things with parents and other family members. Adolescents tend to confide in and seek advice from adults other than their parents.

Teenage interests and activities reflect the need to become independent, to develop relationships with the opposite sex, and to act like males or females. Both sexes are interested in parties, dances, and other social activities. Clothing, makeup, and hairstyles are important. A teenager may babysit or get a part-time job to have extra money for clothes, makeup, and hair-care and skin-care products. Parents and teenagers rarely agree about clothing styles. Teenagers may spend a lot of time experimenting with makeup and hairstyles. They may also spend a lot of time talking to friends on the phone, listening to music, and reading teen magazines.

Dating begins during adolescence. Although the age when dating begins varies, there is usually a dating pattern. "Crowd" dates are common in the seventh and eighth grades. They are usually related to school activities, such as a dance or basketball game. The same group of girls just happens to be with the same group of boys during these social events. In the ninth grade, pairing off is common during crowd dating. The tenth grade is usually when boy-girl couples go to social events together and then join other couples. Double dating occurs in the eleventh grade. Dates involve one couple during the twelfth grade, although there is some double dating.

Many difficult decisions and conflicts result as the adolescent matures physically, psychologically, and emotionally. Parents and teenagers often disagree about dating. Parents worry that dating will lead to sexual activities, pregnancy, and sexually transmitted diseases. Teenagers usually do not understand or appreciate these concerns. "Going steady" helps meet the teenager's need for security, love and belonging, and self-esteem. Teenagers sometimes have difficulty controlling sexual urges and considering the consequences of sexual activity.

Adolescents begin to think about careers and what to do after high school graduation. Interests, skills, and talents are some factors that influence the choice of further education and getting a job. Adolescents also need to develop morals, values, and attitudes for living in society. They need to develop a sense about what is good and bad, right and wrong, and important and unimportant. Parents, peers, culture, religion, television, school, and movies are among the many factors influencing teenagers. Drug abuse, unwanted pregnancy, alcoholism, and criminal acts are common problems of troubled adolescents.

YOUNG ADULTHOOD (18 TO 40 YEARS)

Psychological and social development continue during young adulthood. There is little physical growth. Adult height has been reached. Body systems are fully developed. Developmental tasks of young adulthood include:

- Choosing education and an occupation
- Selecting a partner
- Learning to live with a partner
- Becoming a parent and raising children
- Developing a satisfactory sex life

Education and occupation are so closely related that they can rarely be separated. Most jobs require specific knowledge and skills. The amount and kind of education needed depend on the career choice. Most adults find that job choices are greater with adequate educational preparation. Employment is necessary for economic independence and for supporting a family.

Fig. 7-20 Communication is necessary for a successful partnership and a satisfactory sex life.

Most adults marry at least once. Others choose to remain single. They may live alone, with friends of the same sex, or with a person from the opposite sex. Gay and lesbian persons may commit to a partner.

The many reasons for marriage include love, emotional security, wanting a family, sex, wanting to leave an unhappy home life, social status, companionship, and money. Some marry to feel wanted, needed, and desirable. Many factors also affect selecting a marriage partner. They include age, religion, interests, education, race, personality, and of course, love. Some marriages are happy and successful, whereas others are not. There are no guarantees that a marriage will work. Therefore the two people must work together to build a marriage based on trust, respect, caring, and friendship.

Partners (married or unmarried) must learn to live together. Habits, routines, meal preparation, and pastimes are changed or adjusted to "fit" the other person's needs. They must learn how to solve problems and make decisions together. They need to work toward the same goals. Open and honest communication helps create a successful partnership (Fig. 7-20).

Adults also need to develop a satisfactory sex life. Sexual frequency, desires, practices, and preferences vary. Understanding and accepting the partner's needs are necessary for a satisfying and intimate relationship.

Most couples decide to have children. Modern birth control methods allow planning about the number of children and when to have them. However, many pregnancies are unplanned. Most couples have a child during the first few years of marriage; some wait several years before starting a family. Other couples decide not to have children. Some have difficulty or cannot have children because of physical problems in the man or woman. Those couples having children need to agree on child-rearing practices and discipline methods. They need to adjust to the child and to the child's need for time, energy, and parental attention.

MIDDLE ADULTHOOD
(40 TO 65 YEARS)

This stage of development is more stable and comfortable. Children are usually grown and have moved away. Partners now have time to spend alone together. There are fewer worries about children and money. The developmental tasks of middle adulthood relate to:

- Adjusting to physical changes
- Having grown children
- Developing leisure-time activities
- Relating to aging parents

Several physical changes occur. Many are gradual and go unnoticed; others are seen early. People in their early forties may feel energetic and able to function as they did in their twenties. However, energy and endurance begin to slow down. Weight control becomes a problem as metabolism and physical activities slow down. Facial wrinkles and gray hair appear. The need for eyeglasses is common. Hearing loss may begin. Menstruation stops between the ages of 42 and 55; this is called **menopause**. Ovaries stop secreting hormones, and the woman can no longer have children. Many diseases and illnesses can develop. The disorders can become chronic or life threatening.

Children leave home for college, marry, move to homes of their own, and start their own families. Adults have to cope with letting children go, being in-laws, and becoming grandparents. Parents must let children lead their own lives. However, they need to be available for emotional support in times of need.

Middle-age adults often discover spare time when the demands of parenthood decrease. Hobbies and pastimes such as gardening, fishing, painting, golfing, volunteer work, and membership in clubs and organizations are sources of pleasure (Fig. 7-21). Hobbies and pastimes become even more important after retirement and during late adulthood.

Fig. 7-21 Middle-age adults usually have more time for hobbies.

Some middle-age adults have parents who are aging and developing poor health. Responsibility for aging parents may begin during this stage. Middle-age adults often have to deal with the death of parents.

LATE ADULTHOOD
(65 YEARS AND OLDER)

Many physical, psychological, and social changes occur during later adulthood. Chapter 8 describes the changes that occur in older persons, as well as the care they may need.

The developmental tasks of this stage are:

- Adjusting to decreased physical strength and loss of health
- Adjusting to retirement and reduced income
- Coping with the death of a partner
- Developing new friends and relationships
- Preparing for one's own death

REVIEW

Circle the BEST answer.

1. Changes in psychological and social functioning are called
   A. Growth
   B. Development
   C. A reflex
   D. A stage

2. Which is *false?*
   A. Growth and development occur from the simple to the complex.
   B. Growth and development occur in an orderly pattern.
   C. Growth and development occur at specific rates.
   D. Each stage has its own characteristics.

3. The stage of infancy is the first
   A. 4 weeks of life
   B. 3 months of life
   C. 6 months of life
   D. Year of life

4. Which reflexes are needed for feeding in the infant?
   A. The Moro and startle reflexes
   B. The rooting and sucking reflexes
   C. The grasping and Moro reflexes
   D. The rooting and grasping reflexes

5. Crawling occurs at about
   A. 6 months
   B. 7 months
   C. 8 months
   D. 9 months

6. Solid foods are usually given to a baby during the
   A. Fifth or sixth month
   B. Seventh or eighth month
   C. Ninth or tenth month
   D. Eleventh or twelfth month

7. Toilet training begins
   A. During infancy
   B. During the toddler years
   C. When the primary caregiver is ready
   D. At the age of 3

8. The toddler can
   A. Use a spoon and cup
   B. Ride a bike
   C. Help set the table
   D. Name parts of the body

9. Playing with other children begins during
   A. Infancy
   B. The toddler years
   C. The preschool years
   D. Middle childhood

10. Loss of baby teeth usually begins at the age of
    A. 4
    B. 5
    C. 6
    D. 7

11. Peer group activities become more important at the age of
    A. 6
    B. 7
    C. 8
    D. 9

12. Reproductive organs begin to function and secondary sex characteristics appear during
    A. Late childhood
    B. Preadolescence
    C. Puberty
    D. Early adulthood

13. Which is *false?*
    A. Boys reach puberty earlier than girls.
    B. Most girls reach puberty between the ages of 12 and 13.
    C. Menarche marks the onset of puberty in girls.
    D. A growth spurt occurs during adolescence.

14. Dating usually begins
    A. During late childhood
    B. With "crowd" dating
    C. With "pairing off"
    D. During late adolescence

15. Adolescence is a time when parents and children
    A. Talk openly about sex
    B. Express love and affection
    C. Disagree
    D. Do things as a family

16. Which is *not* a developmental task of young adulthood?
    A. Adjusting to changes in the body and in physical appearance
    B. Selecting a partner
    C. Choosing an occupation
    D. Becoming a parent

17. Middle adulthood is from about
    A. 25 to 35 years
    B. 30 to 40 years
    C. 40 to 50 years
    D. 40 to 65 year

18. Middle adulthood is a time when
    A. Families are started
    B. Physical energy and free time are gained
    C. Children are grown and leave home
    D. People need to prepare for death

Answers to these questions are on p. 834.

CHAPTER

8

CARE OF THE OLDER PERSON

Define the key terms listed in this chapter

Describe the effects of retirement

Identify the social changes common in older adulthood

Describe how a partner's death affects the survivor

Describe the changes that occur in the body's systems during aging and the care required

Describe housing options for older persons

Explain the requirements of the Omnibus Budget Reconciliation Act of 1987

Describe resident rights and how to promote a resident's quality of life

KEY TERMS

geriatrics The care of aging people

gerontology The study of the aging process

involuntary seclusion Separating a person from others against his or her will; keeping the person confined to a certain area or away from his or her room without consent

middle-old Persons between 75 and 84 years of age

old-old Persons older than 85 years

young-old Persons between 60 and 74 years of age

The number of older adults increases every day. People live longer and are healthier and more active than ever before. Most people can expect to live into their 70s. Many live into their 80s and 90s. There also are more 100-year-olds than ever before. Late adulthood is broken down into these age ranges:

- The **young-old**—persons between 60 and 74 years of age
- The **middle-old**—persons between 75 and 84 years of age
- The **old-old**—persons older than 85 years

Gerontology is the study of the aging process. **Geriatrics** is the care of the aged. Aging, or growing old, is a normal process. Normal changes occur in body structure and function. These changes increase the risk for illness, injury, chronic disease, and disability. Usually the changes are gradual. Psychological and social changes also occur. Most older persons adjust to these changes and live healthy and happy lives. They live in their own homes with their partners. Others live with family. Some require long-term care in a nursing center.

As stated in Chapter 7, the developmental tasks of late adulthood are:

- Adjusting to decreased physical strength and loss of health
- Adjusting to retirement and reduced income
- Coping with the death of a partner
- Developing new friends and relationships
- Preparing for one's own death

PSYCHOLOGICAL AND SOCIAL CHANGES

Graying hair, wrinkles, and slow movements are physical reminders of growing old. Retirement and death of a partner, family, and friends are social reminders. Physical and social changes have psychological effects on the person. They affect the basic needs of love and belonging and self-esteem.

RETIREMENT

Most people look forward to retiring. People usually retire at the age of 65. Some retire earlier. Others work until the age of 70. Retirement is a reward for a lifetime of work. The person has earned the right not to work and can now relax and enjoy life (Fig. 8-1). Travel, leisure, and doing what one wants are retirement "benefits." Many people enjoy retirement.

Fig. 8-1 A retired couple enjoying arts and crafts together.

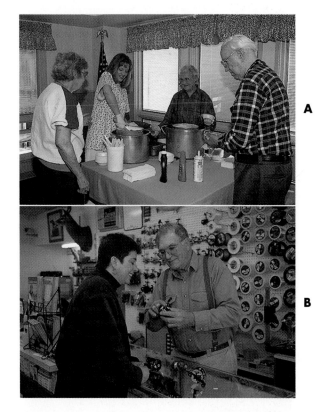

Fig. 8-2 **A,** This retired woman does volunteer work at a nursing center. **B,** This retired man works at a sporting goods shop.

Others are not as lucky. Retirement is often a person's first real experience with aging. Some must retire because of chronic disease or disability. Poor health and medical bills can make retirement very difficult.

Work has social and psychological effects. It helps meet the basic needs of love and belonging and self-esteem. Work brings fulfillment and usefulness. There is pride in a day's work or a job well done. Friendships form, and co-workers share daily events. Leisure time, recreation, and companionship often involve co-workers. Some people need work for psychological and social fulfillment. Retirement can be hard for them. Some retired people have part-time jobs or do volunteer work (Fig. 8-2). Such activities promote usefulness and well-being.

Reduced Income. Retirement income is often less than one half of the person's working income. Social Security may provide the only income. Even that has not kept pace with the high cost of living.

Retirement and aging do not mean fewer expenses. Rent or mortgage payments, food, clothing, utility bills, and taxes are usual expenses. Car expenses, home repairs, medicine, and health care are other costs. So are entertainment and gifts for children, grandchildren, and other family and friends.

Reduced income may force life-style changes. Some retirees limit social and leisure activities. A person may buy cheaper food, clothes, and household items. A move to cheaper housing may be necessary. Some older persons live with children or relatives. Some cannot afford health care or medicine. Some retirees have to rely on children or family for money or needed items.

Retirement can cause severe money problems. Some people plan for retirement through savings, investments, retirement plans, and insurance. Their retirement years are financially comfortable.

Caring About Culture

COMMUNICATING IN A FOREIGN LANGUAGE
Some older persons speak and understand a foreign language. Communication occurs with family and friends who speak the same language. They also share cultural values and practices. These relatives and friends may move away or die. The person may not have anyone to talk to and may not be understood by others. Greater loneliness and isolation for the foreign-speaking person may result.

SOCIAL RELATIONSHIPS

Social relationships change throughout life. *(See Caring About Culture [Communicating in a Foreign Language] box.)* Children grow up, leave home, and have their own families. Many live far away from parents. Older friends and family move away, die, or are disabled. Yet most older people have regular contact with children, grandchildren, brothers and sisters, nieces and nephews, and other relatives and friends. However, many older people are lonely. Separation from children and lack of companionship with people their own age are common causes of loneliness in older persons (Fig. 8-3, p. 148).

Fig. 8-3 Older people enjoy companionship with people their own age.

Fig. 8-4 An older woman plays with her grandchild.

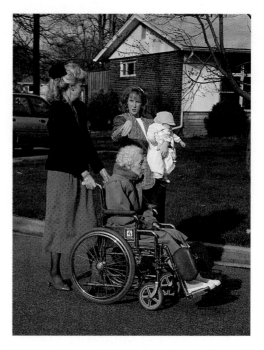

Fig. 8-5 An older woman is included in family activities.

Many older people adjust to these changes. Hobbies, church and community activities, and new friends help prevent loneliness. Being a grandparent brings great love and enjoyment (Fig. 8-4). Taking part in family activities helps prevent loneliness. It also allows the older person to feel useful and wanted (Fig. 8-5).

Children often care for older parents. Parents and children change roles. Instead of the parent caring for the child, the child cares for the parent. This role change and dependency on a child can make the older person feel more secure. However, others feel unwanted, in the way, and useless. Some feel a loss of dignity and self-respect. Tensions may develop among the child, parent, and other family members in the home. Lack of privacy, disagreements, and criticisms about housekeeping, child rearing, cooking, and friends are common causes of tension.

DEATH OF A PARTNER

As a couple grows older, the chances increase that one partner will die. Women usually live longer than men. Therefore many women will become widows.

A person may try to psychologically prepare for a partner's death. When death occurs, the loss is crushing. No amount of preparation is ever enough for the emptiness and changes that result. The person loses a friend, lover, companion, and confidant. The survivor's grief may be very great. Serious physical and mental health problems can result. The surviving partner may lose the will to live or attempt suicide.

PHYSICAL CHANGES

Certain physical changes are a normal part of aging. The changes occur in everyone (Table 8-1). Body processes slow down. Energy level and body efficiency decline. The rate and degree of change vary with each person. Influencing factors include diet, general health, exercise, stress, environment, and heredity. Many changes are gradual and not noticed for a long time. Some older people also have physical changes caused by disease, illness, or injury.

THE INTEGUMENTARY SYSTEM

The skin loses its elasticity, strength, and fatty tissue layer. This causes the skin to thin and sag. Folds, lines, and wrinkles appear. Dry skin develops because of

Table 8-1 Physical Changes During the Aging Process

System	Changes	System	Changes
Integumentary	Skin becomes less elastic Skin loses its strength Brown spots ("age spots" or "liver spots") on the wrists and hands Fewer nerve endings Fewer blood vessels Fatty tissue layer is lost Skin thins and sags Skin is fragile and easily injured Folds, lines, and wrinkles appear Decreased secretion of oil and sweat glands Dry skin develops Itching Increased sensitivity to cold Decreased sensitivity to pain Nails become thick and tough Whitening or graying hair Loss or thinning of hair Facial hair in some women Drier hair	Cardiovascular	Dizziness Changes in sleep patterns Heart pumps with less force Arteries narrow and are less elastic Less blood flows through narrowed arteries Weakened heart has to work harder to pump blood through narrowed vessels
		Respiratory	Respiratory muscles weaken Lung tissue becomes less elastic Difficulty breathing Decreased strength for coughing
Musculoskeletal	Muscle atrophy Decreasing strength Bones become brittle; can break easily Joints become stiff and painful Gradual loss of height Decreased mobility	Digestive	Decreased saliva production Difficulty in swallowing Decreased appetite Decreased secretion of digestive juices Fried and fatty foods difficult to digest Indigestion Loss of teeth Decreased peristalsis causing flatulence and constipation
Nervous	Vision and hearing decrease Decreased senses of taste and smell Reduced sense of touch Reduced sensitivity to pain Reduced blood flow to the brain Progressive loss of brain cells Shorter memory Forgetfulness Slowed ability to respond Confusion	Urinary	Reduced blood supply to kidneys Kidneys atrophy Kidney function decreases Poisonous substances can build up in the blood Urine becomes concentrated Urinary frequency and urgency may occur Urinary incontinence may occur The need to urinate at night may occur

decreases in oil and sweat glands. The skin is fragile and easily injured. Skin breakdown, skin tears, and pressure ulcers are dangers (see Chapter 25).

Brown spots appear on the skin. These often are called "age spots" or "liver spots." The usually occur on the wrists and hands.

The skin has fewer nerve endings. This affects the person's ability to sense heat, cold, and pain. Bruising and delayed healing result from a decreased number of blood vessels.

Loss of fatty tissues beneath the skin increases sensitivity to cold. Sweaters, lap blankets, socks, and extra blankets are often needed for warmth. Older peo-

ple need protection from drafts and extreme cold. Often thermostat settings are higher than normal.

Nails become thick and tough. Feet usually have poor circulation. A nick or cut can lead to a serious infection. Nail and foot care are described in Chapter 15.

Dry skin is easily damaged and causes itching. Daily showers or tub baths are avoided. Usually a complete bath is taken twice a week. Partial baths are taken on the other days. This bathing schedule will maintain hygiene. Only mild soaps are used. Often soap is not used on the arms, legs, back, chest, and abdomen. Lotions, oils, and creams prevent drying and itching.

An older person may complain of cold feet. Socks help provide warmth. Hot water bottles and heating pads are not used. The risk of burns is very great. Fragile skin, poor circulation, and decreased sensitivity to heat and cold increase the risk of burns.

White or gray hair is common. Hair loss occurs in men. Hair thins on both men and women. Thinning occurs on the head, in the pubic area, and under the arms. Growth of facial hair (lip and chin) may occur in women. Hair is drier because of decreased scalp oils. Brushing helps stimulate circulation and oil production. Shampoo frequency depends on personal choice. Usually shampooing is less frequent than when younger. Shampooing should be done as often as necessary for hygiene and comfort.

The person and others can see skin changes. Gray hair, hair loss, brown spots, and sagging skin are some examples. These changes can affect the person's self-esteem and body image.

THE MUSCULOSKELETAL SYSTEM

The number of muscle cells decreases. Muscles atrophy and decrease in strength. Bones lose strength, become brittle, and break easily. Joints become stiff and painful. These changes result in a gradual loss of height, loss of strength, and decreased mobility.

Activity and diet can help slow the rate of these changes. Older persons need to be as active as possible. A regular exercise program is helpful. Bathing, dressing, grooming, and other daily activities are forms of physical activity. Range-of-motion exercises (see Chapter 20) also are helpful. The diet should be high in protein, calcium, and vitamins.

Remember, bones can break easily. The person should be protected from injury. Measures to prevent falls are practiced (see Chapter 9). Turn and move the person gently and carefully. A person may need help and support getting out of bed and in walking.

THE NERVOUS SYSTEM

Changes occur in the senses. Hearing and vision losses occur (see Chapter 29). The senses of taste and smell dull. Touch and sensitivity to pain and pressure are reduced. So is the ability to sense heat and cold. Injuries and diseases that normally cause severe pain may go unnoticed. The person may feel only minor discomfort. Therefore older persons are at risk for injury. They must be protected from injury. Safety measures are practiced when applying heat or cold (see Chapter 26). The skin is carefully inspected for signs of breakdown. Good skin care and the measures to prevent pressure ulcers are practiced.

Blood flow to the brain is reduced. There is also a progressive loss of brain cells. These changes affect personality and mental function. Memory is often shorter, and forgetfulness increases. The ability to respond is slowed. Confusion, dizziness, and fatigue also may occur. Older people often remember events from long ago better than recent events. Many older people are mentally active and involved in current events. They show fewer personality and mental changes. Care of the confused person is described in Chapter 32.

Less sleep is needed. Loss of energy and decreased blood flow cause fatigue. Usually older people rest or nap during the day. They usually go to bed early and get up early. Their sleep periods are shorter.

THE CARDIOVASCULAR SYSTEM

The heart muscle becomes less efficient. Blood is pumped through the body with less force. These changes may not cause problems when the person is resting. Activity, exercise, excitement, and illness increase the body's need for oxygen and nutrients. The heart may be unable to meet these needs.

Arteries lose their elasticity and become narrow. Less blood flows through them, causing poor circulation in many body parts. As a result, a weakened heart has to work harder to pump blood through the narrowed vessels.

Rest periods are needed during the day. Daily activities are planned to avoid overexertion. The person should not walk long distances, climb many stairs, or carry heavy objects. Personal care items, the television, the telephone, and other frequently used items are in handy places.

A moderate amount of daily exercise helps to stimulate circulatory, respiratory, digestive, and musculoskeletal functions. Exercise also helps to prevent blood clots (*thrombi*) in the leg veins. Many older persons engage in exercise programs. Activities include golf, walking, biking, dancing, tennis, swimming, and other forms of exercise. Active or passive range-of-motion exercises are necessary if the person is confined to bed (see Chapter 20). Some people have more severe cardiovascular changes. Doctors may order certain exercises and activity limitations.

THE RESPIRATORY SYSTEM

Respiratory muscles weaken. Lung tissue becomes less elastic and more rigid. Often lung changes are not obvious at rest. However, difficulty in breathing (*dyspnea*) may occur with activity. The person may not have enough strength to cough and clear the upper airway of secretions. Respiratory infections and diseases may develop. These can be life threatening to older persons.

Normal breathing is promoted. Heavy bed linens should not cover the chest. They can prevent normal chest expansion. Turning, repositioning, and deep breathing help prevent respiratory complications from bedrest. Breathing is usually easier in semi-Fowler's position (see Chapter 11). The person should be as active as possible.

THE DIGESTIVE SYSTEM

Many changes occur in the digestive system. Salivary glands produce less saliva. This can cause difficulty swallowing *(dysphagia)*. Taste and smell become dull. This decreases appetite. Secretion of digestive juices decreases. As a result, fried and fatty foods are hard to digest and may cause indigestion. Loss of teeth and ill-fitting dentures affect chewing. This results in digestion problems. Hard to chew foods are avoided—usually high-protein foods such as meat. Peristalsis decreases. Therefore the stomach and colon empty at a slower rate. Flatulence and constipation are common because of decreased peristalsis (see Chapter 17).

Dry, fried, and fatty foods are avoided. This helps swallowing and digestion problems. Good oral hygiene and denture care improve the ability to taste. Some people do not have natural teeth or dentures. Their food is pureed or ground. Often high-fiber foods are avoided even though they help prevent constipation. High-fiber foods are hard to chew and can irritate the intestines. They include apricots, celery, and fruits and vegetables with skins and seeds. Foods providing soft bulk are often ordered for persons with chewing problems or constipation. These foods include whole-grain cereals and cooked fruits and vegetables.

Aging requires certain diet changes. Older people need fewer calories than younger people do. Energy and activity levels are lower. More fluids are needed to aid chewing, swallowing, and digestion and for kidney function. The person needs foods that prevent constipation and bone changes. High-protein foods are needed for tissue growth and repair. However, some older persons do not eat enough protein. High-protein foods usually are costly.

THE URINARY SYSTEM

Kidney function decreases with age. Blood flow to the kidneys is reduced. The kidneys shrink *(atrophy)*. Removal of body wastes is less efficient. Poisonous substances can build up in the blood and cause serious health problems. Urine is more concentrated. This is caused by decreased kidney function and not drinking enough fluids.

Bladder muscles weaken. Bladder size decreases. Therefore the bladder holds less urine. Urinary frequency or urgency may occur. Many older persons have to urinate several times during the night. Urinary incontinence (inability to control the passage of urine from the bladder) may occur (see Chapter 16).

In men, the prostate gland enlarges. This causes pressure on the urethra. Difficulty urinating and frequent urination are common problems.

Older persons are at risk for urinary tract infections. Adequate fluids are necessary. Intake should include water, fruit juices, and milk. Personal choice in beverages is important. Most fluids should be ingested before 1700 (5:00 PM). This reduces the need to urinate during the night. Bladder training programs may be necessary for those with urinary incontinence. Indwelling catheters are sometimes needed. Urinary elimination is discussed in Chapter 16.

THE REPRODUCTIVE SYSTEM

Reproductive changes occur in both men and women. Changes occur in the reproductive structures. Hormonal changes also occur. Reproductive system changes are discussed in Chapter 34.

HOUSING OPTIONS

Most older persons live in their own homes. Many function without help. Others need assistance from family or community agencies. Often simple changes can make a person's home easier and safer to use. *(See Focus on Home Care box at top on p. 152.)*

Many in-home and community-based services are available for older persons. Many are free services funded by the Older Americans Act of 1965. Other services require a modest fee. *(See Focus on Home Care box at bottom on p. 152.)*

Some older persons choose to give up their homes; others are forced to do so. Reduced income, taxes, home repairs, and the inability to do yard work are influencing factors. Some older people retire to warmer climates. Others no longer want a large home when children are gone. Some cannot care for themselves.

Giving up a home is often very hard. Family memories, favorite gardens, neighbors, relatives, friends, churches, parks, and shopping are closely linked to a person's home and neighborhood. Moving, whether across town or to another city, brings many losses. When a person has to move, the losses are even greater.

Many housing options can meet the needs of older persons. Ideally, new living arrangements should maintain or improve the older person's quality of life. Living with family or moving to an apartment are options for some older persons.

The American Association of Retired Persons (AARP) suggests simple changes that can make an older person's home safe and easier to use. If you are working for a home care agency, the nurse will discuss needed changes with the patient and family.

FOR LOSS OF ARM OR LEG STRENGTH
- Install grab bars by showers, tubs, and toilets. These help prevent falls.
- Install non-skid strips in showers and tubs. These help prevent falls.
- Install shower or tub seats. These help prevent falls.
- Install large levers on faucets. These are easier to turn and handle.
- Install large door latches. These are easier to turn and handle.
- Install large knobs on stoves and other appliances. These are easier to turn and handle.

FOR POOR EYESIGHT
- Carpet stairs in red or yellow colors. This helps prevent falls because older people see reds and yellows better than other colors.

- Increase the wattage of light bulbs, or add more lights to rooms. This helps in reading, cooking, sewing, playing cards, and other activities that involve seeing.
- Use shades on windows and lights to avoid glares. Glares interfere with vision and can cause falls.

FOR HEARING LOSS
- Obtain text teletypewriters (TTYs), amplified telephone handsets, and extension bells to make telephone use easier. With TTYs (also called TDDs—telecommunications devices for the deaf), the hearing-impaired person receives written messages (Fig. 8-6). Amplified handsets increase sound. The caller's voice is made louder. Extension bells make the telephone ring louder. Handsets and extension bells are available wherever telephones are sold. TTYs are available through the telephone company.
- Carpet floors. The carpet absorbs noise and reduces echoes.
- Hang curtains over windows. Curtains absorb noise and reduce echoes.

In-home and community-based services assist older persons with activities of daily living. Bathing, dressing, meals, housekeeping, shopping, and transportation are some examples. Many services also provide social interaction. The American Association of Homes and Services for the Aging (AAHSA) describes the following common services available in most communities:
- *Adult day care services*—Some adult day care programs are designed for persons with Alzheimer's disease (see Chapter 32).
- *Case management*—A case manager assesses the needs of the older person and family. Needed services are determined. Then the case manager arranges for the needed services.
- *Meal programs*—Nutritious meals are provided in-home or in a senior center. Home delivery programs are often called "Meals-on-Wheels" programs.
- *Financial counseling*—The person is assisted with balancing a checkbook, paying bills, filing income taxes, and completing insurance forms.
- *Companionship services*—A volunteer makes friendly visits in the older person's home. Supervision and support services are provided as needed.
- *Health maintenance and screening*—Blood pressure, blood sugar, and other measurements are done to promote health. Such services are usually provided at a senior center, church, or other community agency.
- *Home health care*—Nursing, physical therapy, occupational therapy, and speech therapy are provided. So are housekeeping and medical equipment services.

- *Homemaker or chore housekeeper services*—A homemaker or chore housekeeper helps with housekeeping and meals. Some shovel snow and wash floors, windows, and walls.
- *Hospice care*—See Chapter 1. Nursing, comfort, and homemaker services are provided.
- *Personal care*—The older person is assisted in meeting personal care needs. These include eating, hygiene (oral care and bathing), grooming, and dressing.
- *Rehabilitation*—Necessary therapies are given to assist the person to regain or maintain his or her highest level of functioning.
- *Senior centers*—Offer a variety of social and recreational activities. Many centers offer continuing education courses, day trips, travel groups, performing arts, and nature activities. Other services include meals, counseling, legal assistance, health screenings, and transportation.
- *Senior companion program*—Volunteers provide social contact and assist and support frail older persons.
- *Telephone reassurance*—Regular telephone contact is provided. A telephone call is made to check on the older person at various times throughout the day. If the person does not answer, someone is sent to the person's home. Also, the older person can call the service when help is needed.
- *Transportation*—Services help older persons get to and from doctor visits, appointments, shopping, church, and other places.

Fig. 8-6 A hearing-impaired person uses a teletypewriter to communicate with a caller using a standard telephone. Required by the Americans With Disabilities Act of 1990, every state must provide access to Telecommunications Relay Services (TRS). A communications assistant relays messages between the caller and the hearing-impaired person. Messages are typed to the hearing-impaired person. They are relayed orally to the caller. The communications assistant must relay everything that is said and maintain the confidentiality of all conversations.

Fig. 8-7 An adult day care center.

LIVING WITH FAMILY

Sometimes older brothers, sisters, and cousins live together. They provide companionship for each other. They can also share living expenses. They can care for each other during illness or disability. One may have the role of caregiver if the other is ill or disabled.

Some older people live with their adult children. The older parent or parents move in with the child, or the child moves into the parent's home. The parent may be healthy, may need some supervision, or may be ill or disabled. Some adult children are caregivers for ill or disabled parents. Often children assume the caregiver role to avoid nursing home care. They try the caregiver role first. A nursing center is an option if they cannot give needed care.

Living with an adult child is a social change. The parent, the adult child, and the child's family all need to adjust. Sleeping arrangements may change if there is no spare bedroom. The parent may need a hospital bed. It may need to go in a living room, dining room, or bedroom.

The adult child's family still needs time alone. Other brothers, sisters, and family members may help give care. *Respite care* is an option. Respite means a break, rest, or lull. Respite care is when the person is admitted to a nursing center or home care is obtained for a few days or weeks. Caregivers can have a vaca-

tion, rest, or simply take a break from the stress of giving care. Many community and church groups have volunteers who can help give care.

Adult Day Care Centers. Adult children may need to work even though the older parent cannot stay alone. Adult day care centers provide meals, supervision, and activities for older persons. Some provide transportation to and from the center.

Requirements vary. Some may require that the person be able to walk using a cane or walker if needed. Others allow wheelchairs. Most require that the person be capable of some self-care activities.

Many activities are available. Examples include cards, board games, movies, crafts, dancing, walks, and lectures (Fig. 8-7). Some provide bowling and swimming. All activities are supervised. Assistance is given as needed.

ELDER COTTAGE HOUSING OPPORTUNITY

Elder Cottage Housing Opportunity (ECHO) homes are housing options listed by the American Association of Retired Persons (AARP). These small homes are designed to meet the needs of older and disabled persons. The home is a portable unit that is placed in the yard of a single-family home. The older person lives independently but near family or friends.

APARTMENTS

Apartments have some advantages for older persons. The owner is responsible for maintenance, yard work, snow removal, and major appliance repair. The older person is independent. Personal belongings are kept. However, rent and utility bills are costly. Many older persons enjoy gardening and yard work (Fig. 8-8, p. 154). Apartment living usually does not provide those opportunities.

Fig. 8-8 This man enjoys gardening. Apartment living usually does not provide opportunities for gardening or other yard work.

An *accessory apartment* is an apartment in a home. A home is built or remodeled to include an area that includes a bedroom, bathroom, and kitchen. Some have a small living area. The older person lives independently but is very near other people. Sometimes children have accessory apartments for older parents. Or the older person's home may have an accessory apartment. Renting the home or apartment gives the older person additional income.

Senior rental apartments are designed for older persons. They are usually near shopping, churches, and other community services. Many provide security services and transportation. Some provide meals in a central dining room.

SENIOR CITIZEN HOUSING

State and federal funds have helped build apartment complexes for senior citizens. It is often called *congregate housing*. (Congregate means a group, a gathering, or a cluster.) An older person or couple can live independently in an apartment near people of the same age. The buildings have wheelchair access, handrails, elevators, and other safety measures. Some apartments are furnished. Appliances are arranged to meet the special needs of older persons.

Many services are available. A dining room and a nurse or doctor on call are common. A daily telephone call is made to check on each tenant. Transportation is usually available to church, the doctor, or shopping areas. Tenants pay monthly rent. However, the rent is usually less than that for a regular apartment if government funds are involved.

RESIDENTIAL HOTELS

Some cities have residential hotels. Private rooms or efficiency apartments are rented. Food services may include a dining room, cafeteria, or room service. Some hotels provide recreational activities and emergency medical services. Most hotels are close to shopping areas, churches, and other civic services.

ASSISTED LIVING

Assisted living facilities are designed for persons who need help with activities of daily living. A group of residents live together. They have their own rooms but share dining and living room areas. Residents are usually ambulatory (able to walk) but need help with meals, personal care, medications, laundry, and housekeeping. Health care, 24-hour oversight, and social contact with staff and other residents are provided in a homelike setting. Nursing care is not provided.

Some states require that assisted living facilities be licensed. The license helps ensure that the facility meets certain quality, safety, and upkeep standards.

Assisted living facilities may be part of a retirement community, nursing center, or senior citizen housing. Assisted living facilities also are called:

- Board and care homes
- Personal care homes
- Sheltered housing
- Adult care homes
- Residential care

CONTINUING CARE RETIREMENT COMMUNITIES

Continuing care retirement communities (CCRCs) offer a wide range of services from independent living units to 24-hour nursing care. The American Association of Homes and Services for the Aging (AAHSA) describes a CCRC as part housing complex, part activity center, and part health care system. It meets the changing needs of older persons living alone or with a partner. CCRCs usually provide the following:

- Nursing care and other health care services
- Meals (including special diets)
- Housekeeping services
- Transportation
- Personal assistance
- Recreational and educational activities

Independent living units are small apartments. Residents perform self-care activities and take their own medications. Food services are available, and help is nearby if needed. However, each person takes care of himself or herself. Little supervision or help is needed. Many older persons have their own cars. They travel or drive about in the community as desired. Transportation is provided for those without a car or unable to drive.

As the person's needs change, more services are added. When nursing care is needed, the person moves to the nursing center within the community. Many older couples find comfort in this arrangement. When one partner needs nursing care, the other is still very close and can visit often.

Fig. 8-9 The atmosphere of a nursing center is as homelike as possible.

Box 8-1	Features of a Quality Nursing Center

- The center has a current operating license from the state.
- The administrator has a current state license.
- The center is certified for Medicare and Medicaid.
- The location suits the person. Family and friends can visit easily.
- The center has safety features (see Chapter 9). Examples include hand rails in hallways and grab bars in bathrooms and showers.
- The center has clearly marked and unobstructed exits.
- The center meets state and federal fire codes.
- Resident rooms open to the hallway.
- Resident rooms have windows.
- A doctor is available for emergencies.
- No heavy odors are present. The center does not use scented sprays to mask odors.
- Hallways are wide enough so that two wheelchairs can pass with ease.
- Wheelchair ramps provide easy access into and out of the center.
- The kitchen has separate areas for food preparation, garbage, and dishwashing.
- The kitchen has adequate refrigerator space for food.
- Toilet facilities can be accessed by wheelchair.
- Dining rooms are attractive and allow wheelchair use.
- Food looks and smells good.
- Residents receive needed help with eating.
- Residents look clean.
- Residents are dressed appropriately for activities inside or outside the center.
- The center has attractive gardens and landscaping.
- The center has an activity area for resident use.
- Staff are friendly and well groomed.
- The center meets OBRA requirements.

Modified from *Choosing a quality nursing home*, American Association of Homes and Services for the Aging, 1995.

The resident signs a contract with the CCRC. The contract is for a certain period or for the person's lifetime. The contract lists the services provided and the required fees.

NURSING CENTERS

Nursing centers are housing options for persons who cannot care for themselves. Nursing centers offer different levels of care. Some merely provide room, food, and laundry services. Others provide nursing, rehabilitation, dietary, recreational, social, and religious services.

Some people stay in nursing centers the rest of their lives. Others stay until they can return home. The nursing center is the person's temporary or perma-

nent home. The surroundings are as homelike as possible (Fig. 8-9).

Nursing centers are designed to meet the special needs of older and disabled persons. Physical changes of aging and safety needs (see Chapter 9) are considered in the center's design and construction. The programs and services offered meet the person's basic needs. Box 8-1 lists the features of a quality nursing center.

Nursing centers are privately owned or operated by the government. In either case, state and federal agencies monitor the care given. The center must follow the state and federal standards required by law. Surveyors make periodic inspections that are expected or unannounced.

Box 8-2   OBRA Environment Requirements

SUFFICIENT SPACE AND EQUIPMENT

- Dining space with easy access and appropriate tables and chairs
- Program areas with easy access; appropriate exercise and other equipment
- Recreational areas with easy access and sufficient space for movement and storage of equipment and supplies
- Toilet facilities with easy access and located nearby
- Functional and comfortable furniture for residents, families, and visitors
- Tables of proper height
- Chairs that provide comfort and allow ease of sitting and standing
- Halls with handrails and easy access for wheelchairs, walkers, and other space and safety needs

QUALITY OF LIFE AND COMFORT IN THE ENVIRONMENT

- Clean and orderly halls, dining, health services, program and recreational areas, bathroom facilities
- Odor-free environment
- Temperature between 71° and 81° F
- Acceptable noise level
- Adequate ventilation and humidity
- No glare from environment and proper lighting
- Music, television as requested by the resident or family
- Paint color or wallpaper appealing to residents
- Pest-free, hazard-free environment
- Resident's needs and independence accommodated
- Clean, soft, and adequate linens for resident
- Posted signs to identify nonsmoking areas

RESIDENT ROOMS

- See Chapter 12

SAFETY

- See Chapter 9

From Jaffe MS: *The OBRA guidelines for quality improvement,* ed 2, 1996, Skidmore-Roth, Aurora, Colo.

Most nursing centers receive Medicare or Medicaid funds. Such centers must meet the requirements of the Omnibus Budget Reconciliation Act of 1987 (OBRA). Unannounced surveys are conducted to determine if nursing centers are meeting OBRA requirements. Funding is lost if the many requirements are not met. OBRA requirements are described throughout this book. Box 8-2 lists the OBRA requirements for a center's physical environment.

Hospital Long-Term Care Units. Many hospitals have long-term care units. These units are for persons who still need skilled care but not to the extent required previously. At one time these persons went to nursing centers. Now they can receive skilled care on the long-term care unit. Some eventually go home. Others may go to nursing centers.

OBRA REQUIREMENTS

The Omnibus Budget Reconciliation Act of 1987 is concerned with the quality of life, health, and safety of residents. Nursing centers must provide care in a manner and in a setting that maintains or improves each person's quality of life, health, and safety. Nursing assistant training and competency evaluation are OBRA requirements (see Chapter 2). The center must meet many other requirements.

RESIDENT RIGHTS

Nursing center residents have certain rights under federal and state laws. Residents have rights as citizens of the United States. They also have rights relating to their everyday lives and care in a nursing center. Nursing centers must protect and promote resident rights. Residents must be free to exercise their rights without center interference. Some residents are incompetent (not able) and cannot exercise their rights. Legal representatives exercise rights for them.

Nursing centers must inform residents of their rights. They must be informed orally and in writing. Such information is given before or during admission to the center. It must be given in the language used and understood by the resident.

Resident rights that relate to your roles and responsibilities are discussed here.

Information. The right to information means access to all records about the resident. Such records include the person's medical record, contracts, incident reports, and financial records. The request for any record can be oral or written. The record must be available within 24 hours of the request. The center has 2 working days to provide requested photocopies.

The resident or legal representative also has the right to be fully informed of the person's total health condition. Such information is given in language the person can understand. Interpreters are used for those speaking a language other than English. Sign language or other aids are used for those with hearing impairments.

The resident or legal representative must also have information about the resident's doctor. This includes the doctor's name and specialty and how to contact the doctor.

You need to report any request for information to the nurse. Remember, you *do not* give the information just described to the resident or family (see Chapter 2).

Refusing Treatment. The resident has the right to refuse treatment. Like hospital patients, the resident also has the right to refuse to take part in research. OBRA defines treatment as care provided to relieve symptoms, improve functional level, or maintain or restore health. A person who does not give consent or refuses treatment cannot be given the treatment. However, the center must find out what the person is refusing and why. Through teaching and clarifying, the center should try to educate the person about the treatment, problems from not having the treatment, and other treatment choices. Although a person may refuse a specific treatment, the center must provide all other services. Changes in the resident's care plan may be needed.

Advance directives are also part of the right to refuse treatment. They include living wills or other instructions about life support. Advance directives are discussed in Chapter 37.

Like requests for information, you need to report any treatment refusal to the nurse.

Privacy and Confidentiality. The rights to privacy and confidentiality are discussed in Chapter 2. They are also presented under the Patient's Bill of Rights in Chapter 5. OBRA also provides for privacy and confidentiality.

Residents have the right to personal privacy. The resident's body must not be exposed unnecessarily. Only staff directly involved in care, treatments, or examinations are present. The person must give consent for others to be present. For example, a student wants to observe a procedure or treatment. The person's consent is needed for the student to observe. A person also has the right to use the bathroom in private. Privacy also is maintained for personal care activities.

Residents have the right to visit with others in private. They have the right to visit in an area where they cannot be seen or heard by others. The center must try to provide private space when it is requested. Offices, chapels, dining rooms, meeting rooms, activity rooms, and conference rooms are used if available.

The right to visit in privacy also involves telephone conversations (Fig. 8-10). Residents also have the right to send and receive mail without interference by others. Letters sent and received by the resident are not opened by others without the resident's consent. Mail is delivered to the resident within 24 hours of its delivery to the center.

Information about the resident's care, treatment, and condition is kept confidential. Medical and financial records are also confidential. The person must give consent for them to be released to other agencies or persons. However, consent is not needed for the release of medical records when the resident is transferred to another agency. Records also are released

Fig. 8-10 Resident talking privately on a telephone.

Fig. 8-11 Resident choosing what clothing to wear.

without the resident's consent when they are required by law or for insurance purposes.

Throughout this book you are reminded to provide privacy. You are reminded also to keep information about the person confidential. Providing for privacy and confidentiality shows respect for the person. It also protects the person's dignity.

Personal Choice. OBRA requires that residents be free to choose their own doctors. They also have the right to take part in planning their own care and treatment. This means that residents have the right to make decisions about their own care and treatment. It also means that they have the right to choose activities, schedules, and care based on their personal preferences. For example, residents have the right to choose when to get up and go to bed, what to wear, how to spend their time, and what to eat (Fig. 8-11). They are also free to choose companions and visitors inside and outside the center.

Personal choice is important for quality of life, dignity, and self-respect. The individual's personal preference is emphasized throughout this book. You need to allow the person's preferences whenever safely possible.

Disputes and Grievances. Residents have the right to voice concerns, questions, and complaints about treatment or care. The dispute or grievance may involve another resident. It may be about treatment or care that was not given. The center must promptly try to correct the matter. The resident must not be punished in any way for voicing the dispute or grievance.

Work. The resident has rights that relate to performing work for the center. The person does not work to receive care, items, or other things or privileges. There is no requirement that the resident must perform services for the center.

However, the resident *can* work or perform services if the desire or need for work is part of the person's care plan. The resident may like being active—gardening, doing repairs, building, sewing, mending, or cooking. The person may want to work. Another resident may need to work for rehabilitation or activity purposes. In either case, the desire for work or the need for work becomes part of the person's care plan.

The care plan should specify:

- The reason for the work—desire or need
- What work will be done
- If the services are paid or voluntary

Participation in Resident and Family Groups. Residents have the right to take part in resident and family groups. This means that residents have the right to form groups. And a resident's family has the right to meet with the families of other residents. These groups can discuss concerns and offer ideas to improve quality of life in the center. They can also plan activities for residents and families. Or the groups can provide support and reassurance for group members. Residents also have the right to take part in social, cultural, religious, and community activities. They have the right to help in getting to and from activities of their choice.

Care and Security of Personal Possessions. Residents have the right to keep and use personal items. This includes clothing and some furnishings. Available space and the health and safety of other residents affect the type and amount of personal items allowed. A person's property is treated with care and respect. Though the items may not have value to you, they are important to the resident. They also relate to personal choice, dignity, and quality of life.

The center must take reasonable measures to protect the person's property. Items are labeled with the person's name. And the center must investigate reports of lost, stolen, or damaged items. Police help is sometimes needed. The resident and family are usually advised not to keep jewelry and other costly items in the center.

You must protect yourself and the center from being accused of stealing a person's property. Do not go through a resident's closet, drawers, purse, or other space without the person's knowledge and consent. Have a staff member with you and the resident (or legal representative) present if you must inspect closets and drawers. The staff member serves as a witness to your activities.

Freedom From Abuse, Mistreatment, and Neglect. OBRA states that residents have the right to be free from verbal, sexual, physical, or mental abuse (see Chapter 2). They also have the right to be free from involuntary seclusion. **Involuntary seclusion** is separating a person from others against his or her will. It can also mean keeping the person confined to a certain area or away from his or her room without consent. If the person is incompetent, involuntary seclusion occurs against the legal representative's consent.

No one can abuse, neglect, or mistreat the resident. This includes center staff, volunteers, staff from other agencies or groups, other residents, family, visitors, and legal guardians. Nursing centers must have policies and procedures for investigating suspected or reported cases of resident abuse. Also, nursing centers cannot employ persons who were convicted of abusing, neglecting, or mistreating other individuals.

Freedom From Restraints. Residents have the right not to have body movements restricted. Body movements are restricted by the application of restraints or the administration of certain drugs. Some drugs can restrain the person because they affect mood, behavior, and mental function. Sometimes residents require restraints to protect them from harming themselves or others. A doctor's order is necessary for using restraints. Restraints cannot be used for staff convenience or to discipline a resident. Restraints are discussed in Chapter 9.

Box 8-3   OBRA Required Actions to Promote the Resident's Dignity and Privacy

COURTEOUS AND DIGNIFIED INTERACTIONS WITH RESIDENTS
- Use appropriate tone of voice
- Use good eye contact when interacting with the resident
- Stand or sit close enough to the resident as appropriate
- Use proper name and title of resident
- Obtain resident's attention before interacting with the resident
- Use touch if approved by the resident
- Respect the resident's social status, and listen with interest to what the resident is saying
- Do not yell, scold, or embarrass the resident

COURTEOUS AND DIGNIFIED CARE TO RESIDENTS
- Groom hair, beards, and nails as the resident wishes
- Assist with dressing in clothing appropriate to time of day and resident's personal choice
- Promote resident independence and dignity in dining
- Respect resident's private space and property
- Assist with ambulation and transfer without interfering with independence
- Assist with bathing and personal hygiene preferences without interfering with independence
  - Neat and clean appearance
  - Clean shaven or groomed beard
  - Nails trimmed and clean

- Dentures, hearing aid, glasses, and other prostheses used as appropriate
- Clothing clean and properly fitted and fastened
- Shoes and hose properly applied and fastened
- Extra clothing for warmth as needed such as sweater or lap blanket

PRIVACY AND SELF-DETERMINATION OF RESIDENTS
- Drape properly during personal care and procedures to avoid exposure and embarrassment
- Drape properly in chair
- Use curtains or screens during personal care and procedures
- Close door to room during care and procedures or as person desires
- Knock on door before entering, and wait to be asked in
- Provide privacy during doctor examination with draping and curtains or screen
- Close bathroom door when person uses bathroom

MAINTAIN PERSONAL CHOICE AND INDEPENDENCE
- Resident smokes in designated areas
- Resident participates in activities according to interests
- Resident is involved in scheduling activities and care
- Resident gives input into plan of care regarding preferences and independence
- Resident is involved in room or roommate change

QUALITY OF LIFE

OBRA requires that nursing centers care for residents in a manner that promotes dignity, self-worth, and physical, psychological, and emotional well-being. Protecting resident rights is one way to promote quality of life. Personal choice, privacy, participation in group activities, having personal property, and freedom from restraint show respect for the person.

The resident is also spoken to in a polite and courteous manner (see Chapter 5). Giving good, honest, and thoughtful care enhances the person's quality of life.

Box 8-3 lists actions that show concern for the person's dignity and privacy. These actions are required by OBRA. Surveyors check to make sure that these actions are shown in the person's care.

Activities. Activities are important for a resident's quality of life. OBRA requires that nursing centers provide activity programs that meet the interests and physical, mental, and psychosocial needs of each person. Such activities must allow personal choice and promote physical, intellectual, social, and emotional well-being. Many centers also provide religious services for spiritual health. You will assist residents to and from activity programs. You may also be assigned to help residents with activities.

Environment. The center's environment must also promote quality of life. The environment must be clean, safe, and as homelike as possible. Allowing the person to have personal items enhances quality of life. It allows personal choice and promotes a homelike setting. The safe environment is discussed in Chapter 9. The resident's room is discussed in Chapter 12.

Circle the BEST answer.

1. Retirement usually results in
   A. Lowered income
   B. Physical changes from aging
   C. Companionship and usefulness
   D. Financial security

2. Which does *not* cause loneliness in older persons?
   A. Children moving away
   B. The death of family and friends
   C. Problems communicating with others
   D. Contact with other older persons

3. When older people live with their children they often feel
   A. Independent
   B. Wanted and a part of things
   C. Useless
   D. Dignified

4. Death of a partner results in the loss of a
   A. Friend
   B. Lover
   C. Companion
   D. All of the above

5. Changes occur in the skin with aging. Care should include the following *except*
   A. Providing for warmth
   B. Applying lotion
   C. Using soap daily
   D. Providing good skin care

6. An older person has cold feet. You should
   A. Provide socks
   B. Apply a hot water bottle
   C. Soak the feet in hot water
   D. Apply a heating pad

7. Changes occur in the musculoskeletal system with aging. Which is *false?*
   A. Bones become brittle and can break easily.
   B. Bedrest is needed because of loss of strength.
   C. Joints become stiff and painful.
   D. Range-of-motion exercises help to slow the rate of the musculoskeletal changes.

8. Reduced blood supply to the brain can result in the following *except*
   A. Confusion
   B. Dizziness
   C. Improved memory
   D. Fatigue

9. Changes occur in the nervous system. Which is *true?*
   A. More sleep is needed than when younger.
   B. Recent events are remembered better than past events.
   C. Sensitivity to pain is reduced.
   D. Confusion occurs in every older person.

10. Arteries lose their elasticity and become narrow. These changes result in
    A. A slower heart rate
    B. Lower blood pressure
    C. Poor circulation to many body parts
    D. Less blood in the body

11. An older person has cardiovascular changes. Care includes the following *except*
    A. Placing personal items nearby
    B. A moderate amount of daily exercise
    C. Planning activities to avoid exertion
    D. Walking long distances

12. Respiratory changes occur with aging. Which is *false?*
    A. Heavy bed linens prevent normal chest expansion.
    B. The person is turned and repositioned frequently if on bedrest.
    C. The side-lying position is best for breathing.
    D. The person should be as active as possible.

13. Older persons should avoid dry foods because of
    A. Decreases in saliva
    B. Loss of teeth or ill-fitting dentures
    C. Decreased amounts of digestive juices
    D. Decreased peristalsis

14. Changes occur in the digestive system. The older person should avoid the following *except*
    A. Fruits and vegetables with skins and seed
    B. Dry and fatty foods
    C. Raw apricots and celery
    D. Protein foods

15. The doctor ordered increased fluid intake for an older person. You should
    A. Give most of the fluid before 1700 (5:00 PM)
    B. Provide mostly water
    C. Start a bladder training program
    D. Insert an indwelling urinary catheter

16. You are working in a nursing center. You must
    A. Open a resident's mail
    B. Choose what the resident wears
    C. Provide for the resident's privacy
    D. Search the resident's closet and drawers

17. Who decides how to style a resident's hair?
    A. The resident
    B. The nurse
    C. The nursing assistant
    D. The family

18. Which statement is *false?*
    A. Residents can offer suggestions to improve the center.
    B. Residents can be restrained to prevent them from leaving the center.
    C. Residents must be free from abuse, neglect, and mistreatment.
    D. Allowing personal choice is important for the resident's quality of life.

Answers to these questions are on p. 834.

CHAPTER

9

SAFETY

OBJECTIVES

Define the key terms listed in this chapter

Describe accident risk factors

Identify safety precautions for infants and children

Describe the safety measures for preventing falls, burns, poisoning, and suffocation

Explain why a person is identified before receiving care and how to accurately identify a person

Explain how to prevent equipment accidents

Explain the purpose and complications of restraints and how to use them safely

Identify restraint alternatives

Explain how to handle hazardous substances

Describe the safety measures related to fire prevention and the use of oxygen

Explain what to do if a fire occurs

Give examples of natural and human-made disasters

Explain how to protect yourself from workplace violence

Describe your role in risk management

Perform the procedures described in this chapter

KEY TERMS

active physical restraint A restraint attached to the person's body and to a stationary (non-movable) object; movement and access to one's body are restricted

coma A state of being unaware of one's surroundings and being unable to react or respond to people, places, or things

disaster A sudden catastrophic event in which many people are injured and killed and property is destroyed

ground That which carries leaking electricity to the earth and away from an electrical appliance

hazardous substance Any chemical that presents a physical hazard or a health hazard in the workplace

hemiplegia Paralysis on one side of the body

paraplegia Paralysis from the waist down

passive physical restraint A restraint near but not directly attached to the person's body; it does not totally restrict freedom of movement and allows access to certain body parts

quadriplegia Paralysis from the neck down

restraint Any item, object, device, garment, material, or chemical that restricts a person's freedom of movement or access to one's body

suffocation When breathing stops from the lack of oxygen

workplace violence Any physical assault or threatening behavior or verbal abuse that occurs in a work setting

Safety is a basic need. In a safe setting, a person has little risk of illness or injury. The person feels safe and secure physically and mentally. Risk of falling, burns, poisoning, or other injuries is low. The person and the person's property are safe from fire and intruders. The person is not afraid and has few worries and concerns.

ACCIDENT RISK FACTORS

Certain factors increase a person's risk for injury. Age, poor vision, and loss of hearing are some examples. Some people cannot protect themselves. They rely on others for safety.

- *Awareness of surroundings*—People must be aware of their surroundings to protect themselves from injury. Some persons are unconscious or in a **coma**. A person in a coma cannot react or respond to people, places, or things. Other people must protect the person. Confused and disoriented persons may not understand what is happening to and around them (see Chapter 32). They can harm themselves and others.
- *Vision*—People with poor vision are at risk for falls. They can trip on toys, rugs, furniture, or electrical cords. They also may have problems reading labels on medicines, cleaners, and other containers. Taking the wrong medicine, the wrong dose, or poisoning can result.
- *Hearing*—Hearing-impaired persons have problems hearing explanations and instructions. For example, a person does not hear well and takes the wrong drug or takes it the wrong way. The person may not hear fire alarms, sirens, weather warnings, car horns, and oncoming cars. In health care settings, they may not hear approaching meal carts, medicine carts, stretchers, or people in wheelchairs. The person does not know to move to safety.
- *Smell and touch*—Illness and aging affect smell and touch. The person may have problems smelling smoke or gas. Persons with a reduced sense of touch are easily burned. They have problems sensing heat and cold.

- *Paralysis*—**Paraplegia** is paralysis from the waist down. **Quadriplegia** is paralysis from the neck down. **Hemiplegia** is paralysis on one side of the body. Paralyzed persons may not sense pain, heat, or cold. They may be aware of danger but are unable to move to safety.
- *Medications*—Drugs have side effects. Loss of balance, dizziness, light-headedness, difficulty concentrating, vision changes, reduced awareness, confusion, disorientation, drowsiness, and loss of coordination are some examples. The person may be fearful or uncooperative or act in unusual ways as a result.
- *Age*—Children and older persons are at risk for injuries. (*See Focus on Children box and Focus on Older Persons box.*)

Text continued on p. 168

Focus On... CHILDREN

Infants are helpless. Other people must protect them. Young children have not learned the difference between safety and danger. They normally explore their surroundings, put objects in their mouths, and touch and feel new things. Therefore they are at risk for falls, poisoning, choking, burns, and other accidents. Practice the safety measures listed in Box 9-1 when caring for infants and children. Also practice the safety measures to prevent falls, burns, poisoning, and suffocation.

Focus On... OLDER PERSONS

The physical changes of aging increase the older person's risk for injury. Movements are slower and less steady. Balance may be affected. Decreased sensitivity to heat and cold, poor vision, hearing problems, and a decreased sense of smell are common in older persons. Confusion, poor judgment, memory problems, and disorientation may occur (see Chapter 32).

Box 9-1   Safety Measures for Infants and Children

- Do not leave infants or young children unattended. They need supervision when in strollers, walkers, high chairs, infant carrier seats, bathtubs, infant swings, playpens, and wading pools and when playing outside.
- Use baby walkers only on smooth surfaces. Edges on carpets and throw rugs can cause the walker to tip over. So can carpet moldings and raised thresholds.
- Use the safety strap to fasten a child in a high chair or infant carrier seat.
- Lock the high chair tray after putting the child in the chair.
- Keep high chairs away from stoves, tables, and counters.
- Do not leave children unattended while they are eating.
- Check children in cribs often.
- Make sure crib rails are up and locked in place.
- Keep one hand on a child lying in a crib, on a scale, or on a table if you must look away for a moment (Fig. 9-1, p. 166).
- Make sure bunk beds are fastened and supported properly.
- Keep electrical appliances away from sinks, tubs, toilets, and other water sources.
- Unplug all appliances when not in use.
- Place safety plugs in electrical outlets (Fig. 9-2, p. 166). The plugs prevent children from sticking their fingers or small objects into the openings.
- Keep electrical cords and electrical equipment out of the reach of children.
- Keep cords for window drapes, blinds, and shades out of the reach of children. Be careful where you place cribs and playpens.
- Do not hang items with strings, cords, or elastic cords around cribs or playpens.
- Keep childproof caps on medicine containers, cleaners, and other hazardous substances.
- Store cleaners, medicines, and hazardous substances in their original containers.
- Store cleaners, medicines, and hazardous substances in locked storage areas that are beyond the reach of children (Fig. 9-3, p. 167). This includes items stored in basements and garages.
- Store knives (including kitchen knives), razor blades, matches, guns, and other dangerous items in locked storage areas beyond the reach of children.
- Supervise any child who is in or near water. This includes tubs, toilets, sinks, swimming pools, hot tubs, spas, and whirlpools.
- Keep bathroom doors closed to prevent drowning in toilets or bathtubs.
- Keep sinks, tubs, and basins empty when not in use.
- Keep buckets empty and upside down when not in use.
- Keep toilet lids down. Use safety locks that prevent children from lifting the lid.
- Keep diaper pails locked.
- Keep bedroom doors closed. This prevents children from getting into bedrooms of older children and parents. These bedrooms may contain toys, perfumes, and other items that present choking, poisoning, burn, and suffocation hazards to young children.
- Keep a locked safety cover on spas, hot tubs, and whirlpools when not in use.
- Remove pool, spa, hot tub, and whirlpool covers before use. The cover must be completely off. Otherwise the child can get trapped under it.
- Remove steps to above-ground pools when not in use.
- Have a telephone at poolside for emergencies. Also have a phone near spas, hot tubs, and whirlpools.
- Keep rescue equipment near pools.
- Do not allow children to dive into above-ground pools. They are too shallow.
- Do not allow children to dive from the side of an in-ground pool. Children should enter feet first because the area is too shallow.
- Allow children to dive only from the diving board. Children should dive with their hands in front of them.
- Do not allow children to slide down a pool slide head first. Head injuries can occur.
- Prevent hair entanglement or body part entrapment in suction and drain covers in pools, spas, hot tubs, and whirlpools. If hair becomes caught, the person's head is kept underwater. Trapped body parts also can keep the person underwater or cause serious injury. Have suction and drain covers installed that meet current safety standards. Also have missing or broken covers replaced. Do not let children play near drain or suction covers.
- Know where to find the electrical cut-off switch for pools, spas, hot tubs, and whirlpools. This allows you to quickly turn off the electricity in an emergency.
- Keep the temperature of hot tubs, spas, and whirlpools no higher than 104° F. Higher temperatures can cause drowsiness, which can lead to drowning. Higher temperatures also can cause heat stroke and death.
- Keep your car locked, trunk closed, and your car keys in a safe place out of the reach of children. Children can open a car or car trunk with a key that has remote controls. Children like to play hide-and-seek in cars and car trunks. Children can easily suffocate from high temperatures in the car or trunk.
- Do not leave children unattended in a car, truck, van, or other motor vehicle. Children can develop heat related illness, suffocate, and die very quickly from high temperatures in the vehicle. It only takes a few minutes for death to occur.
- Do not prop baby bottles on a rolled towel or blanket. Hold the baby and bottle during feedings.
- Keep plastic bags and wraps away from children. They can cause suffocation.

Continued

Box 9-1 **Safety Measures for Infants and Children—cont'd**

- Use guardrails at the top and bottom of stairs to prevent small children from climbing up and down stairs. Make sure the child cannot get caught in the guardrails.
- Do not use pins on children's clothing.
- Remove drawstrings from jackets, coats, sweaters, and other clothing. This includes drawstrings on the hood, at the neckline, and at the waist. Drawstrings can get tangled or caught in play equipment, furniture, hand rails, car and bus doors, escalators, and other moving devices.
- Do not dress children in loose clothing or clothing that has drawstrings, fringe, strings, or ties if they will play on playground equipment. The clothing can get caught on the playground equipment.
- Do not let children wear necklaces, strings, cords, or other items around the neck. These can get caught on furniture, doorknobs, and playground equipment.
- Do not let children play on curbs or behind parked cars. They should not play in piles of leaves or snow near heavy traffic.
- Make sure children wear helmets when riding tricycles and bicycles.
- Keep children away from exercise bikes. A child's finger can be amputated by touching a moving exercise bike.
- Read all warning labels on toys.
- Check age recommendations on toys. Give children only age-appropriate toys.
- Check toys and other play equipment regularly.
- Use federally approved car restraints that fit the child's size and weight. (Fig. 9-4). *Infant car seats are installed rear-facing only* (Fig. 9-5). Children less than 20 pounds must ride facing the rear of the vehicle. Rear-facing car seats are never used in the front seat of a vehicle with an air bag (Fig. 9-6).
- Follow seat-belt laws.
- Prevent furniture from tipping over onto children. Injuries and deaths can occur from children falling on, leaning on, climbing on, pulling on, sitting on, or trying to move poorly secured furniture. TV carts, bookcases, stands, chest of drawers, and tables present dangers. Make sure TVs are placed on low stands and are as far back on the stand as possible. Make sure that angle braces or anchors are used to secure furniture to walls.
- Do not use tablecloths. This prevents infants and young children from pulling things off the table and onto themselves. Center pieces, items on the table, and hot food and liquids can injure the child.
- Do not use toy chests with free-falling lids. Such a lid can fall on the child's head or neck. The lid should have a spring-loaded lid support or sliding panels.
- Keep children away from open windows. Window screens are not strong enough to prevent children from falling out windows.
- Do not place furniture near windows. This prevents children from climbing from furniture onto a window seat or sill.
- Protect the child from falls (see Box 9-3).
- Protect the child from burns (see Box 9-4).
- Protect the child from poisoning (see Box 9-5).
- Protect the child from choking and suffocating (see Box 9-6).
- See Chapter 35 for other infant safety measures.

Fig. 9-1 Keep one hand on the child if you need to look away momentarily.

Fig. 9-2 Safety plug in an electrical outlet.

A   B

Fig. 9-3 **A,** Household cleaners are within a child's reach when placed in low cabinets. They should be kept in high, locked cabinets not used to store food. **B,** The bathroom medicine chest holds many medicine containers. Like household products, they should be in high, locked places out of the reach of children.

Fig. 9-4 Federally approved infant car restraints carry this label.

Fig. 9-5 Child in a car restraint.

Fig. 9-6 An air bag could injure an infant. (*From* Wong: Whaley and Wong's nursing care of infants and children, *ed 6, 1999, St Louis, Mosby.*)

SAFETY MEASURES

Common sense and simple safety measures can prevent most accidents. You must protect patients and residents, yourself, and co-workers from accidents and injuries. The safety measures in this section apply to everyday life. They also apply to hospital, long-term care, and home settings. The nursing care plan lists other safety measures needed by the person.

PREVENTING FALLS

Most falls occur in bedrooms and bathrooms. They are caused by throw rugs, poor lighting, cluttered floors, furniture that is out of place, and pets underfoot. Slippery floors, bathtubs, and showers are other causes. Needing to urinate also is a major cause of falls. For example, Mrs. Ford has an urgent need to urinate. She falls trying to get out of bed quickly and without help.

The risk of falling increases with age. Most falls are in persons between the ages of 65 and 85. A history of falls increases a person's risk of falling.

Most falls occur in the evening, between 1800 (6:00 PM) and 2100 (9:00 PM). Falls also are more likely during shift changes. Shift changes usually occur between 0600 (6:00 AM) and 0800 (8:00 AM), 1400 (2:00 PM) and 1600 (4:00 PM), and between 2200 (10:00 PM) and 2400 (midnight). During shift changes, staff are busy going off and coming on duty. Often there is confusion about who is providing care and answering signal lights.

Besides the accident risk factors, many people have other problems that increase their risk of falling (Box 9-2). Therefore agencies have fall prevention programs. Box 9-3 lists safety measures that prevent falls. These are part of the agency's fall prevention program and the person's nursing care plan. The nursing care plan also lists measures for the person's specific risk factors.

Box 9-2   Factors That Increase the Risk of Falls

- A history of falls
- Weakness
- Slow reaction time
- Poor vision
- Confusion
- Disorientation
- Decreased mobility
- Foot problems
- Shoes that fit poorly
- Elimination needs
- Urinary incontinence
- Dizziness and lightheadedness
- Dizziness on standing
- Joint pain and stiffness
- Muscle weakness
- Low blood pressure
- Balance problems

- Medication side effects
  - Low blood pressure when standing or sitting
  - Drowsiness
  - Fainting
  - Dizziness
  - Poor muscle coordination
  - Unsteadiness
  - Frequent urination
  - Confusion and disorientation
  - Visual impairment
- Excessive alcohol use
- Depression
- Strange surroundings
- Poor judgment
- Memory problems
- Care equipment (e.g., IV poles, drainage tubes and bags)
- Improper use of wheelchairs, walkers, canes, and crutches

Box 9-3   Safety Measures to Prevent Falls

- Good lighting is provided in rooms, hallways, and bathrooms.
- Light switches (including those in bathrooms) are within reach and easy to find.
- Night-lights are placed in bedrooms, hallways, and bathrooms.
- Hand rails are on both sides of stairs and in bathrooms.
- Safety rails and grab bars are in showers and tubs and by the toilet.
- Floors have wall-to-wall carpeting or carpeting that is tacked down. Avoid scatter, area, and throw rugs.
- Floor coverings are one color. Bold designs can cause dizziness in older persons.
- Floors have nonglare, nonslip surfaces.
- Nonskid wax is used on hardwood, tiled, or linoleum floors.
- Floors and stairs are uncluttered. They are free of toys, electrical cords, and other items that can cause tripping.
- Floors are free of spills and excess furniture.
- Electric and extension cords are out of the way.
- Furniture is arranged for easy movement.
- Rearranging furniture is avoided.
- Chairs have armrests that give support when sitting and standing.
- A telephone and lamp are at the bedside.
- Tubs and showers have nonslip surfaces or nonslip bath mats.
- Nonskid shoes and slippers are worn. Long shoelaces are avoided.
- Clothing fits properly. Clothing is not loose and does not drag on the floor. Belts are tied or secured in place.
- Fluid needs are met.
- Glasses and hearing aids are worn as needed. Reading glasses are not worn when up and about.
- The person is taught how to use the signal light.
- The signal light is always within the person's reach.
- The person is asked to call for assistance when help is needed in getting out of bed or a chair or when walking.
- Signal lights are answered promptly. The person may need immediate assistance or may not wait for help.
- Frequent checks are made on persons with poor judgment or memory.
- Persons at risk for falling are in rooms close to the nurses' station.
- Family and friends are asked to visit during busy times and during the evening and night shifts.
- Companionship is provided. Arrangements are made for sitters, companions, or volunteers to be with the person at risk for falling.
- Electronic warning devices are used. Weight-sensitive alarms for beds and chairs sense when the person tries to get up (Fig. 9-7, p. 170).
- Explanations are given often about medical devices and treatments.
- Pillows or wedge pads or seats keep the person correctly positioned (see Chapter 11).
- Nonslip strips are on the floor next to the bed and in the bathroom.
- The person is assisted to the bathroom as soon as requested. Or the bedpan, urinal, or commode is provided.
- The person is assisted to the bathroom, or the bedpan, urinal, or commode is offered at regular times.
- The bedpan or urinal is kept within easy reach of persons able to use the device without help.
- A warm drink, soft lights, or a back massage is used to calm the agitated person.
- Barriers are used to prevent wandering (Fig. 9-8, p. 170).
- The bed is in the lowest horizontal position, except when giving bedside nursing care. The distance from the bed to the floor is reduced if the person falls or gets out of bed.
- Bed rails are kept up, if ordered by the doctor. They are in the up position when the bed is raised.
- Crutches, canes, and walkers have nonskid tips.
- Wheelchair brakes are in working order.
- Wheels of beds, wheelchairs, and stretchers are locked when transferring persons.
- Caution is used when turning corners, entering corridor intersections, and going through doors. A person coming from the other direction could be injured.
- A safety check is made of the room after visitors leave. They may have lowered a bed rail, removed the signal light, moved a walker out of reach, or brought an item that could present dangers to the person.

Fig. 9-7 Weight-sensitive alarm. (**A,** *Courtesy J.T. Posey Co., Arcadia, Calif.)*

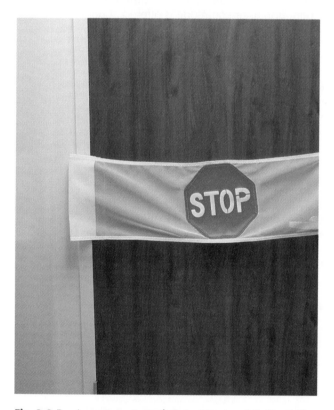

Fig. 9-8 Barriers prevent wandering. *(Courtesy J.T. Posey Co., Arcadia, Calif.)*

Fig. 9-9 Hospital bed with bed rails locked in the raised position.

Bed Rails. Bed rails (side rails) on hospital beds are raised and lowered. They lock in place with levers, latches, or buttons. Bed rails are half, three quarters, or the full length of the bed (Fig. 9-9). When half-length rails are used, usually each side has two rails. One is for the upper part of the bed and the other for the lower part.

The nurse tells you when to raise bed rails. They are necessary for persons who are unconscious or sedated with drugs. Some confused or disoriented people require them. If a person requires bed rails, they are kept up at all times except when giving bedside nursing care.

Bed rails are hazards for a persons trying to get out of bed without help. A person can get caught or entangled in the rail. A person can also get caught or entangled in bed rail gaps. Gaps occur between half-length rails and between the rail and the head or foot of the bed. These hazards are great risks for confused, disoriented, and restrained persons.

Bed rails prevent the person from getting out of bed. Therefore they are considered restraints under the Omnibus Budget Reconciliation Act of 1987 (OBRA). The law forbids the use of bed rails unless they are required to meet the person's medical condition. They also are allowed if the person requests them. Some nursing center residents use the bed rails to change positions. Also, some residents feel safe when bed rails are used. This law applies to nursing centers and hospital long-term care units. Under OBRA, the person or the person's legal representative must give consent for raised bed rails.

The Joint Commission on Accreditation of Healthcare Organizations (JCAHO) has standards for bed rail use. Bed rails are allowed when the person's clinical condition requires them. Bed rails must be in the person's best interests.

The procedures in this book include using bed rails. This helps you to remember their importance and how to use them correctly. The nurse tells you which people require bed rails. If bed rails are not used, you can omit the "raise or lower bed rails" steps. *However, whenever the bed is raised to give care or perform a procedure, the bed rails are raised to prevent the person from falling. The right not to use bed rails applies only when the bed is in its lowest position. Always explain to the person why the bed rails are used. Check persons with raised bed rails often. Report to the nurse that you checked these persons. If you are allowed to chart, record when you check the person and your observations.*

Hand Rails and Grab Bars. Hand rails are in hallways, stairways, and bathrooms (Fig. 9-10). They provide support for persons who are weak or unsteady when walking. They also provide support for sitting down on or getting up from a toilet. Grab bars are along bathtubs for use in getting in and out of the tub.

Wheel Locks. Bed legs have wheels or casters. A caster is a small wheel that lets the bed move easily. Each wheel or caster has a lock to prevent the bed from moving (Fig. 9-11). Lock the bed wheels when giving bedside care. Also lock them when you transfer a person to and from the bed. Wheelchair and stretcher wheels also are locked during transfers. You or the person can be injured if the bed, wheelchair, or stretcher moves.

PREVENTING BURNS

Burns are a leading cause of death, especially among children and older persons. Common causes of fires are smoking in bed, spilling hot liquids, children playing with matches, charcoal grills, fireplaces, and stoves. Box 9-4 on p. 172 lists safety measures to prevent burns.

Fig. 9-10 Hand rails provide support when walking.

Fig. 9-11 Lock on a bed wheel.

PREVENTING POISONING

Poisoning also is a major cause of death. Children are often victims. Aspirin and household products are common poisons. Poisoning in adults may be from carelessness or poor vision when reading labels. Taking too much medicine is another cause. Confused or disoriented persons can take more medicine than the ordered dose. Sometimes poisoning is a suicide attempt. Box 9-5 on p. 172 lists the safety measures that prevent poisoning.

Box 9-4 Safety Measures to Prevent Burns

- Keep matches out of the reach of children.
- Supervise the play of children.
- Do not let children use baby walkers near stoves, space heaters, and fireplaces.
- Never leave children at home alone.
- Teach children fire safety, fire prevention measures, and the dangers of fire.
- Turn pot and pan handles so they point inward. They must point away from where people stand and walk.
- Use the stove's back burners when infants and children are in the kitchen.
- Check metal playground equipment before letting children play on it. Metal surfaces exposed to sunlight can heat to high temperatures and burn hands, arm, legs, and buttocks.
- Supervise the smoking of adults who cannot protect themselves.
- Do not allow smoking in bed.
- Keep space heaters and materials that can catch fire away from children.
- Measure the temperature of bath water (see Chapter 14).
- Do not leave children unattended in bathtubs. They may turn on the hot water.
- Position the child facing away from faucets when bathing a child in a tub or at a sink.
- Place knob covers over faucets to prevent children from turning on the water.
- Supervise children who are eating to prevent spills of hot foods. Also supervise persons who are eating in bed and older persons who are at risk for spilling.
- Apply heat applications correctly (see Chapter 26).
- Use electrical appliances correctly.
- Keep curling irons and electric rollers out of the reach of children. Keep these items turned off when not in use.

Box 9-5 Safety Measures to Prevent Poisoning

- Keep childproof caps on all medicine containers, household products, and hazardous substances.
- Label all medicine containers and household products clearly. Make sure hazardous substances are labeled.
- Use safety latches on kitchen, bathroom, garage, basement, and workshop cabinets.
- Store medicines and poisonous materials in places that are high, locked, and out of the reach of children. Store hazardous substances as directed by the manufacturer.
- Store medicines, poisonous materials, and hazardous substances in their original containers. Do not store them in food containers.
- Do not store medicines, poisonous materials, or hazardous substances near food.
- Keep medicines out of purses, backpacks, briefcases, luggage, and other items where children may find them. Remember that visitors may keep medicines in such places. Keep children away from such items.
- Provide good lighting for reading labels.
- Keep poisonous houseplants out of the reach of children.
- Teach children not to eat plants, unknown foods, or leaves, stems, seeds, berries, nuts, or bark.
- Place poison warning stickers ("Mr. Yuk") on household cleaners and toxic substances (Fig. 9-12).
- Never call medicine candy.
- Read labels and follow directions on household products and other toxic or hazardous substances.
- Keep all baby products and diaper-changing supplies out of the child's reach.
- Keep emergency phone numbers by the telephone: poison control center, police, ambulance, hospital, and doctor.
- Supervise children closely during visits at the homes of family and friends. Look for medicines stored on kitchen counters, kitchen tables, or bathroom counters.

Fig. 9-12 The "Mr. Yuk" warning sticker is placed on poisonous products. *(Courtesy Children's Hospital, Pittsburgh Poison Center, Pittsburgh, Penn.)*

SUFFOCATION

Suffocation is when breathing stops from the lack of oxygen. Death occurs if the person does not start breathing. Common causes include choking on an object, drowning, inhaling gas or smoke, strangulation, and electrical shock. Carbon monoxide poisoning also results in the lack of oxygen. The person breathes in air filled with carbon monoxide rather than oxygen. Faulty exhaust systems on cars and damaged furnaces and chimneys are common causes of carbon monoxide poisoning. Safety measures to help prevent suffocation are listed in Box 9-6.

Box 9-6   Safety Measures to Prevent Suffocation

- Dispose of plastic wrappings, trash bags, and plastic bags (includes those from dry cleaners and produce) properly.
- Do not place a pillow under an infant's head.
- Position infants on their back or sides. *Do not lay infants on their stomachs.*
- Do not use pillows to position infants or to prevent them from falling off beds.
- Check blankets, sheets, and comforters for loose threads or edging. An infant or child could choke on or become entangled in loose threads or edging.
- Do not leave rattles, teethers, or toys in an infant's crib or playpen when the child sleeps.
- Place cribs away from windows. This prevents the child from reaching blinds, shades, and drapes.
- Do not leave an infant in a playpen with the sides down. The child can roll into a space between the mattress and loose mesh side.
- Keep cords for blinds, shades, and drapes out of a child's reach.
- Do not hang items with strings, cords, or elastic cords around cribs or playpens.
- Do not tie pacifiers or other items around a baby's neck. Cords and ribbons can become tightly twisted. Or they can get caught on furniture or other immovable items.
- Remove bibs and other clothing tied around the neck before placing children in cribs. The ties can get caught in the crib.
- Check children's clothes and toys for loose buttons, decals, and other adornments.
- Do not let unsupervised children play with deflated balloons.

- Collect the pieces of broken balloons to keep them out of a child's reach. Pick up the pieces and dispose of them immediately after a balloon breaks.
- Do not let children play on reclining chairs. The leg rest can fold down on the child.
- Do not let children play near ice chests, picnic coolers, clothes dryers, and refrigerators. This includes such items in campers parked outside the home. A child can get trapped inside these items.
- Do not let children play in hammocks. Children can get trapped in them and strangle.
- Take small bites of food. Chew food slowly and thoroughly.
- Make sure dentures fit properly.
- Have exhaust systems on cars checked regularly.
- Have gas odors promptly investigated by competent repairmen.
- Have furnaces and chimneys inspected when persons in the same dwelling have signs and symptoms of carbon monoxide poisoning. Signs and symptoms include headache, confusion, difficulty breathing, dizziness, sleepiness, and cherry-pink skin.
- Open doors and windows if you notice gas odors or signs and symptoms of carbon monoxide poisoning.
- Rest for at least 1 hour after eating and before strenuous activity or swimming.
- Keep all electric cords and appliances in good repair.
- Unplug hair dryers, electric rollers, make-up mirrors, and curling irons when not in use. These can easily fall into bathroom sinks, tubs, and toilets.

IDENTIFYING THE PERSON

Safety also means giving the right care to the right person. Each person has different treatments, therapies, and activity limits. A person's life and health are threatened if the wrong care is given.

Patients and most residents receive identification (ID) bracelets when admitted to a hospital or nursing center (Fig. 9-13). Information on the bracelet includes the person's name, room and bed numbers, age, gender (male or female), and doctor. Known allergies and the agency's name also are included. Some agencies also include the person's religion.

You use the ID bracelet to identify the person before giving care. Treatment cards or assignment sheets state the treatment or therapy ordered by the doctor. To identify the person, compare the identifying information on the treatment card or assignment sheet with that on the ID bracelet (Fig. 9-14, p. 174). This comparison helps ensure that you give the right care to the right person.

Fig. 9-13 Identification bracelet.

Also call the person by name when checking the ID bracelet. Calling the person by name is a courtesy given as you touch the person and before giving care. However, calling the person by name is not a safe way to identify the person. Confused, disoriented, drowsy, hearing-impaired, or distracted persons may answer to any name.

Fig. 9-14 The person's ID bracelet is compared with an assignment sheet to accurately identify the person.

Alert and oriented nursing center residents may choose not to wear ID bracelets. This is noted on the person's care plan. Follow center policy to identify residents who do not wear ID bracelets.

Some nursing centers have identification systems that use photographs. The person's picture is taken on admission. The photo is placed in the person's medical record. If your center uses such a system, you need to learn to use it safely.

PREVENTING EQUIPMENT ACCIDENTS

All equipment is unsafe if broken, not used correctly, or not working properly. Inspect all equipment before use. Check glass and plastic items for cracks, chips, and sharp or rough edges. All these can cause cuts, stabs, or scratches. Follow the Bloodborne Pathogen Standard (see Chapter 10). Do not use or give damaged items to patients or residents.

Electric equipment must work properly and be in good repair. Frayed cords (Fig. 9-15) and overloaded electrical outlets (Fig. 9-16) can cause electrical shocks. Such shocks can cause death and fires. Frayed cords and broken equipment are repaired by a trained person.

Three-pronged plugs (Fig. 9-17) are used on all electrical items. Two prongs carry electrical current. The third prong is the ground. A **ground** carries leaking electricity to the earth and away from the item. If

Fig. 9-15 A frayed electric cord.

Fig. 9-16 An overloaded electrical outlet.

Fig. 9-17 A three-pronged plug.

a ground is not used, leaking electricity can be conducted to a person and cause electrical shocks and possible death. Immediately report any shock received while using a piece of equipment. Send the item for repair immediately.

Warning signs of a faulty electrical item include:

- Shocks
- Loss of power or a power outage
- Dimming or flickering lights
- Sparks
- Sizzling or buzzing sounds
- Burning odor
- Loose plugs

Practice these safety measures when using equipment:

- Follow agency policies and procedures.
- Follow the manufacturer's instruction.
- Read all caution and warning labels.
- Do not use unfamiliar equipment. Ask for needed training. Also ask a nurse to supervise you the first time you use the item.
- Use equipment only for its intended purpose.
- Make sure the item is working before you begin.
- Make sure you have all needed equipment. For example, if you need to plug in an item, you need an outlet.
- Place a "do not use" sticker on broken equipment. Complete a repair request form and explain the problem.
- Notify the nurse about broken equipment.
- Do not try to repair broken equipment yourself.

An incident report is completed if a patient or resident, visitor, or staff member has an equipment-related accident. The Safe Medical Devices Act requires that agencies report equipment-related illnesses, injuries, and deaths.

APPLYING RESTRAINTS

A **restraint** is any item, object, device, garment, material, or chemical that restricts a person's freedom of movement or access to one's body. Freedom from restraint is a resident right under OBRA. Restraints are used only as a last resort to protect persons from harming themselves or others.

REASONS FOR USE

Restraints can cause serious injury and even death. Therefore OBRA has guidelines about using restraints. So does the Joint Commission on Accreditation of Health Care Organizations (JCAHO) and the Food and Drug Administration (FDA).

Restraints are not used to *discipline* a person or for staff convenience. *Discipline* is any action that punishes or penalizes a person. *Convenience* is any action that:

- Controls the person's behavior
- Requires less effort by the agency
- Is not in the person's best interests

According to OBRA, restraints are used only when necessary to treat a person's medical symptoms. The symptoms may relate to physical, emotional, or behavioral problems. Restraints may be needed to ensure the physical safety of the person or other individuals. That is, persons are protected from harming themselves or others. Certain behaviors are harmful to the person or to others in the area. They include:

- Getting out of bed, a chair, or a wheelchair or off of a stretcher when help is needed
- Crawling over bed rails or the foot of the bed
- Interfering with treatment (pulling out tubes, removing dressings, or disconnecting equipment)
- Wandering in or away from the agency
- Agitated or combative behavior toward staff, family, or other persons

Restraints were once used to prevent falls. However, research shows that restraints cause falls. Falls occur when persons try to get free of the restraints. More serious injuries occur from falls in restrained persons than in unrestrained persons.

Restraints were common in persons who were confused, showed poor judgment, or had behavior problems. Older persons were restrained more often than younger persons. *Now, all other alternatives must be tried before using restraints.*

PHYSICAL AND CHEMICAL RESTRAINTS

OBRA's legal definition of *physical restraints* includes the following key points:

- May be any manual method, physical or mechanical device, material, or equipment
- Is attached to or next to the person's body
- Cannot be easily removed by the person
- Restricts freedom of movement or access to one's body

A restraint confines the person to a bed or chair or prevents movement of a body part. Restraints are applied to the chest, waist, elbows, wrists, hands, or legs. Certain furniture or barriers also prevent free movement. Geriatric chairs (Geri-chairs) or chairs with attached trays are examples (Fig. 9-18, p. 176). Such chairs are often used for persons who need support to sit up. Placing any chair so close to a wall that the person cannot move is another form of restraint. Bed rails are also restraints. So are sheets tucked in so tightly that they restrict movement.

Fig. 9-18 A Geri-chair with a tray is considered to be a restraint when used to prevent freedom of movement. *(Courtesy Invacare Corporation, Elyria, Ohio.)*

Chemical restraints are drugs used to prevent a certain behavior or movement. OBRA defines chemical restraints as drugs used for discipline or staff convenience. Drugs are chemical restraints:

- If they are not required for the person's medical treatment
- If they affect the person's physical function
- If they affect the person's mental function

Sometimes doctors order drugs to help confused and disoriented persons. The drugs help control anxious, agitated, or combative behaviors. However, the drugs should not make the person sleepy or unable to function.

COMPLICATIONS OF RESTRAINT USE

Box 9-7 list the many complications from restraint use. Injuries occur as the person tries to get free of the restraint. Cuts, bruises, and fractures are common injuries. Injuries also occur from using the wrong restraint, applying it wrong, or keeping it on too long. *The most serious risk from restraints is death from strangulation.* There are also mental effects. Being restrained affects a person's dignity and self-esteem. Depression, anger, and agitation are common in restrained persons. So are embarrassment, humiliation, and mistrust.

Restraints are medical devices. The Safe Medical Devices Act applies if a restraint causes illness, injury, or death.

RESTRAINT ALTERNATIVES

OBRA, JCAHO, and the FDA do not forbid the use of restraints. Restraints are allowed only after trying all other alternatives. Box 9-8 lists restraint alternatives. Those selected for a person are listed in the person's nursing care plan.

Box 9-7 **Risks of Restraint Use**

- Agitation
- Anal incontinence (see Chapter 17)
- Anger
- Bruises
- Cuts
- Dehydration
- Depression
- Embarrassment
- Fractures

- Humiliation
- Mistrust
- Nerve injuries
- Nosocomial infection (see Chapter 10)
- Pneumonia (see Chapter 30)
- Pressure ulcers (see Chapter 25)
- Strangulation
- Urinary incontinence (see Chapter 16)
- Urinary tract infection (see Chapter 30)

Box 9-8 **Alternatives to Restraints**

- Diversion activities: for example, television, videos, music, games, books, relaxation tapes
- Pillows and positioning aids
- Keeping the signal light within reach
- Meeting food, fluid, and elimination needs
- Visits by family, friends, and volunteers
- Arranging for companions and sitters
- Spending time with the person
- Reminiscing with the person
- A calm, quiet environment
- Allowing wandering in a safe area
- Exercise programs
- Outdoor time
- Jobs or tasks the person consents to

- Electronic warning devices on beds and doors
- Measures to prevent falls (see Box 9-3)
- Reclining chairs
- Frequent observation
- Moving the person closer to the nurses' station
- Explaining all procedures and care measures
- Frequent explanations about required medical equipment or devices
- Orienting confused individuals to person, time, and place; providing calendars and clocks
- Good lighting
- Consistent staff assignments
- Promoting uninterrupted sleep

SAFETY GUIDELINES

If a restraint is used, the least restrictive method is used. Remember the following about using restraints:

- *Restraints are used to protect the person. They are not used for staff convenience.* Restraining a person is thought to be easier for the staff than properly supervising and observing the person. Actually, a restrained person requires more staff time for care, supervision, and observation. A restraint is used only when it is the best safety precaution for the person. It is not used to punish uncooperative persons.
- *Restraints require a doctor's order.* OBRA, JCAHO, state laws, and FDA warnings protect persons from unnecessary restraint. Agencies must have policies and procedures about restraint use. If a person needs restraining for medical reasons, a written doctor's order is required. The doctor gives the reason for the restraint, what to use, and how long to use the restraint. Usually restraint orders are valid only for 24 hours. This information is in the person's nursing care plan. Do not apply a restraint if the order is more than 24 hours old. Always check if the order is current. You need to know the laws and policies about using restraints where you work.
- *The least restrictive method is used.* An **active physical restraint** attaches to the person's body and to a stationary (immovable) object. It restricts the person's movement or body access. Vest, leg, arm, wrist, hand, and some belt restraints are active physical restraints. A **passive physical restraint** is near but not directly attached to the person's body. It allows some movement and access to certain body parts. Passive physical restraints are the least restrictive.
- *Restraints are used only after trying other methods to protect the person.* Some people can harm themselves or others. The nursing care plan must include measures to protect the person and to prevent the person from harming others. Restraints lessen the person's dignity. They are allowed only after other measures fail to provide needed protection (see Box 9-8). Many fall prevention measures are restraint alternatives (see Box 9-3).
- *Unnecessary restraint is false imprisonment (see Chapter 2).* If told to apply a restraint, you must clearly understand the need. If not, politely ask about its use. If you apply a restraint unnecessarily, you face false imprisonment charges.
- *Restraints require informed consent.* The person must understand the reason for the restraint. The person is told how the restraint will help the planned medical treatment. The person also is told about risks of restraint use. If the person cannot give informed consent, the person's legal representative

is given the information. Either the person or legal representative must give consent. Restraints cannot be used without consent. The doctor or RN provides the necessary information and obtains informed consent.

- *The manufacturer's instructions are followed.* The manufacturer gives instructions about applying and securing the restraint. Failure to follow the instructions could affect the person's safety. You could be negligent for improperly applying or securing a restraint.
- *The restrained person's basic needs are met by the nursing and health teams.* The restraint must be snug and firm but not tight. Tight restraints interfere with circulation and breathing. The person must be comfortable and able to move the restrained part to a limited and safe extent. Check the person at least every 15 minutes. Remember to meet the person's food, fluid, elimination, and exercise needs.
- *Restraints are applied with enough help to protect the person and staff from injury.* Persons in immediate danger of harming themselves or others are restrained quickly. Combative and agitated people can hurt themselves and the staff when restraints are applied. Enough staff members are needed to complete the task safely and quickly.
- *Restraints can increase a person's confusion and agitation.* Whether confused or alert, people are aware of restricted body movements. They may try to get out of the restraint or struggle or pull at it. Many restrained persons beg anyone who passes by to set them free or to help release them. These behaviors are often viewed as signs of confusion. Confusion increases in some persons because they do not understand what is happening to them. Restrained persons need repeated explanations and reassurance. Spending time with them has a calming effect.
- *The person's quality of life is protected.* Restraints are used for as short a time as possible. The person's care plan shows how to slowly reduce restraint use. The goal is to meet the person's needs using as little restraint as possible. Besides meeting physical needs, you must meet the person's psychosocial needs. These needs are met by visiting with the person and explaining the purpose of the restraints.

Restraints are dangerous. Improper use and poor supervision have lead to deaths and injuries from restraints. *The person is observed at least every 15 minutes.* Complications from restraints are prevented, such as interferences with breathing and circulation. Practice the safety measures in Box 9-9 on p. 178 when caring for a restrained person. *Remember to release the restraint at least every 2 hours.*

Text continued on p. 182

Box 9-9 Safety Measures for Using Restraints

- Use the restraint specified by the nurse and the care plan. The least restrictive device is used.
- Apply a restraint only after receiving instruction about its proper use. Demonstrate proper application to the nurse before using it on any person.
- Use the correct size as instructed by the nurse. Small restraints are tight. They cause discomfort, agitation, restricted breathing, or reduced circulation. Strangulation is a risk from big or loose restraints.
- Use only restraints that have manufacturer instructions. Read the manufacturer's warning labels. Note the front and back of the restraint.
- Follow the manufacturer's instructions. Some restraints are safe for bed, chair, and wheelchair use. Others are used only with certain equipment.
- Do not use sheets, towels, tape, rope, straps, bandages, or other items to restrain a person.
- Use intact restraints. Look for tears, frayed edges, missing loops or straps, or other damage.
- Do not use restraints to position a person on a toilet. Use them only with the furniture for which they are intended (see the manufacturer's instructions).
- Follow agency policies and procedures when applying restraints.
- Position the person in good body alignment before applying the restraint (see Chapter 11).
- Pad bony areas and skin to prevent pressure and injury from the restraint.
- Secure the restraint. It should be snug but allow some movement of the restrained part. If the restraint is applied to the chest, make sure that the person can breathe easily. A flat hand should slide between the restraint and the person's body (Fig. 9-19).
- Criss-cross vest restraints in front (Fig. 9-20). Do not criss-cross restraints in the back unless part of the manufacturer's instructions. Criss-crossing vests in the back can cause death from strangulation.
- Do not criss-cross the straps of a vest or jacket restraint at the person's back (Fig. 9-21). Improper application can lead to strangulation.
- Tie restraints according to agency policy. The policy should follow the manufacturer's instructions. The knot must be easily released in an emergency. Quick-release knots often are used (Fig. 9-20). Some restraints have quick-release buckles (Fig. 9-23, p. 180).
- Secure straps out of the person's reach.
- Secure the restraint to the movable part of the bed frame or to the bed springs (see Fig. 9-22). Never secure restraints to the bed rails. The person can reach bed rails to release knots or buckles. Also, injury to the person is likely when raising or lowering bed rails. For chairs, secure straps to the wheelchair or the chair frame (Fig. 9-24, p. 180).
- Pad the bed rails as in Figure 9-25 on p. 180. Padded bed rails prevent the person from getting caught between the rails (Fig. 9-26, p. 180). Entrapment can occur between:

- The bars of the bed rail
- The space between half-length (split) bed rails
- The bed rail and mattress
- The headboard or footboard, bed rail, and mattress
- Keep full bed rails up when using a vest or belt restraint if required by the manufacturer's instructions and agency policy. If the bed rails are not up, the person could fall off the bed and strangle on the restraint. Remember to pad the bed rails. Use gap protectors for split bed rails that have built-in bed controls (Fig. 9-27, p. 181). Follow the manufacturer's instructions and agency policy for the use of gap protectors or padded bed rails.
- Position the person in a chair so the hips are well to the back of the chair. If using a belt restraint, apply it at a 45-degree angle over the hips (Fig. 9-28, p. 181).
- Do not use back cushions when a person is restrained in a chair. If the cushion moves out of place, slack occurs in the straps. Strangulation could result if the person slides forward or down because of the extra slack (Fig. 9-29, p. 181).
- Check the person's circulation every 15 minutes if wrist or leg restraints are applied. You should feel a pulse at a pulse site below the restraint. Fingers or toes should be warm and pink. Notify the nurse immediately if:
  - You cannot feel a pulse
  - Fingers or toes are cold, pale, or blue in color
  - The person complains of pain, numbness, or tingling in the restrained part
  - The skin is red or damaged
- Check the person every 15 minutes for safety and comfort. Also check the position of the restraint, especially in the front and back. (Chart that this was done, the care give, and your observations.)
- Keep scissors in your pocket. In an emergency, cutting the tie may be faster than untying the knot. Never leave scissors at the bedside or where the person can reach them.
- Remove the restraint and reposition the person every 2 hours. Give skin care, perform range-of-motion exercises, and meet elimination needs at this time. Remember, injuries often occur when the restrained person tries to get to the bathroom. The person must be free of the restraint for at least 10 minutes every 2 hours. (Chart that this was done, the care give, and your observations.)
- Meet the person's basic needs. The person must have food and fluids. Offer water often to prevent dehydration. (Chart that this was done, the care given, and your observations.)
- Make sure the signal light is always within the person's reach. (Chart that this was done.)
- Report to the nurse every time the restraint is released. Thoroughly and accurately report your observations made and the care given. (Chart that this was done and what you reported to the nurse.)

Fig. 9-19 A flat hand slides between the restraint and the person.

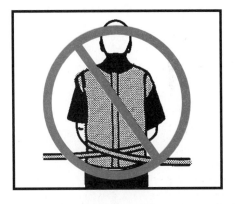

Fig. 9-21 Never criss-cross vest or jacket straps in the back. *(Courtesy J.T. Posey Co, Arcadia, Calif.)*

Fig. 9-20 Vest restraint criss-crosses in front.

Fig. 9-22 The Posey quick-release tie. *(Courtesy J.T. Posey Co, Arcadia, Calif.)*

Fig. 9-23 Quick-release buckle. *(Courtesy J.T. Posey Co, Arcadia, Calif.)*

Fig. 9-24 The restraint straps are secured to the wheelchair frame using a quick-release tie. *(Courtesy J.T. Posey Co, Arcadia, Calif.)*

Fig. 9-25 Padded bed rails. *(Courtesy J.T. Posey Co, Arcadia, Calif.)*

Fig. 9-26 A, Padded bed rails prevent the person from getting caught between the rails. **B,** Half-length bed rails are dangerous for the restrained person. *(Courtesy J.T. Posey Co, Arcadia, Calif.)*

Fig. 9-27 Gap protectors. *(Courtesy J.T. Posey Co, Arcadia, Calif.)*

Fig. 9-28 The safety belt is at a 45-degree angle over the person's hips. *(Courtesy J.T. Posey Co, Arcadia, Calif.)*

Straps to prevent sliding should always be over the thighs—NOT around the waist or chest. Straps should be at a 45° angle and secured to the chair under the seat, not behind the back. They should be snug but comfortable and not restrict breathing. If a belt or vest is too loose or applied around the waist, the person may slide partially off the seat—resulting in the possible suffocation and death.

Tray tables (with or without a belt or vest) pose potential danger if the person should slide partly under the table and become caught. This could result in suffocation and death. Make sure the person's hips are positioned at the back of the chair—this may necessitate the use of an anti-slide material (Posey Grip), a pommel cushion, or a restrictive device if the person shows any tendency to slide forward.

Fig. 9-29 Strangulation could result if the person slides forward or down because of the extra slack in the restraint. *(Courtesy J.T. Posey Co, Arcadia, Calif.)*

REPORTING AND RECORDING

Information about restraints is recorded in the person's medical record. You might apply restraints or care for a restrained person. Report and record the following:

- The type of restraint applied
- The reason for the application
- Safety measures taken (e.g., bed rails padded and up)
- The time you applied the restraint
- The time you removed the restraint
- The care given when the restraint was removed
- The color and condition of the person's skin
- The pulse felt in the restrained extremity
- Complaints of a tight restraint, difficulty breathing, and pain, numbness, or tingling in the restrained part

Recording the care you gave and the observations you made is very important. Should the person die or suffer injuries from restraint use, an investigation is conducted. Legal action may result. Malpractice or criminal charges are possible. Also, if your actions contributed to the person's death or injury, a report is made to the state nursing assistant registry. Therefore your charting helps prove what you did or did not do. It protects you and the person.

TYPES OF RESTRAINTS

Restraints are made of cloth or leather. Cloth restraints (soft restraints) are belts, straps, and vests. They are applied to the wrists, ankles, hands, elbows and forearms, waist, and chest. Leather restraints are applied to the wrists and ankles. They are used in extreme cases of agitation and combativeness.

▶ Wrist Restraints and Ankle Restraints.

Wrist restraints limit the movement of arms and legs. They are often described by their application points:

- *2-Point restraints* are applied to two extremities. The wrists are common sites.
- *3-Point restraints* are applied to three extremities. They are usually applied to both wrists and one ankle.
- *4-Point restraints* are applied to all four extremities. They are applied to both wrists and both ankles. The nurse tells you where to apply the restraints.

Fig. 9-30 The soft part of the restraint is toward the skin.

Fig. 9-31 Two fingers fit between the restraint and the wrist.

Applying Wrist and Ankle Restraints

QUALITY OF LIFE

Remember to:
- Knock before entering the person's room
- Address the person by name
- Introduce yourself by name and title

Pre-Procedure

1 Get the number of restraints you need.

2 Wash your hands.

3 Identify the person. Check the ID bracelet against the assignment sheet.

4 Explain the procedure to the person.

5 Provide for privacy.

Procedure

6 Make sure the person is comfortable and in good body alignment (see Chapter 11).

7 Apply the restraint, following the manufacturer's instructions. Place the soft part toward the skin (Fig. 9-30).

8 Secure the restraint so it is snug but not tight. Make sure that you can slide two fingers under the restraint (Fig. 9-31).

9 Tie the ends to the movable part of the bed frame or to the bed springs. Use an agency-approved knot.

10 Repeat steps 7, 8, and 9 for a 2-point, 3-point, or 4-point application.

Post-Procedure

11 Place the signal light within the person's reach.

12 Unscreen the person.

13 Wash your hands.

14 Check the person and the restraints at least every 15 minutes. Check the pulse, color, and temperature of the restrained parts. Report your observations to the nurse.

15 Do the following at least every 2 hours:
   a Remove the restraints.
   b Reposition the person.
   c Meet the person's food, fluids, and elimination needs.
   d Give skin care.
   e Perform range-of-motion exercises, or ambulate the person. Follow the care plan.
   f Reapply the restraints.

16 Report and record your observations and the care given.

▶ **Mitt Restraints.** Hands are placed in mitt restraints. They prevent finger use but do not prevent hand, wrist, or arm movements. Mitt restraints are thumbless and prevent the person from scratching, pulling out tubes, or removing dressings. The person holds a hand roll to keep the fingers in a normal position. Hand rolls are not needed with padded mitts (Fig. 9-32).

Applying Mitt Restraints

QUALITY OF LIFE

Remember to:
- Knock before entering the person's room
- Address the person by name
- Introduce yourself by name and title

Pre-Procedure

1 Collect the following equipment:
- Two mitt restraints
- Two washcloths or two commercial hand rolls if mitts are not padded
- Tape if washcloths are used for hand rolls

2 Make the hand rolls as in Figure 9-33 or use commercial ones.

3 Wash your hands.

4 Identify the person. Check the ID bracelet against the assignment sheet.

5 Explain the procedure to the person.

6 Provide for privacy.

Procedure

7 Make sure the person's hands are clean and dry. Fingernails should be short so they do not cut into the person's palm.

8 Give the person a hand roll to hold if a padded mitt is not used.

9 Apply the mitt restraint (Fig. 9-34). Follow the manufacturer's instructions.

10 Tie the ends to the movable part of the bed frame or to the bed springs. Use an agency-approved knot.

11 Repeat steps 8, 9, and 10 for the other hand.

Post-Procedure

12 Place the signal light within the person's reach.

13 Unscreen the person.

14 Wash your hands.

15 Check the person and the restraints at least every 15 minutes.

16 Do the following at least every 2 hours:
  a Remove the restraints.
  b Reposition the person.

  c Meet the person's needs for food, fluids, and elimination.
  d Give skin care.
  e Perform range-of-motion exercises, or ambulate the person. Follow the care plan.
  f Reapply the restraints.

17 Report and record your observations and the care given.

Fig. 9-32 Padded mitt restraint. *(Courtesy J.T. Posey Co, Arcadia, Calif.)*

A

B

C

Fig. 9-33 Make a hand roll from a washcloth. **A,** Fold the washcloth in half. **B,** Roll up the washcloth. **C,** Tape the rolled washcloth.

Fig. 9-34 Mitt restraint. Person is holding a hand roll.

▶ **Vest and Jacket Restraints.** Vest and jacket restraints are applied to the chest. They always are applied over a gown, pajamas, or clothes. They are used for persons at risk of a life-threatening fall or to assist in a medical treatment. The person cannot get out of bed or out of a chair.

Jacket restraints have sleeves (Fig. 9-35). They close in the back with zippers or a hook and loop. The closure device is off-center in the back so it does not cause pressure on the spine.

Vest restraints always cross in the front (see Fig. 9-20). The vest must *never* cross in the back. If it crosses in the back, there is only a small neck opening at the front. Strangulation can occur from the small neck opening if the person slides down in the bed or chair.

Vest and jacket restraints carry great risks to the person's life. Death can occur from strangulation. If the person becomes caught in the restraint, it can become so tight that the person's chest cannot expand to inhale air. The person quickly suffocates and dies. Correct application of a restraint is always important. In the case of vest and jacket restraints, it is critical. Therefore you are advised to only assist the nurse in its application. It is best that the nurse assume full responsibility for the application of vest and jacket restraints.

Fig. 9-35 Jacket restraint. *(Courtesy J.T. Posey Co, Arcadia, Calif.)*

Applying a Vest or Jacket Restraint

QUALITY OF LIFE

Remember to:
- Knock before entering the person's room
- Address the person by name
- Introduce yourself by name and title

Pre-Procedure

1. Collect the following:
   - Vest or jacket restraint (the nurse tells you the size)
   - Pads for the bed rails
2. Get help if needed.
3. Wash your hands.
4. Identify the person. Check the ID bracelet against the assignment sheet.
5. Explain the procedure to the person.
6. Provide for privacy.

Procedure

7. Put the pads on the bed rails if the person is in bed.
8. Assist the person to a sitting position.
9. Apply the restraint with your free hand. Follow the manufacturer's instructions. Remember, the vest crosses in front.
10. Make sure the restraint is free of wrinkles in the front and back.
11. Help the person lie down if he or she is in bed.
12. Bring the ties through the slots.
13. Make sure the person is comfortable and in good body alignment (see Chapter 11).
14. Secure the straps to the movable part of the bed frame, the bed springs, or to the chair or wheelchair. Use an agency-approved knot.
15. Slide a flat hand under the restraint (see Fig. 9-19). Adjust the straps as needed so the restraint is snug but not tight.

Post-Procedure

16. Place the signal light within the person's reach.
17. Raise the bed rails.
18. Unscreen the person.
19. Wash your hands.
20. Check the person and the restraint at least every 15 minutes.
21. Do the following at least every 2 hours:
    a. Remove the restraint.
    b. Reposition the person.
    c. Meet the person's needs for food, fluids, and elimination.
    d. Give skin care.
    e. Perform range-of-motion exercises, or ambulate the person. Follow the care plan.
    f. Reapply the restraint.
22. Report your observations to the nurse. Include the care given when the restraint was removed.

Belt Restraints. The belt restraint (Fig. 9-36) is used for the same reasons as the vest restraint. The belt is applied around the waist and secured to the bed or chair. It is applied over clothes, a gown, or pajamas. The person can release the quick-release type. It is less restrictive than those that are released only by a staff member.

Fig. 9-36 Roll belt.

Applying a Belt Restraint

QUALITY OF LIFE

Remember to:
- Knock before entering the person's room
- Address the person by name
- Introduce yourself by name and title

Pre-Procedure

1 Obtain a belt restraint. The nurse tells you the size.
2 Get help if needed.
3 Wash your hands.
4 Identify the person. Check the ID bracelet against the assignment sheet.
5 Explain the procedure to the person.
6 Provide for privacy.

Procedure

7 Assist the person to a sitting position.
8 Apply the restraint with your free hand. Follow the manufacturer's instructions.
9 Remove wrinkles or creases from the front and back of the restraint.
10 Bring the ties through the slots in the belt.
11 Help the person lie down if he or she is in bed.
12 Make sure the person is comfortable and in good body alignment (see Chapter 11).
13 Secure the straps to the movable part of the bed frame, the bed springs, or to the chair or wheelchair. Use an agency-approved knot.

Post-Procedure

14 Place the signal light within the person's reach.
15 Unscreen the person.
16 Wash your hands.
17 Check the person and the restraint at least every 15 minutes.
18 Do the following at least every 2 hours:
    a Remove the restraint.
    b Reposition the person.
    c Meet the person's needs for food, fluids, and elimination.
    d Give skin care.
    e Perform range-of-motion exercises, or ambulate the person. Follow the care plan.
    f Reapply the restraint.
19 Report and record your observations and the care given.

▶ **Elbow Restraints.** Elbow restraints limit arm movements (Fig. 9-37). The person cannot bend the elbows. Elbow restraints are useful in preventing infants and small children from bending their elbows. They prevent children from scratching and touching incisions or pulling out tubes. Both arms are restrained to achieve the desired effect.

Elbow restraints wrap around the arm. They are secured in place with Velcro, hook and loop fasteners, or ties. They can be pinned to clothing to hold the device in position (Fig. 9-38).

Fig. 9-37 Elbow restraint. *(Courtesy J.T. Posey Co, Arcadia, Calif.)*

Fig. 9-38 An elbow restraint is secured to the shirt with safety pins. The pins point down and away from the child.

Applying Elbow Restraints

QUALITY OF LIFE

Remember to:
- Knock before entering the person's room
- Address the person by name
- Introduce yourself by name and title

Pre-Procedure

1 Collect the following:
   - Two elbow restraints
   - Stiffeners
   - Safety pins
2 Insert the stiffeners into the slots (Fig. 9-39).
3 Wash your hands.

4 Identify the person. Check the ID bracelet against the assignment sheet.
5 Explain the procedure to the person. If applying the restraints on a child, explain the procedure to the child and parents.
6 Provide for privacy.

Procedure

7 Wrap the restraint around the person's elbow.
8 Secure the restraint.

9 Pin the restraint to the shirt. Point pins down and away from the child (see Fig. 9-38).
10 Repeat steps 7, 8, and 9 to apply the other restraint.

Post-Procedure

11 Place the signal light within the person's or parents' reach.
12 Unscreen the person.
13 Wash your hands.
14 Check the person and the restraints often.
15 Do the following at least every 2 hours:
   a Remove the restraint.
   b Reposition the person.

   c Meet the person's needs for food, fluids, and elimination.
   d Give skin care.
   e Perform range-of-motion exercises, or ambulate the person. Follow the care plan.
   f Reapply the restraint.
16 Report and record your observations and

Fig. 9-39 Stiffeners keep the elbow restraint rigid.

HANDLING HAZARDOUS SUBSTANCES

The Occupational Safety and Health Administration (OSHA) requires that health care employees understand the risk of hazardous substances and how to handle them safely. A **hazardous substance** is any chemical that presents a physical hazard or a health hazard in the workplace.

Physical hazards can cause fires or explosions. Health hazards are chemicals that can cause acute or chronic health problems. Acute problems occur rapidly and last a short while. They usually occur from a short-term exposure. Chronic problems usually result from long-term exposure and occur over a long period. Health hazards can cause cancer and affect the formation and function of blood cells. They also can damage the kidneys, nervous system, lungs, skin, eyes, or mucous membranes. Birth defects, miscarriages, and fertility problems result from damage to the reproductive system.

Exposure to hazardous substances can occur under normal working conditions or during certain emergencies. Such emergencies include equipment failures, container ruptures, or the uncontrolled release of a hazard into the workplace. Hazardous substances include:

- Drugs used in cancer therapy (chemotherapy, anticancer drugs)
- Gases used to give anesthesia
- Gases used to sterilize equipment
- Oxygen
- Disinfectants and cleaning solutions
- Radiation used for x-rays and cancer treatments

To protect employees, OSHA requires a hazard communication program. The program includes container labeling, material safety data sheets, and employee training about hazards and protective measures.

LABELING

Hazardous substance containers include bags, barrels, bottles, boxes, cans, cylinders, drums, and storage tanks. Such containers need warning labels (Fig. 9-40). The manufacturer applies the labels. Warning labels always identify physical hazards and health hazards. Health hazards relate to the organs affected and potential health problems. Warning labels may include:

- Precaution measures (e.g., "do not use near open flame" or "avoid skin contact")
- What personal protective equipment to wear (Chapter 10)
- Directions about using the substance safely
- Storage and disposal information

Fig. 9-40 Warning label on a hazardous substance.

Words, pictures, and symbols communicate the warnings. A container must have a label. Warning labels must not be removed or damaged in any way. If a warning label is removed or damaged, do not use the chemical. Take the container to the nurse, and explain the problem. Do not leave the container unattended.

MATERIAL SAFETY DATA SHEETS

Every hazardous substance has a material safety data sheet (MSDS). An MSDS provides detailed information about each hazardous chemical:

- The chemical name and any common names
- The ingredients contained in the substance
- Physical and chemical characteristics (appearance, color, odor, boiling point, and others)
- Potential physical effects (fire, explosion)
- Conditions that could cause a chemical reaction
- How the chemical enters the human body (inhalation, ingestion, skin contact, or absorption)
- Health hazards including signs and symptoms
- Protective measures (how to use, handle, and store the substance)
- Emergency and first aid procedures
- Explosion information and firefighting measures (including what type of fire extinguisher to use)
- How to clean up a spill or leak
- Personal protective equipment needed during clean up
- How to dispose of the hazardous material
- Manufacturer information (name, address, and a telephone number for information)

Employees must have ready access to the MSDSs. They are in a binder at a specified location on each

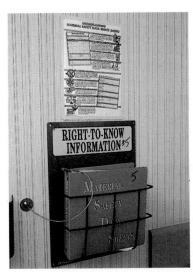

Fig. 9-41 Material safety data sheets (MSDSs) are in a binder. The binder is available for staff use.

unit (Fig. 9-41). Many agencies also have them on computer. Check the MSDS before using a hazardous substance, cleaning up a leak or spill, or disposing of the substance. Also, immediately notify the nurse of a spill or leak. Do not leave a spill or leak unattended.

EMPLOYEE TRAINING

Your employer provides hazardous substance training. Information is given about the hazards, exposure risks, and protection measures. You also learn to read and use warning labels and the MSDSs.

Each hazardous substance requires certain protection measures. Box 9-10 lists general guidelines for the safe handling of hazardous substances.

FIRE SAFETY

Faulty electrical equipment and wiring, overloaded electrical circuits, and smoking are major causes of fire. Fire is a constant danger. The entire health team must prevent fires. They must act quickly and responsibly if a fire occurs.

FIRE AND THE USE OF OXYGEN

Three things are needed for a fire:

- A spark or flame
- A material that will burn
- Oxygen

Air has some oxygen. However, some people need extra oxygen. Doctors order supplemental oxygen for these persons. Supplemental oxygen is supplied in oxygen tanks or through wall outlets (see Chapter 27).

Box 9-10   Safety Measures for Handling Hazardous Substances

- Read all warning labels.
- Follow the safety precautions on the warning label and MSDS.
- Make sure each container has a warning label that is not damaged.
- Use a leak-proof container to carry or transport a hazardous substance.
- Wear personnel protective equipment to clean spills and leaks. The warning label or MSDS tells you what to wear (mask, gown, gloves, eye protection, safety boots).
- Clean up spills immediately. Work from clean to dirty, using circular motions.
- Dispose of hazardous waste in sealed bags or containers.
- Stand behind a lead shield during x-ray or radiation therapy procedures.
- Do not enter a room while a person is having x-rays or radiation therapy.
- Wash your hands after handling hazardous substances.
- Work in well-ventilated areas to avoid inhaling gases.
- Store hazardous substances according to the MSDS.

Oxygen is needed for fires. Therefore special safety precautions are practiced where oxygen is used and stored:

- "No Smoking" signs are placed on the person's door and near the bed.
- Patients, residents, and visitors are politely reminded not to smoke in the person's room.
- Smoking materials (cigarettes, cigars, pipes), matches, and lighters are removed from the room.
- Electrical equipment is turned off *before* being unplugged. Sparks occur when electrical appliances are unplugged while turned on.
- Wool blankets and synthetic fabrics that cause static electricity are removed from the person's room. The person wears a cotton gown or pajamas. Health team members wear cotton uniforms.
- Electrical equipment is removed from the person's room. This includes electric razors, heating pads, and radios.
- Candles and incense are not used in the person's room.
- Materials that ignite easily are removed from the person's room. These include oil, grease, alcohol, nail polish remover, and other hazardous substances that ignite easily.

Many agencies have no-smoking policies and are smoke-free environments. No smoking is allowed inside the buildings. Signs are posted on all entry doors. However, some people ignore such policies. If a person is receiving supplemental oxygen, remind the person, family, and any visitors about the need for no smoking. *(See Focus on Home Care box.)*

Focus On... HOME CARE

Home care patients may require supplemental oxygen. Remind the patient, family, and visitors about needed safety precautions (see Chapter 27).

PREVENTING FIRES

Fire prevention measures were described in relation to children, burns, equipment-related accidents, and the use of oxygen. These and other fire safety measures are summarized in Box 9-11. *(See Focus on Home Care box at left on p. 195.)*

Box 9-11   Fire Prevention Measures

- Follow the fire safety precautions involved in the use of oxygen.
- Smoke only in areas where smoking is allowed. Do not smoke in patient homes.
- Be sure all ashes, cigars, and cigarettes are out before emptying ashtrays.
- Provide ashtrays to persons who are allowed to smoke.
- Empty ashtrays into a metal container partially filled with sand or water. Do not empty ashtrays into plastic containers or wastebaskets lined with paper or plastic bags.
- Supervise the smoking of persons who cannot protect themselves. This includes persons who are confused, disoriented, or sedated.
- Follow safety practices when using electrical equipment.
- Supervise the play of children, and keep matches out of their reach.
- Do not leave cooking unattended on stoves, in ovens, or in microwave ovens.
- Store flammable liquids in their original containers. Keep the containers out of children's reach.
- Do not light matches or lighters or smoke around flammable liquids or materials.
- Do not leave candles unattended.
- Keep candles away from flammable liquids or materials.

Focus On... HOME CARE

Focus On... HOME CARE

Smoke detectors are important for fire safety. Always locate smoke detectors in patient homes. Make sure they are working. Notify the nurse and the family if a smoke detector does not work.

Space heaters present fire hazards. Electric and kerosene heaters are common. These safety measures are important:

- Follow the manufacturer's instructions when using space heaters.
- Keep space heaters at least 3 feet away from curtains, drapes, and furniture.
- Do not place the heater on stairs, in doorways, or where people walk.
- Protect yourself and others from burns. Heaters are hot. Do not touch them. Keep them away from children and persons who cannot protect themselves.
- Prevent electrocution. Keep electric heaters away from water (water conducts electricity). Make sure the cord is in good repair.
- Do not leave space heaters unattended.
- Store kerosene in its original container. Keep the container outside.

Know the exit routes from the home or apartment building. If a fire occurs, get the patient, family, and yourself out as fast as possible. In an apartment building, notify others of the fire. Use the fire alarm system, and yell FIRE in the hallways. Call 911 or the local fire department from a nearby phone. Do not go back into the building.

If your clothing is on fire, do not run. Drop to the floor or ground. Roll to smother the flames. If another person's clothing is on fire, get the person to the floor or ground. Roll the person, or cover the person with a blanket or coat. This smothers the flames.

If smoke is present, cover your nose and mouth with a damp cloth. Do the same for the patient and family. Have everyone crawl to the nearest exit.

Do the following if you cannot get out of the building because of flames or smoke:

- Call 911 or the fire department. Tell the operator where you are. Give precise information: address, phone number, and where you are in the home.
- Cover your nose and mouth with a damp cloth. Do the same for the patient and family.
- Move away from the fire. Go to a room with a window. Close the door to the room, and place wet towels and blankets at the bottom of the door.
- Open the window.
- Hang something from the window (towel, sheet, blanket, clothing). This helps the firefighters find you.

WHAT TO DO IF A FIRE OCCURS

Every agency has policies and procedures for fire emergencies. You must know your agency's policies and procedures. Also know the location of fire alarms, fire extinguishers, and emergency exits. Agencies conduct fire drills to practice emergency fire procedures.

Remember the word *RACE* when a fire occurs. That will help you remember what to do first:

- *R* stands for *rescue.* Rescue persons in immediate danger. Move them to a safe place.
- *A* stands for *alarm.* Sound the nearest fire alarm, and notify the switchboard operator.
- *C* stands for *confine.* Confine the fire by closing doors and windows. Turn off oxygen or electrical equipment in use in the general area of the fire.
- *E* stands for *extinguish.* Use a fire extinguisher on a small fire that has not spread to a larger area.

Also clear equipment from all regular and emergency exists. *Remember, do not use elevators if there is a fire. (See Focus on Home Care box above.)*

▶ **Using a Fire Extinguisher.** Agencies require that all employees demonstrate use of a fire extinguisher. Fire departments give fire extinguisher demonstrations once or twice a year.

Different extinguishers are used for different kinds of fires: oil and grease fires; electrical fires; and paper and wood fires. A general procedure for using a fire extinguisher follows. *(See Focus on Home Care box.)*

Focus On ... HOME CARE

Locate fire extinguishers in the patient's home. Read the manufacturer's instructions. Make sure the fire extinguisher works. Notify the nurse and the family if a fire extinguisher does not work.

Using a Fire Extinguisher

Procedure

1 Pull the fire alarm.
2 Get the nearest fire extinguisher.
3 Carry the extinguisher upright.
4 Take the extinguisher to the fire.

5 Remove the safety pin (Fig. 9-42, *A*).
6 Direct the hose at the base of the fire (Fig. 9-42, *B*).
7 Push the top handle down (Fig. 9-42,C).

Fig. 9-42 A, The safety pin of the fire extinguisher is removed. **B,** The hose is directed at the base of the fire. **C,** The top handle is pushed down.

Evacuating. Agency policies and procedures specify evacuation procedures. If evacuation is necessary, persons closest to the danger are taken out first. Those who can walk are given blankets to wrap around themselves. They are escorted to a safe place by a staff member. Figures 9-43 and 9-44 show how to rescue nonambulatory persons. Once firefighters arrive, they direct rescue efforts.

Fig. 9-43 Swing carry technique. **A,** Assist the person to a sitting position. A co-worker grasps the person's ankles as you both turn the person so that he sits on the side of the bed. **B,** Pull the person's arm over your shoulder. With one arm, reach across the person's back to your co-worker's shoulder. Reach under the person's knees and grasp your co-workers arm. Your co-worker does the same.

Fig. 9-44 One-rescuer carry. **A,** Spread a blanket on the floor. Make sure that the blanket will extend beyond the person's head. Assist the person to sit on the side of the bed. Grasp the person under the arms, and cross your hands over her chest. Lower the person to the floor by sliding her down one of your legs. **B,** Wrap the blanket around the person. Grasp the blanket over the head area, and pull the person to a safe area.

DISASTERS

A **disaster** is a sudden catastrophic event. Many people are injured and killed, and property is destroyed. Natural disasters include tornadoes, hurricanes, blizzards, earthquakes, volcanic eruptions, floods, and some fires. Human-made disasters include auto, bus, train, and airplane accidents. They also include fires, nuclear power plant accidents, riots, explosions, and wars.

Local communities, fire and police departments, and agencies have disaster plans. You should know the disaster plan where you work. Also know the disaster plan of the community where you live and work.

Disaster plans include policies and procedures to deal with great numbers of people needing treatment. The plan generally provides for the discharge of persons who can go home. Certain staff members are assigned to the emergency department. Others are assigned to take equipment to the emergency area and to transport persons from the initial treatment area. Off-duty personnel may be called in to work.

A disaster may damage the agency. Therefore the disaster plan includes policies and procedures for evacuating the agency.

WORKPLACE VIOLENCE

Workplace violence is any physical assault or threatening behavior or verbal abuse that occurs in a work setting. It includes:

- Murders
- Beatings
- Stabbings
- Suicides or near suicides
- Shootings
- Rapes
- Kidnappings
- Robberies
- Psychological traumas—threats, obscene phone calls, a threatening presence, and harassment of any nature (being followed, sworn at, or shouted at)

Workplace violence can occur in any location where an employee performs a work-related duty. It can be a permanent or temporary location. This includes buildings, parking lots, field locations, homes, and travel to and from work assignments.

According to OSHA, more assaults occur in health care settings than in other industries. Risk factors for work-related assaults in health care agencies include:

- Handguns in the possession of patients, residents, families, and friends
- Patients as police holds (persons arrested or convicted of crimes)
- Acutely disturbed and violent persons seeking health care
- Mentally ill persons who do not take medicine, do not receive follow-up care, and are not in hospitals unless they are an immediate threat to themselves or others
- Agency pharmacies being a source of drugs and therefore a target for robberies
- Gang members and substance abusers having access to agencies as patients or visitors
- Upset, agitated, and disturbed family members and visitors
- Long emergency room waits that increase a person's agitation and frustration
- Being alone with patients and residents during care or transport to other agency areas
- Low staff levels during meals, emergencies, and at night
- Poorly lighted parking areas
- Lack of training in recognizing and managing potentially violent situations

OSHA has guidelines for violence prevention programs. The goal is to eliminate or reduce employee exposure to situations that can cause death or injury. The work site is checked for hazards. Prevention strategies are developed and implemented. Also, employees receive safety and health training. Your responsibilities in violence prevention programs include:

- Understanding and following the workplace violence prevention program
- Understanding and following safety and security measures
- Voicing safety and security concerns
- Reporting violent incidents promptly and accurately
- Serving on health and safety committees that review incidents of workplace violence
- Taking part in training programs that focus on recognizing and managing agitation, assaultive behavior, and criminal intent

Box 9-12	Measures to Prevent or Control Workplace Violence

- Alarm systems, closed-circuit video monitoring, panic buttons, hand-held alarms, cellular phones, two-way radios, and telephone systems that have a direct line to police are installed.
- Metal detectors are at entrances to identify guns, knives, or other weapons.
- Curved mirrors are at hallway intersections and hard-to-see areas.
- Bullet-resistant, shatter-proof glass is at the nurses' stations, reception areas, and admitting areas.
- Waiting rooms are comfortable and reduce stress.
- Family and visitors receive information in a timely manner.
- Furniture is arranged to prevent entrapment.
- Pictures, vases, and other items that can serve as weapons are few in number.
- Staff restrooms lock and prevent access to visitors.
- Unused doors are locked, in keeping with local fire codes.
- Bright lights are inside and outside buildings.
- Burned-out lights are replaced or repaired.
- Broken lights, windows, and door locks are replaced or repaired.
- Security escort services are used for walking to cars, bus stops, or train stations.
- Vehicles are locked and in good repair.
- Security officers deal with agitated, aggressive, or disruptive patients, residents, and visitors.
- Patients, residents, and visitors are restrained if they are a threat to themselves or others.
- Visitors sign in and receive a pass to access patient or resident areas.

- Visiting hours and policies are enforced.
- A list of "restricted visitors" is made for patients or residents with a history of violence or who are victims of violence.
- Psychiatric patients are supervised as they move throughout the hospital.
- Access to the pharmacy and drug storage areas is controlled.
- The RN assesses the behavioral history of new and transferred patients and residents.
- Aggressive and agitated persons are treated in open areas. Privacy and confidentiality are maintained.
- Staff is not alone when caring for persons with agitated or aggressive behaviors.
- Jewelry that can serve as weapons is not worn (grabbing earrings and bracelets, strangulating with necklaces).
- Long hair is worn up and off the collar (see Chapter 3). A person can pull long hair and cause head injuries.
- Keys, scissors, pens, and other items that can serve as weapons are not visible.
- Tools or items left by maintenance staff or visitors are removed if they can serve as weapons.
- Staff wear ID badges (without last names) that verify employment.
- A "buddy system" is used when using elevators, restrooms, and low-traffic areas.
- Uniforms fit well. Tight uniforms limit your ability to run. An attacker can grab loose uniforms.
- Shoes have good soles. Shoes that cause slipping limit your ability to run.

Box 9-12 lists some of the many measures that can prevent or control workplace violence. Box 9-13 on p. 202 lists personal safety practices to follow in all activities. In addition, you can practice the following safety measures when dealing with agitated or aggressive persons:

- Stand away from the person. Judge the length of the person's arms and legs. Stand far enough away that the person cannot hit or kick you.
- Position yourself close to the door. Do not become trapped in the room.
- Note the location of panic buttons, call bells, alarms, closed-circuit monitors, and other security devices (Fig. 9-45, p. 203).
- Keep your hands free.

- Stay calm. Talk to the person in a calm manner. Do not raise your voice or argue, scold, or interrupt the person.
- Do not touch the person.
- Tell the person that you will get a nurse to speak to the person.
- Leave the room as soon as you can. Make sure the person is safe.
- Notify the nurse or security officer of the situation.
- Complete an incident report according to agency policy.

(See Focus on Home Care box on p. 203.)

Box 9-13 Personal Safety Practices

- Know the area you will visit. Ask questions about the area.
- Make a "dry run" of the area. Know the route in advance. The shortest route is not always the safest.
- Have plenty of gas in your car.
- Keep your car in good working order.
- Keep a flashlight with working batteries, flares, a fire extinguisher, and a first aid kit in your car.
- Raise the hood and use the flares if the car breaks down. Stay in the car and call the police if you have a cellular phone. If someone stops by to help, ask that person to call the police.
- Check for places to park. Choose a well-lit area. If using a parking garage, park near entrances, exits, and on the lower level. Try to get close to the attendant if possible. Remember, the closest space to your destination is not always the safest for parking.
- Park your car so that you can leave quickly and easily. Park at street corners so no one can park in front of you. In parking lots, back in. You can see more from your front windshield than from the back window.
- Lock your car. However, there are times you may consider leaving your car unlocked. If you need to get in the car fast, you do not want to fumble with keys. Use your judgment. Do not leave anything in the car if you leave it unlocked.
- Have your car key ready so you can get into the car quickly. Do not fumble for keys on the way to or at the car.
- Check the back seat before getting into the car. Make sure no one is in the car. Leave immediately if someone is in the car.
- Check under the car. A person hiding under the car can grab your ankle or leg. Leave immediately if someone is under the car.
- Lock car doors when you get in the car, and keep windows rolled up.
- Keep purses and other valuables under the seat or near your side. Do not leave them on the seat. They are an easy target for smash-and-grab robberies.
- Use well-lit and busy streets if you have to walk. Avoid vacant lots, alleys, wooded areas, and construction sites. Again, the shortest way is not always the safest.

- Note the location of phone booths, or carry a cellular phone. Know your location, and keep phone calls simple.
- Go to a police or fire station or a store if you think someone is following you.
- Carry money for phone calls and for bus, train, or taxi fares. Have money in your pocket to avoid fumbling with a purse or wallet.
- Stand with others and near the ticket booth if using public transportation. Sit near the driver or conductor.
- Do not hitchhike or pick up hitchhikers.
- Let someone know where you are at all times. Let someone know when you leave and when you arrive at your destination. If you do not call in when expected, the person knows something is wrong.
- Make it known that you do not carry drugs, needles, or syringes.
- Do not carry valuables with you. Leave them at home or in the car trunk. If someone wants what you have, give it. The only thing of value is *you*.
- Carry wallets and purses safely. A wallet should be in an inside coat or pants pocket. Never carry a wallet in the rear pocket. Keep a firm grip on a purse ,and keep it close to your body.
- Do not wear headphones when walking. They keep you from hearing cars and people around you.
- Carry a whistle or shriek alarm.
- Scream as loud and as long as you can. Keep screaming. Both men and women should scream.
- Use your car keys as a weapon. Carry them in your strong hand, and have one key extended (Fig. 9-46). Hold the key firmly. If you are attacked, go for the person's face. Use the key to slash the person's face. Do not use poking motions. Also, do not try for a specific target because you might miss. Do not be shy because your attacker will not be.
- Remember, you have two arms, two hands, two feet, and two knees. This means that you can attack from four directions at once. Do not be shy—your attacker will not be. Push, pull, yank, and so on. You can attack the genital area of either a man or woman.
- Use your thumbs as weapons. Go for the eyes, and push hard.
- Carry a travel size of aerosol hair spray. Go for the face.

Modified from McLean County Sheriff's Department, Bloomington, Ill, and the Illinois Criminal Justice Information Authority, Chicago, Ill.

Fig. 9-45 The closed-circuit TV allows staff to monitor persons entering and leaving the agency.

Fig. 9-46 Car keys are held to use a car key as a weapon.

Focus On... HOME CARE

Additional measures are needed for home safety. Always keep doors locked. Do not let strangers into the home or apartment building. Also remember not to give information over the phone. Do not let any stranger know that you are with an older, ill, or disabled person.

Physical, emotional, verbal, and sexual abuse are possible in the home setting. If you feel uncomfortable or threatened in any way, you must report the situation to the nurse. Give as much information as you can. Failure to report the situation does not help you or the patient. Leave the home, and call your supervisor if you feel that there is an immediate threat to your health or well-being.

The following are examples of threats to your safety. Report these and other threats to the nurse:
- Sexual abuse or harassment by the patient or by any person in the patient's home (husband, wife, sister, brother, boyfriend, girlfriend, son, daughter, and other relatives and friends) (see Chapter 2)
- Hitting, kicking, slapping, spitting, biting, scratching, pinching, pushing, or other bodily attacks by the patient or anyone in the person's home
- Attacks or threatened attacks with any weapon (knife, gun, baseball bat, rope, tool [hammer, screwdriver, and so on], razor, scissors, aerosol spray, pot, pan, cane, chair, and so on)
- Denial of meal breaks, drinking water, bathroom use, toilet paper, or handwashing facilities
- Denial of adequate sleeping conditions if you are in a live-in situation
- Inadequate heating or ventilation
- Being subject to name calling, obscene language, or racial or cultural slurs
- Exposure to unsafe household conditions (blocked fire escapes, broken stairways, vermin infestations, and so on)

RISK MANAGEMENT

Risk management involves identifying and controlling risk and safety hazards affecting the agency. The intent is to protect everyone in the agency (patients and residents, visitors, and staff) and all agency property from harm or danger. The person's valuables also are protected. Safety, accident and fire prevention, negligence and malpractice, and federal and state requirements are among the many issues within the scope of risk management.

Risk managers work with all agency departments to prevent accidents and injuries. They study incident reports, patient and resident complaints, staff complaints, and accident and injury investigations. They look at these reports for patterns and trends. Risk managers also look for and correct unsafe situations. They also make policy and procedures changes and training recommendations as needed.

CLOTHING AND VALUABLES

The person's valuables must be kept safe. Often they are sent home with the family. A clothing list is completed. Each item is identified and described. The staff member and person sign the completed list.

A valuables envelope is used for money and jewelry. Each jewelry item is listed and described on the envelope. Describe what you see. For example, describe a ring as having a white stone with six prongs in a yellow setting. Do not assume the stone is a diamond in a gold setting. Place each jewelry item in the envelope while the person watches. Count money with the person. Then put it in the envelope. The envelope is sealed and signed like the clothing checklist. Give the envelope to the nurse. The nurse takes it to the safe or sends it home with the family.

Focus On... LONG-TERM CARE

Clothing and shoes are labeled with the person's name. Radios, blankets, and other items brought from home also are labeled.

Dentures, eyeglasses, contact lenses, watches, and radios are kept at the bedside. Valuables kept at the bedside are listed in the person's record. Some people keep money for newspapers and gift cart items. The amount of money kept by the person is noted in the person's record. *(See Focus on Long-Term Care box.)*

REPORTING ACCIDENTS AND ERRORS

Accidents and errors are reported immediately to your supervisor. This includes accidents involving patients and residents, visitors, and staff. You must report errors in care. Such errors include giving a person a wrong treatment, giving a treatment to the wrong person, or forgetting to give a treatment. Broken items owned by the person, such as dentures or eyeglasses, are reported. Lost money or clothing is also reported. So are hazardous substance accidents and workplace violence incidents.

An *incident report* is completed. The report is completed as soon as possible after the incident. The following information is required:

- Names of those involved
- Date and time of the accident or error
- Location of the accident or error
- A complete description of what happened
- Names of witnesses
- Any other requested information

Incident reports are reviewed by risk management and a committee of health care workers. They look for patterns and trends of accidents or errors. For example, are falls occurring on the same shift and on the same unit? Are there reports of lost or missing items on the same shift or same unit? The committee may recommend new policies or procedures to prevent future incidents.

REVIEW

Circle T if the answer is true and F if it is false.

1. T F Only medicine containers need childproof caps.

2. T F Household cleaners are kept in locked storage areas out of the reach of children.

3. T F Safety plugs in electrical outlets protect children from electrical shocks.

4. T F The "Mr. Yuk" sticker indicates a poisonous substance.

5. T F Keeping electrical cords and appliances in good repair prevents suffocation.

6. T F The person is called by name to accurately identify the person before giving care.

7. T F Persons between the ages of 65 and 85 years are at risk of falling.

8. T F Falls are more likely to occur during the evening hours.

9. T F Restraints prevent falls.

10. T F The need to urinate is a major cause of falls.

11. T F Bed rails are restraints.

12. T F Bed rails are always raised when the bed is raised.

13. T F The signal light must always be within the person's reach.

14. T F A person is in a coma. Bed rails are required for safety.

15. T F A restraint restricts freedom of movement or access to one's body.

16. T F Restraints require a nurse's order.

17. T F Restraints are used only to prevent persons from harming themselves or others.

18. T F Some drugs are chemical restraints.

19. T F Unnecessary restraint is false imprisonment.

20. T F Restraints are applied so that they are tight.

21. T F Restraints are removed every 2 hours to reposition the person and give care.

22. T F Elbow restraints prevent children from scratching and touching incisions.

23. T F Hazardous substances must have warning labels.

24. T F Many people are injured and killed and property is destroyed in a disaster.

Circle the BEST answer.

25. Why is age a factor in safety?
    A. Young children have not learned what is safe and what is dangerous.
    B. Infants are helpless.
    C. Physical changes from aging can affect balance and movements.
    D. All of the above

26. Which is not a risk for accidents?
    A. The need for eyeglasses
    B. Hearing impairment
    C. Memory problems
    D. Oriented to person, time, and place

27. You are caring for an infant and young children. Which measure is unsafe?
    A. Checking children in cribs often
    B. Keeping one hand on a child in a crib if you need to look away
    C. Propping a baby bottle on a rolled towel or blanket
    D. Keeping plastic bags away from children

28. A paraplegic is paralyzed
    A. From the waist down
    B. From the neck down
    C. On the right side of the body
    D. On the left side of the body

29. Safety measures are needed so Mrs. Ford does not fall. Which is unsafe?
    A. Nonglare, waxed floors
    B. One-color floor coverings
    C. Safety rails and grab bars in the bathroom
    D. Nonskid shoes

30. Burns can be caused by the following *except*
    A. Smoking in bed and space heaters
    B. Leaving children unattended or home alone
    C. Bath water that is too hot
    D. Oxygen

31. Mrs. Ford often tries to get up without help. You should do the following *except*
    A. Remind her to use her signal light when she needs help
    B. Check on her often
    C. Help her to the bathroom at regular intervals
    D. Place her chair by a wall

32. The following can occur because of restraints. Which is the most serious?
    A. Fractures
    B. Strangulation
    C. Pressure ulcers
    D. Urinary tract infection

33. A belt restraint is applied to a person in bed. Where should you tie the straps?
    A. To the bed rails
    B. To the head board
    C. To the movable part of the bed frame
    D. To the foot board

34. A vest restraint is ordered. Which statement is *false?*
    A. The vest should criss-cross in back.
    B. You should be able to slide a flat hand under the restraint.
    C. The restraint is tied according to agency policy.
    D. The bed rails must be up and padded.

35. Mrs. Ford has a restraint. How often should you check her and the position of the restraint?
    A. Every 15 minutes
    B. Every 30 minutes
    C. Every hour
    D. Every 2 hours

36. To prevent equipment accidents, you should
    A. Fix broken equipment
    B. Use two-pronged plugs to ground electrical equipment
    C. Check glass and plastic items for damage
    D. All of the above

37. You gave Mrs. Ford the wrong treatment. Which is *true?*
    A. The error is reported to the nurse at the end of the shift.
    B. Action is taken only if Mrs. Ford was injured.
    C. You will be found guilty of negligence.
    D. You must complete an incident report.

38. All the following are needed to start a fire *except*
    A. A spark or flame
    B. A material that will burn
    C. Oxygen
    D. Carbon monoxide

39. You spilled a hazardous substance. You should do the following *except*
    A. Read the material safety data sheet
    B. Cover the spill and go tell the nurse
    C. Wear any needed personnel protective equipment to clean up the spill
    D. Complete an incident report

40. The fire alarm sounds. The following are done *except*
    A. Turning off oxygen
    B. Using elevators
    C. Closing doors and windows
    D. Moving patients and residents to a safe place

41. Your agency has a violence prevention program. You need to do the following *except*
    A. Follow safety and security measures
    B. Take part in training programs
    C. Wear personnel protective equipment
    D. Report safety and security concerns

42. A person is agitated and aggressive. You should do the following *except*
    A. Stand away from the person
    B. Stand close to the door
    C. Use touch to show you care
    D. Talk to the person without raising your voice

Answers to these questions are on p. 834.

Preventing Infection

OBJECTIVES

Define the key terms listed in this chapter
Identify what microbes need to live and grow
List the signs and symptoms of infection
Explain the chain of infection
Describe nosocomial infection and the persons at risk
Describe the practices of medical asepsis
Describe common disinfection and sterilization methods
Explain how to care for equipment and supplies
Carry out Standard Precautions and Transmission-Based Precautions
Explain the Bloodborne Pathogen Standard
Explain the principles and practices of surgical asepsis
Perform the procedures described in this chapter

KEY TERMS

asepsis Being free of disease-producing microbes

autoclave A pressure steam sterilizer

biohazardous waste Items contaminated with blood, body fluids, secretions, and excretions and that may be harmful to others; *bio* means life, and *hazardous* means dangerous or harmful

carrier A human or animal that is a reservoir for microbes but does not have signs and symptoms of infection

clean technique Medical asepsis

communicable disease A disease caused by pathogens that spread easily; a contagious disease

contagious disease Communicable disease

contamination The process of becoming unclean

disinfection The process of destroying pathogens

immunity Protection against a certain disease

infection A disease state resulting from the invasion and growth of microorganisms in the body

medical asepsis The practices used to remove or destroy pathogens and to prevent their spread from one person or place to another person or place; clean technique

microbe A microorganism

microorganism A small *(micro)* living plant or animal *(organism)* seen only with a microscope; a microbe

nonpathogen A microbe that usually does not cause an infection

normal flora Microbes that usually live and grow in a certain location

nosocomial infection An infection acquired during a stay in a health care agency

pathogen A microbe that is harmful and can cause an infection

personal protective equipment Special clothing or equipment worn to protect against a hazard

reservoir The environment in which a microbe lives and grows

spore A bacterium protected by a hard shell that forms around the microbe

sterile The absence of *all* microbes

sterile field A work area free of all pathogens and nonpathogens (including spores)

sterile technique Surgical asepsis

KEY TERMS *continued*

sterilization The process of destroying *all* microbes

surgical asepsis The practices that keep equipment and supplies free of all microbes; sterile technique

vaccination The administration of a vaccine to produce immunity

vaccine A preparation that contains dead or weakened microbes and is given to produce immunity against an infectious disease

Infection is a major safety and health hazard. Some infections are minor and cause short illnesses. Others are serious and can cause death. Infections are serious for infants and older persons. The health team protects patients, residents, visitors, and themselves from infection. They prevent the cause of the infection from spreading.

MICROORGANISMS

A **microorganism (microbe)** is a small *(micro)* living plant or animal *(organism)* seen only with a microscope. Microbes are everywhere. They are in the air, food, mouth, nose, respiratory tract, stomach, intestines, skin, soil, water, and animals. They are on clothing and furniture. Some microbes cause infections and are harmful. They are called **pathogens**. **Nonpathogens** are microbes that usually do not cause an infection.

TYPES OF MICROBES

There are five types of microbes:

- *Bacteria*—microscopic plant life that multiply rapidly. Often called *germs,* they consist of one cell. They can cause infection in any body system.
- *Fungi*—plants that live on other plants or animals. Mushrooms, yeasts, and molds are common fungi. In humans, fungi can infect the mouth, vagina, skin, feet, and other body areas.
- *Protozoa*—microscopic one-cell animals. They can infect the blood, brain, intestines, and other body areas.
- *Rickettsiae*—microscopic forms of life found in fleas, lice, ticks, and other insects. They are transmitted to humans by insect bites. Rocky Mountain spotted fever and similar infections are caused by these microbes. The person has fever, chills, headache, rash, and other signs and symptoms.
- *Viruses*—extremely small microscopic organisms that grow in living cells. They cause many diseases including the common cold, herpes, acquired immunodeficiency syndrome (AIDS), and hepatitis.

REQUIREMENTS OF MICROBES

Microbes require a **reservoir** to live and grow. The reservoir *(host)* is the environment where the microbe lives and grows. People, plants, animals, the soil, food, and water are common reservoirs. Microbes must get *water* and *nourishment* from the reservoir. They also need *oxygen* to live. A *warm, dark* environment is needed. Most microbes grow best at body temperature and are destroyed by heat and light.

NORMAL FLORA

Normal flora are microbes that usually live and grow in a certain area. Certain microbes are found in the respiratory tract, in the intestines, and on the skin. They are nonpathogens when in or on a natural reservoir. When a nonpathogen is transmitted from its natural site to another site or host, it becomes a pathogen. *Escherichia coli* is normally found in the large intestine. If the *E. coli* enters the urinary system, it can cause an infection.

INFECTION

An **infection** is a disease state resulting from the invasion and growth of microbes in the body. A *local infection* is in a body part. A *systemic infection* involves the whole body. (Systemic means entire.) The person has certain signs and symptoms of infection. Some or all of the signs and symptoms listed in Box 10-1 on p. 210 are present. Pathogens do not always cause an infection. The development of an infection depends on many factors.

THE CHAIN OF INFECTION

The chain of infection (Fig. 10-1, p. 210) is a process involving a:

- Source
- Reservoir
- Portal of exit
- Method of transmission
- Portal of entry
- Susceptible host

Box 10-1	Signs and Symptoms of Infection

- Fever
- Increased pulse and respiratory rates
- Pain or tenderness
- Fatigue and loss of energy
- Loss of appetite *(anorexia)*
- Nausea
- Vomiting
- Diarrhea
- Rash
- Sores on mucous membranes
- Redness and swelling of a body part
- Discharge or drainage from the infected area

The *source* is a pathogen. The pathogen must have a *reservoir* where it can grow and multiply. Humans and animals are common reservoirs for microbes. If they do not have signs and symptoms of infection, they are **carriers**. Carriers can pass the pathogen to others. The pathogen must leave the reservoir. That is, it needs a *portal of exit*. Exits are the respiratory, gastrointestinal, urinary, and reproductive tracts, breaks in the skin, and the blood.

When a pathogen leaves the reservoir, it must be *transmitted* to another host. Methods of transmission are shown in Figure 10-2. The pathogen must enter

the body through a *portal of entry*. Portals of entry and exit are the same. A *susceptible host* (a person at risk for infection) is needed for the microbe to grow and multiply. The human body can protect itself from infection. A person's ability to resist infection relates to age, nutritional status, stress, fatigue, general health, medications, and the presence of disease or injury.

NOSOCOMIAL INFECTION

Persons can develop infections in health care settings. A **nosocomial infection** is an infection acquired during a stay in an agency. (*Nosocomial* comes from the Greek word for hospital.)

Nosocomial infections are caused by normal flora or by pathogens transmitted to the person from another source. Remember, normal flora become pathogens when transmitted from their natural location to another site or host. For example, *E. coli* is normally in the large intestine. Feces (bowel movements) contain *E. coli*. Poor wiping after bowel movements can cause *E. coli* to enter the urinary system. The hands can also transmit *E. coli* to other body areas. If handwashing is poor, *E. coli* spreads to any body part or anything the hands touch. In turn, the *E. coli* can be transmitted to other people.

Microbes can enter the body through equipment used in treatments, therapies, and diagnostic tests. Therefore equipment must be free of microbes. Staff

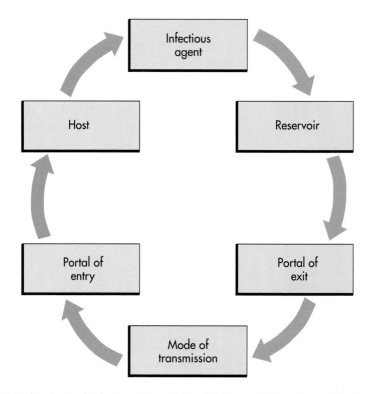

Fig. 10-1 The chain of infection. (*From Potter PA, Perry, AG:* Fundamentals of nursing: concepts, process, and practice, *ed 4, St Louis, 1997, Mosby.*)

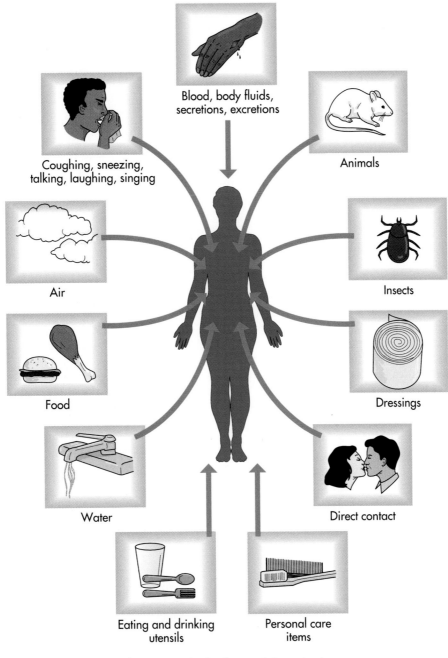

Fig. 10-2 Methods of transmitting microbes.

also can transfer microbes from one person to another and from themselves to others. The urinary and respiratory systems, wounds, and the bloodstream are common sites for nosocomial infections.

Patients and residents are already weak from disease or injury. Surgical wounds or open skin areas are often present. Infants and older persons cannot fight infections like other persons. Therefore the health team must prevent the spread of infection. Medical and surgical asepsis, isolation precautions, and the Bloodborne Pathogen Standard all help prevent nosocomial infections.

MEDICAL ASEPSIS

Asepsis is being free of disease-producing microbes. Microbes are everywhere. Therefore practices are needed to achieve asepsis. **Medical asepsis (clean technique)** is the practices used to remove or destroy pathogens and to prevent their spread from one person or place to another person or place. The number of pathogens is reduced.

Microbes cannot be present during surgery or when instruments are inserted into the body. Also, open wounds (cuts, burns, surgical incisions) require the absence of microbes. These provide portals of entry for microbes. **Surgical asepsis (sterile technique)** is the practices that keep equipment and supplies free of all microbes. **Sterile** means the absence of *all* microbes—both pathogenic and nonpathogenic. **Sterilization** is the process that destroys *all* microbes. Both pathogens and nonpathogens are destroyed. Surgical asepsis is discussed on p. 234.

Contamination is the process of becoming unclean. In medical asepsis, an item or area is *clean* when it is free of pathogens. The item or area is contaminated if pathogens are present. A sterile item or area is contaminated when pathogens or nonpathogens are present.

COMMON ASEPTIC PRACTICES

Aseptic practices break the chain of infection. To prevent the spread of microbes:

- Wash your hands after urinating or having a bowel movement. Also wash your hands after changing tampons or sanitary pads.
- Wash your hands after contact with your own or another person's blood, body fluids, secretions, or excretions. This includes saliva, vomitus, urine, feces, vaginal discharge, mucus, semen, wound drainage, pus, and respiratory secretions.
- Provide all persons with their own toothbrush, drinking glass, towels, washcloths, and other personal care items.
- Cover your nose and mouth when coughing, sneezing, or blowing your nose.
- Bathe, wash hair, and brush your teeth regularly. See Chapter 3 for the practices for a professional appearance.
- Wash your hands before and after handling, preparing, or eating food.
- Wash fruits and raw vegetables before eating or serving them.
- Wash cooking and eating utensils with soap and water after use.

(See Focus on Home Care box.)

Fig. 10-3 Safe-handling instructions for meat and poultry. These are required by the U.S. Department of Agriculture.

Fig. 10-4 Dishes are rinsed and loaded into the dishwasher.

Focus On... HOME CARE

You must prevent the spread of microbes in the home. Also protect the person from microbes brought into the home. Besides the measures just listed, other infection control measures are needed in the home setting:

- Handle meat and poultry safely as instructed on safe-handling labels (Fig. 10-3).
- Cook meats and poultry adequately.
- Protect leftover food. Place leftover food in small containers. Cover containers with lids, foil, or plastic wrap. Date and refrigerate containers as soon as possible. Use the food within the next 2 to 3 days.
- Wash dishes and other eating and cooking utensils. Use liquid detergent and hot water. Wash glasses and cups first. Follow with silverware, plates, bowls, and then pots and pans. Rinse items well with hot water and place them in a drainer to dry. Air drying is more aseptic than towel drying. If using a dishwasher, rinse dishes before loading them into the dishwasher (Fig. 10-4). Use dishwasher soap. Do not wash pots and pans and cast iron, wood, and most plastic items in a dishwasher.
- Clean kitchen appliances, counters, tables, and other surfaces after each meal. Use a sponge or dishcloth moistened with warm water and detergent. Thoroughly remove grease, spills, and splashes. Use a liquid surface cleaner. Clean sinks with scouring powder.
- Dispose of garbage, leftover food, and other soiled supplies after each meal. Place paper, boxes, and cans in a paper or plastic bag or in recycle bins. A garbage disposal is preferred for food and liquid garbage. Otherwise put food or wet items in a container lined with a plastic bag. Do not put bones in the garbage disposal. Some homes have trash compactors that crush garbage. Some cities recycle paper, glass, plastic, and other substances. Follow required recycling procedures.
- Empty garbage at least once a day.
- Dust furniture and vacuum and mop floors. Damp-mop uncarpeted floors at least weekly. Wipe up spills right away. Use a dust mop or broom for sweeping and a dustpan to collect dust and crumbs. Sweep daily or more often if needed.
- Wash clothes and linens.

Bathrooms need special attention. Microbes easily grow and spread in bathrooms. Every family member must help keep the bathroom clean. Aseptic measures are needed whenever the bathroom is used. These include:

- Flushing the toilet after each use
- Rinsing the sink after washing, shaving, or oral hygiene
- Wiping out the tub or shower after each use
- Removing and disposing of hair from the sink, tub, or shower
- Hanging towels out to dry or placing them in a hamper
- Wiping up water spills

Your job may include cleaning bathrooms every day. Use a disinfectant or water and detergent to clean all surfaces:

- The toilet bowl, seat, and outside areas
- The floor
- The sides, walls, and curtain or door of the shower or tub
- Towel racks
- Toilet tissue, toothbrush, and soap holders
- The mirror
- The sink
- Windowsills

Cleaning the bathroom also includes:

- Mopping uncarpeted floors; vacuuming carpeted floors
- Emptying wastebaskets
- Putting out clean towels and washcloths
- Opening bathroom windows for a short time and using air fresheners, these help eliminate odors and give a fresh smell to the bathroom
- Washing bath mats, the wastebasket, and the laundry hamper every week
- Replacing toilet and facial tissue as needed

▶ HANDWASHING

Handwashing with soap and water is the easiest and most important way to prevent the spread of infection. You use your hands in almost every task. They are easily contaminated. Without handwashing, microbes on the hands spread to other persons or items. *Wash your hands before and after giving care.* The rules for handwashing are in Box 10-2.

Fig. 10-5 The uniform does not touch the sink. Soap and water are within reach. Hands are lower than the elbows.

Box 10-2	Rules of Handwashing

- Wash your hands under warm running water.
- Stand away from the sink. Do not let your hands touch the sink. The sink is contaminated (Fig. 10-5).
- Hold your hands and forearms lower than your elbows throughout the procedure. Your hands are dirtier than your elbows and forearms. If you hold your hands and forearms up, dirty water runs from hands to elbows. Those areas become contaminated.
- Rub your palms together to work up a good lather (Fig. 10-6). The rubbing action helps remove microbes and dirt.
- Pay attention to areas often missed during handwashing: thumbs, knuckles, sides of the hands, little fingers, and under the nails.
- Clean fingernails by rubbing the tips against your palms (Fig. 10-7). Also use a nail file or orange stick to clean under fingernails (Fig. 10-8). Microbes easily grow under the fingernails.
- Check agency policy for how long to wash your hands. At least a 10- to 15-second handwash is required. Wash your hands longer if they are visibly soiled with blood, body fluids, secretions, or excretions. Your judgment is important.
- Dry your hands starting at the fingers and working up to your forearms. You will dry the cleanest area first.
- Use a clean paper towel for each faucet to turn off water (Fig. 10-9). Faucets are contaminated. Using paper towels prevents clean hands from becoming contaminated again.
- Use a lotion after handwashing to prevent skin chapping and drying. Skin breaks can occur in chapped and dry skin. Remember, skin breaks are portals of entry for microbes.

Fig. 10-6 The palms are rubbed together to work up a good lather.

Fig. 10-7 The tips of the fingers are rubbed against the palms to clean underneath the fingernails.

Fig. 10-8 A nail file is used to clean under the fingernails.

Fig. 10-9 A paper towel is used to turn off the faucet.

Handwashing

NNAAP™

Procedure

1   Make sure you have soap, paper towels, orange stick or nail file, and a wastebasket. Collect missing items.

2   Push your watch up 4 to 5 inches. Also push up uniform sleeves.

3   Stand away from the sink so your clothes do not touch the sink. Stand so the soap and faucet are easy to reach (see Fig. 10-5).

4   Turn on the faucet. Adjust the water until it feels warm and comfortable.

5   Wet your wrists and hands thoroughly under running water. Keep your hands lower than your elbows during the procedure (see Fig. 10-5).

6   Apply about 1 teaspoon of soap to your hands.

7   Rub your palms together and interlace your fingers to work up a good lather (see Fig. 10-6). This step should last 10 to 15 seconds.

8   Wash each hand and wrist thoroughly. Clean well between the fingers. Clean under the fingernails by rubbing the tips of your fingers against your palms (see Fig. 10-7).

9   Use a nail file or orange stick to clean under the fingernails (see Fig. 10-8). This step is necessary for the first handwashing of the day and when your hands are highly soiled.

10 Rinse your wrists and hands well. Water should flow from the arms to the hands.

11 Repeat steps 6 through 10 if needed.

12 Dry your wrists and hands with paper towels. Pat dry starting at your fingertips.

13 Discard the paper towels.

14 Turn off faucets with clean paper towels to avoid contaminating your hand. Use a clean paper towel for each faucet.

15 Discard paper towels.

CARE OF SUPPLIES AND EQUIPMENT

Supply departments disinfect, sterilize, and distribute equipment. Many items are disposable. They help reduce the spread of infection. Single-use disposable items are discarded after use. The same person uses multi-use disposable items many times. Multi-use items include bedpans, urinals, wash basins, water pitchers, and drinking cups.

Large and costly equipment is not disposable. It is disinfected or sterilized before reuse. Before disinfection or sterilization, equipment is cleaned.

Cleaning. Cleaning removes debris and organic material. It also reduces the number of microbes present. Organic material includes blood, body fluids, secretions, and excretions. Follow these guidelines when cleaning equipment:

- Wear personal protective equipment (gloves, mask, gown, and protective eyewear) when cleaning items contaminated with organic material—blood, body fluids, secretions, or excretions.
- Rinse the item in cold water first. Rinsing removes organic material. Heat causes organic matter to become thick, sticky, and hard to remove.
- Wash the item with soap and hot water.
- Scrub thoroughly. Use a brush if necessary.
- Rinse the item in warm water.
- Dry the item.
- Disinfect or sterilize the item.
- Disinfect equipment and the sink used in the cleaning procedure.
- Discard personal protective equipment.

Disinfection. **Disinfection** is the process of destroying pathogens. However, spores are not destroyed. **Spores** are bacteria protected by a hard shell. Spores are killed by extremely high temperatures.

Germicides are disinfectants applied to skin, tissues, and nonliving objects. Alcohol is a common germicide.

> ### Focus On... HOME CARE
>
> Detergent and hot water are common disinfectants. They are used for eating and drinking utensils, linens, and clothes. Many commercial products are available for household surfaces. Such surfaces include sinks, countertops, floors, toilets, tubs, and showers. You need to use the products preferred by the family or as instructed by the nurse.
>
> Vinegar is also an effective and cheap disinfectant. You can use it to clean bedpans, urinals, commodes, and toilets. To make a vinegar solution, you need 1 cup of white vinegar and 3 cups of water. Make sure you label the container as "vinegar solution." Also put the date on the container and your name.

Chemical disinfectants are used to clean nondisposable items. Such items include glass thermometers, metal bedpans, blood pressure cuffs, commodes, chairs, counter tops, wheelchairs, stretchers, and room furniture. Chemical disinfectants can burn and irritate the skin. Wear utility gloves or rubber household gloves to prevent skin irritation. These gloves are *waterproof*. Do not wear disposable gloves when using disinfectants. Some chemical disinfectants have special precautions for use or storage. Check the material safety data sheet before handling a disinfectant (see Chapter 9). (*See Focus on Home Care box above.*)

Sterilization. Sterilization procedures destroy all nonpathogens and pathogens, including spores. Very high temperatures are used. Remember, microbes grow best at body temperature. They are destroyed by heat.

Boiling water, radiation, liquid or gas chemicals, dry heat, and *steam under pressure* are sterilization methods. An autoclave (Fig. 10-10) is a pressure steam sterilizer. Glass, surgical linens, and metal objects (such as surgical instruments and basins) are autoclaved. High temperatures destroy plastic and rubber items. Therefore they are not autoclaved. Steam under pressure usually sterilizes objects in 30 to 45 minutes. (*See Focus on Home Care box on p. 217.*)

Fig. 10-10 An autoclave.

Focus On... HOME CARE

Boiling water is a simple way to sterilize items in the home (Fig. 10-11).
- Get a pot with a lid that is large enough to hold the items.
- Place the items in the pot.
- Fill the pot with cold water so that all items are completely covered with water.
- Place the lid on the pot.
- Bring the water to a full boil. When the water is boiling, steam escapes from under the lid.
- Boil the items for at least 15 minutes.
- Turn off the heat.
- Let the water and items cool.
- Remove the item onto a clean towel. Use tongs to remove the items.
- Let the items air dry.
- Put the items away as preferred by the family or as instructed by the nurse.

Fig. 10-11 Boiling water is used to sterilize these baby bottles. The water completely covers the bottles.

OTHER ASEPTIC MEASURES

Handwashing, cleaning, disinfection, and sterilization are important aseptic measures. However, other aseptic measures also prevent the spread of infection and microbes. These measures are listed in Box 10-3. The measures are useful in home, work, and everyday activities.

Box 10-3   Aseptic Measures

CONTROLLING RESERVOIRS (HOSTS—YOU OR THE PERSON)
- Provide for the person's hygiene needs (Chapter 14).
- Wash contaminated areas with soap and water. Feces, urine, blood, pus, and other body fluids, secretions, or excretions may contain microbes.
- Use leakproof plastic bags for soiled tissues, linen, and other materials.
- Keep tables, counter tops, wheelchair trays, and other surfaces clean and dry.
- Label bottles with the person's name and the date the bottle was opened.
- Keep bottles and fluid containers tightly capped or covered.
- Keep drainage containers below drainage site (see Chapters 16 and 25).
- Empty drainage containers and dispose of drainage following agency policy. Usually drainage containers are emptied every shift. Follow the nurse's instructions.

CONTROLLING PORTALS OF EXIT
- Cover your nose and mouth when coughing or sneezing.
- Provide the person with tissues to use when coughing or sneezing.
- Wear personal protective equipment as needed.

CONTROLLING TRANSMISSION
- Make sure all persons have their own personal care equipment. This includes wash basins, bedpans, urinals, commodes, glass thermometers, and eating and drinking utensils.
- Do not take equipment from one person's room to use for another person. Even if the item is unused, do not take it from one room to another.
- Hold equipment and linens away from your uniform (Fig. 10-12).
- Wash your hands:
  - Before and after contact with every person
  - Whenever they are visibly soiled
  - After contact with blood, body fluids, secretions, or excretions
  - After removing gloves
  - Before assisting the nurse with any sterile procedure
- Assist the person with handwashing:
  - Before and after eating
  - After elimination
  - After changing tampons, sanitary napkins, or other personal hygiene products

- After contact with blood, body fluids, secretions, or excretions
- Prevent dust movement. Do not shake linens or equipment. Use a damp cloth for dusting.
- Clean from the cleanest area to the dirtiest. This prevents soiling a clean area.
- Clean away from your body. If you dust, brush, or wipe toward yourself, you transmit microbes to your skin, hair, and clothing.
- Flush urine and feces down the toilet. Avoid splatters and splashes.
- Pour contaminated liquids directly into sinks or toilets. Avoid splashing onto other areas.
- Avoid sitting on a person's bed. You will pick up microbes and transfer them to the next surface that you sit on.
- Do not use items that are on the floor. The floor is contaminated.
- Clean tubs, showers, and shower chairs after each use. Follow the agency's disinfection procedures.
- Clean bedpans, urinals, and commodes after each use. Follow the agency's disinfection procedures.

CONTROLLING PORTALS OF ENTRY
- Provide for good skin care (see Chapter 14). This promotes intact skin.
- Provide for good oral hygiene (see Chapter 14). This promotes intact mucous membranes.
- Do not let the person lie on tubes or other items. This protects the skin from injury.
- Make sure linens are dry and wrinkle-free (see Chapter 13). This protects the skin from injury.
- Turn and reposition the person as directed by the nurse. This protects the skin from injury.
- Assist with or clean the genital area after elimination (see Chapter 14). This is called perineal care. Wipe and clean from the urethra (the cleanest area) to the rectum (the dirtiest area). This helps prevent urinary tract infections.
- Make sure drainage tubes are properly connected. If drainage tubes are not connected properly, microbes can enter the drainage system.

PROTECTING THE SUSCEPTIBLE HOST
- Follow the nursing care plan to meet the person's hygiene needs. This protects the skin and mucous membranes.
- Following the nursing care plan to meet the person's nutrition and fluid needs. Good nutrition and adequate fluid intake help prevent infection.
- Assist the person with coughing and deep breathing exercises as directed. This helps prevent respiratory infections.

ISOLATION PRECAUTIONS

Sometimes barriers are needed to prevent the escape of pathogens. The pathogens are kept within a certain area, usually the person's room. This requires isolation procedures.

Fig. 10-12 Hold equipment away from your uniform.

The Centers for Disease Control and Prevention (CDC) has guidelines for isolation precautions. The guidelines recognize that all body fluids (including blood), secretions, and excretions can transmit pathogens. Two tiers of precautions are practiced—Standard Precautions and Transmission-Based Precautions.

Standard Precautions and Transmission-Based Precautions prevent the spread of **communicable** or **contagious diseases.** Communicable diseases are caused by pathogens that are spread easily. Common communicable diseases include measles, mumps, chickenpox, syphilis, gonorrhea, and acquired immunodeficiency syndrome (AIDS) (see Chapter 30). Persons may have respiratory, wound, skin, gastrointestinal, or blood infections that are highly contagious.

Isolation precautions are based on *clean* and *dirty.* *Clean* areas or objects are not contaminated. Uncontaminated areas are free of pathogens. *Dirty* areas or objects are contaminated. If a *clean* area or object has contact with something *dirty,* the clean item is now dirty. *Clean* and *dirty* also depend on how the pathogen is spread.

STANDARD PRECAUTIONS

Standard Precautions (Box 10-4) reduce the risk of spreading pathogens and known and unknown infec-

---

Box 10-4	Standard Precautions

HANDWASHING
- Wash your hands after touching blood, body fluids, secretions, excretions, and contaminated items. Wash your hands even if you wore gloves.
- Wash your hands immediately after removing gloves and between patient or resident contacts. Also wash your hands whenever needed to avoid transferring microbes to other persons or environments.
- Wash your hands between tasks and procedures on the same person. This prevents cross-contamination of different body sites.
- Use plain soap for routine handwashing. (The nurse tells you when other agents are needed. The nurse also tells you what to use.)

GLOVES
- Wear gloves when touching blood, body fluids, secretions, excretions, and contaminated items.
- Put on clean gloves just before touching mucous membranes and nonintact skin.
- Change gloves between tasks and procedures on the same person. Also change gloves after contacting material that may be highly contaminated.

- Remove gloves promptly after use. Remove gloves before touching uncontaminated items and surfaces. Also remove gloves before going to another person.
- Wash your hands immediately after removing gloves. This prevents the transfer of microbes to other persons or environments.

MASKS, EYE PROTECTION, AND FACE SHIELDS
- Wear masks, eye protection, and face shields during procedures and tasks that are likely to cause splashes or sprays of blood, body fluids, secretions, and excretions. Masks, eye protection, and face shields protect the mucous membranes of the mouth, eyes, and nose from splashes or sprays (Fig. 10-13, p. 220).

GOWNS
- Wear a gown during procedures and care activities that are likely to cause splashes or sprays of blood, body fluids, secretions, or excretions. The gown protects the skin and prevents soiling of clothing.
- Remove a soiled gown as promptly as possible.
- Wash your hands after gown removal. This prevents transferring microbes to other persons or environments.

Continued

Box 10-4 Standard Precautions—cont'd

CARE OF EQUIPMENT
- Handle used care equipment carefully. Equipment may be soiled with blood, body fluids, secretions, and excretions. Prevent skin and mucous membrane exposure and clothing contamination. Also prevent the transfer of microbes to other persons and environments.
- Do not use reusable equipment for another person. The item must be cleaned and disinfected or sterilized.
- Discard disposable (single-use) items properly.

ENVIRONMENTAL CONTROL
- Follow agency procedures for the routine care, cleaning, and disinfection of surfaces. This includes environmental surfaces, bed rails, bedside equipment, and other frequently touched surfaces.

LINEN
- Follow agency policy for used linen that is soiled with blood, body fluids, secretions, or excretions. The policy describes how to handle, transport, and process soiled linen. Prevent skin and mucous membrane exposures and clothing contamination. Also prevent the transfer of microbes to other persons and environments.

OCCUPATIONAL HEALTH AND BLOODBORNE PATHOGENS
- Prevent injuries when handling needles, scalpels, and other sharp instruments or devices.
- Prevent injuries when handling sharp instruments after procedures and when cleaning used instruments.
- Prevent injuries when disposing of used needles.
- Never recap used needles. Do not handle them with both hands. Do not use any technique that involves directing the needle point toward any body part. Use a one-handed "scoop" technique or a mechanical device that holds the needle sheath.
- Do not remove used needles from disposable syringes by hand.
- Do not bend, break, or otherwise handle used needles by hand.
- Place used disposable syringes and needles, scalpel blades, and other sharp items in puncture-resistant containers.
- Place reusable syringes and needles in a puncture-resistant container for transport to the reprocessing area.
- Use resuscitation devices for mouth-to-mouth resuscitation (see Chapter 36).

PATIENT OR RESIDENT PLACEMENT
- A private room is used if the person:
  - Contaminates the environment
  - Does not or cannot assist in maintaining hygiene or environmental control
- Follow the nurse's instructions if a private room is not available.

Fig. 10-13 Goggles and a face mask protect the eyes and mucous membranes of the mouth.

tions. *Standard Precautions are used in the care of all persons.* They prevent the spread of infection from:

- Blood
- All body fluids, secretions, and excretions (except sweat) even if blood is not visible
- Nonintact skin (skin with open breaks)
- Mucous membranes

TRANSMISSION-BASED PRECAUTIONS

Some infections require precautions in addition to the Standard Precautions. Transmission-Based Precautions (Table 10-1) depend on how the pathogen is spread. You must understand how certain infections are spread (see Fig. 10-2). This helps you understand the different types of Transmission-Based Precautions.

Table 10-1   Transmission-Based Precautions

AIRBORNE PRECAUTIONS

For known or suspected infections involving microbes transmitted by airborne droplets—measles, chickenpox, tuberculosis

Practices:
- Standard Precautions are followed.
- A private room is preferred.
- Keep the room door closed and the person in the room.
- Wear respiratory protection (tuberculosis respirator) when entering the room of a person with known or suspected tuberculosis.
- Do not enter the room of a person with known or suspected measles or chickenpox if you are susceptible to these diseases.
- Wear respiratory protection (mask) if you must enter the room of a person with known or suspected measles or chickenpox if you are susceptible to these diseases. (Respiratory protection is not needed for persons immune to measles or chickenpox.)
- Limit moving and transporting the person from the room. The person wears a mask if moving or transporting from the room is necessary.

DROPLET PRECAUTIONS

For known or suspected infections involving microbes transmitted by droplets produced by coughing, sneezing, talking, or procedures—meningitis, pneumonia, epiglottitis, diphtheria, pertussis (whooping cough), influenza, mumps, rubella, streptococcal pharyngitis, or scarlet fever

Practices:
- Standard Precautions are followed.
- A private room is preferred.
- Wear a mask when working within 3 feet of the person. (Wear a mask on entering the room if required by agency policy.)
- Limit moving and transporting the person from the room. The person wears a mask if moving or transporting from the room is necessary.

CONTACT PRECAUTIONS

For known or suspected infections involving microbes transmitted by:
- Direct contact with the person (hand or skin-to-skin contact that occurs during care activities)
- Indirect contact (touching surfaces or care items in the person's room)—gastrointestinal, respiratory, skin, or wound infections

Practices:
- Standard Precautions are followed.
- A private room is preferred.
- Wear gloves when entering the room.
- Change gloves after having contact with infective material that may contain high concentrations of microbes.
- Remove gloves before leaving the person's room.
- Wash your hands immediately with an agent specified by the nurse.
- Make sure your hands do not touch potentially contaminated surfaces or items after removing gloves and handwashing.
- Wear a gown on entering the room if you will have substantial contact with the person, environmental surfaces, or items in the room.
- Wear a gown on entering the room if the person is incontinent or has diarrhea, an ileostomy, a colostomy, or wound drainage not contained by a dressing.
- Remove the gown before leaving the person's room. Make sure your clothing does not contact potentially contaminated surfaces in the person's room.
- Limit moving or transferring the person from the room. Maintain precautions if the person is moved or transferred from the room.

Box 10-5	Rules for Isolation Precautions

- Collect all needed equipment before entering the room.
- Prevent contamination of equipment and supplies. Floors are contaminated. So is any object on the floor or that falls to the floor.
- Use mops wetted with a disinfectant solution to clean floors. Floor dust is contaminated.
- Prevent drafts. Pathogens are carried in the air by drafts.
- Use paper towels to handle contaminated items.
- Remove items from the room in sturdy, leakproof plastic bags.
- Double bag items if the outer part of the bag is or can be contaminated.
- Follow agency policy for removing and transporting disposable and reusable items.
- Return reusable dishes, eating utensils, and trays to the food service department. Discard disposable dishes, eating utensils, and trays in the waste container in the person's room.
- Do not touch your hair, nose, mouth, eyes, or other body parts when caring for a person in isolation.
- Do not touch any clean area or object if your hands are contaminated.
- Wash your hands if they become contaminated.
- Place clean items or objects on paper towels.
- Do not shake linen.
- Use paper towels to turn faucets on and off.
- Tell the nurse if you have any cuts, open skin areas, a sore throat, vomiting, or diarrhea.

PROTECTIVE MEASURES

Agency policies may differ from those in this text. The rules in Box 10-5 are a guide for giving safe care when isolation precautions are used.

Isolation precautions involve wearing gloves, a gown, a mask, or protective eyewear. Removing linens, trash, and equipment from the room may require double-bagging. Special measures are needed to collect specimens and to transport persons on isolation precautions.

Wearing Gloves. The skin is a natural barrier. It prevents microbes from entering the body. Small skin breaks on the hands and fingers are common. Some are very small and hard to see. Disposable gloves give added protection. They protect you from pathogens in the person's blood, body fluids, secretions, and excretions. They also protect the person from microbes on your hands.

Wear gloves whenever contact with blood, body fluids, secretions, excretions, mucous membranes, and nonintact skin is likely. Contact may be direct. Or contact may be with items or surfaces contaminated with blood, body fluids, secretions, or excretions.

Do not tear gloves when putting them on. Carelessness, long fingernails, and rings can tear gloves. Blood, body fluids, secretions, and excretions can enter the glove through the tear. This contaminates the hand. Remember the following about wearing gloves:

- Gloves are easier to put on when your hands are dry.
- You need a new pair for every person.
- Remove and discard torn, cut, or punctured gloves immediately. Wash your hands, and put on a new pair.
- Wear gloves only once. Discard them after use.
- Put on clean gloves just before touching mucous membranes or nonintact skin.
- Put on new gloves whenever gloves become contaminated with blood, body fluids, secretions, or excretions. You may need more than one pair of gloves for a task.
- Make sure gloves cover your wrists. If you wear a gown, gloves must cover the cuffs (Fig. 10-14).
- Remove gloves so the inside part is on the outside. The inside is considered *clean*.
- Wash your hands after removing gloves.

Fig. 10-14 The gloves cover the cuffs of the gown.

Removing Gloves

Procedure

1 Make sure that glove touches only glove. Do not let gloves touch skin on your wrists or arms.

2 Grasp a glove just below the cuff (Fig. 10-15, *A*).

3 Pull the glove down over your hand so it is inside out (Fig. 10-15, *B*).

4 Hold the removed glove with your other gloved hand.

5 Reach inside the other glove with the first two fingers of your ungloved hand (Fig. 10-15, *C*).

6 Pull the glove down (inside out) over your hand and the other glove (Fig. 10-15, *D*).

7 Discard the gloves. Follow agency policy.

8 Wash your hands.

A

B

C

D

Fig. 10-15 Removing gloves. **A,** The glove is grasped below the cuff.
B, The glove is pulled down over the hand. The glove is inside out.
C, The fingers of the ungloved hand are inserted inside the other glove.
D, The glove is pulled down and over the hand and glove. The glove is inside out.

▶ **Wearing Protective Apparel.** Gowns, plastic aprons, shoe covers, boots, and leg coverings are barriers that prevent the transmission of microbes. They protect your clothes, wrists, and arms from contact with blood, body fluids, secretions, or excretions. They also protect against splashes and sprays.

Gowns must be long and large enough to completely cover clothing. The sleeves are long with tight cuffs. The gown opens at the back. It is tied at the neck and waist. The inside and neck are *clean.* The outside and waist strings are contaminated.

Gowns are used once. A wet gown is contaminated. A wet gown is removed and a dry one put on. Disposable gowns are made of paper. They are discarded after use. Reusable gowns are made of cloth. Laundering is necessary before reuse.

▶ Donning and Removing a Gown

Procedure

1 Remove your watch and all jewelry.
2 Roll up uniform sleeves.
3 Wash your hands.
4 Put on a face mask if required.
5 Pick up a clean gown. Hold it out in front of you, and let it unfold. Do not shake the gown.
6 Put your hands and arms through the sleeves (Fig. 10-16, *A*).
7 Make sure the gown covers the front of your uniform. It should be snug at the neck.
8 Tie the strings at the back of the neck (Fig. 10-16, *B*).
9 Overlap the back of the gown. Make sure the gown covers your uniform. The gown should be snug and not hang loosely (Fig. 10-16, *C*).
10 Tie the waist strings at the back.
11 Put on the gloves.
12 Provide necessary care.

13 Remove and discard the gloves.
14 Remove the gown:
   a Untie the waist strings.
   b Wash your hands.
   c Untie the neck strings. Do not touch the outside of the gown.
   d Pull the gown down from the shoulder.
   e Turn the gown inside out as it is removed. Hold the gown at the inside shoulder seams and bring your hands together (Fig. 10-16, *D*).
15 Roll up the gown away from you. Keep it inside out.
16 Discard the gown. Follow agency policy.
17 Wash your hands.
18 Remove the face mask. Discard it following agency policy.
19 Wash your hands.
20 Open the door using a paper towel. Discard it as you leave.

Fig. 10-16 Gowning technique. **A,** The arms and hands are put through the sleeves. **B,** The strings are tied at the back of the neck. **C,** The gown is overlapped in the back to cover the entire uniform. **D,** The gown is turned inside out as it is removed.

▶ Wearing Masks and Respiratory Protection. Masks prevent the spread of microbes from the respiratory tract. They are used for Airborne and Droplet Precautions. Masks are worn by patients and residents, visitors, and staff. Disposable masks are used. A wet or moist mask is contaminated. Breathing can cause masks to become wet or moist. Apply a new mask when contamination occurs.

A mask should fit snugly over your nose and mouth. Wash your hands before putting on a mask. To remove the mask, first remove your gloves. Touch only the ties during removal. The front of the mask is contaminated.

Tuberculosis respirators (Fig. 10-17) are worn when caring for persons with tuberculosis (TB) (see Chapter 30). Such protection is used for Airborne Precautions.

Wearing Eye Protection and Face Shields. Goggles and face shields protect the mucous membranes of your eyes from the person's pathogens. You wear goggles or face shields with face masks (see Fig. 10-13). Together they protect your eyes, nose, and mouth from splashing or spraying of blood, body fluids, secretions, or excretions. You may need such protection when giving care, cleaning instruments, or disposing of contaminated fluids.

Discard disposable eyewear after use. Reusable eyewear is cleaned before reuse. After being washed with soap and water, a disinfectant is used.

Fig. 10-17 Tuberculosis respirator.

▶ Wearing a Mask

Procedure

1 Wash your hands.
2 Pick up the mask by its upper ties. Do not touch the part that will cover your face.
3 Place the mask over your nose and mouth (Fig. 10-18, *A*).
4 Place the upper strings over your ears. Tie the strings in the back toward the top of your head (Fig. 10-18, *B*).
5 Tie the lower strings at the back of your neck (Fig. 10-18, *C*). The lower part must be under your chin.
6 Pinch the metal band around your nose if you wear glasses. The top of the mask must be snug over your nose and under the bottom edge of the glasses.
7 Wash your hands.

8 Provide necessary care. Avoid coughing, sneezing, and unnecessary talking.
9 Change the mask if it becomes moist or contaminated.
10 Remove the mask as follows:
  a Remove the gloves.
  b Untie the lower strings.
  c Untie the top strings.
  d Hold the top strings, and remove the mask.
  e Bring the strings together. The inside of the mask folds together (Fig. 10-19, *D*). Do not touch the inside of the mask.
11 Discard the mask. Follow agency policy.
12 Wash your hands.

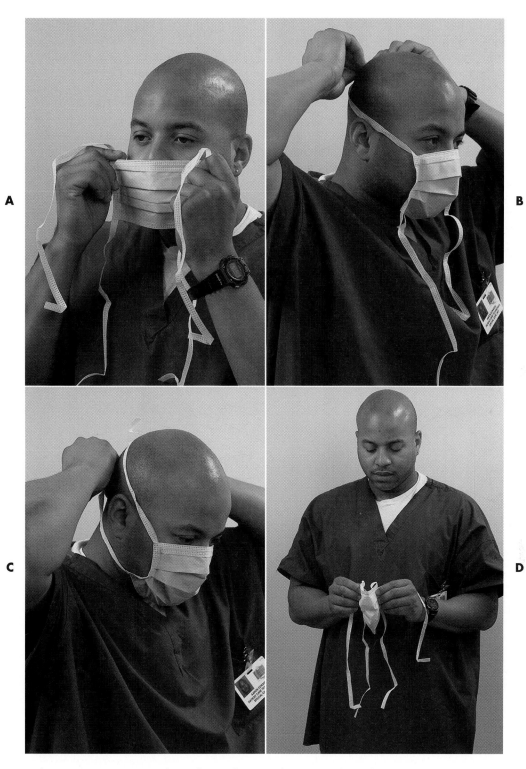

Fig. 10-18 Donning a mask. **A,** The mask covers the nose and mouth. **B,** Upper strings are tied at the back of the head. **C,** Lower strings are tied at the back. **D,** The inside of the mask is folded together after removal.

▶ **Bagging Items.** Contaminated items are bagged to remove them from the person's room. Leakproof plastic bags are used. These bags are labeled with the *BIOHAZARD* symbol (Fig. 10- 19). **Biohazardous waste** is items contaminated with the person's blood, body fluids, secretions, or excretions. (*Bio* means life. *Hazardous* means dangerous or harmful.)

Linen is bagged and transported following agency policy. Usually melt-away bags are used. These bags dissolve in hot water. Once the soiled linen is in the bag, no one else has to handle it. This helps prevent the transmission of microbes. Do not overfill the bag with linen. Tie the bag securely. All linen bags must have a *BIOHAZARD* label. The linen bag is placed in the laundry hamper. The hamper is lined with a biohazard plastic bag.

Trash also is placed in a container labeled with the *BIOHAZARD* symbol. Follow agency policy for bagging and transporting trash, equipment, and supplies.

One bag is usually adequate. Double bagging involves two bags. The CDC does not recommend double bagging unless the outside of the bag is soiled. Two staff members are needed for double bagging. One is inside the room. The other is at the doorway outside the room. The person in the room places contaminated items into a bag. Then the bag is sealed securely. The person outside the room holds open another bag. This bag is clean. A wide cuff is made on the clean bag to protect the hands from contamination (Fig. 10-20). The contaminated bag is placed in the clean bag at the doorway (Fig. 10-21).

Fig. 10-19 BIOHAZARD symbol.

Fig. 10-20 A cuff is made on a clean bag.

Fig. 10-21 Two nursing assistants double bagging. One nursing assistant is in the room inside the doorway. The other is outside the room. The "dirty" bag is placed inside the "clean" bag.

Double Bagging

Procedure

1 Ask a co-worker to help you. The co-worker stands outside the room.

2 Placed soiled linen, reusable equipment, disposable supplies, and trash in the right containers. These containers are lined with leakproof plastic bags. They have the *BIO-HAZARD* label.

3 Seal the bags securely with ties.

4 Ask your co-worker to make a wide cuff on the clean bag and then hold it wide open. The cuff protects the hands from contamination (see Fig. 10-20.)

5 Place the contaminated bag into the clean bag held by your co-worker. Do not touch the outside of the clean bag.

6 Ask your co-worker to seal the bag. Also have the bag labeled according to agency policy.

7 Repeat steps 4, 5, and 6 as needed for other contaminated bags.

8 Ask your co-worker to take or send the bags to the appropriate department for disposal, disinfection, or sterilization.

Collecting Specimens. Specimen containers are labeled following agency policy. Then the container and lid are placed on a paper towel in the person's bathroom. Gloves are worn. Do not contaminate the outside of the container when collecting the specimen. Also avoid contamination when transferring the specimen from the collecting vessel to the container. Put the lid on securely. Then wash your hands.

Once outside the room, place the specimen in a biohazard bag for transport to the laboratory. The bag must be labeled with the person's identifying information. Check agency policy about applying warning labels.

Transporting Persons. Persons on isolation precautions usually do not leave their rooms. However, special treatments or tests may require transporting the person to another area. Transporting procedures vary among agencies. Some require transport by bed. This prevents contaminating wheelchairs and stretchers. Other agencies use wheelchairs and stretchers.

A safe transport means that other persons, staff, and visitors are protected from the infection. Follow these guidelines for safely transporting persons on isolation precautions:

- The person wears a clean gown or pajamas and an isolation gown.
- The person wears a mask if on Airborne or Droplet Precautions.
- Cover any draining wounds.
- Give the person tissues and a leakproof bag. Used tissues are placed in the bag.
- Wear a clean gown, mask, and gloves as required by the isolation precaution.
- Place an extra layer of sheets and absorbent pads on the stretcher or wheelchair. This protects against draining body fluids.
- Do not let anyone else on the elevator. This reduces exposure to the infection.
- Alert staff in the receiving area about the isolation precautions. They wear gowns, masks, protective eyewear, and gloves as needed.
- Disinfect the stretcher or wheelchair after use.

Psychological Impact of Isolation Precautions

The person has love, belonging, and self-esteem needs. Too often these needs are unmet when isolation precautions are used. Visitors and staff often avoid the person. They may need to wear gowns, masks, protective eyewear, and gloves. This takes extra effort before entering the room. Some are unsure about what to touch. Fears about getting the disease are common. Loneliness, feeling unloved and unwanted, and rejection can occur.

Self-esteem easily suffers. The person knows the disease can be spread to others. The person may feel dirty and undesirable. Sometimes visitors and staff unknowingly make the person feel ashamed and guilty about having a contagious disease.

The nurse helps the person, visitors, and staff understand the need for isolation precautions and how they affect the person. You can help meet the person's need for love, belonging, and self-esteem. The following actions are helpful. Remember to disinfect or discard items that become contaminated with infected material:

- Remember, the pathogen is undesirable, not the person.
- Treat the person with respect, kindness, and dignity.
- Provide newspapers, magazines, and other reading matter.
- Provide hobby materials if possible.
- Place a clock in the room.
- Encourage the person to telephone family and friends.
- Provide a current television schedule.
- Organize your work so you can stay to visit with the person.
- Say hello from the doorway often.

(See Focus on Children box; Focus on Older Persons box; and Focus on Home Care box.)

BLOODBORNE PATHOGEN STANDARD

The AIDS (HIV) and hepatitis B viruses are found in blood (see Chapter 30). Therefore they are bloodborne pathogens. The viruses exit the body through blood and are transmitted to others by blood. *Potentially infectious materials* also transmit the viruses. Such materials are contaminated with blood or with a body fluid that may contain blood. Potentially infectious materials also include needles, suction equipment, soiled linens, dressings, and other items used in the person's care.

The Bloodborne Pathogen Standard is a regulation of the Occupational Safety and Health Administration (OSHA). The standard is intended to protect the health team from exposure to the viruses. Box 10-6 contains the definitions used in OSHA's Bloodborne Pathogen Standard.

EXPOSURE CONTROL PLAN

Employers must have a written exposure control plan. The plan identifies employees at risk for exposure to blood or other potentially infectious materials. Staff at risk include all caregivers, surgical staff, central supply staff, laundry and housekeeping staff, laboratory

Box 10-6	Bloodborne Pathogen Standard Definitions

Blood Human blood, human blood components, and products made from human blood

Bloodborne pathogens Pathogens that are present in human blood and can cause disease in humans; these pathogens include, but are not limited to, hepatitis B virus (HBV) and human immunodeficiency virus (HIV)

Contaminated The presence or reasonably anticipated presence of blood or other potentially infectious materials on an item or surface

Contaminated laundry Laundry soiled with blood or other potentially infectious materials or that may contain sharps

Contaminated sharps Any contaminated object that can penetrate the skin including, but not limited to, needles, scalpels, broken glass, broken capillary tubes, and exposed ends of dental wires

Decontamination The use of physical or chemical means to remove, inactivate, or destroy bloodborne pathogens on a surface or item to the point where they can no longer transmit infectious particles and the surface or item is safe for handling, use, or disposal

Engineering controls Controls that isolate or remove the bloodborne pathogen hazard from the workplace (sharps disposal containers, self-sheathing needles)

Exposure incident A specific eye, mouth, other mucous membrane, nonintact skin, or parenteral contact with blood or other potentially infectious materials that results from the performance of an employee's duties

Handwashing facilities The adequate supply of running water, soap, single-use towels, or hot-air drying machines

HBV Hepatitis B virus

HIV Human immunodeficiency virus

Occupational exposure Reasonably anticipated skin, eye, mucous membrane, or parenteral contact with blood or other potentially infectious materials that may result from the performance of an employee's duties

Other potentially infectious materials
- The following human body fluids: semen, vaginal secretions, cerebrospinal fluid, synovial fluid, pleural fluid, pericardial fluid, peritoneal fluid, amniotic fluid, saliva in dental procedures, any body fluid that is visibly contaminated with blood, and all body fluids in situations where it is difficult or impossible to differentiate between body fluids
- Any tissue or organ (other than intact skin) from a human (living or dead)
- HIV-containing cell or tissue cultures, organ cultures, and HIV- or HBV-containing culture medium or other solutions; and blood, organs, or other tissues from experimental animals infected with HIV or HBV

Parenteral Piercing mucous membranes or the skin barrier through events such as needlesticks, human bites, cuts, and abrasions

Personal protective equipment Specialized clothing or equipment worn by an employee for protection against a hazard

Regulated waste
- Liquid or semiliquid blood or other potentially infectious materials
- Contaminated items that would release blood or other potentially infectious materials in a liquid or semiliquid state if compressed
- Items that are caked with dried blood or other potentially infectious materials that are capable of releasing these materials during handling
- Contaminated sharps; pathological and microbiological wastes containing blood or other potentially infectious materials

Source individual Any person (living or dead) whose blood or other potentially infectious materials may be a source of occupational exposure to employees; examples include, but are not limited to:
- Hospital and clinical patients
- Clients in institutions for the developmentally disabled
- Trauma victims
- Clients of drug and alcohol treatment facilities
- Residents of hospices and nursing homes
- Human remains
- Persons who donate or sell blood or blood components

Sterilize The use of a physical or chemical procedure to destroy all microbial life, including spores

Work practice controls Controls that reduce the likelihood of exposure by altering the way the task is performed staff, and others. The plan includes actions to take when an exposure incident occurs.

Staff at risk for exposure must receive free information and training. Training occurs upon employment and yearly. Training is also required for new or changed tasks involving exposure to bloodborne pathogens. OSHA requires that training include:

- An explanation of the Bloodborne Pathogen Standard and where to get a copy
- The causes, signs, and symptoms of bloodborne diseases
- How bloodborne pathogens are transmitted
- An explanation of the exposure control plan and where to get a copy
- How to know which tasks might cause occupational exposure
- The use and limits of safe work practices, engineering controls, and personal protective equipment
- Information on the hepatitis B vaccination
- Who to contact and what to do in an emergency
- Information on reporting an exposure incident, postexposure evaluation, and follow-up
- Information on warning labels and color coding

PREVENTIVE MEASURES

Preventive measures reduce the risk of occupational exposure. Such measures include hepatitis B vaccination and Standard Precautions.

Hepatitis B Vaccination.
Hepatitis B is a liver disease caused by the hepatitis B virus (HBV). HBV is transmitted by blood and sexual contact. The hepatitis B vaccine is given to produce immunity against hepatitis B. **Immunity** means that a person has protection against a certain disease. The immune person will not get the disease.

A **vaccination** involves giving a vaccine to produce immunity. A **vaccine** is a preparation that contains dead or weakened microbes. There are vaccines for many diseases, including measles, mumps, polio, and smallpox.

The hepatitis B vaccination involves 3 injections (shots). The second injection is given 1 month after the first one. The third injection is given 6 months after the second one. The vaccination can be given before or after exposure to HBV.

The hepatitis B vaccination is available to employees within 10 working days of being hired. The vaccination is free. The employer pays for the cost. An employee can refuse the vaccination. If refused, the employee signs a statement refusing the vaccine. The employee can have the vaccination at a later date.

OSHA requires engineering and work practice controls and personal protective equipment. Guidelines also are given for handling equipment and laundry.

Engineering and Work Practice Controls.
Engineering controls reduce employee exposure in the workplace. Special containers for contaminated sharps (needles, broken glass) and specimens remove and isolate the hazard from staff. Containers are puncture-resistant, leakproof, and color coded in red. Or they are labeled with the *BIOHAZARD* symbol (see Fig. 10-19).

Work practice controls also reduce exposure risks. All tasks involving blood or other potentially infectious materials are done in ways that limit splattering, splashing, and spraying. Producing droplets also is avoided. OSHA requires these work practice controls:

- Do not eat, drink, smoke, apply cosmetics or lip balm, or handle contact lenses in areas of occupational exposure.
- Do not store food or drinks in refrigerators or other areas where blood or potentially infectious materials are kept.
- Wash hands after removing gloves. Wash hands as soon as possible after skin contact with blood or other potentially infectious materials.
- Never recap, bend, or remove needles by hand. When a medical procedure requires recapping, bending, or removing contaminated needles, use mechanical means (forceps) or a one-handed method.
- Never shear or break contaminated needles.
- Discard contaminated needles and sharp instruments in containers that are closable, puncture-resistant, and leakproof. Containers are color coded red or have the *BIOHAZARD* symbol. Containers must be upright and not allowed to overfill.

Personal Protective Equipment. Personal protective equipment includes gloves, goggles, face shields, masks, laboratory coats, gowns, shoe covers, and surgical caps. Blood or other potentially infectious material must not pass through the equipment. The equipment protects clothes, undergarments, skin, eyes, mouth, and other mucous membranes.

Personal protective equipment is free to employees. Correct sizes are available. The employer makes sure that equipment is properly cleaned, laundered, repaired, replaced, or discarded. OSHA requires these measures for safely handling and using personal protective equipment:

- Remove protective equipment before leaving the work area and when a garment becomes contaminated.
- Place used protective equipment in marked areas or containers when being stored, washed, decontaminated, or discarded.
- Wear gloves when you expect contact with blood or other potentially infectious materials. Also wear gloves when handling or touching contaminated items or surfaces. Replace worn, punctured, or contaminated gloves.
- Never wash or decontaminate disposable gloves for reuse.
- Discard utility gloves that show signs of cracking, peeling, tearing, or puncturing. Utility gloves are decontaminated for reuse if the process will not ruin them.

Equipment. Contaminated equipment is cleaned and decontaminated. Decontaminate work surfaces with an appropriate disinfectant:

- Upon completing tasks
- Immediately when there is obvious contamination
- After any spill of blood or other potentially infectious material
- At the end of the work shift when surfaces became contaminated since the last cleaning

Use a brush and dustpan or tongs to clean up broken glass. Never pick up broken glass with your hands, not even if wearing gloves. Discard broken glass into a puncture-resistant container.

Waste. Federal, state, and local laws regulate the removal of waste from the agency. The Bloodborne Pathogen Standard requires special measures when discarding contaminated sharps and other regulated waste. Regulated waste includes:

- Liquid or semi-liquid blood or other potentially infectious materials
- Items contaminated with blood or other potentially infectious materials
- Items caked with blood or other potentially infectious materials
- Contaminated sharps

Closable, puncture-resistant, and leakproof containers are required for regulated waste. Containers are color coded in red or labeled with the *BIOHAZARD* symbol. *(See Focus on Home Care box.)*

Focus On... HOME CARE

Dressings, gloves, syringes, needles, and other sharps are used by home care patients and caregivers. Although you will not use syringes, needles, and other sharps, you will assist the family in disposing of these items. Proper disposal of care items is necessary to protect trash handlers from infection. The United States Environmental Protection Agency (EPA) offers these suggestions:
- Place needles, syringes, and other sharp items into hard plastic or metal containers. The container should have a screw-on lid or other secure lid. A plastic detergent bottle and lid are examples. Do not use glass or clear plastic containers.
- Tape the lid in place with a heavy tape. This adds more protection by reinforcing the lid.
- Keep the sharps container out of the reach of children and pets.
- Place dressings, gloves, soiled bed protectors, disposable sheets, and other care items in plastic bags. Close the bags securely.
- Label containers and plastic bags with a "Not for Recycling" label.
- Place plastic bags and sharps containers in a garbage can that has a lid.
- Make sure animals cannot get into the garbage can. Scents from the trash can attract animals.

Housekeeping. The Bloodborne Pathogen Standard requires that the agency be kept clean and sanitary. The employer must have a cleaning schedule. The schedule must include methods of decontamination to be used and the tasks and procedures to be done.

Laundry. OSHA requires these precautions for contaminated laundry:

- Handle contaminated laundry as little as possible.
- Wear gloves or other needed personal protective equipment when handling contaminated laundry.
- Bag contaminated laundry where it was used.
- Mark laundry bags or containers with the *BIOHAZARD* symbol for laundry sent offsite.
- Place wet contaminated laundry in leakproof containers before transporting. The containers are color coded in red or labeled with the *BIOHAZARD* symbol.

EXPOSURE INCIDENTS

An *exposure incident* is any eye, mouth, other mucous membrane, nonintact skin, or parenteral contact with blood or other potentially infectious materials. *Parenteral* means piercing the mucous membranes or the skin barrier. Piercing occurs through needlesticks, human bites, cuts, and abrasions.

Report exposure incidents at once. Medical evaluation and follow-up are free. This includes required laboratory tests. The employee's blood is tested for HBV and HIV. If the employee refuses testing, the blood sample is kept for at least 90 days. Testing is done later if the employee changes his or her mind.

Confidentiality is important. The employee is told of evaluation results. The employee is also told of any medical conditions that may need further treatment. The employee receives a written opinion of the medical evaluation within 15 days after its completion.

The source individual's blood is tested for HIV or HBV. The *source individual* is the person whose blood or body fluids are the source of an exposure incident. State laws vary about releasing the results. The employer informs the employee about any laws affecting the source's identity and test results.

SURGICAL ASEPSIS

Surgical asepsis (sterile technique) is the practices that keep equipment and supplies free of all microbes. **Sterile** means the absence of *all* microbes, including spores. Surgical asepsis is required any time the skin or sterile tissues are penetrated. The operating room and labor and delivery areas require surgical asepsis. So do many tests and nursing procedures. If any break occurs in sterile technique, pathogens and nonpathogens can enter the body. An infection can develop.

Some states allow assistive personnel to perform selected sterile procedures. Examples include urinary catheterizations, sterile dressing changes, suctioning, and collecting blood specimens. In other states, assistive personnel can only assist nurses with sterile procedures. Do not perform any sterile procedure unless:

- Your state allows assistive personnel to perform the procedure.
- The procedure is in your job description.
- You received the necessary education and training.
- You review the procedure with the nurse.
- A nurse is available for questions and guidance.

PRINCIPLES OF SURGICAL ASEPSIS

Operating room and labor and delivery staff must follow certain procedures. They wear masks and surgical caps for handwashing. This handwashing is called a surgical "scrub." It takes at least 5 minutes. Then they put on sterile gowns and sterile gloves. For sterile nursing procedures, regular handwashing and sterile gloves are needed. You also wear personal protective equipment as needed to prevent contact with blood, body fluids, secretions, and excretions.

For a sterile procedure, all items in contact with the person are kept sterile. If any item is contaminated, the person is at risk for infection. Therefore you must maintain a sterile field. A **sterile field** is a work area free of pathogens and nonpathogens (including spores). Box 10-7 lists the principles and practices of surgical asepsis. Follow them to maintain a sterile field. (*See Focus on Home Care box.*)

Focus On... HOME CARE

You may need to clean a work surface before you practice surgical asepsis. Use soap and water and practice Standard Precautions. Always clean from the cleanest area to the dirtiest. Also clean away from your body and uniform. Dry the surface after cleaning.

Box 10-7 | Principles and Practices for Surgical Asepsis

- A sterile item can touch only another sterile item.
- If a sterile item touches a clean item, the sterile item is contaminated.
  - If a clean item touches a sterile item, the sterile item is contaminated.
  - A sterile package that is open, torn, punctured, wet, moist, or has a water mark is contaminated.
  - A sterile package is contaminated after the expiration date on the package.
  - Place only sterile items on a sterile field.
  - Use sterile gloves or sterile forceps to handle other sterile items (Fig. 10-22).
  - Consider any item as contaminated if unsure of its sterility.
  - Do not use contaminated items. They are discarded or resterilized.
- Sterile items or a sterile field are always kept within your vision and above your waist.
  - If you cannot see an item, the item is contaminated.
  - If the item is below your waist, the item is contaminated.
  - Keep sterile gloved hands above your waist and within your sight.
  - Do not leave a sterile field unattended.
  - Do not turn your back on a sterile field.
- Airborne microorganisms can contaminate sterile items or a sterile field.
  - Prevent drafts by closing the door and avoiding extra movements. Ask other staff in the room to avoid extra moving.
  - Avoid coughing, sneezing, talking, or laughing over a sterile field. Turn your head away from the sterile field if you must talk.
  - Wear a mask if you need to talk during the procedure.
  - Do not perform or assist with sterile procedures if you have a respiratory infection.
  - Do not reach over a sterile field.
- Fluid flows downward, in the direction of gravity.
  - Hold wet items down (see Fig. 10-22). If held up, fluid flows down into a contaminated area. The contaminated fluid flows back into the sterile field when the item is held down.
  - Hold your hands higher than your elbows during a surgical scrub. Water from your elbows will not flow onto your clean hands and fingers.
- The sterile field is kept dry, unless the area below it is sterile.
  - The sterile field is contaminated if it gets wet and the area below it is not sterile.
  - Avoid spilling and splashing when pouring sterile fluids into sterile containers.
- The edges of a sterile field are contaminated.
  - A 1-inch (2.5 cm) margin around the sterile field is contaminated (Fig. 10-23).
  - Place all sterile items inside the 1-inch (2.5 cm) margin of the sterile field.
  - Items outside the 1-inch (2.5 cm) margin are contaminated.
- Honesty is essential to sterile technique.
  - You know when you contaminate an item or sterile field. Be honest with yourself even if other staff members are not present.
  - Remove the contaminated item, and correct the situation. If necessary, start over with sterile supplies.
  - Report the contamination to the nurse.

Fig. 10-22 Sterile forceps are used to handle sterile items.

Fig. 10-23 A 1-inch (2.5 cm) margin around the sterile field is considered contaminated.

▷ DONNING AND REMOVING STERILE GLOVES

Sterile gloves are put on after setting up the sterile field. After putting on sterile gloves, you can handle sterile items within the sterile field. You cannot touch anything outside the sterile field.

In operating rooms and delivery areas, the closed method of sterile gloving is followed. A sterile gown is donned and then sterile gloves. You will learn sterile gowning and closed gloving if you work in those areas. The open gloving method is used for sterile procedures at the bedside.

Sterile gloves are disposable. They come in peelback packaging. A variety of sizes let them fit each person snugly. The insides are powdered for ease in donning the gloves. Also, the right glove and left glove are marked on the package.

Always keep sterile gloved hands above your waist and within your vision. You can touch only items within the sterile field. If your gloves become contaminated, you must remove the gloves and put on a new pair. Also replace gloves that are torn, cut, or punctured.

Fig. 10-24 Donning sterile gloves. **A,** Open the inner wrapper to expose the gloves. **B,** Pick up the glove at the cuff with your thumb and index finger. **C,** Slide your fingers and hand into the glove. **D,** Reach under the cuff of the other glove with your fingers. **E,** Pull on the glove. **F,** Adjust each glove for comfort. **G,** Slide your fingers under the cuffs to pull them up.

Donning and Removing Sterile Gloves

Procedure

1 Inspect the package for sterility:
   a Check the expiration date
   b See if the package is dry
   c Check for tears, holes, punctures, and watermarks
2 Arrange a work surface:
   a Make sure you have enough room
   b Arrange the work surface at waist level and within your vision
   c Clean and dry the work surface
   d Do not reach or turn your back on the work surface
3 Open the package. Grasp the flaps, and gently peel the flaps back.
4 Remove the inner package. Place it on a clean work surface. Have your work surface at waist height.
5 Read any manufacturer's instructions or information on the inner package. The package may be labeled with left, right, up, and down.
6 Arrange the inner package for left, right, up, and down. Have the left glove on your left and the right glove on your right. Have the cuffs near you with the fingers pointing away.
7 Use the thumb and index finger of each hand to grasp the folded edges of the inner package.
8 Fold back the inner package to expose the gloves (Fig. 10-24, *A*). Do not touch or otherwise contaminate the inside of the package or the gloves. The inside of the inner package is a sterile field.
9 Note that each glove has a cuff about 2 to 3 inches wide. The cuffs and insides of the gloves are not sterile.

10 Put on the right glove if you are right-handed. Put on the left glove if you are left-handed:
   a Pick up the glove with your other hand. Use your thumb and index and middle fingers (Fig. 10-24, *B*).
   b Touch only the cuff and the inside of the glove.
   c Turn the hand to be gloved palm side up.
   d Lift the cuff up. Slide your fingers and hand into the glove (Fig. 10-24, *C*).
   e Pull the glove up over your hand. If some fingers get stuck, leave them that way until the other glove is on. *Do not use your ungloved hand to straighten the glove. Do not let the outside of the glove touch any nonsterile surface.*
   f Leave the cuff turned down.
11 Put on the other glove with your gloved hand:
   a Reach under the cuff of the second glove with the four fingers of your gloved hand (Fig. 10-24, *D*). Keep your gloved thumb close to your gloved palm.
   b Pull on the second glove (Fig. 10-24, *E*). Your gloved hand cannot touch the cuff or any other surface. Hold the thumb of your first gloved hand away from your gloved palm.
12 Adjust each glove with the other hand. The gloves should be smooth and comfortable (Fig. 10-24, *F*).
13 Slide your fingers under the cuffs to pull them up (Fig. 10-24, *G*).
14 Touch only sterile items.
15 Remove the gloves as in Figure 10-15.

CROSS-TRAINING OPPORTUNITIES

Other health workers are involved in infection control. They work in the central supply department and the housekeeping department. Infection control measures and the Bloodborne Pathogen Standard are followed. Personal protective equipment is worn as needed. You may be asked to cross-train to work in one or both of these areas.

CENTRAL SUPPLY

Staff in the central supply department disinfect and sterilize supplies and equipment. These procedures may be done for new items bought by the agency. Used equipment and supplies are also disinfected or sterilized before being used for another person. Central supply staff also make sure that each nursing unit is stocked with items needed for care. They also bring special equipment to nursing units as requested.

HOUSEKEEPING

The housekeeping staff clean patient or resident rooms, the nursing units, hallways, bathrooms, and other departments and parts of the agency. They have special cleaning methods and procedures for cleaning and disinfecting floors, furniture, bathrooms, and equipment.

REVIEW

Circle T if the answer is true and F if it is false.

1. T F Microbes are pathogens in their natural environments.

2. T F An infection results from the invasion and growth of microbes in the body.

3. T F An item is sterile if nonpathogens are present.

4. T F You hold your hands and forearms up during the handwashing procedure.

5. T F Unused items in a person's room are used for another person.

6. T F A person has immunity against hepatitis B. The person will develop the disease.

7. T F The 1-inch edge around a sterile field is contaminated.

8. T F A sterile package has a watermark. The package is contaminated.

9. T F The inside and cuffs of sterile gloves are contaminated.

Circle the BEST answer.

10. Pathogens need the following to grow *except*
    A. Water
    B. Light
    C. Oxygen
    D. Nourishment

11. The person with an infection may have
    A. Fever, nausea, vomiting, rash, and/or sores
    B. Pain or tenderness, redness, and/or swelling
    C. Fatigue, loss of appetite, and/or a discharge
    D. All of the above

12. Microbes enter and leave the body through the following *except*
    A. Respiratory tract and/or breaks in the skin
    B. Gastrointestinal system and/or the blood
    C. Reproductive system and/or urinary system
    D. Intact skin

13. Which does not prevent nosocomial infections?
    A. Handwashing before and after giving care
    B. Sterilizing all items used for care
    C. Surgical asepsis
    D. Standard Precautions

14. When cleaning equipment, do the following *except*
    A. Rinse the item in cold water before cleaning
    B. Wash the item with soap and hot water
    C. Use a brush if necessary
    D. Clean from the dirtiest area to the cleanest

15. Isolation precautions
    A. Prevent infection
    B. Destroy pathogens
    C. Keep pathogens within a certain area
    D. Destroy pathogens and nonpathogens

16. Standard Precautions
    A. Are used for all persons
    B. Prevent the spread of pathogens through the air
    C. Require gowns, masks, gloves, and protective eyewear
    D. Involve medical and surgical asepsis

17. Gloves are worn when in contact with
    A. Blood
    B. Body fluids
    C. Secretions and excretions
    D. All of the above

18. A mask
    A. Can be reused
    B. Is clean on the inside
    C. Is contaminated when moist
    D. Should fit loosely for breathing

19. Proper use of personal protective equipment involves the following *except*
    A. Washing disposable gloves for reuse
    B. Removing protective equipment before leaving the work area
    C. Discarding cracked or torn utility gloves
    D. Wearing gloves when touching contaminated items or surfaces

20. When are contaminated work surfaces cleaned?
    A. After completing a task
    B. Immediately when there is obvious contamination
    C. After blood or other potentially infectious material is spilled
    D. All of the above

21. The Bloodborne Pathogen Standard involves the following *except*
    A. Washing hands after removing gloves
    B. Discarding sharp items into containers with the *BIOHAZARD* symbol
    C. Storing food and blood in different places
    D. Eating and drinking in areas of occupational exposure

22. You were exposed to a bloodborne pathogen. Which is *true?*
    A. You do not have to report the incident.
    B. You pay for any required laboratory tests.
    C. You can refuse HBV and HIV testing.
    D. The source individual can refuse testing.

23. These statements are about surgical asepsis. Which is *false?*
    A. A sterile item can touch only another sterile item.
    B. Wet items are held up.
    C. If you cannot see an item, it is contaminated.
    D. Sterile items are kept above your waist.

24. You have on sterile gloves. You can touch
    A. Anything on the sterile field
    B. Anything on your work surface
    C. Anything below your waist
    D. Any part of your uniform

Answers to these questions are on p. 835.

BODY

MECHANICS

OBJECTIVES

Define the key terms listed in this chapter

Explain the purpose and rules of using good body mechanics

Identify comfort and safety measures for lifting, turning, and moving persons in bed

Know the basic bed positions

Explain the purpose of a transfer belt

Explain why good body alignment and position changes are important

Identify the comfort and safety measures for positioning persons in bed

Position persons in the basic bed positions and in a chair

Perform the procedures described in this chapter

KEY TERMS

base of support The area on which an object rests

body alignment The way in which body parts are aligned with one another; posture

body mechanics Using the body in an efficient and careful way

dorsal recumbent position The back-lying or supine position

Fowler's position A semisitting position; the head of the bed is elevated 45 to 60 degrees

friction The rubbing of one surface against another

gait belt A transfer or safety belt

lateral position The side-lying position

logrolling Turning the person as a unit, in alignment, with one motion

posture The way in which body parts are aligned with one another; body alignment

prone position Lying on the abdomen with the head turned to one side

safety belt A transfer belt or gait belt

shearing When skin sticks to a surface and muscles slide in the direction the body is moving

side-lying position The lateral position

Sims' position A left side-lying position in which the upper leg is sharply flexed so that it is not on the lower leg and the lower arm is behind the person

supine position The back-lying or dorsal recumbent position

transfer belt A belt used to hold onto a person during a transfer or when walking with the person; a gait belt or safety belt

You will turn and reposition patients and residents in bed. You also transfer them to and from chairs, wheelchairs, and stretchers. During these and other activities, you must use your body correctly. This protects you and the person from injury.

Box 11-1 contains a review of the structure and function of the musculoskeletal system. For more detailed information, see Chapter 6.

BODY MECHANICS

Body mechanics means using the body in an efficient and careful way. It involves good posture and balance and using the strongest and largest muscles for work. Fatigue, muscle strain, and injury can result from improper use and positioning of the body during activity or rest. You must focus on the person's and your

Box 11-1	Musculoskeletal System: Review of Body Structure and Function

The musculoskeletal system provides the framework for the body and allows the body to move. It also protects and gives the body shape.

BONES

Bones are hard, rigid structures that are made up of living cells. *Long bones* (leg bones) bear the weight of the body. *Short bones* allow skill and ease in movement. Bones in the wrists, fingers, ankles, and toes are short bones. *Flat bones* protect the organs. Such bones include the ribs, skull, pelvic bones, and shoulder blades. *Irregular bones* are the vertebrae in the spinal column. They allow various degrees of movement and flexibility.

JOINTS

A *joint* is the point at which two or more bones meet. Joints allow movement (joint movement is discussed in Chapter 20). There are three types of joints (Fig. 11-1). A *ball-and-socket* joint allows movement in all directions. The joints of the hips and shoulders are ball-and-socket joints. A *hinge joint* allows movement in one direction. The elbow and knee are hinge joints. A *pivot joint* allows turning from side to side. The skull is connected to the spine by a pivot joint.

MUSCLES

There are more than 500 muscles in the human body (Fig. 11-2, p. 244). *Voluntary* muscles can be consciously controlled. Muscles that are attached to bones *(skeletal muscles)* are voluntary. Arm muscles do not work unless you move your arm; likewise for leg muscles. *Involuntary* muscles work automatically and cannot be consciously controlled. Involuntary muscles control the action of the stomach, intestines, blood vessels, and other body organs. *Cardiac muscle* is in the heart. It is an involuntary muscle.

Muscles perform three important body functions:
- Movement of body parts
- Maintenance of posture
- Production of body heat

Some muscles constantly contract to maintain the body's posture. When muscles contract, they burn food for energy, resulting in the production of heat. The greater the muscular activity, the greater the amount of heat produced in the body. Shivering is a way the body produces heat when exposed to cold. The shivering sensation is from rapid, general muscle contractions.

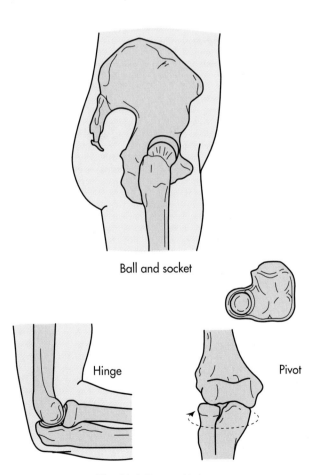

Ball and socket

Hinge

Pivot

Fig. 11-1 Types of joints.

A

Frontalis
Orbicularis oculi
Orbicularis oris
Sternocleidomastoid
Rectus abdominis
Deltoid
Pectoralis major
Brachoradialis
Biceps brachii
Pronator teres
Brachialis
Flexor carpi radialis
Iliopsoas
Sartorius
Gracilis
Vastus lateralis
Vastus medialis
Pectineus
Rectus femoris
Gastrocnemius
Peroneus longus
Soleus
Tibialis anterior

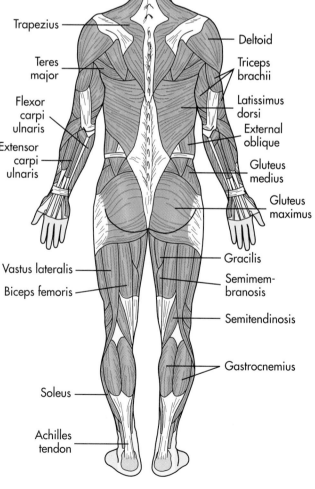

B

Trapezius
Deltoid
Teres major
Triceps brachii
Flexor carpi ulnaris
Latissimus dorsi
Extensor carpi ulnaris
External oblique
Gluteus medius
Gluteus maximus
Gracilis
Vastus lateralis
Semimembranosis
Biceps femoris
Semitendinosis
Gastrocnemius
Soleus
Achilles tendon

Fig. 11-2 A, Anterior (front) view of muscles. **B,** Posterior (back) view of muscles.

A   B

Base of support

Fig. 11-3 A, Anterior (front) view of an adult in good body alignment with feet apart for a wide base of support. **B,** Lateral (side) view of an adult with good posture and alignment.

own body mechanics. Good body mechanics reduce the risk of injury.

Posture (body alignment) is the way body parts (head, trunk, arms, and legs) are aligned with one another. Good body alignment (posture) lets the body move and function with strength and efficiency. Standing, sitting, and lying down require good alignment.

Base of support is the area on which an object rests. A good base of support is needed for balance (Fig. 11-3). When standing, your feet are your base of support. Stand with your feet apart for a wider base of support and more balance.

The strongest and largest muscles are in the shoulders, upper arms, hips, and thighs. Use these muscles to lift and move heavy objects. Otherwise, you place strain and exertion on smaller and weaker muscles. This causes fatigue and injury. *Back injuries are a major risk.* Good body mechanics involve:

- Bending your knees and squatting to lift a heavy object (Fig. 11-4, p. 246). Do not bend from your waist. Bending from the waist places strain on small back muscles.
- Holding items close to your body and base of support (see Fig. 11-4). This involves upper arm and shoulder muscles. Holding objects away from your body places strain on small muscles in your lower arms.

All activities require good body mechanics. Follow the rules in Box 11-2 on p. 246 to safely and efficiently lift and move persons and heavy objects.

Text continued on p. 248

Fig. 11-4 Picking up a box using good body mechanics.

Box 11-2   Rules for Body Mechanics

- Keep your body in good alignment with a wide base of support.
- Use the stronger and larger muscles in your shoulders, upper arms, thighs, and hips.
- Keep objects close to your body when you lift, move, or carry them (see Fig. 11-4).
- Avoid unnecessary bending and reaching. Raise the bed so it is close to your waist. Adjust the overbed table so it is at your waist level.
- Face your work area. This prevents unnecessary twisting.
- Push, slide, or pull heavy objects whenever you can, rather than lifting them.
- Widen your base of support when pushing or pulling. Move your front leg forward when pushing. Move your rear leg back when pulling (Fig. 11-5).
- Use both hands and arms to lift, move, or carry heavy objects.

- Turn your whole body when changing the direction of your movement. Move your feet in the direction of the turn instead of twisting your body.
- Work with smooth and even movements. Avoid sudden or jerky motions.
- Get help from a co-worker if the person cannot assist with turning or moving.
- Get help from a co-worker to move heavy objects or persons. Avoid lifting or moving a person by yourself.
- Bend your hips and knees to lift heavy objects from the floor (see Fig. 11-4). Straighten your back as the object reaches thigh level. Your leg and thigh muscles work to raise the item off the floor and to waist level.
- Do not lift objects higher than chest level. Do not lift above your shoulders. Use a step stool to reach an object higher than chest level.
- Wear a body support (Fig. 11-6) to help you use good body mechanics.

Fig. 11-5 Move your rear leg back when pulling an item.

Fig. 11-6 A body support helps in using good body mechanics.

LIFTING AND MOVING PERSONS IN BED

Some persons can move and turn in bed themselves. Others need help from at least one person. Those who are unconscious, paralyzed, on complete bedrest, in a cast, or weak from surgery or injury need help. Sometimes 2 or 3 people are needed.

COMFORT AND SAFETY

The person's skin is protected during lifting and moving. Friction and shearing injure the skin. Both cause infection and pressure ulcers (see Chapter 25). **Friction** is the rubbing of one surface against another. When moved in bed, the person's skin rubs against the sheet. **Shearing** is when the skin sticks to a surface and muscles slide in the direction the body is moving (Fig. 11-7). Shearing occurs when the person slides down in bed or is moved in bed. Reduce friction and shearing by rolling or lifting the person. A cotton drawsheet (see Chapter 13) serves as a *lift sheet (turning or pull sheet)* to move the person in bed and reduce friction. Some agencies use turning pads for this purpose. *(See Focus on Older Persons box.)*

Other comfort and safety measures for moving persons in bed include the following:

- Ask the nurse about limits or restrictions in positioning or moving the person.
- Decide how to move the person and how much help you need.
- Ask co-workers to help *before* starting the procedure.
- Cover and screen the person to protect the right to privacy.
- Protect tubes or drainage containers connected to the person.
- Use caution when moving persons with severe arthritis or osteoporosis (see Chapter 30). Ask a co-worker to help you move these persons. This protects such persons from pain or injury.

Focus On... OLDER PERSONS

Older persons are at great risk for shearing. Their skin is fragile and easily torn. Use a lift or turning sheet or turning pad when lifting and moving older persons.

Fig. 11-7 When the head of the bed is raised to a sitting position, skin on the buttocks stays in place. However, internal structures move forward as the person slides down in bed. Skin is pinched between the mattress and hip bones.

▶ RAISING THE PERSON'S HEAD AND SHOULDERS

You may have to raise a person's head and shoulders to give care. Simply removing or straightening a pillow requires this procedure. You can raise the person's head and shoulders easily and safely by locking arms with the person. Figure 11-8 on p. 250 shows the procedure being done by one nursing assistant. Figure 11-9 on p. 251 shows two nursing assistants doing the procedure. *(See Focus on Older Persons box.)*

Text continued on p. 252

Focus On... OLDER PERSONS

Older persons have fragile bones and joints. When raising the older person's head and shoulders, it is best that two staff members perform the procedure. This protects the older person from pain and injury.

Raising the Person's Head and Shoulders

QUALITY OF LIFE

Remember to:
- Knock before entering the person's room
- Address the person by name
- Introduce yourself by name and title

Pre-Procedure

1 Ask a co-worker to help you if you need assistance.
2 Wash your hands.
3 Identify the person. Check the ID bracelet, and call the person by name.
4 Explain what you are going to do.
5 Provide for privacy.
6 Lock the bed wheels.
7 Raise the bed to the best level for good body mechanics. Make sure bed rails are up.

Procedure

8 Ask your co-worker to stand on the other side of the bed. Lower the bed rails.
9 Ask the person to put the near arm under your near arm and behind your shoulder. His or her hand rests on top of your shoulder. If you are standing on the right side, the person's right hand rests on your right shoulder (Fig. 11-8, *A*, p. 250). If you have help, the person does the same with your co-worker. The person's left hand rests on your co-workers left shoulder (Fig. 11-9, *A*, p. 251).
10 Put your arm nearest to the person under his or her arm. Your hand is on the person's shoulder. Have your co-worker do the same.
11 Put your free arm under the person's neck and shoulders (Fig. 11-8, *B*, p. 250). Your co-worker does the same (Fig. 11-9, *B*, p. 251).
12 Help the person pull up to a sitting or semi-sitting position on the count of "3" (Figs. 11-8, *C* and 11-9, *C*, p. 250).
13 Use the arm and hand that supported the person's neck and shoulders to give care (Fig. 11-8, *D*). Your co-worker supports the person (Fig. 11-9, *D*, p. 251).
14 Help the person lie down. Provide support with your locked arms. Support the person's neck and shoulders with your other arm.

Post-Procedure

15 Provide for comfort. Position the person in good body alignment.
16 Place the signal light within reach.
17 Raise or lower bed rails. Follow the care plan.
18 Lower the bed to its lowest position.
19 Unscreen the person.

Fig. 11-8 Raise the person's head and shoulders by locking arms with the person. **A,** The person's near arm is under the nursing assistant's near arm and behind the shoulder. **B,** The nursing assistant's far arm is under the person's neck and shoulders, with the near arm under the person's nearest arm. **C,** The person is raised to a semisitting position by locking arms. **D,** The nursing assistant lifts the pillow while the person is in a semisitting position.

Fig. 11-9 Raising the person's head and shoulders with assistance. **A,** Two nursing assistants lock arms with the person. **B,** The nursing assistants have their arms under the person's head and neck. **C,** The nursing assistants raise the person to a semisitting position. **D,** One nursing assistant supports the person in the semisitting position while the other gives care.

▶ MOVING THE PERSON UP IN BED

When the bed is raised, it is easy to slide down toward the middle and foot of the bed (Fig. 11-10). The person is moved up in bed for good body alignment and comfort. At least two caregivers are needed to move heavy, weak, and very old persons up in bed. You can usually move children up in bed alone. You can sometimes move lightweight adults up in bed alone if they use a trapeze. However, it is best to have help. This protects you and the person from injury.

Fig. 11-10 A person in poor alignment after sliding down in bed.

Fig. 11-11 A person is moved up in bed by two nursing assistants. Each has one arm under the person's shoulders and the other under the thighs. They have locked arms under the person. The person's knees are flexed. The nursing assistants will shift their weight from the rear leg to the front leg as the person is moved up in bed.

Fig. 11-12 The person grasps a trapeze and flexes the knees. The nursing assistants' body weight is shifted from the rear leg to the front leg as the person is moved up in bed. NOTE: Although you can move children and light weight adults alone using this method, it is best to have help.

Moving the Person Up in Bed

QUALITY OF LIFE

Remember to:
- Knock before entering the person's room
- Address the person by name
- Introduce yourself by name and title

Pre-Procedure

1 Ask a co-worker to help you.
2 Wash your hands.
3 Identify the person. Check the ID bracelet, and call the person by name.
4 Explain what you are going to do.
5 Provide for privacy.
6 Lock the bed wheels.
7 Raise the bed to the best level for body mechanics. Make sure the bed rails are up.

Procedure

8 Lower the head of the bed to a level appropriate for the person. It is as flat as possible.
9 Stand on one side of the bed. Your co-worker stands on the other side.
10 Lower the bed rail near you. Your co-worker does the same.
11 Place the pillow against the headboard if the person can be without it. This prevents the person's head from hitting the headboard when being moved up.
12 Stand with a wide base of support. Point the foot near the head of the bed toward the head of the bed. Face the head of the bed.
13 Bend your hips and knees. Keep your back straight.
14 Place one arm under the person's shoulder and one arm under the thighs. Your co-worker does the same. Grasp each other's forearms (Fig. 11-11).
15 Ask the person to grasp the trapeze. (Omit this step if the person does not have one.)
16 Have the person flex both knees.
17 Explain that you will move on the count of "3." The person should push against the bed with the feet if able.
18 Move the person to the head of the bed on the count of "3." Shift your weight from your rear leg to your front leg (Fig. 11-12).
19 Repeat steps 12 through 18 if necessary.

Post-Procedure

20 Put the pillow under the person's head and shoulders. Straighten linens.
21 Provide for comfort. Position the person in good body alignment.
22 Place the signal light within reach.
23 Raise or lower bed rails. Follow the care plan.
24 Raise the head of the bed to a level appropriate for the person.
25 Lower the bed to its lowest position.
26 Unscreen the person.
27 Wash your hands.

► MOVING THE PERSON UP IN BED WITH A LIFT SHEET

With a co-worker's help, you can easily and safely move a person up in bed with a *lift sheet*. (It is called a *turning sheet* when used to turn the person.) Friction and shearing are reduced, and the person is lifted more evenly. You can use a flat sheet folded in half, a drawsheet, or a turning pad (Fig. 11-13). It is placed under the person from the head to above the knees.

Use this procedure to move persons who are unconscious, paralyzed, or recovering from spinal surgery or who have spinal cord injuries. Also use it for older persons.

Fig. 11-13 Turning pad.

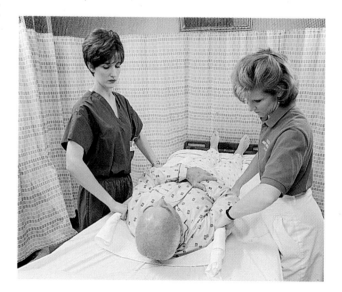

Fig. 11-14 A lift sheet is used to move the person up in bed. The lift sheet extends from the person's head to above the knees. The lift sheet is rolled close to the person and held near the shoulders and buttocks.

Moving the Person Up in Bed With a Lift Sheet

QUALITY OF LIFE

Remember to:
- Knock before entering the person's room
- Address the person by name
- Introduce yourself by name and title

Pre-Procedure

1 Ask a co-worker to help you.

2 Wash your hands.

3 Identify the person. Check the ID bracelet, and call the person by name.

4 Explain what you are going to do.

5 Provide for privacy.

6 Lock the bed wheels.

7 Raise the bed to the best level for good body mechanics. Make sure the bed rails are up.

Procedure

8 Lower the head of the bed to a level appropriate for the person. It is as flat as possible.

9 Stand on one side of the bed. Your helper stands on the other side.

10 Lower the bed rails.

11 Place the pillow against the headboard if the person can be without it.

12 Stand with a broad base of support. Point the foot near the head of the bed toward the head of the bed. Face that direction.

13 Roll the sides of the lift sheet up close to the person.

14 Grasp the rolled-up lift sheet firmly near the person's shoulders and buttocks (Fig. 11-14). Make sure you support the person's head.

15 Bend your hips and knees.

16 Slide the person up in bed on the count of "3". Shift your weight from your rear leg to your front leg.

17 Unroll the lift sheet.

Post-Procedure

18 Put the pillow under the person's head and shoulders. Straighten linens.

19 Provide for comfort. Position the person in good body alignment.

20 Place the signal light within reach. ·

21 Raise or lower bed rails. Follow the care plan.

22 Raise the head of the bed to a level appropriate for the person.

23 Lower the bed to its lowest position.

24 Unscreen the person.

25 Wash your hands.

► MOVING THE PERSON TO THE SIDE OF THE BED

Repositioning and care procedures require moving the person to the side of the bed. The person is moved to the side of the bed before turning. Otherwise, after turning, the person lies on the side of the bed—not in the middle.

Sometimes you have to reach over the person. Giving a bed bath is an example. You have to reach less if the person is close to you.

One method involves moving the person in segments. One person can sometimes do this. The lift sheet method is used for persons with spinal cord injuries or recovering from spinal surgery. Using a lift shift helps prevent pain, skin damage, and injury to the bones, joints, and spinal cord. When using a lift sheet, you need a co-worker to help you. *(See Focus on Older Persons box.)*

Focus On... **OLDER PERSONS**

A lift sheet is used to move older persons in bed. It is also used to move persons with arthritis. The lift sheet helps prevent pain and bone and joint injuries.

Fig. 11-15 The person is moved to the side of the bed in segments.

Moving the Person to the Side of the Bed

QUALITY OF LIFE

Remember to:
- Knock before entering the person's room
- Address the person by name
- Introduce yourself by name and title

Pre-Procedure

1 Ask a co-worker to help if you will use a lift sheet.
2 Wash your hands.
3 Identify the person. Check the ID bracelet, and call the person by name.
4 Explain the procedure to the person.
5 Provide for privacy.
6 Lock the bed wheels.
7 Raise the bed to the best level for good body mechanics. Make sure the bed rails are up.

Procedure

8 Lower the head of the bed to a level appropriate for the person. It is as flat as possible.
9 Stand on the side of the bed to which you will move the person.
10 Lower the bed rail near you. (Both bed rails are lowered for Step 14).
11 Stand with your feet about 12 inches apart and with one foot in front of the other. Flex your knees.
12 Cross the person's arms over the person's chest.
13 *Method 1:* Moving the person in segments
  a Place your arm under the person's neck and shoulders. Grasp the far shoulder.
  b Place your other arm under the midback.
  c Move the upper part of the person's body toward you. Rock backward and shift your weight to your rear leg (Fig. 11-15, *A*).
  d Place one arm under the person's waist and one under the thighs.
  e Rock backward to move the lower part of the person toward you (Fig. 11-15, *B*).
  f Repeat the procedure for the legs and feet (Fig. 11-15, *C*). Your arms should be under the person's thighs and calves.
Method 2: Moving the person with a lift sheet
  a Roll the lift sheet up close to the person (see Fig. 11-14).
  b Grasp the rolled-up lift sheet near the person's shoulders and buttocks. Make sure you support the head.
  c Rock backward on the count of "3," moving the person toward you. Your co-worker rocks backward slightly and then forward toward you while keeping the arms straight.
  d Unroll the lift sheet.

Post-Procedure

14 Provide for comfort.
15 Position the person in good alignment. Follow the nurse's directions and the care plan. Reposition the pillow under the person's head and shoulders.
16 Place the signal light within the person's reach.
17 Raise or lower bed rails. Follow the care plan.
18 Lower the bed to its lowest position.
19 Unscreen the person.
20 Wash your hands.

TURNING PERSONS

Turning persons onto their sides helps prevent complications from bedrest. Certain medical and nursing procedures require the side-lying position. Persons are turned toward or away from you. The direction depends on the person's condition and the situation. *(See Focus on Older Persons box.)*

Focus On... OLDER PERSONS

Many older persons suffer from arthritis in their spines and knees. When turning these persons it is best to logroll the person using a turning sheet (lift sheet). Logrolling is less painful for these persons.

Turning a Person   NNAAP™

QUALITY OF LIFE

Remember to:
- Knock before entering the person's room
- Address the person by name
- Introduce yourself by name and title

Pre-Procedure

1 Wash your hands.
2 Identify the person. Check the ID bracelet, and call the person by name.
3 Explain the procedure to the person.
4 Provide for privacy.
5 Lock the bed wheels.
6 Raise the bed to the best level for body mechanics. Make sure bed rails are up.

Procedure

7 Lower the head of the bed to a level appropriate for the person. It is as flat as possible.
8 Stand on the side of the bed opposite to where you will turn the person. The far bed rail is up.
9 Lower the bed rail near you.
10 Move the person to the side near you. (See *Moving the Person to the Side of the Bed,* p. 257.)
11 Cross the person's arms over the person's chest. Cross the leg near you over the far leg.
12 *Moving the person away from you:*
  a Stand with a wide base of support. Flex your knees.
  b Place one hand on the person's shoulder and the other on the buttock near you.
  c Push the person gently toward the other side of the bed (Fig. 11-16). Shift your weight from your rear leg to your front leg.
  Moving the person toward you:

  a Raise the bed rail.
  b Go to the other side. Lower the bed rail.
  c Stand with a wide base of support. Flex your knees.
  d Place one hand on the person's far shoulder and the other on the far hip.
  e Roll the person toward you gently (Fig. 11-17).
13 Provide for comfort. Position the person in good body alignment as directed by the nurse and the care plan. The following is common:
  a Place a pillow under the head and neck.
  b Position the upper leg in front of the lower leg.
  c Support the upper leg and thigh with pillows.
  d Place a small pillow under the upper hand and arm.
  e Position a pillow against the back.

Post-Procedure

14 Place the signal light within reach.
15 Raise or lower bed rails. Follow the care plan.
16 Lower the bed to its lowest position.
17 Unscreen the person.
18 Wash your hands.

Fig. 11-16 Turning the person away from you.

Fig. 11-17 Turning the person toward you.

◢ Logrolling

Logrolling is turning the person as a unit, in alignment, with one motion. The spine is kept straight. The procedure is used to turn:

- Older persons with arthritic spines or knees
- Persons recovering from hip fractures
- Persons with spinal cord injuries (the spine is kept straight at all times following spinal cord injury)

- Persons recovering from spinal surgery (the spine is kept straight at all times following spinal surgery)

Two or three staff members are needed to logroll a person. Three are needed if the person is tall or heavy. Sometimes a turning sheet is used.

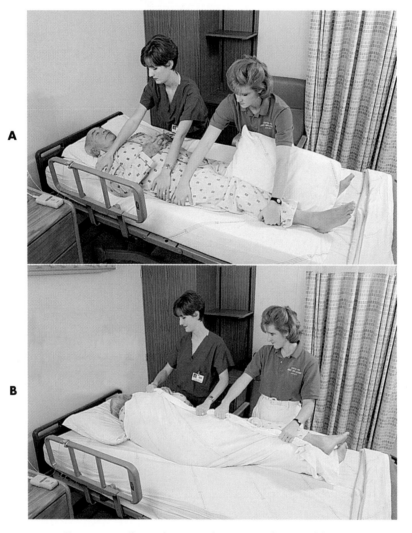

Fig. 11-18 Logrolling. **A,** A pillow is between the person's legs, and the arms are crossed on the chest. The person is on the far side of the bed. **B,** A turning sheet is used to logroll a person.

Logrolling The Person

QUALITY OF LIFE

Remember to:
- Knock before entering the person's room
- Address the person by name
- Introduce yourself by name and title

Pre-Procedure

1. Ask a co-worker to help you.
2. Wash your hands.
3. Identify the person. Check the ID bracelet, and call the person by name.
4. Explain the procedure to the person.
5. Provide for privacy.
6. Lock the bed wheels.
7. Raise the bed to the best level for good body mechanics. Make sure the bed rails are up.

Procedure

8. Make sure the bed is flat.
9. Stand on the side opposite to which you will turn the person. Have your co-worker stand on the other side.
10. Lower the bed rails.
11. Move the person as a unit to the side of the bed near you. Use the turning sheet.
12. Place the person's arms across the chest. Place a pillow between the knees (Fig. 11-18, A).
13. Raise the side rail. Go to the other side, and lower the bed rail.
14. Position yourself near the shoulders and chest. Your co-worker stands near the buttocks and thighs.
15. Stand with a broad base of support. One foot is in front of the other.
16. Ask the person to hold his or her body rigid.
17. Roll the person toward you as in Fig. 11-18, A. Or use a turn sheet as in Fig. 11-18, B. Turn the person as a unit.

Post-Procedure

18. Provide for comfort. Use pillows as directed by the nurse and care plan. The following is common:
    a. One pillow against the back for support
    b. One pillow under the head and neck if allowed
    c. One pillow or folded bath blanket between the legs
    d. A small pillow under the arm and hand
19. Place the signal light within reach.
20. Raise or lower bed rails. Follow the care plan.
21. Lower the bed to its lowest position.
22. Unscreen the person.
23. Wash your hands.

▶ SITTING ON THE SIDE OF THE BED

Persons sit on the side of the bed *(dangle)* for many reasons. Some increase activity in stages. They progress from bedrest to sitting on the side of the bed and then to sitting in a chair. Walking is the next step. Surgical patients sit on the side of the bed some time after surgery. While dangling their legs, they cough and deep breathe. They also move their legs back and forth and in circles to stimulate circulation. The procedure is also part of preparing a person to walk or for transfer to a chair or wheelchair.

Two staff members may be needed. Support the person if he or she has problems with balance or coordination. *(See Focus on Older Persons box.)*

Focus On... OLDER PERSONS

Circulatory changes cause older persons to become dizzy or faint if they get out of bed too fast. They may need to sit on the side of the bed for a few minutes before a transfer or walking.

Also, problems with sitting and balance are common after a stroke. The person is supported when dangling to prevent falling and other injuries.

Fig. 11-19 Helping the person sit on the side of the bed. **A,** The person is supported under the shoulders and under the thighs. **B,** The person sits upright as the legs and feet are pulled over the edge of the bed.

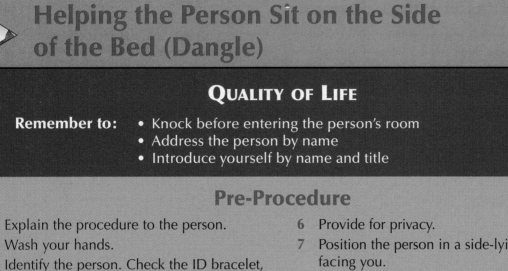

Helping the Person Sit on the Side of the Bed (Dangle)

QUALITY OF LIFE

Remember to:
- Knock before entering the person's room
- Address the person by name
- Introduce yourself by name and title

Pre-Procedure

1. Explain the procedure to the person.
2. Wash your hands.
3. Identify the person. Check the ID bracelet, and call the person by name.
4. Decide what side of the bed to use.
5. Move furniture to provide moving space.
6. Provide for privacy.
7. Position the person in a side-lying position facing you.
8. Lock the bed wheels.
9. Raise the bed to the best level for body mechanics. Make sure bed rails are up.

Procedure

10. Raise the head of the bed so the person is in a sitting position.
11. Stand near the person's waist.
12. Lower the bed rail.
13. Stand by the person's hips. Turn so you face the far corner of the foot of the bed.
14. Slide one arm under the person's neck and shoulders. Grasp the far shoulder. Place your other hand under the thighs near the knees (Fig. 11-19, *A*).
15. Pivot toward the foot of the bed while pulling the person's feet and legs over the edge of the bed. As the legs go over the edge of the mattress, the trunk is upright (Fig. 11-19, *B*).
16. Ask the person to hold onto the edge of the mattress. This supports the person in the sitting position.
17. Do not leave the person alone. Provide support if necessary.
18. Ask how the person feels. Check pulse and respirations. Observe for difficulty breathing, pale skin, or *cyanosis* (bluish skin color). Also note complaints of dizziness or lightheadedness. Help the person lie down if necessary.
19. Reverse the procedure to return the person to bed.
20. Lower the head of the bed after the person returns to bed. Help him or her move to the center of the bed.

Post-Procedure

21. Provide for comfort. Position the person in good alignment.
22. Place the signal light within reach.
23. Lower the bed to its lowest position.
24. Raise or lower bed rails. Follow the care plan.
25. Return furniture to its proper location.
26. Unscreen the person.
27. Wash your hands.
28. Report the following to the nurse:
    - How well the activity was tolerated
    - The length of time the person dangled
    - Pulse and respiratory rates
    - The amount of assistance needed
    - Other observations or complaints

TRANSFERRING PERSONS

Persons are often moved from beds to chairs, wheelchairs, or stretchers. Some need little help in transferring. Sometimes 2 or 3 people are needed. The nurse and care plan tell you how much help a person needs. The rules of body mechanics apply to transfers. So do the safety and comfort measures for lifting and moving persons. Always make sure that you have enough room for a safe transfer. You may have to move furniture to make room for a chair, wheelchair, or stretcher.

▶ APPLYING TRANSFER BELTS

A **transfer belt (gait belt or safety belt)** is used to transfer unsteady and disabled persons. It helps prevent falls and other injuries. The belt goes around the person's waist. You grasp the belt to support the person during the transfer. The belt is called a *gait belt* when used for walking with a person. Many agencies require staff to use these belts when transferring or walking a person. *(See Focus on Long-Term Care box.)*

Focus On... **LONG-TERM CARE**

Transfer belts are used routinely in nursing centers. The belts help to prevent falls.

Applying a Transfer Belt

QUALITY OF LIFE

Remember to:
- Knock before entering the person's room
- Address the person by name
- Introduce yourself by name and title

Procedure

1 Wash your hands.
2 Identify the person. Check the ID bracelet, and call the person by name.
3 Explain the procedure to the person.
4 Provide for privacy.
5 Assist the person to a sitting position.
6 Apply the belt around the person's waist over clothing. Do not apply it over bare skin.

7 Tighten the belt so it is snug. It should not cause discomfort or impair breathing. You should be able to slide your fingers under the belt.
8 Make sure that a woman's breasts are not caught under the belt.
9 Place the buckle off center in the front or in the back for the person's comfort (Fig. 11-20).

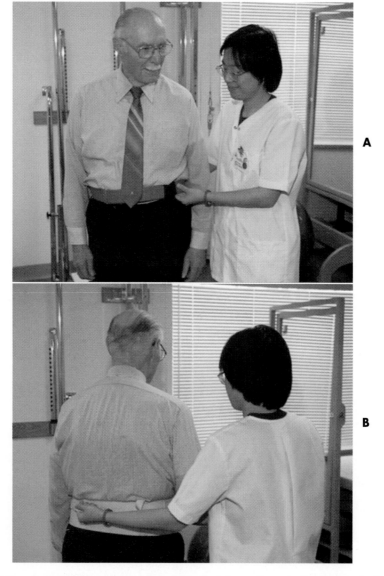

Fig. 11-20 Transfer belt (gait or safety belt). **A,** The belt is positioned off center in the front. **B,** The belt buckle is positioned at the back.

TRANSFERRING THE PERSON TO A CHAIR OR WHEELCHAIR

Safety is important for chair and wheelchair transfers. You must prevent falls. The person wears shoes with nonskid soles to prevent sliding or slipping on the floor. The chair or wheelchair must support the person's weight. The number of staff members needed for a transfer depends on the person's physical capabilities, condition, and size. *(See Focus on Long-Term Care box below.)*

Focus On... LONG-TERM CARE

Some residents cannot assist in transfers to or from chairs or wheelchairs. For those residents, a mechanical lift is used (see p. 272).

The person is helped out of bed on his or her strong side. If the left side is weak, get the person out of bed on the right side. When transferring, the strong side moves first and pulls the weaker side along. Transfers from the weak side are awkward and unsafe.

Most bedside chairs and wheelchairs have vinyl seats and backs. Vinyl holds body heat. The person becomes warm and perspires more. To promote comfort, you can cover the back and seat with a folded bath blanket. Some people rely on wheelchairs for mobility. They may have special cushions to prevent pressure ulcers (see Chapter 25), to maintain posture, or to prevent them from sliding forward (see pp. 278-279). Ask the nurse about the proper use and placement of these cushions. *(See Focus on Long-Term Care box below.)*

Text continued on p. 272

Focus On... LONG-TERM CARE

Most nursing centers require the use of transfer belts when assisting residents to transfer to or from chairs or wheelchairs.

Transferring the Person to a Chair or Wheelchair

NNAAP™

QUALITY OF LIFE

Remember to:
- Knock before entering the person's room
- Address the person by name
- Introduce yourself by name and title

Pre-Procedure

1　Explain the procedure to the person.
2　Collect:
- Wheelchair or arm chair
- One or two bath blankets
- Robe and nonskid shoes
- Paper or sheet
- Transfer belt if needed
- Seat cushion if used by the person

3　Wash your hands.
4　Identify the person. Check the ID bracelet, and call the person by name.
5　Provide for privacy.
6　Decide which side of the bed to use. Move furniture to provide moving space.

Procedure

7 Place the chair back even with the head-board (Fig. 11- 21, *A*, p. 268).

8 Place a folded bath blanket or cushion on the seat. Lock wheelchair wheels and raise the footrests.

9 Lower the bed to its lowest position. Lock the bed wheels.

10 Fanfold top linens to the foot of the bed.

11 Place the paper or sheet under the person's feet. Put shoes on the person.

12 Help the person dangle. Make sure his or her feet touch the floor.

13 Help the person put on a robe.

14 Apply the transfer belt if it will be used.

15 *Method 1:* Using a transfer belt

  a Stand in front of the person.

  b Have the person hold onto the mattress. Or ask the person to place his or her fists on the bed by the thighs.

  c Make sure the person's feet are flat on the floor.

  d Have the person lean forward.

  e Grasp the transfer belt at each side.

  f Brace your knees against the person's knees. Block his or her feet with your feet (Fig. 11-21, *B*, p. 268).

  g Ask the person to push down on the mattress and to stand on the count of "3." Pull the person into a standing position as you straighten your knees (Fig. 11-21, *C*, p. 268).

16 *Method 2:* A transfer belt is not used

  a Follow Step 15 a–c.

  b Place your hands under the person's arms. Your hands are around the person's shoulder blades (Fig. 11-22, *A*, p. 269).

  c Have the person lean forward.

  d Brace your knees against the person's knees. Block his or her feet with your feet.

  e Ask the person to push down on the mattress and to stand on the count of "3." Pull the person up into a standing position as you straighten your knees.

17 Support the person in the standing position. Hold the transfer belt, or keep your hands around the person's shoulder blades. Continue to block the person's feet and knees with your feet and knees.

18 Turn the person so he or she can grasp the far arm of the chair. The legs will touch the edge of the chair as in Figure 11-22, *B* on p. 269.

19 Continue to turn the person until the other armrest is grasped.

20 Lower him or her into the chair as you bend your hips and knees. The person assists by leaning forward and bending the elbows and knees (Fig. 11-22, *C*, p. 269).

21 Make sure the buttocks are to the back of the seat. Position the person in good alignment.

22 Position the person's feet on the wheelchair footrests.

23 Cover the person's lap and legs with a bath blanket. Keep the blanket off the floor and the wheels.

24 Remove the transfer belt if used.

25 Position the chair as the person prefers.

Post-Procedure

26 Make sure the signal light and other necessary items are within reach.

27 Unscreen the person.

28 Wash your hands.

29 Report the following to the nurse:
  • The pulse rate if taken
  • How well the activity was tolerated
  • Complaints of lightheadedness, pain, discomfort, difficulty breathing, weakness, or fatigue
  • The amount of assistance required to transfer the person

30 Reverse the procedure to return the person to bed.

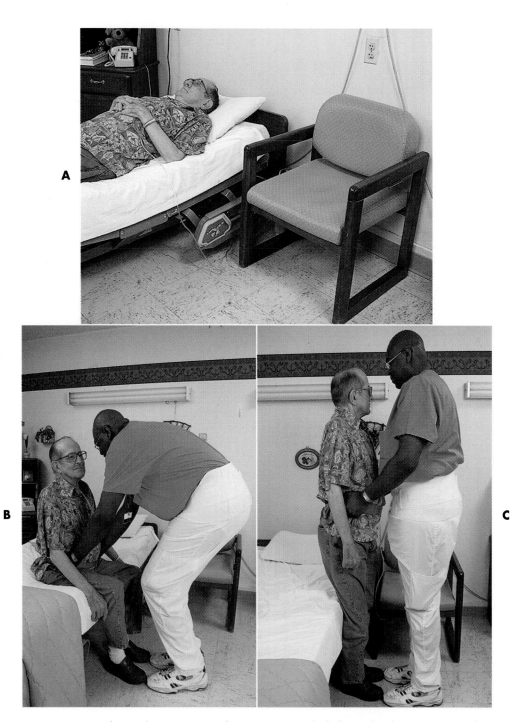

Fig. 11-21 Transferring the person to a chair using a transfer belt. **A,** The chair is positioned next to and even with the headboard. **B,** The person's feet and knees are blocked by the nursing assistant's feet and knees. This prevents the person from sliding or falling. **C,** The person is pulled up to a standing position and supported by holding the transfer belt and blocking the person's knees and feet.

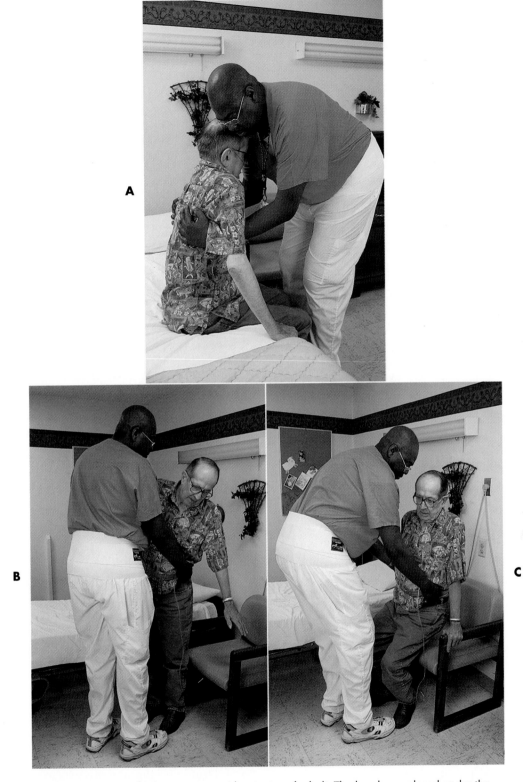

Fig. 11-22 A, Transferring a person without a transfer belt. The hands are placed under the person's arms and around the shoulder blades. **B,** The person is supported as he grasps the far arm of the chair. The legs are against the chair. **C,** The person holds the armrests, leans forward, and bends the elbows and knees while being lowered into the chair.

Transferring the Person to a Wheelchair With Assistance

QUALITY OF LIFE

Remember to:
- Knock before entering the person's room
- Address the person by name
- Introduce yourself by name and title

Pre-Procedure

1 Ask a co-worker to help you.
2 Explain the procedure to the person.
3 Collect:
- Wheelchair with removable armrests
- Bath blankets
- Shoes
- Cushion if used

4 Wash your hands.
5 Identify the person. Check the ID bracelet, and call the person by name.
6 Provide for privacy.
7 Decide which side of the bed to use. Move furniture to provide moving space.

Procedure

8 Fanfold top linens to the foot of the bed.
9 Assist the person to the side of the bed near you. Help him or her to a sitting position by raising the head of the bed.
10 Place the wheelchair at the side of the bed, even with the person's hips.
11 Remove the armrest near the bed. Put the cushion or a folded bath blanket on the seat.
12 Lock wheelchair and bed wheels.
13 Stand behind the wheelchair. Put your arms under the person's arms, and grasp the person's forearms (Fig. 11-23, *A*).
14 Have your co-worker grasp the person's thighs and calves (Fig. 11-23, *B*).

15 Bring the person toward the chair on the count of "3." Lower him or her into the chair as in Figure 11-23, *C*.
16 Make sure the person's buttocks are to the back of the seat. Position the person in good alignment.
17 Put the armrest back on the wheelchair.
18 Put the shoes on the person. Position the person's feet on the footrests.
19 Cover the person's lap and legs with a blanket. Keep the blanket off the floor and wheels.
20 Position the chair as the person prefers.

Post-Procedure

21 Make sure the signal light and other necessary items are within reach.
22 Unscreen the person.
23 Wash your hands.
24 Report the following to the nurse:
- The pulse rate if taken
- Complaints of lightheadedness, pain, discomfort, difficulty breathing, weakness, or fatigue
- How well the activity was tolerated

25 Reverse the procedure to return the person to bed.

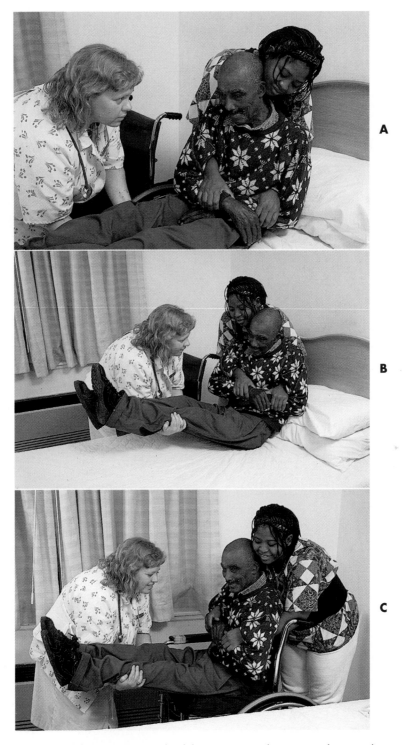

Fig. 11-23 Transferring the person to a wheelchair. **A,** Grasp the person's forearms by putting your arms under the person's arms. **B,** Hold the thighs and calves to support the lower extremities during a transfer. **C,** Lower the person into the chair.

▶ USING A MECHANICAL LIFT

Persons who cannot help themselves are transferred with mechanical lifts. Lifts are used for transfers to chairs, stretchers, tubs, shower chairs, toilets, whirlpools, and cars.

There are manual and electric mechanical lifts. Before using a lift:

- Make sure you are trained it its use
- Make sure the lift works
- Compare the person's weight and the lift's weight limit. Do not use the lift if a person's weight exceeds the lift's capacity.

At least two staff members are needed. The manufacturer's instructions are followed for a safe transfer. The following procedure is used as a guide.

▶ Transferring a Person Using a Mechanical Lift

QUALITY OF LIFE

Remember to:
- Knock before entering the person's room
- Address the person by name
- Introduce yourself by name and title

Pre-Procedure

1 Ask a co-worker to help you.
2 Explain the procedure to the person.
3 Collect:
   - Mechanical lift
   - Arm chair or wheelchair
   - Slippers
   - Bath blanket
   - Seat cushion if used by the person
4 Wash your hands.
5 Identify the person. Check the ID bracelet, and call the person by name.
6 Provide for privacy.

Procedure

7 Center the sling under the person (Fig. 11-24, *A*). Turn the person from side to side as if making an occupied bed to position the sling (see Chapter 13). Position the sling according to the manufacturer's instructions.

8 Position the chair next to the bed. It should be about 1 foot away from the bed. Place a folded bath blanket or seat cushion in the chair.

9 Lock the bed wheels and lower the bed to its lowest position.

10 Raise the lift so it can be positioned over the person.

11 Position the lift over the person (Fig. 11-24, *B*).

12 Lock the lift wheels in position.

13 Attach the sling to the swivel bar (Fig. 11-24, *C*).

14 Raise the head of the bed to a sitting position.

15 Cross the person's arms over the chest. Let him or her hold onto the straps or chains, but not the swivel bar.

16 Pump the lift high enough until the person and sling are free of the bed (Fig. 11-24, *D*).

17 Ask your co-worker to support the person's legs as you move the lift and person away from the bed (Fig. 11-24, *E*).

18 Position the lift so that the person's back is toward the chair.

19 Lower the person into the chair. (Follow the manufacturer's instructions for lowering the lift.) Guide the person into the chair as in Figure 11-24, *F*.

20 Lower the swivel bar to unhook the sling. Leave the sling under the person unless otherwise indicated.

21 Put the slippers on the person. Position the person's feet on wheelchair footrests.

22 Cover the person's lap and legs with a blanket. Keep the blanket off the floor and wheels.

23 Position the chair as the person prefers.

Post-Procedure

24 Make sure the signal light and other necessary items are within reach.

25 Wash your hands.

26 Report the following to the nurse:
- The pulse rate if taken
- Complaints of lightheadedness, pain, discomfort, difficulty breathing, weakness, or fatigue
- How well the activity was tolerated

27 Reverse the procedure to return the person to bed.

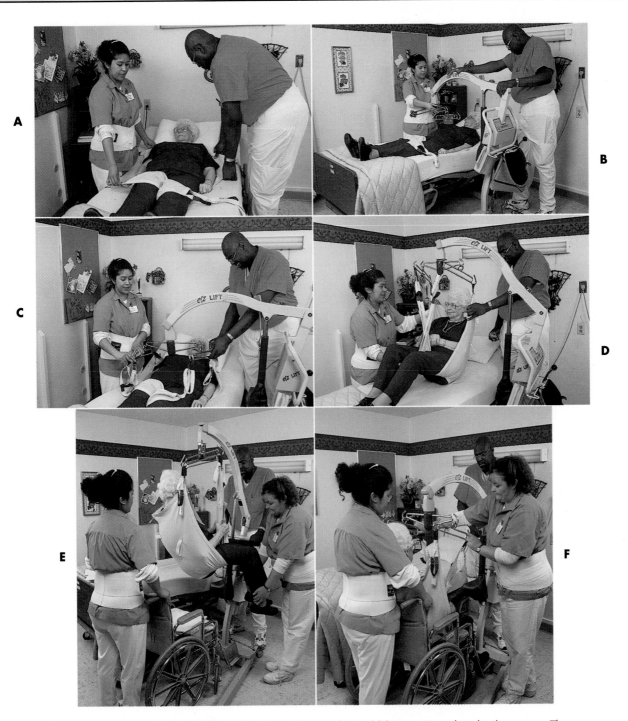

Fig. 11-24 Using a mechanical lift. **A,** The sling of the mechanical lift is positioned under the person. The lower edge of the sling is behind the person's knees. **B,** The lift is over the person. The lift's legs are spread to widen the base of support. **C,** The sling is attached to a swivel bar. **D,** The lift is raised until the sling and person are off of the bed. **E,** The person's legs are supported as the person and lift are moved away from the bed. **F,** The person is guided into a chair.

► MOVING THE PERSON TO A STRETCHER

Stretchers are used to transport persons to other areas. They are used for persons who:

- Cannot sit up
- Must stay in a lying position
- Are seriously ill

The stretcher is covered with a folded flat sheet or bath blanket. A pillow and extra blankets are available. With the nurse's permission, raise the head of the stretcher to Fowler's or semi-Fowler's position. This increases the person's comfort.

Safety straps are used when the person is on the stretcher. The stretcher's side rails are kept up during the transport. Move the person feet first so the co-worker at the head of the stretcher can watch the person's breathing and color during the transport. Never leave a person on a stretcher unattended.

A drawsheet or lift sheet is used. At least 3 staff members are needed for a safe transfer. Remember, keep the person in good body alignment and use good body mechanics.

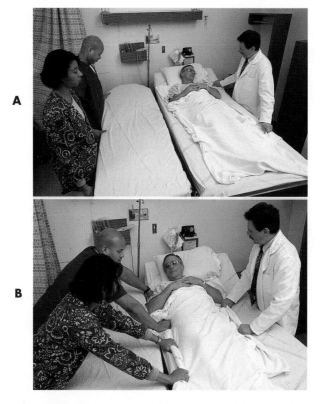

Fig. 11-25 Transferring the person to a stretcher. **A,** The stretcher is against the bed and is held in place. **B,** A drawsheet is used to transfer the person from the bed to a stretcher.

Transferring a Person to a Stretcher

QUALITY OF LIFE

Remember to:
- Knock before entering the person's room
- Address the person by name
- Introduce yourself by name and title

Pre-Procedure

1 Ask two co-workers to help you.
2 Explain the procedure to the person.
3 Collect:
- Stretcher covered with a sheet or bath blanket
- Bath blanket
- Pillow(s) if needed
4 Wash your hands.
5 Identify the person. Check the ID bracelet, and call the person by name.
6 Provide for privacy.
7 Raise the bed to its highest level.

Procedure

8 Cover the person with a bath blanket. Fan-fold top linens to the foot of the bed.
9 Loosen the cotton drawsheet on each side.
10 Lower the head of the bed so it is as flat as possible.
11 Lower the bed rail on the side to which you will move the person.
12 Ask your co-workers to help move the person to the side of the bed. Use the drawsheet.
13 Go to the other side of the bed. Lower the bed rail. Protect the person from falling by holding the far arm and leg.
14 Have your co-workers position the stretcher next to the bed, and stand behind the stretcher (Fig. 11-25, A).
15 Lock the bed and stretcher wheels.
16 Roll up and grasp the drawsheet at the hip and midchest levels.
17 Ask your co-workers to roll up and grasp the drawsheet. This supports the entire length of the person's body.
18 Transfer the person to the stretcher on the count of "3" by lifting and pulling him or her (Fig. 11-25, B). Make sure the person is centered on the stretcher.
19 Place a pillow or pillows under the person's head and shoulders if allowed.
20 Cover the person. Provide for comfort.
21 Fasten safety straps. Raise the bed rails.
22 Unlock the stretcher's wheels. Transport the person.

Post-Procedure

23 Wash your hands.
24 Report the following to the nurse:
- The time of the transport
- Where the person was transported to
- Who accompanied him or her
- How the transfer was tolerated
25 Reverse the procedure to return the person to bed.

POSITIONING

The person must be properly positioned at all times. Regular position changes and good alignment promote comfort and well-being. Breathing is easier, and circulation is promoted. Proper positioning also helps prevent many complications. These include pressure ulcers (see Chapter 25) and contractures (see Chapter 20). Some persons are repositioned every hour or every 2 hours. You need to follow the person's care plan.

The doctor may order certain positions or position restrictions. This is common after certain surgeries or diagnostic procedures. Follow these guidelines to safely position a person:

- Ask the nurse about position changes for a person.
- Know how often to turn a person and to what positions.
- Use good body mechanics.
- Ask a co-worker to help you if indicated.
- Explain the procedure to the person.
- Be gentle when moving the person.
- Provide for privacy.
- Place the signal light within the person's reach after positioning.
- Use pillows as directed for support and alignment.

FOWLER'S POSITION

Fowler's position involves raising the head of the bed 45 to 60 degrees. Good alignment involves keeping the spine straight, supporting the head with a small pillow, and supporting the arms with pillows (Fig. 11-26). The nurse may have you place a small pillow under the lower back, thighs, and ankles. Persons with heart and respiratory disorders usually breathe easier in Fowler's position.

SUPINE POSITION

The **supine (dorsal recumbent) position** is the back-lying position. The bed is flat, the head and shoulders are supported on a pillow, and arms and hands are at the person's sides. The hands may be supported on small pillows with the palms down (Fig. 11-27).

The nurse may ask you to place a rolled towel under the lower back. Often a small pillow is under the thighs or ankles.

PRONE POSITION

Persons in the **prone position** lie on their abdomens with their heads turned to one side. Small pillows are placed under the head, abdomen, and lower legs (Fig. 11-28). Arms are flexed at the elbows with the hands near the head.

You also can position a person with the feet hanging over the end of the mattress (Fig. 11-29). If that is done, a pillow is not needed under the feet. *(See Focus on Older Persons box.)*

LATERAL POSITION

A person in the **lateral (side-lying) position** lies on one side or the other (Fig. 11-30). A pillow is under the head and neck. The upper leg is placed in front of the lower leg. (The nurse may ask you to position the upper leg behind the lower leg.) The upper leg and thigh are supported with pillows. A small pillow is under the upper hand and arm, and a pillow is positioned against the person's back.

Focus On... **OLDER PERSONS**

Most older persons cannot tolerate the prone position. They often have limited range of motion in their necks. Check with the nurse before positioning any older person in the prone position.

Fig. 11-26 Fowler's position.

Fig. 11-27 Supine position.

Fig. 11-28 Prone position.

Fig. 11-29 Prone position with feet hanging over the edge of the mattress.

Fig. 11-30 Lateral position.

SIMS' POSITION

The **Sims' position** is a left side-lying position. The upper leg is sharply flexed so it is not on the lower leg, and the lower arm is behind the person (Fig. 11-31). Good alignment involves placing a pillow under the person's head and shoulder, supporting the upper leg with a pillow, and placing a pillow under the upper arm and hand. *(See Focus on Older Persons box.)*

 Focus On... **OLDER PERSONS**

The Sims' position usually is not comfortable for older persons. Check with the nurse before positioning any older person in Sims' position.

CHAIR POSITION

Persons who sit in chairs must hold their upper bodies and heads erect. The person's back and buttocks are against the back of the chair. Feet are flat on the floor or on wheelchair footrests. Backs of the knees and calves are slightly away from the edge of the seat (Fig. 11-32). The nurse may ask you to put a small pillow between the person's lower back and the chair. *(Remember, a pillow is not used behind the back if restraints are used.)*

Paralyzed arms are supported on pillows. Some residents have special foam positioners (Fig. 11-33). Ask the nurse about their proper use. Wrists are positioned at a slight upward angle.

Some people require postural supports if they cannot keep their upper bodies erect (Fig. 11-34). Postural supports help keep them in good alignment. The health team selects the best product for the person's needs. The person's safety, dignity, and function are considered.

Fig. 11-31 Sims' position.

Fig. 11-32 Person positioned in a chair. The person's feet are flat on the floor, the calves do not touch the chair, and the back is straight and against the back of the chair.

Fig. 11-33 Elevated armrest. (Courtesy J.T. Posey Co, Aracadia, Calif.)

Fig. 11-34 Torso support. (Courtesy J.T. Posey Co, Aracadia, Calif.)

Circle T if the answer is true and F if it is false.

1. T F Body mechanics means the way body segments are aligned with one another.

2. T F Good body mechanics help protect you and the person from injury.

3. T F Body mechanics involve using small muscles.

4. T F Base of support is the area on which an object rests.

5. T F Objects are kept away from the body when lifting, moving, or carrying them.

6. T F Face the direction you are working to prevent unnecessary twisting.

7. T F Push, slide, or pull heavy objects rather than lift them.

8. T F Sliding the person reduces friction and shearing.

9. T F Ask the nurse about limits or restrictions in positioning or moving a person.

10. T F The right to privacy is protected when moving, lifting, or transferring persons.

11. T F A lift sheet should extend from the shoulders to above the knees.

12. T F A person is moved to the side of the bed before being turned to the side-lying position.

13. T F Logrolling is rolling the person in segments.

14. T F Persons with spinal cord injuries are logrolled.

15. T F A transfer belt is part of a mechanical lift.

16. T F Mr. Parker is being transferred from the bed to a chair. He needs nonskid shoes.

17. T F You are going to transfer Mrs. Jones from the bed to a chair. Move her from the direction of the weak side of her body.

18. T F Repositioning prevents deformities and pressure on body parts.

19. T F The head of the bed is elevated 45 to 60 degrees for the supine position.

20. T F The Sims' position is a left side-lying position.

Answers to these questions are on p. 835.

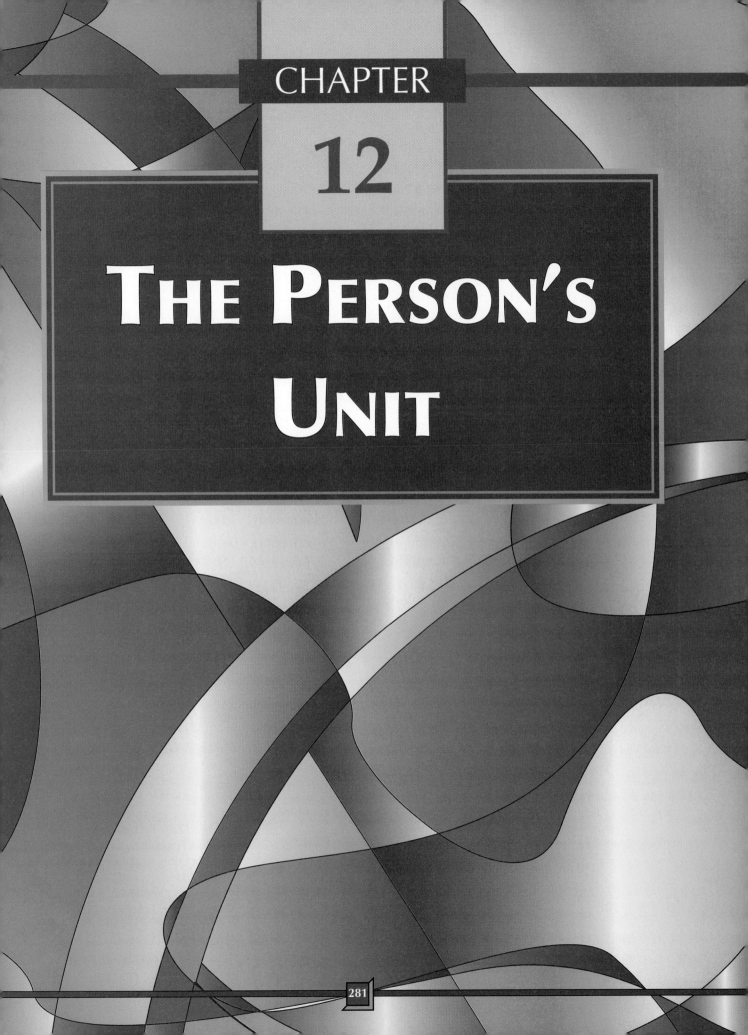

CHAPTER

12

THE PERSON'S UNIT

Define the key terms listed in this chapter

Identify the temperature range comfortable for most people

Identify the temperature range required by OBRA

Describe how to protect the person from drafts

List ways to prevent or reduce odors in the person's room

Describe how to decrease noise in health care agencies

Explain how lighting affects comfort

Know the basic bed positions

Describe the use of furniture and equipment found in the person's unit

Describe how a bathroom is equipped

Explain how to maintain the person's unit

Know the OBRA requirements for resident rooms

KEY TERMS

full visual privacy Having the means to be completely free from public view while occupying a bed

patient/resident pack Personal care equipment provided by the health care agency (wash basin, emesis or kidney basin, bedpan, urinal, water pitcher and glass, soap, and soap dish)

reverse Trendelenburg's position The head of the bed is raised, and the foot of the bed is lowered

semi-Fowler's position The head of the bed is raised 45 degrees, and the knee portion is raised 15 degrees; or the head of the bed is raised 30 degrees and the knee portion is *not* raised

Trendelenburg's position The head of the bed is lowered, and the foot of the bed is raised

Hospital patients and nursing center residents spend a lot of time in their rooms. Rooms may be private (for one person). Semiprivate rooms, furnished for two people, are more common. Rooms must be comfortable and safe and allow enough space for activities of daily living. This chapter describes the furnishings in the person's unit—the furniture and equipment provided for the person by the health care agency (Fig. 12-1).

The agency must follow health and safety standards. Therefore rooms are designed to provide comfort, safety, and privacy.

COMFORT

Age, illness, and activity affect comfort. So do factors like temperature, ventilation, noise, odors, and light-ing. Those factors are controlled to meet the person's needs.

TEMPERATURE AND VENTILATION

Health care agencies have heating, air conditioning, and ventilation systems. The systems maintain a comfortable temperature and provide fresh air in the rooms. A temperature range of 68° F to 74° F is usually comfortable for most healthy people. A comfortable temperature for one person may be too hot or too cold for another. Infants, older persons, and ill persons generally need higher room temperatures for comfort. Therefore higher temperatures are usually needed in hospitals and nursing centers. (*See Focus on Long-Term Care box.*)

Stale room air and lingering odors affect comfort and rest. A good ventilation system provides fresh air and moves room air. Drafts can occur as air moves.

Fig. 12-1 Furniture and equipment in a typical unit.

Infants, older persons, and ill persons are sensitive to drafts and need protection from them. To protect them from drafts:

- Make sure they wear enough clothing.
- Cover them with blankets. Some people like extra blankets.
- Provide lap robes (blankets, afghans) to cover their legs when in chairs or wheelchairs.
- Move them from drafty areas.

(See Focus on Older Persons box.)

ODORS

Many odors occur in health care agencies. Some are pleasant, like food aromas and flower scents. Others are unpleasant. Draining wounds, vomitus, bowel movements, and urine have unpleasant smells that can embarrass the person. Body, breath, and smoking odors may offend patients, residents, visitors, and staff. Good nursing care, good ventilation, and good housekeeping practices help eliminate odors. To reduce odors:

- Empty and clean bedpans, urinals, commodes, and kidney basins promptly.
- Change soiled linens and clothing promptly.
- Dispose of soiled linens and clothing.
- Clean persons who are wet or soiled from urine, feces, vomitus, or wound drainage.
- Dispose of incontinent products promptly (see Chapter 16).
- Dispose of ostomy products promptly (see Chapter 17).

- Keep soiled laundry containers closed.
- Provide the person with good personal hygiene to prevent body and breath odors (see Chapter 14).
- Use room deodorizers when necessary and if allowed by the agency.

Smoke odors cause special problems. Many agencies ban smoking. No one can smoke anywhere in the building. However, nursing centers may let residents smoke in certain areas. If you smoke, you must follow the employer's policy. Wash your hands after handling smoking materials and before giving care. Give careful attention to your uniforms, hair, and breath because of clinging smoke odors.

NOISE

Ill people are sensitive to noises and sounds around them. They are often disturbed by common health care sounds. The clanging of metal bedpans, urinals, and wash basins can be annoying. So can the clatter of dishes and trays. Loud talking and laughing in hallways and at the nurses' station, loud televisions and radios, ringing telephones, and buzzing intercoms can be irritating. So is noise from equipment needing repair or oil. Wheels on stretchers, wheelchairs, carts, and other equipment must be oiled properly.

When in a strange place, people want to know the cause and meaning of new sounds. This is part of the basic need to feel safe and secure. Patients and residents may find sounds dangerous, frightening, or irritating. They may become upset, anxious, and uncomfortable. Remember, noise to one person may not be noise to another. For example, loud stereo music may please a teenager but bother adults.

Health care agencies are designed to reduce noise. Drapes, carpeting, and acoustical tiles help absorb noise. Plastic items have replaced some metal equipment (bedpans, urinals, and wash basins). Staff can reduce noise by controlling the loudness of their voices and handling equipment carefully. Keeping equipment working properly and promptly answering telephones and intercoms also decrease noise.

LIGHTING

Good lighting is needed for the safety and comfort of the person and staff. Glares, shadows, and dull lighting can cause falls, headaches, and eyestrain. People usually relax and rest better in dim light. However, a bright room is more cheerful and stimulating.

Lighting is adjusted to meet the person's changing needs. Shades are pulled or drapes drawn to control natural light. The overbed light is adjusted to provide soft, medium, and bright lighting. Some agencies have ceiling lights over beds. These provide low to very bright light. Bright lighting is helpful when giving care. Light controls should be within the person's reach.

ROOM FURNITURE AND EQUIPMENT

Rooms are furnished and equipped for the person's basic needs. There is furniture and equipment for comfort, sleep, elimination, nutrition, personal hygiene, and activity. There is also equipment for communicating with the nursing team, family, and friends. The right to privacy is considered when equipping the room. *(See Focus on Long-Term Care box.)*

THE BED

Hospital beds have electrical or manual controls. Beds are raised horizontally to give care. This reduces bending and reaching. The lowest horizontal position lets the person get out of bed with ease (Fig. 12-2). The head of the bed can be kept flat or raised to varying degrees.

Most beds are electric. Controls are on a side panel, bed rail, or panel at the foot of the bed (Fig. 12-3). Patients and residents are taught how to safely use the controls. They are warned not to raise the bed to the high position and not to adjust the bed to harmful positions. They are told of any position limits or restrictions.

Most electric beds "lock" into any position by the staff. This prevents the person from raising or lowering the head or foot of the bed. Persons restricted to certain positions may need to have their beds locked. The locking feature is useful for confused persons.

Manually operated beds are still in use in some places. *(See Focus on Home Care box.)*

Fig. 12-2 One bed in the highest horizontal position and the other bed in the lowest horizontal position.

Fig. 12-3 Controls for an electric bed.

> ### Focus On... HOME CARE
>
> Some home care patients have hospital beds. Electric beds are common. Some are operated manually. Manually operated beds have cranks at the foot of the bed (Fig. 12-4). The left crank raises or lowers the head of the bed. The right crank adjusts the knee portion. The center crank raises or lowers the entire bed. The cranks are pulled up for *use*. They are kept down at all other times. Cranks in the up position are safety hazards. Anyone walking past may bump into them.
>
> Other home care patients use their regular beds. You cannot raise regular beds to give care. Therefore you will bend more when giving care. You must use good body mechanics to avoid injuring yourself.

> ### Focus On... LONG-TERM CARE
>
> OBRA requires that nursing center rooms be as homelike as possible. Therefore the resident is allowed to have and use personal items. To the extent possible, residents can bring furniture and personal items from home. This promotes the person's dignity and esteem.

Fig. 12-4 Manually operated hospital bed.

Fig. 12-5 Fowler's position.

Fig. 12-6 Semi-Fowler's position.

Bed Positions. There are five basic bed positions: flat, Fowler's, semi-Fowler's, Trendelenburg's, and reverse Trendelenburg's:

- **Flat**—the usual sleeping position. The position also is used after spinal cord injury or surgery and for cervical traction.
- **Fowler's position**—a semisitting position. The head of the bed is elevated 45 to 60 degrees (Fig. 12-5). The reasons for positioning a person in Fowler's position are described in Chapter 11.

- **Semi-Fowler's position**—the head of the bed is raised 45 degrees and the knee portion is raised 15 degrees (Fig. 12-6). This position is comfortable and prevents the person from sliding down in bed. However, raising the knee portion can interfere with leg circulation. Check with the nurse before positioning a person in semi-Fowler's position. Many agencies define semi-Fowler's position as when the head of the bed is raised 30 degrees and the knee portion is *not* raised. You must know which definition your employer uses so you give safe care.

Fig. 12-7 Trendelenburg's position.

Fig. 12-8 Reverse Trendelenburg's position.

Fig. 12-9 Backrests for regular beds. **A,** Wedge pillow. **B,** Study pillow with armrests.

- **Trendelenburg's position**—the head of the bed is lowered, and the foot of the bed is raised (Fig. 12-7). A doctor's order is required for this position. Blocks are placed under the legs at the foot of the bed. Some beds allow the entire bed frame to be tilted into Trendelenburg's position.
- **Reverse Trendelenburg's position**—the opposite of Trendelenburg's position. The head of the bed is raised, and the foot of the bed is lowered (Fig. 12-8). Blocks are put under the legs at the head of the bed, or the bed frame is tilted. This position requires a doctor's order.

(See Focus on Home Care box.)

Focus On... HOME CARE

Backrests are used with regular beds for Fowler's and semi-Fowler's positions (Fig. 12-9). Check the headboard to make sure it is sturdy. It needs to provide support when the person leans against the backrest. Large, sturdy, sofa pillows are useful if a backrest is not available.

SAFETY CONSIDERATIONS

Bed legs have wheels or casters that are locked when you give bedside care (see Chapter 9). They are also locked when you transfer a person to and from the bed. The person can be injured if the bed moves.

The importance of bed rails on hospital beds is discussed in Chapter 9.

THE OVERBED TABLE

The overbed table (see Fig. 12-1) is positioned over the bed by sliding the base under the bed. The height is adjusted for the person in bed or in a chair. Turn the side handle or lever to raise or lower the table. The overbed table is used for meal trays and for eating, writing, reading, and other activities.

Many overbed tables have movable tops with a storage area underneath. The storage area is often used for beauty, hair care, shaving, or other personal items. Many also have a flip-up mirror.

The nursing team uses the overbed table as a work area. Only clean and sterile items are placed on the table. The table is cleaned after being used as a working surface. Never place bedpans, urinals, or soiled linen on the overbed table.

THE BEDSIDE STAND

The bedside stand is next to the bed. The stand is a storage area for personal items and personal care equipment. It has 2 or 3 drawers or 1 drawer at the top and a lower cabinet with a shelf (Fig. 12-10). The top drawer can be used for money, eyeglasses, books, and other personal items. The first shelf (or second drawer) is used for the wash basin, which can hold personal care items. These include soap and soap dish, powder, lotion, deodorant, towels, washcloth, bath blanket, and a clean gown or pajamas. An emesis or kidney basin (shaped like a kidney) is often used to hold oral hygiene items. The kidney basin is stored on the top shelf or in the top drawer. The bedpan and its cover, the urinal, and toilet paper are on the lower shelf (or third drawer).

The top of the stand is often used for tissues and the telephone. The person may put a radio, flowers, gifts, cards, and other important items there. Some stands have a rod at the side or back for towels and washcloths.

CHAIRS

The person's unit usually has 1 or 2 chairs. One is a straight-back chair without arms. The other is an upholstered chair with armrests. It is used by the person and visitors and is placed near the bed. Nursing center residents may bring their own chairs from home (Fig. 12-11).

PRIVACY CURTAINS

Rooms have privacy curtains. The curtain is pulled around the bed to provide privacy for the person (see Fig. 2-3). The curtain is *always* pulled completely around the bed while care is given. Privacy curtains prevent others from seeing the person. However, they do not block sound or prevent conversations from being heard. *(See Focus on Long-Term Care box and Focus on Home Care box.)*

Fig. 12-10 The bedside stand is used to store personal care items.

Fig. 12-11 Resident's chair from home.

Focus On ... LONG-TERM CARE

According to OBRA, residents have the right to full visual privacy. **Full visual privacy** means that a resident has a means to be completely free from public view while occupying his or her bed. The privacy curtain is a means to full visual privacy.

Focus On ... HOME CARE

Portable screens can be used to provide privacy in the home setting (Fig. 12-12, p. 288).

Fig. 12-12 Portable screen used to provide privacy in the home.

Fig. 12-13 A patient pack.

PERSONAL CARE ITEMS

Personal care items are used for hygiene and elimination. The agency provides a **patient pack.** It usually has a wash basin, emesis or kidney basin, bedpan, urinal, water pitcher and glass, and soap and soap dish (Fig. 12-13). Some provide powder, lotion, toothbrush, toothpaste, mouthwash, tissues, and a comb. Often patients and residents bring their own oral hygiene equipment, hair care supplies, and deodorant. Some prefer their own soap, lotion, and powder. Be sure to respect the individual's choice of personal care products.

THE CALL SYSTEM

The call system lets the person signal when help is needed. A common call system involves a signal light at the bedside that is connected to a light above the room door. The signal light also is connected to a light panel or intercom system at the nurses' station (Fig. 12-14). The signal light is at the end of a long cord (Fig. 12-15). It attaches to the bed or chair so it is always within the person's reach and vision. The person presses the signal light when help is needed. The staff member turns off the signal light at the bedside when responding to the signal for help.

An intercom system lets a nursing team member talk with the person from the nurses' station. It also allows the light to be turned off from the station. Be careful when using intercom systems. Remember confidentiality. Persons nearby can overhear what you say. Also remember that hearing-impaired persons may have difficulty using an intercom.

Fig. 12-14 A, The light above the door of the person's room. **B,** Light panel or intercom system at the nurses' station.

Sometimes people have limited hand mobility. They may need a special signal light that is turned on by tapping it with a hand or fist (Fig. 12-16). *The call system must always be within the person's reach. Therefore controls must be on the person's good side.*

Patients are shown how to use the call system when admitted to the agency. Some people cannot use the signal light. Examples included persons who are confused or in a coma. Check them often to make sure their needs are met. *(See Focus on Home Care box.)*

Some home care patients are confined to bed or to a certain part of the home. They need a way to call caregivers for help. Tap bells, dinner bells, baby monitors, and other devices are useful (Fig. 12-17).

Fig. 12-16 Signal light for a person with limited hand mobility.

Fig. 12-17 A, Tap bell. **B,** Dinner bell. **C,** Baby monitor.

Fig. 12-15 The person presses the button of the signal light when assistance is needed.

THE BATHROOM

Many agencies have a bathroom in each room. Some have a bathroom between two rooms. A toilet, sink, call system, and mirror are standard equipment (Fig. 12-18). Some bathrooms have showers. Hand rails are installed by the toilet for the person's safety. Toilets in some agencies are higher than the standard toilet. Higher toilets make transfers to and from wheelchairs easier. They also are helpful for persons with joint problems.

Towel racks, toilet paper, soap, a paper towel dispenser, wastebasket, and call system are in the bathroom. They are placed within easy reach of the person.

CLOSET AND DRAWER SPACE

Closet and drawer space are provided for the person's clothing. OBRA (see Chapter 8) requires closet space for each nursing center resident. Such closet space must have shelves and a clothes rack (Fig. 12-19). The resident must have free access to the closet and its contents.

Items in the closet or drawers are the person's private property. You must not search the closet or drawers without the person's permission.

Sometimes people hoard items like napkins, straws, sugar, salt and pepper, and food in their drawers. Such hoarding can cause safety or health risks. Agency representatives can inspect a person's closet or drawers if hoarding is suspected. The person must be informed of the inspection and be present when it takes place.

OTHER EQUIPMENT

Many agencies furnish rooms with other equipment. A television, radio, and clock are often included for comfort and relaxation. Many rooms have telephones. Residents may bring favorite furniture and items from home.

Blood pressure equipment is often mounted on the walls. There are also wall outlets for oxygen and suction. Oxygen tanks and portable suction equipment are common in long-term care and home care settings. An IV pole (IV standard) is used to hang an intravenous infusion bottle or bag or a feeding bag. Some hospital beds have an IV pole stored in the bed frame. The IV pole may be a separate piece of equipment that

Fig. 12-18 Bathroom in a health care agency.

Fig. 12-19 The resident can access items in her closet.

 Focus On... LONG-TERM CARE

Nursing center residents have left their homes. Each once had a home or apartment with furniture, appliances, a private bathroom, and many personal belongings and treasures. Now the person lives in a strange place and probably shares a room with another resident. Leaving one's home is a difficult part of growing old with poor health. Therefore it is important to make the person's unit as homelike as possible.

The person may bring some furniture and personal belongings. A chair, footstool, lamp, or small table is often allowed. Residents can always bring such things as family photos, religious items, and books. Some may have plants to care for.

The resident is allowed personal choice in arranging personal items. The health care team must make sure that such choices are safe and will not cause falls or other accidents. Also, the resident's choices must not interfere with the rights of others. You may have to help the person choose the best place for personal items.

Remember, the center is now the person's home. You and other health team members must help the person feel safe, secure, and comfortable. A homelike setting is important for the person's quality of life. OBRA serves to promote quality of life. Box 12-1 lists OBRA's requirements for resident rooms.

is brought to the bedside when needed. Figure 12-20 shows blood pressure equipment, an IV pole, and oxygen and suction outlets.

(See Focus on Long-Term Care box.)

GENERAL RULES

The person's unit is kept clean, neat, and safe. This is a responsibility of everyone involved in the person's care. The rules in Box 12-2 are followed to maintain the person's unit.

Fig. 12-20 This room has blood pressure equipment, an IV pole, and oxygen and suction outlets.

Box 12-1	**OBRA Requirements for Resident Rooms**

- Designed for 1 to 4 residents
- Direct access to exit corridor
- Full visual privacy (privacy curtain that extends around the bed, movable screens, doors)
- At least one window to the outside
- Individual closet space with racks and shelves
- Toilet facilities in the room or nearby (includes bathing facilities)
- Call system in the room and in toilet and bathing facilities
- Bed of proper height and size
- Clean, comfortable mattress with bedding appropriate to the weather and climate
- Furniture to accommodate clothing, personal items, and a chair for visitors
- Clean and orderly room
- Odor-free room
- Room temperature between 71° and 81° F
- Acceptable noise level
- Adequate ventilation and room humidity
- Appropriate lighting
- No glares from floors, windows, and lighting
- Clean, orderly drawers, shelves, and personal items
- Pest-free room
- Hand rails in needed areas
- Side rails only if needed
- Clean, dry floor; pathways are free of clutter and furniture
- Bed in low position and locked
- Personal supplies and items labeled and stored appropriately
- Drawers free of unwrapped food
- Items within reach for use in bed or bathroom
- Space for wheelchair or walker use
- Raised toilet seat
- Stool and skidproof tub or shower

Box 12-2	**Maintaining the Person's Unit**

- Make sure the person can reach the overbed table and the bedside stand.
- Arrange personal items as the individual prefers. Make sure they are easily reached.
- Keep the signal light within the person's reach at all times.
- Make sure the person can reach the telephone, television, and light controls.
- Provide the person with enough tissues and toilet paper.
- Adjust lighting, temperature, and ventilation for the person's comfort.
- Handle equipment carefully to prevent noise.
- Explain the causes of strange noises to the person.
- Empty the person's wastebasket as often as needed.
- Respect the person's belongings. An item may not be important or valuable to you yet it has great meaning for the person. Even a scrap of paper can have great meaning to the person.
- Do not throw away any items belonging to the person.
- Do not move furniture or the person's belongings. Persons with poor vision rely on memory or feel for the location of items.
- Straighten bed linens as often as needed.

Circle the BEST answer.

1. Which is a comfortable temperature range for most people?
    A. 60° F to 66° F
    B. 68° F to 74° F
    C. 74° F to 80° F
    D. 80° F to 86° F

2. Mr. Sale is protected from drafts by the following *except*
    A. Wearing enough clothing
    B. Being covered with adequate blankets
    C. Being moved out of a drafty area
    D. Sitting by the air conditioner

3. Which does *not* prevent or reduce odors?
    A. Placing fresh flowers in the room
    B. Emptying bedpans promptly
    C. Using room deodorizers
    D. Practicing good personal hygiene

4. Which does *not* control noise?
    A. Using plastic equipment
    B. Handling dishes with care
    C. Speaking softly
    D. Talking with others in the hallway

5. Which is Fowler's position?
    A. The head of the bed is raised 45 degrees.
    B. The head of the bed is raised 45 degrees, and the knee portion is raised 15 degrees.
    C. The head of the bed is lowered, and the foot of the bed is raised.
    D. The head of the bed is raised, and the foot of the bed is lowered.

6. The overbed table is *not* used
    A. For eating
    B. As a working surface
    C. To store the urinal
    D. To store shaving articles

Circle T if the answer is true and F if it is false.

7. T F   Soft, dim lighting is usually relaxing and comfortable.

8. T F   The privacy curtain prevents others from hearing conversations.

9. T F   The call system is used by Mr. Sale to signal when help is needed.

10. T F   The signal light must always be within Mr. Sale's reach except when he is in the bathroom.

11. T F   The overbed table and bedside stand should be within the person's reach.

12. T F   You should explain the cause of strange noises to Mr. Sale.

13. T F   Nursing center residents must be able to reach items in their closets.

14. T F   You can adjust the person's room temperature for your comfort.

The answers to these questions are on p. 835.

CHAPTER

13

BEDMAKING

Define the key terms listed in this chapter

Describe the differences between open, closed, occupied, and surgical beds

Explain the purposes of plastic drawsheets and cotton drawsheets

Handle linens according to the rules of medical asepsis

Perform the procedures described in this chapter

KEY TERMS

drawsheet A small sheet placed over the middle of the bottom sheet; it helps keep the mattress and bottom linens clean and dry; can be used to turn and move the person in bed; the cotton drawsheet

plastic drawsheet A drawsheet placed between the bottom sheet and the cotton drawsheet to keep the mattress and bottom linens clean and dry

Bedmaking is an important function. A clean, dry, and wrinkle-free bed helps the person's comfort. It also helps prevent skin breakdown and pressure ulcers (see Chapter 25).

Beds are usually made in the morning after baths. They are also made while the person is taking a shower or out of the room. People like their beds made and rooms clean before visitors arrive.

Linens are straightened whenever loose or wrinkled and at bedtime. Check linens for crumbs after meals, and remove them. Linens are changed whenever they become wet, soiled, or damp. Follow Standard Precautions and the Bloodborne Pathogen Standard for contact with the person's blood, body fluids, secretions, or excretions.

Beds are made in the following ways:

- A *closed bed* is not in use. Top linens are not folded back, and the bed is ready for a new person (Fig. 13-1).
- An *open bed* is in use. Top linens are folded back so the person can get into bed. A closed bed becomes an open bed when the top linens are folded back (Fig. 13-2).
- An *occupied bed* is made with the person in it (Fig. 13-3).
- A *surgical bed* is made so that a person can be moved from a stretcher to the bed. It also is called a postoperative bed, recovery bed, or anesthesia bed (Fig. 13-4).

(See Focus on Long-Term Care box.)

LINENS

When handling linens and making beds, follow the rules of medical asepsis. Your uniform is considered dirty. Therefore always hold linens away from your body and uniform (Fig. 13-5). Never shake linens in the air. Shaking them spreads microbes. Clean linens are placed on a clean surface. Never put clean or dirty linens on the floor.

Collect clean linens in the order of use. Be sure to collect enough linens. If the person has 2 pillows, get 2 pillowcases. The person may need extra blankets for warmth. Do not bring unneeded linens to a person's room. Extra linen is considered contaminated and is not used for another person.

Collect linens in the following order:

- Mattress pad
- Bottom sheet (flat sheet or contour sheet)
- Plastic drawsheet (optional)
- Cotton drawsheet
- Top sheet (flat sheet)
- Blanket
- Bedspread
- Pillowcase(s)
- Bath towel(s)
- Hand towel
- Washcloth
- Hospital gown
- Bath blanket

Fig. 13-1 Closed bed.

Fig. 13-2 Open bed. Top linens are folded to the foot of the bed.

Fig. 13-3 Occupied bed.

Fig. 13-4 Surgical bed.

 Focus On... LONG-TERM CARE

In long-term care, most residents are out of bed most of the day. A closed bed is made until bedtime. Then an open bed is made.

Fig. 13-5 Hold linens away from your body and uniform.

Fig. 13-6 Collecting linens. **A,** The arm is placed over the top of the stack of linens. **B,** The stack of linens is turned over onto the arm. Note that linens are held away from the body.

Fig. 13-7 Roll linens away from you when removing them from the bed.

Use one arm to hold the linens and the other hand to pick them up. The item you will use first is at the bottom of your stack. (You picked up the mattress pad first. It is at the bottom. The bath blanket is on top.) You need the mattress pad first. To get it on top, simply place your arm over the bath blanket. Then turn the stack over onto the arm on the bath blanket (Fig. 13-6). The arm that held the linens is now free. Place the clean linens on a clean surface.

When removing dirty linens, remove each piece separately. The piece of linen is rolled away from you. That way the side that touched the person is inside the roll. The side that has not touched the person is outside (Fig. 13-7).

Top and bottom sheets, drawsheets, and pillowcases are changed daily in hospitals. The mattress pad, plastic drawsheet, blanket, and bedspread are reused for the same person. They are reused if not soiled, wet, or wrinkled. If a person was discharged, remove all linens and make a closed bed. *Remember, wet, damp, or soiled linens are changed right away.*

(See Focus on Long-Term Care box and Focus on Home Care box.)

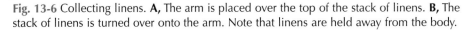

Focus On... LONG-TERM CARE

Policies about linen changes vary among nursing centers. Generally, linens are not changed every day. Remember, the center is the person's home. People do not change linens every day in their homes. A complete linen change is usually done weekly. Pillowcases, top and bottom sheets, and drawsheets (if used) may be changed twice a week. However, linens are changed if wet, soiled, or very wrinkled.

Some residents bring their own bedspreads, pillows, blankets, or afghans from home. Remember to use them when making the bed. Remember, these items are the person's property. Always handle them with care and respect. Make sure the items are labeled with the person's name to prevent them from becoming lost or confused with another resident's property.

Some centers use white, blue, yellow, pink, or other colored or printed linens. If so, let the resident choose what color to use. Also let the person decide how many pillows or blankets to use. If possible, the person also chooses the time when you make the bed. Remember, the resident has the right to personal choice.

Focus On... HOME CARE

Linen changes in the home are usually done weekly. However, follow the person's routine. Change linens more often if the person asks you to do so. Always change linens that are wet, soiled, or very wrinkled. Contact the RN if the person refuses to have linens changed.

A **drawsheet** is a small sheet placed over the middle of the bottom sheet. It helps keep the mattress and bottom linens clean and dry. A **plastic drawsheet** is waterproof. It protects the mattress and bottom linens from dampness and soiling. It is placed between the bottom sheet and cotton drawsheet. The cotton drawsheet protects the person from contact with the plastic and absorbs moisture. However, discomfort and skin breakdown may occur. The plastic retains heat, and plastic drawsheets are hard to keep tight and wrinkle-free.

Many agencies use waterproof pads instead of plastic drawsheets. Plastic drawsheets are usually used only for persons with bowel or bladder control problems or those with excessive wound drainage.

Cotton drawsheets are often used without plastic drawsheets. Plastic-covered mattresses cause some persons to perspire heavily. This increases discomfort. A cotton drawsheet reduces heat retention and absorbs moisture. Cotton drawsheets are often used as lift or turning sheets (see Chapter 11). When used for this purpose, they are not tucked in at the sides.

The bedmaking procedures that follow include plastic and cotton drawsheets so you learn how to use them. Ask the nurse about their use.

(See Focus on Home Care box.)

GENERAL RULES

Your job description will include making beds. No matter what type of bed you make, safety and medical asepsis are important. Standard Precautions and the Bloodborne Pathogen Standard also are followed. Box 13-1 lists the rules for bedmaking. *(See Focus on Home Care box at top left on p. 298 and Focus on Children box on p. 298.)*

Box 13-1   Rules for Bedmaking

- Use good body mechanics at all times.
- Follow the rules of medical asepsis.
- Practice Standard Precautions.
- Follow the Bloodborne Pathogen Standard.
- Wash your hands before handling clean linen and after handling dirty linen.
- Bring enough linen to the person's room.
- Do not use torn linen.
- Never shake linens. Shaking linens spreads microbes.
- Extra linen in a person's room is considered contaminated. Do not use it for other people. Put it with the dirty laundry.
- Hold linens away from your uniform. Dirty linen and clean linen must not touch your uniform.
- Never put dirty linens on the floor or on clean linens. Handle and dispose of linen following agency policy (see Chapter 10).
- Keep bottom linens tucked in and wrinkle-free.
- Cover a plastic drawsheet with a cotton drawsheet. A plastic drawsheet must not touch the person's body.
- Straighten and tighten loose sheets, blankets, and bedspreads whenever necessary.
- Make as much of one side of the bed as possible before going to the other side. This saves time and energy.

Focus On... HOME CARE

A flat sheet folded in half can serve as a cotton drawsheet. Usually a twin-size sheet is easier to use for this purpose. The RN tells you what to use.

Medical supply stores sell plastic drawsheets and waterproof pads. The RN discusses the need for these items with the person and family. Some people place plastic mattress protectors on their beds. These do not protect the bottom linens (cotton drawsheet, bottom sheet, and mattress pad). Some place a piece of plastic under the drawsheet. Again, the RN tells you what is safe to use for the person. Do not use plastic trash bags or dry cleaning bags. These are not strong enough to protect the linens and mattress. They slide easily and can move out of place. The danger of suffocation is great if the bag covers the person's nose and mouth.

Focus On... HOME CARE

Many home care patients do not have hospital beds. You will see twin-, regular-, queen-, and king-size beds. Water beds, sofa sleepers, cots, and recliners also are common. Remember, you are in the person's home. Make the bed according to the person's wishes. No matter the type of bed, follow the rules in Box 13-1. If the person's wishes are unsafe, contact the nurse.

Your assignment may include doing laundry. Remember to wear gloves when handling linen that may contain blood, body fluids, secretions, or excretions. Washing soiled linen when stains are fresh helps prevent staining. Urine, feces, vomit, and blood can stain linens. Always rinse the item with cold water to remove the body fluid or substance. Then treat the stain. The person may use a stain-removing agent. Always read and following the manufacturer's instructions when using a stain remover. Or the nurse may direct you to soak the item in an ammonia solution:

- 1 quart warm water
- $\frac{1}{2}$ teaspoon liquid handwashing detergent
- 1 tablespoon ammonia

After soaking, the item is rinsed with cool water. Then it is machine washed with a detergent.

Remember, ammonia is a poison. Do not inhale the fumes or let the ammonia have contact with your skin or eyes. Always follow the manufacturer's instructions when using ammonia. Do not mix it with other chemicals.

Focus On... CHILDREN

Cribs and crib linens present safety hazards. Mattresses, linens, and bumper pads pose many dangers. They can lead to strangulation and suffocation. Report any safety hazard to the nurse. Always follow these safety rules:

- The crib mattress must be firm. A soft mattress can cover the baby's nose and mouth. This prevents breathing.
- The mattress must fit snugly in the crib frame. Otherwise the baby's head can get caught between the mattress and the frame. The baby can strangulate.
- The space between the mattress and crib sides should be no more than 2 inches. Only two adult fingers should fit in the space. If more than two fingers fit, the mattress does not fit.
- The mattress must be at least 26 inches lower than the top of the crib rails. This protects the baby from falling out of the crib. The mattress is lowered when the baby can stand in the crib.
- Plastic trash bags and dry cleaning bags are not used to protect the mattress.
- Bumper pads must fit snugly against the slats. Otherwise the baby's head can get caught between the bumper pads and the slats. Strangulation can occur.
- Bumper pads are secured in place with at least 6 ties.
- Bumper pad ties must be away from the baby. Avoid long ties. The baby can get entangled in the ties and strangulate.
- Bumper pads are removed when the baby can stand in the crib.
- Do not tuck blankets and top sheets under the crib. A baby can get caught in them.
- Pillows are not used for babies. The pillow can cover the baby's nose and mouth. The baby can suffocate in the pillow.
- Blankets, comforters, and other linens are checked for loose threads and loose trim. Loose threads and trim can cause strangulation.
- Comforters are checked for loose stitching. Stuffing can come out if not stitched properly. The child can inhale the stuffing and suffocate.

Focus On... LONG-TERM CARE

In long-term care, a closed bed also means that the linens are not folded back as in the open bed. Closed beds are made for residents who are up for most or all of the day. Clean linens are used as needed.

Focus On... HOME CARE

In home care, a closed bed also means that linens are not folded back. Closed beds are made for patients who are up for most or all of the day. Clean linens are used as needed.

▶ THE CLOSED BED

A closed bed is made after a person is discharged. It is made ready for a new patient or resident. The bed is made after the bed frame and mattress are cleaned and disinfected. *(See Focus on Long-Term Care and Focus on Home Care boxes at bottom on p. 298.)*

Text continued on p. 304

Making a Closed Bed

QUALITY OF LIFE

Remember to:
- Knock before entering the person's room
- Address the person by name
- Introduce yourself by name and title

Pre-Procedure

1 Wash your hands.
2 Collect clean linen:
   - Mattress pad
   - Bottom sheet (flat sheet or contour sheet)
   - Plastic drawsheet (optional)
   - Cotton drawsheet
   - Top sheet
   - Blanket
   - Bedspread
   - Two pillowcases
   - Bath towel(s)
   - Hand towel
   - Washcloth
   - Hospital gown
   - Bath blanket
   - Gloves
3 Place linen on a clean surface.
4 Raise the bed for good body mechanics.
5 Make sure the bed and bed frame were cleaned if the person was discharged.

Procedure

6 Put on the gloves.
7 Remove linen. Roll each piece away from you. Place each piece in a laundry bag.
8 Remove and discard the gloves. Wash your hands.
9 Move the mattress to the head of the bed.
10 Put the mattress pad on the mattress. It is even with the top of the mattress.
11 Place the bottom sheet on the mattress pad (Fig. 13-8, p. 301):
   a Unfold it lengthwise.
   b Place the center crease in the middle of the bed.
   c Position the lower edge even with the bottom of the mattress.
   d Place the large hem at the top and the small hem at the bottom.
   e Face hem-stitching downward.
12 Pick the sheet up from the side to open it. Fanfold it toward the other side of the bed (Fig. 13-9, p. 301).
13 Go to the head of the bed. Tuck the top of the sheet under the mattress. Make sure the sheet is tight and smooth.
14 Make a mitered corner if using a flat sheet (Fig. 13-10, p. 301).

Continued

Making a Closed Bed—cont'd

Procedure—cont'd

15 Place the plastic drawsheet on the bed about 14 inches from the top of the mattress.

16 Open the plastic drawsheet, and fanfold it toward the other side of the bed.

17 Place a cotton drawsheet over the plastic drawsheet. It must cover the entire plastic drawsheet (Fig. 13-11, p. 302).

18 Open the cotton drawsheet, and fanfold it toward the other side of the bed.

19 Tuck both drawsheets under the mattress. Or tuck each in separately.

20 Go to the other side of the bed.

21 Miter the top corner of the bottom sheet.

22 Pull the bottom sheet tight so there are no wrinkles. Tuck in the sheet.

23 Pull the drawsheets tight so there are no wrinkles. Tuck both in together or pull each tight and tuck them in separately (Fig. 13-12, p. 302).

24 Go to the other side of the bed.

25 Put the top sheet on the bed:
   a Unfold it lengthwise.
   b Place the center crease in the middle.
   c Place the large hem at the top, even with the top of the mattress.
   d Open the sheet, and fanfold the extra part toward the other side.
   e Face hem-stitching outward.
   f Do not tuck the bottom in yet.
   g Never tuck top linens in on the sides.

26 Place the blanket on the bed:
   a Unfold it so the center crease is in the middle.
   b Put the upper hem about 6 to 8 inches from the top of the mattress.
   c Open the blanket, and fanfold the extra part toward the other side.

   d If steps 32 and 33 are not done, turn the top sheet down over the blanket. Hem-stitching is down.

27 Place the bedspread on the bed:
   a Unfold it so the center crease is in the middle.
   b Place the upper hem even with the top of the mattress.
   c Open the bedspread, and fanfold the extra part toward the other side.
   d Make sure the bedspread facing the door is even and covers all the top linens.

28 Tuck in top linens together at the foot of the bed. They should be smooth and tight. Make a mitered corner.

29 Go to the other side.

30 Straighten all top linen, working from the head of the bed to the foot.

31 Tuck in the top linens together. Make a mitered corner.

32 Turn the top hem of the bedspread under the blanket to make a cuff (Fig. 13-13, p. 302).

33 Turn the top sheet down over the spread. Hem-stitching is down. (Steps 32 and 33 are not done in some agencies. The bedspread covers the pillow. Be sure to tuck the spread under the pillow.)

34 Place the pillow on the bed.

35 Open the pillowcase so it is flat on the bed.

36 Put the pillowcase on the pillow as in Figure 13-14 on p. 303. Fold extra pillowcase material under the pillow at the seam end of the pillowcase.

37 Place the pillow on the bed so the open end is away from the door. The seam of the pillowcase is toward the head of the bed.

Post-Procedure

38 Attach the signal light to the bed.

39 Lower the bed to its lowest position.

40 Put towels, washcloth, gown, and bath blanket in the bedside stand.

41 Wash your hands.

Fig. 13-8 The bottom sheet is on the bed with the center crease in the middle. The lower edge of the sheet is even with the bottom of the mattress.

Fig. 13-9 The bottom sheet is fanfolded to the other side of the bed.

Fig. 13-10 Making a mitered corner. **A,** Bottom sheet is tucked under the mattress, and the side of the sheet is raised onto the mattress. **B,** The remaining portion of the sheet is tucked under the mattress. **C,** The raised portion of the sheet is brought off the mattress. **D,** The entire side of the sheet is tucked under the mattress.

Fig. 13-11 A cotton drawsheet over the plastic drawsheet. The cotton drawsheet completely covers the plastic drawsheet.

Fig. 13-12 The drawsheet is pulled tight to remove wrinkles.

Fig. 13-13 The top hem of the bedspread is turned under the top hem of the blanket to make a cuff.

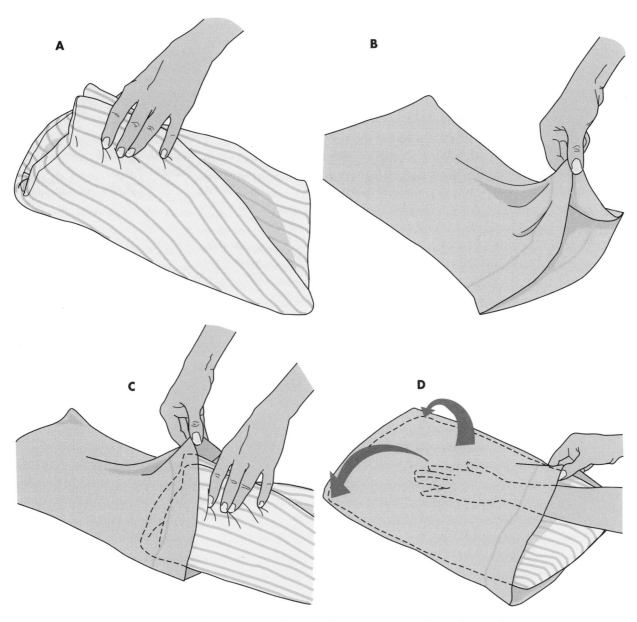

Fig. 13-14 Putting a pillowcase on a pillow. **A,** Grasp the corners of the pillow at the seam end and form a "V" with the pillow. **B,** The pillowcase is flat on the bed; the pillowcase is opened with the free hand. **C,** The "V" end of the pillow is guided into the pillowcase. **D,** The "V" end of the pillow falls into the corners of the pillowcase.

▶ THE OPEN BED

A closed bed becomes an open bed by folding the top linens back. Open beds are made for newly admitted persons arriving by wheelchair. They are also made for persons who are out of bed when their beds are being made.

Making an Open Bed

QUALITY OF LIFE

Remember to:
- Knock before entering the person's room
- Address the person by name
- Introduce yourself by name and title

Procedure

1 Wash your hands.
2 Collect linen for a closed bed.
3 Make a closed bed.
4 Fanfold top linens to the foot of the bed (see Fig. 13-2).
5 Attach the signal light to the bed.
6 Lower the bed to its lowest position.
7 Put towels, washcloth, gown, and bath blanket in the bedside stand.
8 Follow agency policy for dirty linen.
9 Wash your hands.

THE OCCUPIED BED

An occupied bed is made when a person cannot get out of bed because of illness or injury. You must keep the person in good body alignment. You must know about restrictions or limits in the person's movement or positioning. Explain each step of the procedure to the person before it is done. Always explain what you are doing even if the person cannot respond to you or is in a coma.

Making an Occupied Bed

NNAAP™

QUALITY OF LIFE

Remember to:
- Knock before entering the person's room
- Address the person by name
- Introduce yourself by name and title

Pre-Procedure

1 Explain the procedure to the person.
2 Wash your hands.
3 Collect the following:
   - Gloves
   - Linen bag
   - Clean linen (see *Making a Closed Bed,* p. 299.)
4 Place linen on a clean surface.
5 Provide for privacy.
6 Remove the signal light.
7 Raise the bed for good body mechanics. Make sure bed rails are up.
8 Lower the head of the bed to a level appropriate for the person. It should be as flat as possible.
9 Lower the bed rail near you.

Procedure

10 Put on gloves. Follow Standard Precautions and the Bloodborne Pathogen Standard.
11 Loosen top linens at the foot of the bed.
12 Remove the bedspread and blanket separately. Fold them as in Figure 13-15 on p. 307 if you will reuse them.
13 Cover the person with a bath blanket for warmth and privacy:
   a Unfold a bath blanket over the top sheet.
   b Ask the person to hold onto the bath blanket. If he or she cannot, tuck the top part under the person's shoulders.
   c Grasp the top sheet under the bath blanket at the shoulders. Bring the sheet down to the foot of the bed. Remove the sheet from under the blanket (Fig. 13-16, p. 308).
14 Move the mattress to the head of the bed.
15 Position the person on the side of the bed away from you. Move the pillow to the far side of the bed. Adjust the pillow for the person's comfort.
16 Loosen bottom linens from the head to the foot of the bed.
17 Fanfold bottom linens one at a time toward the person: cotton drawsheet, plastic drawsheet, bottom sheet, and mattress pad (Fig. 13-17, p. 308). Do not fanfold the mattress pad if it will be reused.
18 Place a clean mattress pad on the bed. Unfold it lengthwise so the center crease is in the middle. Fanfold the top part toward the person. If reusing the mattress pad, straighten and smooth any wrinkles.

Continued

Making an Occupied Bed—cont'd

Procedure—cont'd

19   Place the bottom sheet on the mattress pad so hem-stitching is away from the person. Unfold the sheet so the crease is in the middle. The small hem should be even with the bottom of the mattress. Fanfold the top part toward the person.

20   Make a mitered corner at the head of the bed if using a flat sheet. Tuck the sheet under the mattress from the head to the foot.

21   Pull the fanfolded plastic drawsheet toward you over the bottom sheet. Tuck excess material under the mattress. Do the following if you are using a clean plastic drawsheet (Fig. 13-18, p. 308):

   a   Place the plastic drawsheet on the bed about 14 inches from the mattress top.

   b   Fanfold the top part toward the person.

   c   Tuck in the excess material.

22   Place the cotton drawsheet over the plastic drawsheet. It must cover the entire plastic drawsheet. Fanfold the top part toward the person. Tuck in excess material.

23   Raise the bed rail. Go to the other side, and lower the bed rail.

24   Explain to the person that he or she will roll over a bump. Assure the person that he or she will not fall.

25   Position the person on the side of the bed away from you. Adjust the pillow for the person's comfort.

26   Loosen bottom linens. Remove soiled linen one piece at a time. Place linen in a laundry bag.

27   Remove and discard the gloves.

28   Straighten and smooth the mattress pad.

29   Pull the clean bottom sheet toward you. Make a mitered corner at the top. Tuck the sheet under the mattress from the head to the foot of the bed.

30   Pull the drawsheets tightly toward you. Tuck both under together, or tuck each in separately.

31   Position the person supine in the center of the bed. Adjust the pillow for comfort.

32   Put the top sheet on the bed. Unfold it lengthwise. Make sure the crease is in the middle, the large hem is even with the top of the mattress, and hem-stitching is on the outside.

33   Ask the person to hold onto the top sheet so you can remove the bath blanket. You may have to tuck the top sheet under the person's shoulders. Remove the bath blanket.

34   Place the blanket on the bed. Unfold it so the crease is in the middle. Unfold the blanket so it covers the person. The upper hem should be 6 to 8 inches from the top of the mattress.

35   Place the bedspread on the bed. Unfold it so the center crease is in the middle and it covers the person. The top hem is even with the mattress top.

36   Turn the top hem of the bedspread under the blanket to make a cuff.

37   Bring the top sheet down over the bedspread to form a cuff.

38   Go to the foot of the bed.

39   Lift the mattress corner with one arm. Tuck all top linens under the mattress together. Be sure the linens are loose enough to allow movement of the person's feet. Make a mitered corner.

40   Raise the bed rail. Go to the other side, and lower the bed rail.

41   Straighten and smooth top linens.

42   Tuck the top linens under the mattress as in step 39. Make a mitered corner.

43   Change the pillowcase(s).

44   Place the signal light within reach.

45   Raise or lower bed rails. Follow the care plan.

Making an Occupied Bed—cont'd

NNAAP™

Post-Procedure

46 Raise the head of the bed to a level appropriate for the person. Make sure the person is comfortable.

47 Lower the bed to its lowest position.

48 Put towels, washcloth, gown, and bath blanket in the bedside stand.

49 Unscreen the person. Thank him or her for cooperating.

50 Follow agency policy for dirty linen.

51 Wash your hands.

Fig. 13-15 Folding linen for reuse. **A,** The top edge of the blanket is folded down to the bottom edge. **B,** The blanket is folded from the far side of the bed to the near side. **C,** The top edge of the blanket is folded down to the bottom edge again. **D,** The folded blanket is placed over the back of a straight chair.

Fig. 13-16 The person holds onto the bath blanket. The top sheet is removed from under the bath blanket.

Fig. 13-17 Occupied bed. **A,** The cotton drawsheet is fanfolded and tucked under the person. **B,** All bottom linens are tucked under the person.

Fig. 13-18 A clean bottom sheet and plastic drawsheet are on the bed, with both fanfolded and tucked under the person. The clean cotton drawsheet is put in place in step 22.

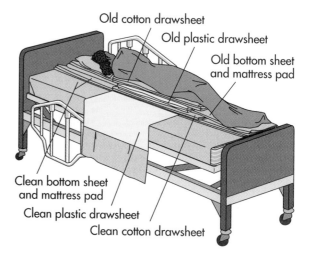

THE SURGICAL BED

The surgical bed (recovery bed, postoperative bed, or anesthesia bed) is a form of the open bed. Top linens are folded for transferring the person from a stretcher to the bed. The term *surgical bed* and its other names imply that the person had surgery. However, this bed is used for persons who arrive on a stretcher. If the bed is made for a postoperative (surgical) patient, a complete linen change is done.

Making a Surgical Bed

QUALITY OF LIFE

Remember to:
- Knock before entering the person's room
- Address the person by name
- Introduce yourself by name and title

Procedure

1 Wash your hands.
2 Collect the following:
   - Clean linen (see *Making a Closed Bed*, p. 299.)
   - IV pole
   - Tissues
   - Kidney basin
   - Gloves
   - Laundry bag
   - Other equipment as requested by the nurse
3 Place linen on a clean surface.
4 Remove the signal light.
5 Raise the bed for good body mechanics.
6 Remove all linen from the bed. Wear gloves for contact with the person's blood, body fluids, secretions, or excretions. Place linen in a laundry bag.
7 Make a closed bed (see *Making a Closed Bed*, p. 299). Do not tuck the top linens under the mattress.
8 Fold all top linens at the foot of the bed back onto the bed. The fold is even with the edge of the mattress (Fig. 13-19, p. 310).
9 Fanfold linen lengthwise to the side of the bed farthest from the door (Fig. 13-20, p. 310).
10 Put the pillowcase(s) on the pillow(s).
11 Place the pillow(s) on a clean surface.
12 Leave the bed in its highest position.
13 Make sure both bed rails are down.
14 Put the towels, washcloth, gown, and bath blanket in the bedside stand.
15 Place the tissues and kidney basin on the bedside stand. Place the IV pole near the head of the bed.
16 Move all furniture away from the bed. Allow enough room for the stretcher and for the staff to move about.
17 Do not attach the signal light to the bed.
18 Follow agency policy for soiled linen.
19 Wash your hands.

Fig. 13-19 Surgical bed. The bottom of the top linens is folded back onto the bed. The fold is even with the edge of the mattress.

Fig. 13-20 A surgical bed with the top linens fanfolded lengthwise to the opposite side of the bed.

REVIEW

Circle the BEST answer.

1. Which does not require a linen change?
   A. Soiled linen
   B. Wet linen
   C. Wrinkled linen
   D. Crumbs in the bed

2. You will transfer a person from a stretcher to the bed. Which bed should you make?
   A. A closed bed
   B. An open bed
   C. An occupied bed
   D. A surgical bed

3. When handling linens
   A. Put dirty linens on the floor
   B. Hold linens away from your body and uniform
   C. Shake linens to remove crumbs
   D. Take extra linen to another person's room

4. A resident is out of the room most of the day. What type of bed should you make?
   A. A closed bed
   B. An open bed
   C. An occupied bed
   D. A surgical bed

5. A complete linen change is done when
   A. The bottom linens are wet or soiled
   B. The bed is made for a new patient or resident
   C. The person will be transferred from a stretcher to the bed
   D. The person is in the shower

6. You are using a plastic drawsheet. Which is *true*?
   A. A cotton drawsheet must completely cover the plastic drawsheet.
   B. Disposable bed protectors are needed.
   C. The person's consent is needed.
   D. The plastic must be in contact with the person's skin.

7. When making an occupied bed, you do the following *except*
   A. Cover the person with a bath blanket
   B. Screen the person
   C. Raise the far side rail
   D. Fanfold top linens to the foot of the bed

8. A surgical bed is kept
   A. In Fowler's position
   B. In the lowest position
   C. In the highest position
   D. In the supine position

Answers to these questions are on p. 835.

CHAPTER

14

PERSONAL HYGIENE

Define the key terms listed in this chapter

Explain the importance of cleanliness and skin care

Describe the routine care given before and after breakfast, after lunch, and in the evening

Describe the importance of oral hygiene and the observations to report

Describe the rules for bathing and the observations to make

Identify the safety precautions for persons taking tub baths or showers

Explain the purposes of a back massage

Identify the purposes of perineal care

Perform the procedures described in this chapter

KEY TERMS

AM care Routine care performed before breakfast; early morning care

aspiration Breathing fluid or an object into the lungs

early morning care AM care

evening care HS care or PM care

HS care Care given in the evening at bedtime (hour of sleep [HS]); evening care or PM care

morning care Care given after breakfast; cleanliness and skin care measures are more thorough at this time

oral hygiene Measures performed to keep the mouth and teeth clean; mouth care

pericare Perineal care

perineal care Cleansing the genital and anal areas

plaque A thin film that sticks to the teeth; it contains saliva, microbes, and other substances

PM care HS care or evening care

tartar Hardened plaque on teeth

Cleanliness and skin care promote comfort, safety, and health. The skin is the body's first line of defense against disease. Intact skin prevents microbes from entering the body and causing an infection. Likewise, mucous membranes of the mouth, genital area, and anus must be clean and intact. Besides cleansing, good hygiene prevents body and breath odors. It also promotes relaxation and increases circulation. (See Box 14-1 on p. 314 for a review of the body structures and functions related to this chapter.)

Culture and personal choice affect hygiene. *(See Caring About Culture [Personal Hygiene Practices of East Indian Hindus] box, p. 314.)* Some people take showers. Others take tub baths. Some bathe at bedtime. Others bathe in the morning. Bathing frequency also varies. Some bathe daily or twice a day—such as before work and after work or exercise. Some people do not have water for bathing. Others cannot afford soap, deodorant, shampoo, toothpaste, or other hygiene products.

Patients and residents usually need some help with personal hygiene. Illness, age, and the changes of aging affect the ability to practice hygiene. Many factors affect hygiene and skin care needs. They include perspiration, vomiting, urinary and bowel elimination, drainage from wounds or body openings, bedrest, and activity. The RN uses the nursing process to meet the person's hygiene needs. The nurse and the nursing care plan tell you how to meet the person's hygiene needs. *(See Focus on Older Persons box on p. 314.)*

Box 14-1   Review of Body Structure and Function

THE TEETH AND GUMS

The teeth cut, chop, and grind food into small bits for digestion and swallowing. A tooth has three parts: the crown, neck, and root (Fig. 14-1). The crown is the outer part. It is covered by enamel. The neck is surround by the gums (gingivae). The root fits into the bone of the lower or upper jaw.

THE SKIN

The skin is the largest system of the body. The skin is the body's natural covering. There are two skin layers: the epidermis and the dermis (Fig. 14-2). The *epidermis* is the outer layer; it contains living cells and dead cells. Dead cells constantly flake off and are replaced by living cells. Living cells also die and flake off. The epidermis has no blood vessels and few nerve endings. The *dermis* is the inner layer of the skin and is made up of connective tissue. Blood vessels, nerves, sweat and oil glands, and hair roots are found in the dermis.

Sweat glands help regulate body temperature. Sweat is secreted through the skin's pores. The body is cooled as sweat evaporates. Oil glands secrete an oily substance into the space near the hair shaft. Oil travels to the skin surface, helping to keep the hair and skin soft and shiny.

The skin is the protective covering of the body. Intact skin prevents bacteria and other substances from entering the body. It also prevents excessive amounts of water from leaving the body and protects organs from injury. Nerve endings in the skin sense both pleasant and unpleasant stimulation. Cold, pain, touch, and pressure can be sensed. The skin also helps regulate body temperature. Blood vessels dilate (widen) when temperature outside the body is high. More blood is brought to the body surface for cooling during evaporation. When blood vessels constrict (narrow), the body retains heat because less blood reaches the skin.

Caring About Culture

PERSONAL HYGIENE PRACTICES OF EAST INDIAN HINDUS

Personal hygiene is very important to East Indian Hindus. Their religious duty requires a bath at least once a day. Some believe it is harmful to bathe after a meal. Another belief of some Hindus is that a cold bath prevents blood disease. Some believe that eye injuries can occur if a bath is too hot. Hot water can be added to cold water, but cold water is not added to hot water. After bathing, the body is carefully rubbed dry with a towel.

Remember, individuals may not follow every belief and practice of their culture and religion. Each person is unique. Do not judge the person by your own standards.

Modified from Giger JN, Davidhizar RE: *Transcultural nursing: assessment and interventions,* St Louis, 1995, Mosby.

Focus On... OLDER PERSONS

Some older persons may resist your efforts to assist with hygiene. Common reason include illness, disability, dementia, and personal choice. The health care team assesses each person's needs. You must know how to approach each person. The care plan explains the best way to work with the person.

Persons with dementia may require special approaches to resistive behaviors (see Chapter 32.)

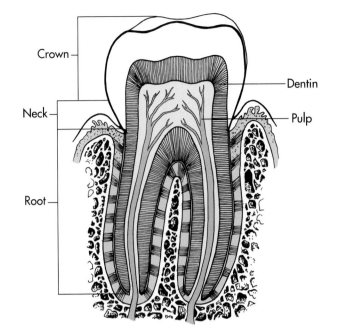

Fig. 14-1 Parts of the tooth. *(From Potter PA, Perry AG: Fundamentals of nursing: concepts, process, and practice, ed 4, St Louis, 1997, Mosby).*

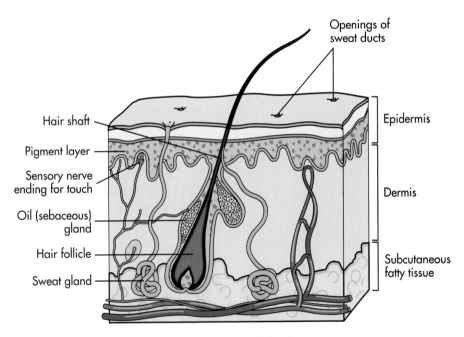

Fig. 14-2 Structure of the skin.

DAILY CARE

People usually have hygiene routines and habits. For example, teeth are brushed and the face and hands washed on awakening. These and other hygiene measures may be done routinely before and after meals and at bedtime.

Infants, young children, and some weak or disabled adults need help with hygiene. Routine care is given at certain times. However, you assist with personal hygiene whenever necessary.

BEFORE BREAKFAST

Routine care before breakfast is **early morning care** or **AM care**. Night shift or day shift staff give AM care. They get patients and residents ready for breakfast or morning tests. Personal hygiene measures at this time include:

- Assisting persons to the bathroom or offering commodes, bedpans, or urinals
- Cleaning incontinent persons and changing any wet or soiled linen
- Helping persons wash their faces and hands
- Assisting with oral hygiene
- Positioning persons in Fowler's position or in chairs for breakfast
- Brushing and combing hair (see Chapter 15)
- Straightening bed linens
- Straightening the person's unit
  (See Focus on Long-Term Care box below.)

Focus On... LONG-TERM CARE

In long-term care, most residents eat in dining rooms. For these persons, AM care includes assisting them to dress. You also assist them to dining rooms.

AFTER BREAKFAST

Morning care is given after breakfast. Hygiene and skin care measures are more thorough. Routine morning care usually involves:

- Assisting persons to the bathroom or offering commodes, bedpans, or urinals
- Cleaning incontinent persons and changing any wet or soiled linen
- Helping persons wash their faces and hands
- Assisting with oral hygiene
- Shaving patients and residents (see Chapter 15)
- Providing showers, tub baths, or bed baths
- Giving perineal care
- Giving back massages
- Performing range-of-motion exercises (see Chapter 20)
- Changing gowns or pajamas or helping the person dress (see Chapter 15)
- Brushing and combing hair
- Changing bed linens
- Straightening the person's unit

AFTERNOON CARE

Routine hygiene is performed after lunch and the evening meal. If it is done before visiting hours, the person feels more refreshed and can visit with family and friends without interruption. Afternoon care involves:

- Assisting persons to the bathroom or offering commodes, bedpans, or urinals
- Helping persons wash their faces and hands
- Assisting with oral hygiene
- Changing gowns, pajamas, or clothes
- Brushing or combing hair if needed
- Changing damp or soiled bed linens
- Straightening the person's unit
  (See Focus on Long-Term Care box below.)

Focus On... LONG-TERM CARE

In long-term care centers, residents often nap in the afternoon. You assist the person in lying down for the nap and in getting up afterwards. Range-of-motion exercises are also done in the afternoon.

EVENING CARE

Care given at bedtime is **HS care**, **evening care**, or **PM care**. (HS stands for *hour of sleep*.) Hygiene measures are performed before the person is ready for sleep. HS care promotes comfort and relaxation. It involves:

- Assisting persons to the bathroom or offering commodes, bedpans, or urinals
- Cleaning incontinent persons and changing wet or soiled linens
- Helping persons wash their faces and hands
- Assisting with oral hygiene
- Changing damp or soiled linens and straightening all other linens
- Changing gowns or pajamas if needed or assisting the person to undress and put on a gown or pajamas
- Giving back massages
- Straightening the person's unit

ORAL HYGIENE

Oral hygiene (mouth care) keeps the mouth and teeth clean. This prevents mouth odors and infections. It also increases comfort and makes food taste better. *Cavities (dental caries)* are prevented. So is *periodontal disease (gum disease, pyorrhea)*. Periodontal disease is an inflammation of the tissues around the teeth. Poor oral hygiene allows the buildup of plaque and tartar. **Plaque** is a thin film that sticks to teeth. It contains saliva, microbes, and other substances. Plaque leads to tooth decay, or cavities. When plaque hardens it is called **tartar.** Tartar builds up at the gum line near the neck of the tooth. Tartar buildup leads to periodontal disease. The gums are red, swollen, and bleed easily. As the disease progresses, bone is destroyed and teeth loosen. Tooth loss is common.

Illness and disease often cause a bad taste in the mouth. Some drugs and diseases cause a whitish coating on the mouth and tongue. Others cause redness and swelling of the mouth and tongue. Dry mouth is common from oxygen, smoking, decreased fluid intake, and anxiety. Some drugs cause dry mouth.

The nurse assesses the person's need for mouth care. The speech/language pathologist and the dietitian also may assess the person's mouth care needs. The nurse tells you the type of mouth care and assistance needed. Oral hygiene is given on awakening, after each meal, and at bedtime. Many people also practice oral hygiene before meals.

EQUIPMENT

A toothbrush, toothpaste, dental floss, and mouthwash are needed. The toothbrush should have soft bristles. Persons with dentures need a denture cleaner, denture cup, and denture brush or regular toothbrush. Use only those products that are recommended for cleaning dentures. Otherwise you could damage the dentures.

Sponge swabs are used for persons with sore, tender mouths and for unconscious persons. Be careful when using sponge swabs. Always check the foam pad to make sure it is tight on the stick. The person could choke on the foam pad if it comes off the stick.

Follow Standard Precautions and the Bloodborne Pathogen Standard when giving oral hygiene. You have contact with the person's mucous membranes. Gums may bleed during oral care. Also, the mouth contains many microbes. Pathogens spread through sexual contact may be in the mouths of some persons.

OBSERVATIONS

The following are reported to the nurse if observed during oral hygiene:

- Dry, cracked, swollen, or blistered lips
- Redness, swelling, irritation, sores, or white patches in the mouth or on the tongue
- Bleeding, swelling, or redness of the gums
- Loose teeth

► BRUSHING TEETH

Many people perform oral hygiene themselves. Others need help gathering and setting up equipment. You may have to brush the teeth of persons who are very weak or who cannot use or move their arms. Some people are too weak or confused to brush their own teeth. You need to provide oral hygiene for them. (*See Focus on Children box.*)

Focus On... CHILDREN

Children learn to brush their teeth around 3 years of age. However, they may not be thorough. They need help brushing. Older children can do a thorough job. Reminding them to brush is often necessary.

► Assisting the Person to Brush the Teeth

QUALITY OF LIFE

Remember to:
- Knock before entering the person's room
- Address the person by name
- Introduce yourself by name and title

Pre-Procedure

1 Explain the procedure to the person.
2 Wash your hands.
3 Collect the following:
   - Toothbrush
   - Toothpaste or dentifrice
   - Mouthwash (or solution specified on the care plan)
   - Dental floss
   - Water glass with cool water
   - Straw
   - Kidney basin
   - Face towel
   - Paper towels
4 Place the paper towels on the overbed table. Arrange items on top of them.
5 Identify the person. Check the ID bracelet, and call the person by name.
6 Provide for privacy.
7 Raise the head so the person can brush with ease.

Procedure

8 Lower the bed rail (if used).
9 Place the towel over the person's chest. This protects the gown and linens from spills.
10 Place the overbed table in front of the person. Adjust table height for the person.
11 Allow the person to perform oral hygiene. This includes brushing the teeth, rinsing the mouth, and using mouthwash or other specified solution.
12 Remove the towel when the person is done.
13 Move the overbed table next to the bed. Lower it to a level appropriate for the person.

Post-Procedure

14 Provide for comfort.
15 Place the signal light within reach.
16 Raise or lower bed rails. Follow the care plan.
17 Clean and return items to their proper place. Wear gloves for this step.
18 Wipe off the overbed table with the paper towels, and discard them.
19 Unscreen the person.
20 Follow agency policy for dirty linen.
21 Wash your hands.
22 Report your observations to the nurse.

Brushing the Person's Teeth

QUALITY OF LIFE

Remember to:
- Knock before entering the person's room
- Address the person by name
- Introduce yourself by name and title

Pre-Procedure

1   Explain the procedure to the person.
2   Wash your hands.
3   Collect gloves and items listed in *Assisting the Person to Brush the Teeth,* p. 318.
4   Place the paper towels on the overbed table. Arrange items on top of them.
5   Identify the person. Check the ID bracelet, and call the person by name.
6   Provide for privacy.
7   Raise the bed to the best level for good body mechanics. Make sure bed rails are up.

Procedure

8   Lower the bed rail near you.
9   Raise the head of the bed so the person can sit comfortably. Position the person in a side-lying position on the side near you if he or she cannot sit up.
10 Place the towel over the person's chest. This protects the gown and linens from spills.
11 Position the overbed table so you can reach it with ease. Adjust the height as needed.
12 Put on the gloves.
13 Apply toothpaste to the toothbrush.
14 Hold the toothbrush over the kidney basin. Pour some water over the brush.
15 Brush the person's teeth gently as shown in Figure 14-3 on p. 320.
16 Let the person rinse the mouth with water. Hold the kidney basin under the person's chin (Fig. 14-4, p. 320). Repeat this step as necessary.
17 Floss the person's teeth (see *Flossing the Person's Teeth,* p. 321).
18 Let the person use mouthwash or other specified solution. Hold the kidney basin under the chin.
19 Remove the towel when done.
20 Remove and discard the gloves.

Post-Procedure

21 Provide for comfort.
22 Place the signal light within reach.
23 Lower the bed to its lowest position.
24 Raise or lower bed rails. Follow the care plan.
25 Clean and return equipment to its proper place. Wear gloves for this step.
26 Wipe off the overbed table with the paper towels and discard them.
27 Lower the overbed table to a level appropriate for the person.
28 Unscreen the person.
29 Follow agency policy for dirty linen.
30 Wash your hands.
31 Report your observations to the nurse.

Fig. 14-3 Brushing teeth. **A,** Position the brush at a 45-degree angle to the gums. Brush with short strokes. **B,** Position the brush at 45-degree angle against the inside of the front teeth. Brush from the gum to the crown of the tooth with short strokes. **C,** Hold the brush horizontally against the inner surfaces of the teeth. Brush back and forth. **D,** Position the brush on the biting surfaces of the teeth. Brush back and forth.

Fig. 14-4 The kidney basin is held under the person's chin.

▶ FLOSSING

Flossing is a preventive measure. It removes plaque and tartar from the teeth. These substances cause serious gum disease that leads to loosening and loss of teeth. Flossing also removes food from between the teeth. It is usually done after brushing but can be done at other times. Some people floss after meals. If flossing is done only once a day, bedtime is the best time to floss.

You need to floss for persons who cannot tend to oral hygiene. (See Focus on Children and Focus on Older Persons boxes on p. 322.)

▶ Flossing the Person's Teeth

QUALITY OF LIFE

Remember to:
- Knock before entering the person's room
- Address the person by name
- Introduce yourself by name and title

Pre-Procedure

1 Explain to the person what you are going to do.
2 Wash your hands.
3 Collect the following:
- Kidney basin
- Water glass with cool water
- Dental floss
- Face towel
- Paper towels
- Gloves
4 Place the paper towels on the overbed table. Arrange items on top of them.
5 Identify the person. Check the ID bracelet, and call the person by name.
6 Provide for privacy.
7 Raise the bed to the best level for good body mechanics. Make sure bed rails are up.

Procedure

8 Lower the bed rail near you.
9 Raise the head of the bed so the person can sit comfortably. Position the person in a side-lying position near you if he or she cannot sit up.
10 Place the towel over the person's chest.
11 Position the overbed table so you can reach it with ease. Adjust the height as needed.
12 Put on the gloves.
13 Break off an 18-inch piece of floss from the dispenser.
14 Hold the floss between the middle fingers of each hand (Fig. 14-5, A, p. 322).
15 Stretch the floss with your thumbs.
16 Start at the upper back tooth on the right side, and work around to the left side.
17 Move the floss gently up and down between the teeth (Fig. 14-5, B, p. 322). Move floss up and down from the top of the crown to the gum line.
18 Move to a new section of floss after every second tooth.
19 Floss the lower teeth. Hold the floss with your index fingers (Fig. 14-5, C, p. 322). Use up and down motions and go under the gums as for the upper teeth. Start on the right side, and work around to the left side.
20 Let the person rinse his or her mouth. Hold the kidney basin under the chin. Repeat rinsing as necessary.
21 Remove the towel when done.
22 Remove and discard the gloves.

Post-Procedure

23 Follow steps 21 through 31 for *Brushing the Person's Teeth.*

Fig. 14-5 Flossing. **A,** Dental floss is held between the middle fingers to floss the upper teeth. **B,** Floss is moved in up-and-down motions between the teeth. Floss is moved up and down from the crown to the gum line. **C,** Floss is held with the index fingers to floss the lower teeth.

Focus On... **CHILDREN**

Preschoolers and older children need to floss. You need to floss for preschoolers. Older children can floss themselves. However, they need reminding and some supervision.

Focus On... **OLDER PERSONS**

Flossing was not a common oral hygiene measure many years ago. Therefore some older persons have never flossed their teeth. A person may refuse to floss or to let you do it. Respect the person's wishes, and tell the nurse. The nurse will change the person's care plan as needed.

► MOUTH CARE FOR THE UNCONSCIOUS PERSON

Unconscious persons need special mouth care. They cannot eat or drink, and they breathe with their mouths open. Many receive oxygen (see Chapter 27). These factors cause mouth dryness. They also cause crusting on the tongue and mucous membranes. Good mouth care helps keep the mouth clean and moist. It is also prevents infection.

Fig. 14-6 The head of the unconscious person is turned well to the side to prevent aspiration. A padded tongue blade is used to keep the mouth open while cleaning the mouth with swabs.

The care plan tells you what cleaning agent to use. Use sponge swabs to apply the cleaning agent. Apply a lubricant (check the care plan) to the lips after cleaning to prevent cracking.

Unconscious persons usually cannot swallow. Protect them from choking and aspiration. **Aspiration** is the breathing of fluid or an object into the lungs. It can cause pneumonia and death. To prevent aspiration, position the person on one side with the head turned well to the side (Fig. 14-6). In this position, excess fluid runs out of the mouth. This reduces the risk of aspiration. Using only a small amount of fluid also reduces the risk of aspiration. Sometimes oral suctioning (see Chapter 27) is part of the procedure.

The person's mouth is kept open with a padded tongue blade. If there are none in the supply area, make a padded tongue blade as in Figure 14-7. Do not use your fingers to hold the mouth open. The person can bite down on them. The bite breaks the skin and creates a portal of entry for microbes. An infection could develop.

Unconscious persons cannot speak or respond to what is happening. However, some can hear. Always assume that unconscious persons can hear. Explain what you are doing step by step. Also tell the person when you are done and when you are leaving the room.

Mouth care is given at least every 2 hours. The RN and health team assess the person's needs and write a care plan. Check with the nurse and the nursing care plan. They tell you how often to do oral hygiene and what to use. Unconscious persons are also repositioned at least every 2 hours. Combining mouth care, skin care, and other comfort measures increases their comfort and safety.

Fig. 14-7 Making a padded tongue blade. **A,** Place two wooden tongue blades together, and wrap gauze around the top half. **B,** Tape the gauze in place.

Providing Mouth Care for an Unconscious Person

QUALITY OF LIFE

Remember to:
- Knock before entering the person's room
- Address the person by name
- Introduce yourself by name and title

Pre-Procedure

1 Wash your hands.
2 Collect the following:
   - Cleaning agent (check the care plan)
   - Sponge swabs
   - Padded tongue blade
   - Water glass with cool water
   - Face towel
   - Kidney basin
   - Lip lubricant
   - Paper towels
   - Gloves
3 Place the paper towels on the overbed table. Arrange items on top of them.
4 Identify the person. Check the ID bracelet, and call the person by name.
5 Explain the procedure to the person.
6 Provide for privacy.
7 Raise the bed to the best level for good body mechanics. Make sure bed rails are up.

Procedure

8 Lower the bed rail near you.
9 Put on the gloves.
10 Position the person in a side-lying position on the side toward you. Turn his or her head well to the side.
11 Place the towel under the person's face.
12 Place the kidney basin under the chin.
13 Position the overbed table so you can reach it. Adjust the height as needed.
14 Separate the upper and lower teeth with the padded tongue blade. Be gentle. Do not use force. If you have problems, ask the nurse for help.
15 Clean the mouth using the sponge swabs moistened with the cleaning agent (see Fig. 14-6):
   a Clean the chewing and inner surfaces of the teeth.
   b Clean the outer surfaces of the teeth.
   c Swab the roof of the mouth, inside of the cheeks, and the lips.
   d Swab the tongue.
   e Moisten a clean swab with water, and swab the mouth to rinse.
   f Place used swabs in the kidney basin.
16 Apply lubricant to the lips.
17 Remove the towel.
18 Remove and discard the gloves.
19 Explain that the procedure is done and that you will reposition him or her.
20 Reposition the person, and provide for comfort.
21 Raise the bed rail. Make sure both bed rails are up.

Post-Procedure

22 Make sure the signal light is within reach.
23 Lower the bed to its lowest position.
24 Clean and return equipment to its proper place. Discard disposable items.
25 Unscreen the person.
26 Tell the person that you are leaving the room.
27 Follow agency policy for dirty linen.
28 Wash your hands.
29 Report your observations to the nurse.

► DENTURE CARE

Dentures are cleaned for persons who cannot do so themselves. Mouth care is given and dentures are cleaned as often as natural teeth. Remember, dentures are the person's property. They are costly. You must handle them carefully. Losing or damaging dentures is negligent conduct.

Dentures are slippery when wet. They easily break or chip if dropped onto hard surfaces such as floors or sinks. You must hold them firmly. During cleaning, firmly hold them over a basin of water lined with a towel. The water and towel prevent dentures from falling onto the hard surface of the sink. Hot water causes them to warp. Do not use hot water to clean or store dentures. If not worn, store dentures in a container of cool water. Otherwise, dentures can dry out and warp.

Dentures are generally removed at bedtime. Some people choose not to wear their dentures. Others wear dentures for eating and remove them after meals. Remind these people s not to wrap dentures in tissues or napkins. Otherwise they are easily discarded.

Many people clean their own dentures. However, they may need help collecting and cleaning items. They may also need help getting to the bathroom.

Providing Denture Care   NNAAP™

QUALITY OF LIFE

Remember to:
- Knock before entering the person's room
- Address the person by name
- Introduce yourself by name and title

Pre-Procedure

1   Explain the procedure to the person.
2   Wash your hands.
3   Collect the following:
- Denture brush or toothbrush
- Denture cup labeled with the person's name and room number
- Denture cleaner or toothpaste
- Water glass with cool water
- Straw
- Mouthwash (or other specified solution)
- Kidney basin
- Two face towels
- Gauze squares
- Gloves

4   Identify the person. Check the ID bracelet, and call the person by name.
5   Provide for privacy.

Procedure

6   Lower the bed rail if used.
7   Place a towel over the person's chest.
8   Put on the gloves.
9   Ask the person to remove the dentures. Carefully place them in the kidney basin.
10 Remove the dentures using gauze if the person cannot do so. (The gauze lets you get a good grip on the slippery dentures.)
  a Grasp the upper denture with your thumb and index finger (Fig. 14-8, p. 327). Move the denture up and down slightly to break the seal. Gently remove the denture once the seal is broken. Place it in the kidney basin.
  b Remove the lower denture by grasping it with your thumb and index finger. Turn it slightly, and lift it out of the person's mouth. Place it in the kidney basin.
11 Follow the care plan for raising bed rails.
12 Take the kidney basin, denture cup, brush, and denture cleaner or toothpaste to the sink.
13 Line the sink with a towel, and fill it with water.
14 Rinse each denture under warm running water. Return them to the denture cup.
15 Apply denture cleaner or toothpaste to the brush.

Continued

Providing Denture Care—cont'd

NNAAP™

Procedure—cont'd

16   Brush the dentures as in Figure 14-9.

17   Rinse dentures under cool running water. Handle them carefully; do not drop them.

18   Place them in the denture cup. Fill it with cool water until the dentures are covered.

19   Clean the kidney basin.

20   Bring the denture cup and kidney basin to the bedside table.

21   Lower the bed rail if up.

22   Position the person for oral hygiene.

23   Assist the person to rinse his or her mouth with mouthwash or specified solution. Hold the kidney basin under the chin.

24   Ask the person to insert the dentures. Insert them if the person cannot:

   a   Grasp the upper denture firmly with your thumb and index finger. Raise the upper lip with the other hand, and insert the denture. Use your index fingers to gently press on the denture to make sure it is securely in place.

   b   Grasp the lower denture securely with your thumb and index finger. Pull down slightly on the lower lip, and insert the denture. Gently press down on it to make sure it is in place.

25   Put the denture cup in the top drawer of the bedside stand if the dentures are not reinserted.

26   Remove the towel.

27   Remove the gloves.

Post-Procedure

28   Provide for comfort.

29   Place the signal light within reach.

30   Raise or lower bed rails. Follow the care plan.

31   Unscreen the person.

32   Clean and return equipment to its proper place. Discard disposable items.

33   Follow agency policy for dirty linen.

34   Wash your hands.

35   Report your observations to the nurse.

Fig. 14-8 Remove the upper denture by grasping it with the thumb and index finger of one hand. Use a piece of gauze to grasp the slippery denture.

Fig. 14-9 Cleaning dentures. **A,** Outer surfaces of the upper denture are brushed with back-and-forth motions. Note that the denture is held over the sink, which is filled halfway with water and lined with a towel. **B,** Position the brush vertically to clean the inner surfaces of the denture. Use upward strokes.

BATHING

Bathing cleans the skin. It also cleans the mucous membranes of the genital and anal areas. Microbes, dead skin, perspiration, and excess oils are removed. A bath also is refreshing and relaxing. Circulation is stimulated and body parts exercised. You make observations during the bath. The bath also gives you time to get to know the person.

A person may get a complete or partial bed bath, a tub bath, or a shower. The method depends on the person's condition, self-care abilities, and personal choice. Bathing usually occurs after breakfast. However, a person who normally bathes at bedtime should continue the practice if possible.

Bathing frequency is a personal matter. Some people bathe daily. Others take a complete bath only once or twice a week. Personal choice, weather, physical activity, and illness affect how often a person bathes. Illness usually increases the need for bathing because of fever and increased perspiration. Other illnesses and dry skin may require bathing every 2 or 3 days.

The rules for bed baths, showers, and tub baths are listed in Box 14-2. Table 14-1 describes common skin care products. *(See Focus on Children box and Focus on Older Persons box.)*

OBSERVATIONS

Observe the skin during bathing procedures. Report the following observations to the nurse:

- The color of the skin, lips, nail beds, and sclera (whites of the eyes)
- The location and description of rashes
- Dry skin
- Bruises or open skin areas
- Pale or reddened areas, particularly over bony parts
- Drainage or bleeding from wounds or body openings
- Skin temperature
- Complaints of pain or discomfort

Box 14-2 Rules for Bathing

- Follow Standard Precautions and the Bloodborne Pathogen Standard. Wear gloves whenever contact with blood, body fluids, secretions, or excretions is likely.
- Ask the nurse what type of bath a person is to have.
- Find out which skin care products to use. Allow personal choice when possible.
- Assist the person to the bathroom, or offer the commode, bedpan, or urinal. Bathing stimulates the need to urinate. Comfort and relaxation increase if urination needs are met.
- Collect equipment before starting the procedure.
- Protect the person's privacy. Properly screen the person, and close doors.
- Cover the person for warmth and privacy.
- Reduce drafts by closing doors and windows.
- Protect the person from falling.
- Use good body mechanics at all times.
- Make sure water temperature is not too hot, particularly for older persons.
- Keep soap in the soap dish between latherings. This prevents soapy water. If a tub bath or shower is taken, the person will not slip on the soap.
- Wash from the cleanest to the dirtiest areas.
- Encourage the person to help as much as is safely possible.
- Rinse the skin thoroughly to remove all soap.
- Pat the skin dry to avoid irritating or breaking the skin. Remember to dry under the breasts, between skin folds, in the perineal area, and between the toes.
- Bathe the skin whenever feces or urine is on the skin. This prevents skin breakdown and odors.

Focus On... CHILDREN

Younger and school-age children may not bathe every day. The nurse collects information about the child's bathing practices on admission. The child's nursing care plan reflects the child's normal practices and needs during illness.

Table 14-1   Common Skin Care Products

Type	Purpose	Nursing Care Considerations
Soaps	Clean the skin Remove dirt, dead skin, skin oil, some microbes, and perspiration	Tend to dry and irritate the skin Dry skin is easily injured and causes itching and discomfort Skin must be rinsed well to remove all soap Not needed for every bath; plain water can clean the skin Plain water is often used for older persons because of dry skin People with dry skin may prefer soaps containing bath oils Not used if a person has very dry skin
Bath oils	Keep the skin soft and prevent drying	Some soaps contain bath oil Liquid bath oil can be added to bath water Showers and tubs become slippery from bath oils; safety precautions are necessary to prevent falls
Creams and lotions	Protect the skin from the drying effect of air and evaporation	Do not feel greasy but leave an oily film on the skin Most are scented
Powders	Absorb moisture and prevent friction when two skin surfaces rub together	Usually applied under the breasts, under the arms, in the groin area, and sometimes between the toes Applied to dry skin in a thin, even layer Excessive amounts cause caking and crusts that can irritate skin
Deodorants	Mask and control body odors	Applied to the axillae (under arms) Not applied to irritated skin Do not take the place of bathing
Antiperspirants	Reduce the amount of perspiration	Applied to the axillae (under arms) Not applied to irritated skin Do not take the place of bathing

Focus On... OLDER PERSONS

Age affects bathing frequency. Dry skin occurs with aging. Soap also dries the skin. Dry skin is easily damaged. Therefore older persons usually need a complete bath once a week. Partial baths are taken the other days. Some bathe daily but do not always use soap. Thorough rinsing is essential when using soap. Lotions and oils help keep the skin soft.

Some older persons have dementia. Persons with dementia are often threatened by bathing procedures. They do not understand what is happening or why. They may fear harm or danger. Therefore persons with dementia may resist care and become agitated and combative. They may shout at the caregiver and cry for help.

The rules in Box 14-2 apply when bathing persons with dementia. The person's care plan will also include measures to help the person through the bathing procedure. Such measures include:

- Not rushing the person
- Using a calm, pleasant voice
- Diverting the person's attention (see Chapter 32)
- Calming the person and trying the bath later

▶ THE COMPLETE BED BATH

The *complete bed bath* involves washing the person's entire body in bed. Persons who are unconscious, paralyzed, in a cast or traction, or weak from illness or surgery generally require bed baths. You give complete bed baths to persons who cannot bathe themselves.

Ask the nurse about the person's ability to assist with the bath. Also ask about any activity or position limits. Remember to follow Standard Precautions and the Bloodborne Pathogen Standard. Also, remember to allow personal choice during the bath.

A bed bath is often a new experience for some people. Some are embarrassed to have another person see their bodies. Some persons fear exposure. Every person must get an explanation about the bed bath procedure and how the body is covered to protect privacy.

The following bed bath procedure is for adults. (*See Focus on Children box and Focus on Older Persons box.*)

Equipment. A bath basin, soap and water, and bath towels are commonly used to give a bed bath. However, some agencies are now using *bag baths.* Eight to ten washcloths are packaged in a plastic bag. The washcloths are premoistened with a cleaning agent that does not require rinsing. Before use, the wash-

cloths are warmed in the microwave for the person's comfort. A new washcloth is used for each body part. The skin air-dries, so towels are not needed. Commercial bag baths are available. Some agencies prepare their own in the central supply area.

Text continued on p. 336

> ### Focus On... CHILDREN
>
> See Chapter 35 for bathing infants. Follow the adult procedure for bathing toddlers and older children. Infants and young children have fragile skin. Lower water temperatures are used. Ask the nurse about what water temperature to use.

> ### Focus On... OLDER PERSONS
>
> Older persons also have fragile skin. Lower water temperatures are used. Ask the nurse about what water temperature to use.

Giving a Complete Bed Bath

QUALITY OF LIFE

Remember to:
- Knock before entering the person's room
- Address the person by name
- Introduce yourself by name and title

Pre-Procedure

1. Identify the person. Check the ID bracelet, and call the person by name.
2. Explain the procedure to the person.
3. Offer the bedpan or urinal (see Chapter 16). Provide for privacy.
4. Wash your hands.
5. Collect clean linen for a closed bed. Place linen on a clean surface.
6. Collect the following:
   - Wash basin
   - Soap dish with bar or liquid soap
   - Bath thermometer
   - Orange stick or nail file

- Washcloth
- Two bath towels and two face towels
- Bath blanket
- Gown or pajamas
- Items for oral hygiene
- Body lotion
- Talcum powder
- Deodorant or antiperspirant
- Brush and comb
- Other toilet articles if requested
- Paper towels
- Gloves (wear when contact with blood, body fluids, secretions, or excretions is likely)

Giving a Complete Bed Bath—cont'd

NNAAP™

Procedure

7   Arrange items on the overbed table. Adjust the height as needed. Use the bedside stand if necessary.

8   Close doors and windows to prevent drafts.

9   Provide for privacy.

10 Raise the bed to the best level for good body mechanics. Make sure bed rails are up.

11 Remove the signal light. Lower the bed rail near you.

12 Provide oral hygiene. Wear gloves for this step.

13 Remove top linens. Cover the person with a bath blanket (see *Making an Occupied Bed,* p. 305).

14 Lower the head of the bed to a level appropriate for the person. Keep it as flat as possible. Let the person have at least one pillow.

15 Place paper towels on the overbed table.

16 Raise the bed rail near you. Go fill the wash basin. (Both bed rails must be up.)

17 Fill the wash basin ²/₃ full with water. Water temperature should be 110° to 115° F (43.3° to 46° C) for adults. These higher water temperatures are needed because the water cools rapidly. Measure water temperature with the bath thermometer. (Some states allow you to test bath water by dipping your elbow or inner wrist into the basin.)

18 Place the basin on the overbed table on top of the paper towels.

19 Lower the bed rail.

20 Place a face towel over the person's chest.

21 Make a mitt with the washcloth (Fig. 14-10, p. 333). Use a mitt throughout the procedure.

22 Wash around the person's eyes with water. Do not use soap. Gently wipe from the inner aspect with a corner of the mitt (Fig. 14-11, p. 333). Clean around the far eye first. Repeat this step for around the near eye.

23 Ask the person if you should use soap to wash the face.

24 Wash the face, ears, and neck. Rinse and dry the skin well using the towel on the chest.

25 Help the person move to the side of the bed near you.

26 Remove the gown. Do not expose the person. (Waiting to remove the gown at this time helps the person feel less exposed and more comfortable with the procedure.)

27 Place a bath towel lengthwise under the far arm.

28 Support the arm with your palm under the person's elbow. His or her forearm rests on your forearm.

29 Wash the arm, shoulder, and underarm with long, firm strokes (Fig. 14-12, p. 333). Rinse and pat dry.

30 Place the basin on the towel. Put the person's hand into the water (Fig. 14-13, p. 334). Wash it well. Clean under fingernails with an orange stick or nail file.

31 Encourage the person to exercise the hand and fingers.

32 Remove the basin, and dry the hand well. Cover the arm with the bath blanket.

33 Repeat steps 27 to 32 for the near arm.

34 Place a bath towel over the chest crosswise. Hold the towel in place, and pull the bath blanket from under the towel to the waist.

35 Lift the towel slightly, and wash the chest (Fig. 14-14). Do not expose the person. Rinse and pat dry, especially under breasts.

36 Move the towel lengthwise over the chest and abdomen. Do not expose the person. Pull the bath blanket down to the pubic area.

37 Lift the towel slightly, and wash the abdomen (Fig. 14-15, p. 335). Rinse and pat dry.

38 Pull the bath blanket up to the shoulders, covering both arms. Remove the towel.

39 Change the water if it is soapy or cool. Measure bath water temperature as in step 17. Raise the bed rail before you leave the bedside. Lower it when you return.

40 Uncover the far leg. Do not expose the genital area. Place a towel lengthwise under the foot and leg.

Continued

Giving a Complete Bed Bath—cont'd

NNAAP™

Procedure—cont'd

41 Bend the knee and support the leg with your arm. Wash it with long, firm strokes. Rinse and pat dry.

42 Place the basin on the towel near the foot.

43 Lift the leg slightly. Slide the basin under the foot.

44 Place the foot in the basin (Fig. 14-16, p. 335). Use an orange stick or nail file to clean under toenails if necessary.

45 Remove the basin, and dry the leg. Cover the leg with the bath blanket. Remove the towel.

46 Repeat steps 40 to 45 for the near leg.

47 Change the water. Measure bath water temperature as in step 17. Raise the bed rail before leaving the bedside. Lower it when you return.

48 Turn the person onto the side away from you. Keep him or her covered with the bath blanket.

49 Uncover the back and buttocks. Do not expose the person. Place a towel lengthwise on the bed along the back.

50 Wash the back, working from the back of the neck to the lower end of the buttocks. Use long, firm, continuous strokes (Fig. 14-17, p. 335). Rinse and dry well.

51 Give a back massage. (The person may prefer to have the back massage after the bath.)

52 Turn the person onto his or her back.

53 Change the water for perineal care. Measure bath water temperature as in step 17. Raise the bed rail before you leave the bedside. Lower it when you return.

54 Let the person wash the genital area. Adjust the overbed table so he or she can reach the wash basin, soap, and towels with ease. Place the signal light within reach. Ask the person to signal when finished. Make sure the person understands what to do. Answer the signal light promptly. Provide perineal care if the person cannot do so (see *Perineal Care*).

55 Give a back massage if you have not already done so.

56 Apply deodorant or antiperspirant. Apply lotion and powder as directed by the nurse or as requested by the person. Use only a thin layer of powder.

57 Put a clean gown or pajamas on the person.

58 Comb and brush the hair (see Chapter 15).

59 Make the bed. Attach the signal light.

Post-Procedure

60 Provide for comfort.

61 Lower the bed to its lowest position.

62 Raise or lower bed rails. Follow the care plan.

63 Empty and clean the wash basin. Return it and other supplies to their proper place.

64 Wipe off the overbed table with the paper towels, and discard them.

65 Unscreen the person.

66 Follow agency policy for dirty linen.

67 Wash your hands.

68 Report your observations to the nurse.

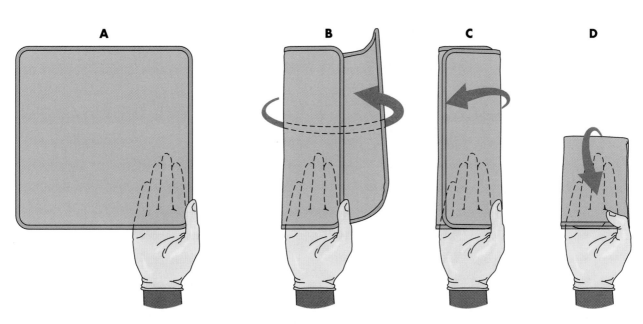

Fig. 14-10 Making a mitted washcloth. **A,** Grasp the near side of the washcloth with your thumb. **B,** Bring the washcloth around and behind your hand. **C,** Fold the side of the washcloth over your palm as you grasp it with your thumb. **D,** Fold the top of the washcloth down and tuck it under next to your palm.

Fig. 14-11 Wash around the person's eyes with a mitted washcloth. Wipe from the inner to the outer aspect of the eye.

Fig. 14-12 Wash the person's arm with firm, long strokes using a mitted washcloth.

Fig. 14-13 The person's hands are washed by placing the wash basin on the bed.

Fig. 14-14 The person's breasts are not exposed during the bath. A bath towel is placed horizontally over the chest area. The towel is lifted slightly to reach under to wash the breasts and chest.

Fig. 14-15 The bath towel is turned so that it is vertical to cover the breasts and abdomen. The towel is lifted slightly to bathe the abdomen. The bath blanket covers the pubic area.

Fig. 14-16 The foot is washed by placing it in the wash basin on the bed.

Fig. 14-17 The back is washed with long, firm, continuous strokes. Note that the person is in a side-lying position. A towel is placed lengthwise on the bed to protect the linens from water.

▷ THE PARTIAL BATH

The *partial bath* involves bathing the face, hands, axillae (underarms), back, buttocks, and perineal area. These areas develop odors or cause discomfort if not clean. You give partial bed baths to persons who cannot bathe themselves. Persons who are able bathe themselves in bed or at the bathroom sink. You assist as needed, especially with washing the back.

The rules for bathing (see Box 14-2) apply for partial bed baths. The considerations involved in giving a complete bed bath also apply.

Fig. 14-18 The person is bathing himself in bed. Necessary equipment is within his reach.

Giving a Partial Bath

QUALITY OF LIFE

Remember to:
- Knock before entering the person's room
- Address the person by name
- Introduce yourself by name and title

Pre-Procedure

1 Follow steps 1 through 9 in *Giving a Complete Bed Bath*, p. 330.

Procedure

2 Make sure the bed is in the lowest position.

3 Assist with oral hygiene. Adjust the height of the overbed table to an appropriate level.

4 Remove top linen. Cover the person with a bath blanket.

5 Place the paper towels on the overbed table.

6 Fill the wash basin with water. Water temperature should be 110° to 115° F (43.3° to 46° C) for adults. (Measure water temperature with the bath thermometer. Some states allow you to test bath water by dipping your elbow or inner wrist into the basin.)

7 Place the basin on the overbed table on top of the paper towels.

8 Raise the head of the bed so the person can bathe comfortably. Assist him or her to sit at the bedside if allowed this position.

9 Position the overbed table so the person can easily reach the basin and supplies.

10 Help the person remove the gown or pajamas.

11 Ask the person to wash easy-to-reach body parts (Fig. 14-18). Explain that you will wash the back and those areas that cannot be reached.

12 Place the signal light within reach. Ask him or her to signal if help is needed or when bathing is complete.

13 Leave the room after washing your hands.

14 Return when the signal light is on. Knock before entering.

15 Change the bath water. Measure bath water temperature as in step 6.

16 Raise the bed to a level for good body mechanics. Make sure bed rails are up.

17 Lower the bed rail near you.

18 Ask what was washed. Wash and dry areas the person could not reach. The face, hands, axillae, back, buttocks, and perineal area are washed for the partial bath. Wear gloves if contact with blood, body fluids, secretions, or excretions is likely.

19 Give a back massage.

20 Apply lotion, powder, and deodorant or antiperspirant.

21 Help the person put on a clean gown or pajamas.

22 Assist with hair care and other grooming needs.

23 Lower the bed if the person will get up.

24 Assist him or her to a chair. Otherwise, turn the person onto the side away from you.

25 Make the bed. Make sure you raise the bed for good body mechanics. The far bed rail is up for an occupied bed.

26 Lower the bed to its lowest position.

27 Assist the person to return to bed.

Post-Procedure

28 Provide for comfort.

29 Place the signal light within reach.

30 Raise or lower bed rails. Follow the care plan.

31 Empty and clean the basin. Return the basin and supplies to their proper place.

32 Wipe off the overbed table with the paper towels, and discard them.

33 Unscreen the person.

34 Follow agency policy for dirty linen.

35 Wash your hands.

36 Report your observations to the nurse

► Tub Baths and Showers

Many people prefer tub baths or showers. However, burns from hot water and falls are risks. The nurse's approval is needed for tub baths and showers. Safety measure for tub baths and showers are listed in Box 14-3. The measures in Box 14-2 also apply.

Tub Baths. Tub baths are relaxing for many people. A tub bath can cause a person to feel faint, weak, or tired. These are greater risks for persons who were on bedrest. A bath lasts no longer than 20 minutes.

You reserve the tub room for the person. The tub is cleaned before and after use. This prevents the spread of microbes and infection. Safety is important. Follow the measures in Box 14-3 to prevent slipping, falls, and chills.

Some agencies have portable tubs. The sides are lowered to transfer the person from bed to the tub (Fig. 14-19). The sides are raised after the transfer. The person is transported to the tub room in the portable tub. There the tub is filled and the person bathed in the usual manner. Remember to cover the person with a blanket for privacy and warmth during the transfers and transports.

Whirlpool tubs have hydraulic lifts (Fig. 14-20). The person is transferred to a special wheelchair in his or her room. The person is transported to the tub room where the chair is attached to the lift. The chair and person are lifted into the tub. The whirlpool action cleans the person's lower body. You wash the upper body. Carefully wash under breasts, between skin folds, and in the perineal area. Dry the person after the bath.

Some tubs have special stretchers for persons who cannot sit up. The person is transferred from bed to the stretcher and transported to the tub room. The person is lowered into the tub on the stretcher (Fig. 14-21). Remember to cover the person with a bath blanket during the transports and transfers.

Box 14-3 Safety Measures for Tub Baths and Showers

- Make sure the tub or shower is clean before and after use.
- Make sure the floor of the bathroom or shower room is dry.
- Check to see that hand rails, grab bars, hydraulic lifts, and other safety aids are in working order.
- Place a bath mat in the tub or on the shower floor unless there are nonskid strips or a nonskid surface.
- Cover the person for warmth and privacy. This includes during transport to and from the shower room or tub room.
- Place needed items within the person's reach. This includes the signal light.
- Show the person how to use the signal light in the shower or tub room.
- Drain the tub before the person gets out of the tub. Keep the person covered to protect from exposure and chilling.

- Have the person use safety bars when getting into and out of the tub.
- Adjust water temperature and pressure before the person gets into the shower. Otherwise you can chill or burn the person. If the person uses a shower chair, position the chair before adjusting the water. Use the hand-held nozzle to direct the water away from the person. Adjust water temperature and pressure.
- Avoid using bath oils. They make tub and shower surfaces slippery.
- Do not leave weak or unsteady persons unattended.
- Stay within hearing distance of the shower or tub if the person can be left alone. Wait outside the shower curtain or door. You will be nearby if the person calls for you or has an accident.
- Have the person use safety bars for support when getting into or out of the tub or shower. Do not let the person use towel bars for support.

Fig. 14-19 Portable tub. *(Courtesy Arjo, Inc, Morton Grove, Ill.)*

Fig. 14-20 Whirlpool tub with a hydraulic lift.

Fig. 14-21 The stretcher and person are lowered into the tub.

Showers. Some rooms have private baths or showers. If not, reserve the tub or shower room. Also clean the tub or shower before use. This prevents the spread of microbes and infection. The person is protected from falls and chilling (see Box 14-3).

Some patients and residents use shower chairs (Fig. 14-22). Shower chairs are made of plastic or metal and have wheels on the legs. The shower chair is wheeled into the shower stall or shower cabinet (Fig. 14-23). Water drains through a round open area in the seat. The wheels are locked during the shower so the chair does not move.

Some shower rooms may have more than one stall or cabinet. You must protect the person's privacy. Remember, the person has the right not to have his or body seen by others. You must properly screen and cover the person.

Shower stalls and cabinets are easier to get into than a shower that is part of the bathtub unit. The person does not have to step over the tub to get into the shower. *(See Focus on Home Care box and Focus on Children box.)*

Focus On... HOME CARE

Shower stalls are common in most homes. So are bathtub-shower units. If the person has to step into the bathtub to take a shower, make sure there are safety bars for the person's use. Assist the person in getting into and out of the shower as needed.

The person can buy or rent a shower chair for home use. Or a sturdy chair can be used. A sturdy lawn chair is an example. The nurse will assist the person or family in finding a safe chair for shower use.

Focus On... CHILDREN

Many older children enjoy showers. The RN tells you how much help and supervision to give the child. Remember, independence is important to older children.

Fig. 14-22 Shower chair in a shower stall.

Fig. 14-23 Shower cabinet. NOTE: This shower cabinet has a built-in shower chair.

Assisting With a Tub Bath or Shower

QUALITY OF LIFE

Remember to:
- Knock before entering the person's room
- Address the person by name
- Introduce yourself by name and title

Pre-Procedure

1. Reserve the bathtub or shower if necessary.
2. Identify the person. Check the ID bracelet, and call the person by name.
3. Explain the procedure to the person.
4. Wash your hands.
5. Collect the following:
   - Washcloth and two bath towels
   - Soap
   - Bath thermometer (for a tub bath)
   - Clean gown or pajamas
   - Deodorant and other toilet articles as requested
   - Robe and nonskid slippers or shoes
   - Rubber bath mat if needed
   - Disposable bath mat

Procedure

6. Place items in the bathroom or shower room in the space provided or on a chair.
7. Clean the tub or shower if needed.
8. Place a rubber bath mat in the tub or on the shower floor. Do not block the drain.
9. Place a disposable bath mat on the floor in front of the tub or shower.
10. Put the *occupied* sign on the door.
11. Return to the person's room. Provide for privacy.
12. Help the person sit on the side of the bed.
13. Help the person put on a robe and slippers or shoes.
14. Assist the person to the bathroom or shower room. Use a wheelchair if necessary.
15. *For a tub bath:*
    a. Have the person sit on the chair by the tub.
    b. Fill the tub halfway with warm water (105° F; 40.5° C). See Figure 14-24 on p. 342. Measure water temperature with the bath thermometer, or check the digital display (Fig. 14-25, p. 342).
    For a shower:
    a. Turn on the shower.
    b. Adjust water temperature and pressure.
16. Help the person remove slippers, robe, and gown.
17. Assist the person into the tub or shower. If using a shower chair, place it in position and lock the wheels.
18. Assist with washing if necessary.
19. Ask the person to use the signal light when done or when help is needed.
20. Remind the person not to stay in the tub longer than 20 minutes.
21. Place a towel across the chair.
22. Leave the room only if the person can be left unattended. Otherwise stay in the room or remain nearby. Wash your hands if you leave the room.
23. Check the person every 5 minutes.
24. Return when he or she signals for you. Knock before entering.
25. Turn off the shower.
26. Help the person out of the tub or shower and onto the chair.
27. Help the person dry off. Pat gently. Remember to dry under the breasts, between skin folds, in the perineal area, and between the toes.
28. Assist with lotion, powder, and deodorant or antiperspirant as needed.
29. Help the person put on a clean gown or pajamas, a bathrobe, and slippers or shoes.
30. Help the person return to the room and to bed.

Continued

Assisting With a Tub Bath or Shower—cont'd

Procedure—cont'd

31 Provide for privacy.
32 Provide a back massage.
33 Assist with hair care and other grooming measures.
34 Make the bed.

Post-Procedure

35 Provide for comfort.
36 Raise or lower bed rails. Follow the care plan.
37 Place the signal light within reach.
38 Unscreen the person.
39 Clean the tub or shower. Remove soiled linen, and discard disposable items. Put the *unoccupied* sign on the door. Return supplies to their proper place.
40 Follow agency policy for dirty linen.
41 Wash your hands.
42 Report your observations to the nurse.

Fig. 14-24 A bath mat is in the tub, the tub is filled halfway with water, and a floor mat is in front of the tub.

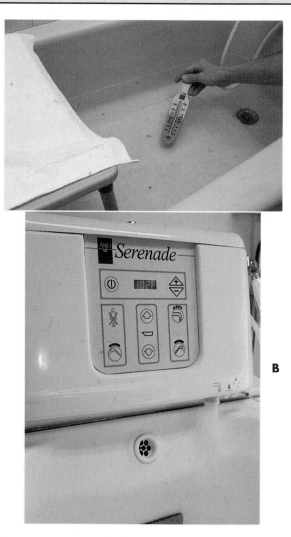

Fig. 14-25 Measuring bath water temperature. **A,** Bath thermometer is used to measure water temperature. **B,** The digital display shows water temperature.

▷ THE BACK MASSAGE

The back massage (back rub) relaxes muscles and stimulates circulation. A massage is normally given after the bath and with HS care. It should last 3 to 5 minutes. Observe the skin before starting the procedure. Look for breaks in the skin, bruises, reddened areas, and other signs of skin breakdown.

Lotion reduces friction when giving the massage. It is warmed before being applied. Warm lotion by placing the bottle in the bath water or holding it under warm water. Or rub some lotion between your hands.

The prone position is best for a massage. The side-lying position is often used. Use firm strokes, and always keep your hands in contact with the person's skin. After the massage, apply some lotion to the elbows, knees, and heels to keep the skin soft. These bony areas are at risk for skin breakdown.

Some persons should not have back massages as described in this procedure. They are dangerous for those with certain heart diseases, back injuries, back surgeries, skin diseases, and some lung disorders. Check with the nurse and nursing care plan before giving back massages to persons with these conditions.

▷ Giving a Back Massage

QUALITY OF LIFE

Remember to:
- Knock before entering the person's room
- Address the person by name
- Introduce yourself by name and title

Pre-Procedure

1. Identify the person. Check the ID bracelet, and call the person by name.
2. Explain the procedure to the person.
3. Wash your hands.
4. Collect the following:
   - Bath blanket
   - Bath towel
   - Lotion
5. Provide for privacy.
6. Raise the bed to the best level for good body mechanics. Make sure bed rails are up.

Procedure

7. Lower the bed rail near you.
8. Position the person in the prone or side-lying position with the back toward you.
9. Expose the back, shoulders, upper arms, and buttocks. Cover the rest of the body with the bath blanket.
10. Lay the towel on the bed along the back.
11. Warm some lotion between your hands.
12. Explain that the lotion may feel cool and wet.
13. Apply lotion to the lower back area.
14. Stroke up from the buttocks to the shoulders. Then stroke down over the upper arms. Stroke up the upper arms, across the shoulders, and down the back to the buttocks (Fig. 14-26, p. 344). Use firm strokes. Keep your hands in contact with the person's skin.
15. Repeat step 14 for at least 3 minutes.
16. Knead by grasping skin between your thumb and fingers (Fig. 14-27, p. 344). Knead half of the back, starting at the buttocks and moving up to the shoulder. Then knead down from the shoulder to the buttocks. Repeat on the other half of the back.
17. Apply lotion to bony areas. Use circular motions with the tips of your index and middle fingers. (Do not massage bony areas that are reddened. See Chapter 25.)
18. Use fast movements to stimulate and slow movements to relax the person.
19. Stroke with long, firm movements to end the massage. Tell the person you are finishing.
20. Cover the person. Remove the towel and bath blanket.

Continued

Giving a Back Massage—cont'd

Post-Procedure

21 Provide for comfort.

22 Lower the bed to its lowest position.

23 Raise or lower bed rails. Follow the care plan.

24 Place the signal light within reach.

25 Return lotion to its proper place.

26 Unscreen the person.

27 Follow agency policy for dirty linen.

28 Wash your hands.

29 Report your observations to the nurse.

Fig. 14-26 The person lies in the prone position for a back massage. Stroke upward from the buttocks to the shoulders, down over the upper arms, back up the upper arms, across the shoulders, and down the back to the buttocks.

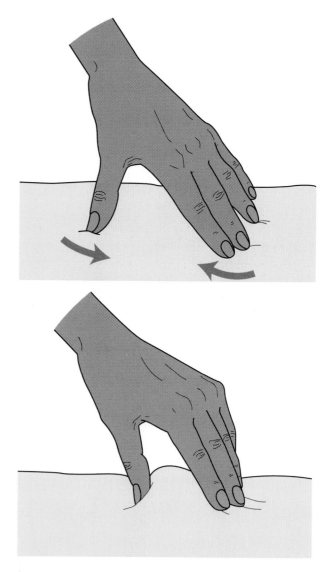

Fig. 14-27 Kneading is done by picking up tissue between the thumb and fingers.

▶ PERINEAL CARE

Perineal care (pericare) involves cleaning the genital and anal areas. These areas are warm, moist, and dark. They provide a place for microbes to grow. The genital and anal areas are cleaned to prevent infection and odors and to promote comfort.

Perineal care is done at least daily during the bath. The procedure is also done whenever the area is soiled with urine or feces. Persons with certain disorders need perineal care more often. It is given before and after some surgeries and after childbirth.

Patients and residents do their own perineal care if able. Otherwise it is given by nursing staff. Many people and nursing staff find the procedure embarrassing, especially when given to the other sex. People may not know the terms *perineum* and *perineal*. Most understand *privates, private parts, crotch, genitals,* or the *area between your legs*. Use terms the person understands. The term must also be in good taste professionally.

Standard Precautions, medical asepsis, and the Bloodborne Pathogen Standard are followed. Work from the cleanest area to the dirtiest. The urethral area is the cleanest, the anal area the dirtiest. Therefore clean from the urethra to the anal area. The perineal area is very delicate and easily injured. Use warm water, not hot. Washcloths are used if pericare is part of the bath. The nurse may have you use cotton balls or swabs at other times. The area is rinsed thoroughly. Pat dry after rinsing to reduce moisture and promote comfort. *(See Focus on Children box.)*

Text continued on p. 350

Focus On... CHILDREN

Children of all ages need perineal care. In children who wear diapers, the perineal area is often exposed to urine and feces. Inadequate wiping after urinating and bowel movements is a common problem in younger children. Older children may hesitate to clean the genital and anal areas.

▶ Giving Female Perineal Care   NNAAP™

QUALITY OF LIFE

Remember to:
- Knock before entering the person's room
- Address the person by name
- Introduce yourself by name and title

Pre-Procedure

1. Explain the procedure to the person.
2. Wash your hands.
3. Collect the following:
   - Soap dish with soap
   - At least four washcloths
   - Bath towel
   - Bath blanket
   - Bath thermometer
   - Waterproof pad
   - Gloves
   - Paper towels
4. Arrange items on the overbed table.
5. Identify the person. Check the ID bracelet, and call her by name.
6. Provide for privacy.
7. Raise the bed to the best level for good body mechanics. Make sure bed rails are up.

Procedure

8. Lower the bed rail near you.
9. Cover the person with a bath blanket. Move top linens to the foot of the bed.
10. Position the person on her back.
11. Position the waterproof pad under her buttocks.
12. Drape the person as in Figure 14-28, p. 347.
13. Raise the bed rail.
14. Fill the wash basin. Water temperature is about 105° to 109° F (40.5° to 43° C).

Continued

Giving Female Perineal Care—cont'd

NNAAP™

Procedure—cont'd

15   Place the basin on the overbed table on top of the paper towels.

16   Lower the bed rail.

17   Help the person flex her knees and spread her legs. If she cannot flex her knees, help her spread her legs as much as possible with her knees straight.

18   Put on the gloves.

19   Fold the corner of the bath blanket between the person's legs onto her abdomen.

20   Wet the washcloths. Squeeze out excess water from washcloths before using them.

21   Apply soap to a washcloth.

22   Separate the labia. Clean downward from front to back with one stroke (Fig. 14-29).

23   Repeat steps 21 and 22 until the area is clean. Use a different part of the washcloth for each stroke. Use more than one washcloth if needed.

24   Rinse the perineum with a clean washcloth. Separate the labia. Stroke downward from front to back. Repeat the step as necessary.

Use a different part of the washcloth for each stroke. Use more than one washcloth if needed.

25   Pat the area dry with the towel.

26   Fold the blanket back between her legs.

27   Help the person lower her legs and turn onto her side away from you.

28   Apply soap to a washcloth.

29   Clean the rectal area. Clean from the vagina to the anus with one stroke (Fig. 14-30).

30   Repeat steps 28 and 29 until the area is clean. Use a different part of the washcloth for each stroke. Use more than one washcloth if needed.

31   Rinse the rectal area with a washcloth. Stroke from the vagina to the anus. Repeat the step as necessary using a different part of the washcloth for each stroke. Use more than one washcloth if needed.

32   Pat the area dry with the towel.

33   Remove and discard the gloves.

Post-Procedure

34   Provide for comfort.

35   Return linens to their proper position, and remove the bath blanket.

36   Lower the bed to its lowest position.

37   Raise or lower bed rails. Follow the care plan.

38   Place the signal light within reach.

39   Empty and clean the wash basin.

40   Return the basin and supplies to their proper place.

41   Wipe off the overbed table with the paper towels, and discard them.

42   Unscreen the person.

43   Follow agency policy for dirty linen.

44   Wash your hands.

45   Report your observations to the nurse:
   • Any odors
   • Redness, swelling, discharge, or irritation
   • Complaints of pain, burning, or other discomfort

Fig. 14-28 Draping for perineal care. **A,** Drape the person for perineal care by positioning the bath blanket like a diamond: one corner is at the neck, there is a corner at each side, and one corner is between the person's legs. **B,** Wrap the blanket around the leg by bringing the corner around under the leg and over the top. Tuck the corner under the hip.

Fig. 14-29 Separate the labia with one hand to give female perineal care. Use a mitted washcloth to cleanse between the labia with downward strokes.

Fig. 14-30 The rectal area is cleaned by wiping from the vagina to the anus. The side-lying position allows the anal area to be cleaned more thoroughly.

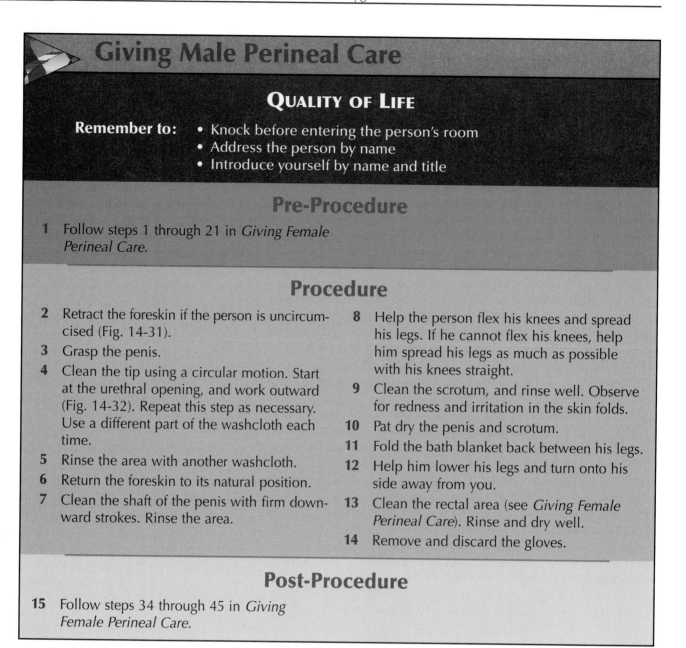

Giving Male Perineal Care

QUALITY OF LIFE

Remember to:
- Knock before entering the person's room
- Address the person by name
- Introduce yourself by name and title

Pre-Procedure

1   Follow steps 1 through 21 in *Giving Female Perineal Care.*

Procedure

2   Retract the foreskin if the person is uncircumcised (Fig. 14-31).

3   Grasp the penis.

4   Clean the tip using a circular motion. Start at the urethral opening, and work outward (Fig. 14-32). Repeat this step as necessary. Use a different part of the washcloth each time.

5   Rinse the area with another washcloth.

6   Return the foreskin to its natural position.

7   Clean the shaft of the penis with firm downward strokes. Rinse the area.

8   Help the person flex his knees and spread his legs. If he cannot flex his knees, help him spread his legs as much as possible with his knees straight.

9   Clean the scrotum, and rinse well. Observe for redness and irritation in the skin folds.

10 Pat dry the penis and scrotum.

11 Fold the bath blanket back between his legs.

12 Help him lower his legs and turn onto his side away from you.

13 Clean the rectal area (see *Giving Female Perineal Care*). Rinse and dry well.

14 Remove and discard the gloves.

Post-Procedure

15 Follow steps 34 through 45 in *Giving Female Perineal Care.*

Fig. 14-31 The foreskin of the uncircumcised male is pulled back for perineal care. It is returned to the normal position immediately after cleaning.

Disposable washcloth

Fig. 14-32 The penis is cleaned with circular motions starting at the urethra.

PRESSURE ULCERS

A *pressure ulcer (decubitus ulcer, bedsore, pressure sore)* is any injury caused by unrelieved pressure. It usually occurs over a bony prominence. (Prominence means to stick out.) Therefore a bony prominence is an area where the bone sticks out or projects out from the flat surface of the body. The shoulder blades, elbows, hip bones, sacrum, knees, ankle bones, heels, and toes are bony prominences.

Pressure, friction, and shearing are common causes of skin breakdown and pressure ulcers. Other factors include breaks in the skin, poor circulation to an area, moisture, dry skin, and irritation by urine and feces. That is why personal hygiene is so important. Pressure ulcers are discussed in Chapter 25.

REVIEW

Circle T if the answer is true and F if it is false.

1. T F Cleanliness and skin care are needed for comfort, safety, and health.

2. T F During the afternoon Mrs. Bell asks for a back massage. You can tell her that back massages are given during HS care.

3. T F Mrs. Bell's toothbrush has hard bristles. They are good for oral hygiene.

4. T F Unconscious persons are supine for mouth care.

5. T F You use your fingers to keep an unconscious person's mouth open for oral hygiene.

6. T F Mrs. Bell has a lower denture. It is washed in warm water over a hard surface.

7. T F Bath oils cleanse and soften the skin.

8. T F Powders absorb moisture and prevent friction.

9. T F Deodorants reduce the amount of perspiration.

10. T F The nurse says that Mrs. Bell can have a tub bath. Mrs. Bell says that she usually takes half-hour baths at home. You can let her take a 30-minute bath.

11. T F You can give permission for showers but not tub baths.

12. T F Weak persons can be left alone in the shower if they are sitting.

13. T F A back massage relaxes muscles and stimulates circulation.

14. T F Perineal care helps prevent infection.

Circle the BEST answer.

15. You brush Mrs. Bell's teeth and note the following. Which do you report to the nurse?
   A. Bleeding, swelling, or redness of the gums
   B. Irritations, sores, or white patches in the mouth or on the tongue
   C. Lips that are dry, cracked, swollen, or blistered
   D. All of the above

16. Which is *not* a purpose of bathing?
   A. Increasing circulation
   B. Promoting drying of the skin
   C. Exercising body parts
   D. Refreshing and relaxing the person

17. Soaps do the following *except*
   A. Remove dirt and dead skin
   B. Remove pigment
   C. Remove skin oil and perspiration
   D. Dry the skin

18. Which action is *wrong* when bathing Mrs. Bell?
   A. Cover her for warmth and privacy.
   B. Rinse her skin thoroughly to remove all soaps.
   C. Wash from the dirtiest to the cleanest area.
   D. Pat her skin dry.

19. Water for Mrs. Bell's complete bed bath should be at least
   A. 100° F
   B. 105° F
   C. 110° F
   D. 120° F

20. You are going to give Mrs. Bell a back massage. Which is *false?*
   A. The massage should last 3 to 5 minutes.
   B. Lotion is warmed before being applied.
   C. Your hands are always in contact with the skin.
   D. The side-lying position is best.

Answers to these questions are on p. 835.

PERSONAL CARE AND GROOMING

Define the key terms listed in this chapter

Explain the importance of hair care and shaving

Identify the factors that affect hair care

Explain how to care for matted and tangled hair

Describe how to shampoo hair

Describe the measures that are practiced when shaving a person

Explain why nail and foot care are important

Describe the rules for changing hospital gowns and clothing

Perform the procedures described in this chapter

KEY TERMS

alopecia Hair loss

dandruff Excessive amount of dry, white flakes from the scalp

hirsutism Excessive body hair in women and children

pediculosis (lice) Infestation with lice

pediculosis capitis Infestation of the scalp *(capitis)* with lice

pediculosis corporis Infestation of the body *(corporis)* with lice

pediculosis pubis Infestation of the pubic *(pubis)* hair with lice

Cleanliness and skin care meet basic physical and safety and security needs. Clean and intact skin protects against infection. Bathing and back massage promote circulation, exercise, comfort, and relaxation. For many people, being clean is necessary for love and belonging and self-esteem needs.

Hair care, shaving, and nail care also are important to many people. People vary in how much attention they give to such matters. Some want only clean hair. Others want hair styled in a certain way. Clean hands are enough for some people. Others want nails clean, manicured, and polished. Shaving and beard grooming are important to many men. Likewise, many women shave their legs and underarms.

HAIR CARE

How the hair looks and feels affects mental well-being. Illness and disability can interfere with hair care. The person is assisted with hair care whenever necessary. *(See Focus on Long-Term Care box on p. 354.)*

The RN uses the nursing process to meet the person's hair care needs. Culture, personal choice, skin and scalp condition, health history, and self-care ability are considered by the RN. These terms are common in nursing care plans:

- **Alopecia** means hair loss. Hair loss may be complete or partial. Male pattern baldness occurs with aging and is the result of heredity. Hair also thins in some women with aging. Cancer treatments (radiation therapy to the head and chemotherapy) often cause alopecia in both men and women. Skin disease is another cause. Other causes include stress, poor nutrition, pregnancy, some drugs, and hormone changes. Except for hair loss from aging, the hair grows back in many cases.

- **Hirsutism** is excessive body hair in women and children. It is the result of heredity and abnormal amounts of male hormones.
- **Dandruff** is the excessive amount of dry, white flakes from the scalp. Itching often occurs. Sometimes the eyebrows and ear canals are involved. Medicated shampoos correct the problem.
- **Pediculosis (lice)** is the infestation with lice. Lice are parasites. Lice bites cause severe itching in the affected body area. **Pediculosis capitis** is the infestation of the scalp *(capitis)* with lice. **Pediculosis pubis** is the infestation of the pubic *(pubis)* hair with lice. Both head and pubic lice attach their eggs to hair shafts. **Pediculosis corporis** is the infestation of the body *(corporis)* with lice. Lice eggs attach to clothing and furniture. Lice easily spread to other persons through clothing, furniture, bed linen, and sexual contact. Medicated shampoos, lotions, and creams are used to treat lice. Thorough bathing is necessary. So is washing clothing and linen in hot water. Report signs of lice to the nurse immediately.

▶ BRUSHING AND COMBING HAIR

Brushing and combing hair are part of early morning care, morning care, and afternoon care. They also are done as needed during the day. Many people want their hair styled before visitors arrive. Encourage patients and residents to do their own hair care. Assist as needed. Perform hair care for those who cannot do so. Let the person choose how to brush, comb, and style hair.

Long hair easily matts and tangles. Daily brushing and combing prevent the problem. So does braiding. Do not braid hair unless the person gives consent. *Never cut hair to remove matted or tangled hair.*

Brushing brings scalp oils along the hair shaft. Scalp oils help keep hair soft and shiny. Brushing and combing keep hair from tangling and matting. When brushing and combing hair, start at the scalp. Then brush or comb to the hair ends.

Talk to the nurse if the person has matted or tangled hair. The nurse may have you comb or brush through the matting and tangling. To do this, take a small section of hair near the ends. Then comb or brush through to the hair ends. Working up to the scalp, add small sections of hair. Comb or brush through each longer section to the hair ends. Finally, brush or comb from the scalp to the hair ends. *Never cut matted or tangled hair.*

Special measures are needed for curly, coarse, and dry hair. Use a wide-toothed comb for curly hair. Start at the neckline. Work upward, lifting and fluffing hair outward. Continue until you reach the forehead. Wetting the hair or applying a conditioner or petroleum jelly makes combing easier. The person may have certain practices or use special hair care products. The nurse asks the individual about personal preferences and routine hair care measures. These become part of the person's care plan. The person can guide you when giving hair care.

When giving hair care, place a towel across the shoulders to protect the person's gown or clothing. If the person is in bed, give hair care before changing the pillowcase. If done after a linen change, place a towel across the pillow to collect falling hair. *(See Focus on Children box.)*

Brushing and Combing a Person's Hair

QUALITY OF LIFE

Remember to:
- Knock before entering the person's room
- Address the person by name
- Introduce yourself by name and title

Pre-Procedure

1 Identify the person. Check the ID bracelet, and call the person by name.
2 Explain the procedure to the person. Ask the person how to style hair.
3 Collect the following:
   - Comb and brush
   - Bath towel
   - Hair care items as requested by the person
4 Arrange items on the bedside stand.
5 Wash your hands.
6 Provide for privacy.

Procedure

7 Lower the bed rail if used.
8 Help the person to a chair or to Fowler's position if possible. The person puts on a robe and shoes or nonskid slippers when up. (If the person is in bed, make sure both bed rails are up. Raise the bed to a level for good body mechanics. Lower the bed rail near you.)
9 Place a towel across the shoulders or across the pillow.
10 Ask the person to remove eyeglasses. Put them in the glass case. Put the case inside the bedside stand.
11 Part hair into 2 sections (Fig. 15-1, *A*, p. 356). Divide one side into 2 sections (Fig. 15-1, *B*, p. 356).
12 Brush the hair. Start at the scalp and brush toward the hair ends (Fig. 15-2, p. 356).
13 Style the hair as the person prefers.
14 Remove the towel.
15 Let the person put on the eyeglasses.

Post-Procedure

16 Provide for comfort.
17 Raise or lower bed rails. Follow the care plan.
18 Lower the bed to its lowest position.
19 Place the signal light within reach.
20 Unscreen the person.
21 Clean and return items to their proper place.
22 Follow agency policy for dirty linen.
23 Wash your hands.

Fig. 15-1 Parting hair. **A,** Part hair down the middle, and divide it into two main sections. **B,** Then part the main section into two smaller sections.

Fig. 15-2 Brush hair by starting at the scalp and brushing down to the hair ends.

► SHAMPOOING

Most people shampoo at least once a week. Some shampoo 2 or 3 times a week. Others shampoo every day. Many factors affect frequency. These include the condition of the hair and scalp, hairstyle, and personal choice. Shampoo and hair conditioner also involve personal choice. *(See Focus on Children box.)*

Patients and residents often need help shampooing. Personal choice is followed whenever possible. However, safety is important and the nurse's approval is needed. Tell the nurse if a shampoo is requested. Do not wash a person's hair unless a nurse asks you to do so.

The shampooing method depends on the person's condition, safety factors, and personal choice if possible. The nurse decides which method to use. Dry and style hair as quickly as possible after shampooing. Women may want hair curled or rolled up before drying. Consult with the nurse before curling or rolling up a person's hair. *(See Focus on Long-Term Care box.)*

Focus On... CHILDREN

Oil gland secretion increases during puberty. Therefore adolescents tend to have oily hair. Frequent shampooing is often necessary.

Focus On... LONG-TERM CARE

Shampooing is usually done weekly on the resident's bath or shower day. If a woman has her hair done in the beauty shop, do not shampoo her hair. Protect her hair with a shower cap during the tub bath or shower.

Fig. 15-3 Shampooing while the person is on a stretcher. The stretcher is in front of the sink.

Fig. 15-4 A trough is used when shampooing a person in bed. The trough is directed to the side of the bed so water drains into a collecting basin.

Shampooing During the Shower or Tub Bath.
Persons who shower can usually shampoo at the same time. A hand-held nozzle is used for those using shower chairs or taking tub baths. A spray of water is directed to the hair. Place an extra towel, shampoo, and hair conditioner within the person's reach. Assist as necessary.

Shampooing at the Sink.
The chair or wheel-chair is placed so the person faces away from the sink. The person's head is tilted back over the edge of the sink. A folded towel is placed over the sink edge to protect the neck. A water pitcher or hand-held nozzle is used to wet and rinse the hair.

Shampooing a Person on a Stretcher.
The stretcher is positioned in front of a sink. A pillow is placed under the head and neck, and the head is tilted over the edge of the sink (Fig. 15-3). A water pitcher or hand-held nozzle is used to wet and rinse the hair. Safety measures include locking the stretcher wheels, using the safety straps, and raising the far rail.

Shampooing a Person in Bed.
This method is for those who cannot be out of bed. The person's head and shoulders are moved to the edge of the bed if the position is allowed. A rubber or plastic trough is placed under the head to protect the linens and mattress from water. The trough also drains water into a basin placed on a chair by the bed (Fig. 15-4). A water pitcher is used to wet and rinse the hair. (See Focus on Older Persons box, and Focus on Home Care box.)

Focus On... OLDER PERSONS

Oil gland secretion decreases with aging. Older persons may shampoo less often than younger adults.

When shampooing during the tub bath or shower, the person needs to tip his or her head back to keep shampoo and water out of the eyes. You need to support the back of the person's head with one hand as you shampoo with the other. Some older people cannot tip their heads back. They need to lean forward and hold a washcloth over the eyes. Support the person's forehead with one hand as you shampoo with the other. Make sure the person can breathe easily.

Shampooing at the sink or on a stretcher is difficult for older people who have limited range of motion in their necks. They cannot tolerate these shampooing methods.

Focus On... HOME CARE

You can make a trough from a plastic shower curtain or tablecloth. A plastic drop cloth for painting is also useful. Avoid plastic trash bags. They slip and slide easily and are not sturdy. To make a trough, place the plastic under the person's head. Make a raised edge around the plastic to prevent water from spilling over the sides. Direct the ends of the plastic into the basin. This directs water into the basin.

Shampooing the Person's Hair

QUALITY OF LIFE

Remember to:
- Knock before entering the person's room
- Address the person by name
- Introduce yourself by name and title

Pre-Procedure

1 Explain the procedure to the person.
2 Wash your hands.
3 Collect the following:
- Two bath towels
- Face towel or washcloth folded lengthwise
- Shampoo
- Hair conditioner if requested
- Bath thermometer
- Pitcher or hand-held nozzle
- Gloves (optional)

- Equipment for the shampoo in bed (if needed)
- Trough
- Basin or pail
- Bath blanket
- Waterproof pad
- Comb and brush
- Hair dryer

4 Arrange items nearby.
5 Identify the person. Check the ID bracelet against the assignment sheet.
6 Provide for privacy.

Procedure

7 Position the person for the method you are going to use. (If the person is in bed, make sure both bed rails are up. Raise the bed to a level for good body mechanics. Lower the bed rail near you.)
8 Place a bath towel across the shoulders or across the pillow under the person's head.
9 Brush and comb the hair to remove snarls and tangles.
10 Raise the bed rail if down.
11 Obtain warm water. Water temperature should be about 105° F (40.5° C).
12 Lower the bed rail near you.
13 Ask the person to hold the face towel or washcloth over the eyes. Make sure it does not cover the person's nose and mouth.
14 Apply water until the hair is completely wet. Use the pitcher or nozzle.

15 Apply a small amount of shampoo.
16 Work up a lather with both hands. Start at the hairline, and work toward the back.
17 Massage the scalp with your fingertips. Do not scratch the scalp.
18 Rinse the hair.
19 Repeat steps 15 through 18.
20 Apply conditioner and rinse as directed on the container.
21 Wrap the person's head with a bath towel.
22 Dry his or her face with the towel or washcloth used to protect the eyes.
23 Help the person raise the head if appropriate.
24 Rub the hair and scalp with the towel. Use the second towel if the first is wet.
25 Comb the hair to remove snarls and tangles. A woman may want hair curled or rolled up.
26 Dry the hair as quickly as possible.

Post-Procedure

27 Provide for comfort.
28 Place the signal light within reach.
29 Raise or lower bed rails. Follow the care plan.
30 Lower the bed to its lowest position.

31 Clean and return equipment to its proper place. Discard disposable items.
32 Follow agency policy for dirty linen.
33 Unscreen the person.
34 Wash your hands.

► SHAVING

Many men want a clean-shaven face for comfort and mental well-being. Likewise, many women shave their legs and underarms. *(See Focus on Older Persons box.)*

Some people use electric shavers. These shavers are cleaned between each use. You must follow the safety precautions for using electrical equipment (see Chapter 9).

Other people prefer blade shavers. Razor blades can cause nicks or cuts. Follow Standard Precautions and the Bloodborne Pathogen Standard to prevent contact with the person's blood. Razor blades and disposable shavers are discarded into the sharps container.

Blade shavers are not used for persons receiving anticoagulant drugs. An *anticoagulant* prevents or slows down (anti) blood clotting (coagulate). Bleeding occurs easily. A nick or cut can cause serious bleeding problems. Electric shavers are used for persons receiving anticoagulant drugs.

The beard and skin are softened before shaving with a blade. Apply a warm washcloth or face towel to the face for a few minutes. Then lather the face with soap and water or a shaving cream. Take care not to cut or irritate the skin while shaving. Follow the rules listed in Box 15-1 when shaving the person's face.

CARING FOR MUSTACHES AND BEARDS

Beards and mustaches need daily care. Food can collect in hair. So can mouth and nose drainage. Daily washing and combing usually is enough. Ask the person how to groom his beard or mustache. *Never trim or shave a beard or mustache without the person's consent.*

SHAVING FEMALE LEGS AND UNDERARMS

Many women shave their legs and underarms. This practice varies among cultures. Some women shave only the lower legs. Others shave to mid-thigh, and others shave the entire leg.

Women's legs and underarms are shaved after bathing, when the skin is soft. Soap and water or a shaving cream is used for lather. Needed shaving items are collected with the bath items. Use the kidney basin to rinse the razor rather than using the bath water.

Shaving underarms and legs is similar to shaving the male face. Practice the measures in Box 15-1.

Focus On... OLDER PERSONS

Many older women have coarse facial hair. They may want such hair shaved off.

Box 15-1   Rules for Shaving

- Follow Standard Precautions and the Bloodborne Pathogen Standard.
- Protect the bed linens by placing a towel under the part being shaved. Or place a towel across the shoulders to protect the person's clothes.
- Soften the skin before shaving.
- Encourage the person to do as much for himself or herself as safely possible.
- Hold the skin taut as necessary.
- Shave in the direction of hair growth when shaving the male face and female underarms.
- Shave upward, starting at the ankle, when shaving legs.
- Rinse the body part thoroughly.
- Apply direct pressure to any nicks or cuts.
- Report nicks and cuts to the nurse immediately.

Shaving a Person

Pre-Procedure

1. Explain the procedure to the person.
2. Wash your hands.
3. Collect the following:
   - Wash basin
   - Bath towel
   - Face towel
   - Washcloth
   - Bath thermometer
   - Blade shaver
   - Mirror
   - Shaving cream, soap, or lotion
   - Shaving brush
   - After-shave lotion (for men only)
   - Tissues
   - Paper towel
   - Gloves
4. Arrange items on the overbed table.
5. Identify the person. Check the ID bracelet against the assignment sheet.
6. Provide for privacy.
7. Raise the bed to the best level for good body mechanics. Raise the bed rails.

Procedure

8. Fill the wash basin with warm water.
9. Place the basin on the overbed table on top of the paper towels.
10. Lower the bed rail.
11. Position the person in semi-Fowler's position if allowed or in the supine position.
12. Adjust lighting to clearly see the person's face.
13. Place the bath towel over the chest.
14. Position the overbed table within easy reach and at a comfortable working height.
15. Tighten the razor blade to the shaver.
16. Wash the person's face. Do not dry.
17. Place a washcloth or face towel in the water and wet it thoroughly. Wring it out.
18. Apply the washcloth or towel to the face for a few minutes.
19. Put on the gloves.
20. Apply shaving cream to the face with your hands. Use a shaving brush if using soap for lather.
21. Hold the skin taut with one hand.
22. Hold the shaver so the blade is at a 45-degree angle to the skin.
23. Shave in the direction of hair growth. Use shorter strokes around the chin and lips (Fig. 15-5).
24. Rinse the razor often, and wipe with tissues.
25. Apply direct pressure to any bleeding areas.
26. Wash off any remaining shaving cream or soap. Dry with a towel.
27. Apply after-shave lotion if requested.
28. Remove the towel.
29. Remove the gloves.
30. Move the overbed table to the side of the bed.

Post-Procedure

31. Provide for comfort.
32. Place the signal light within reach.
33. Lower the bed to its lowest position.
34. Raise or lower bed rails. Follow the care plan.
35. Clean and return equipment and supplies to the proper place. Discard disposable items.
36. Wipe off the overbed table with the paper towels. Discard the paper towels.
37. Position the table as appropriate for the person.
38. Unscreen the person.
39. Follow agency policy for dirty linen.
40. Wash your hands.
41. Report any nicks or bleeding to the nurse.

Fig. 15-5 Shave in the direction of hair growth. Use longer strokes on the larger areas of the face. Use short strokes around the chin and lips.

▶ CARE OF NAILS AND FEET

Nails and feet need special attention to prevent infection, injury, and odors. Hangnails, ingrown nails (nails that grow in at the side), and nails torn away from the skin cause skin breaks. These breaks are portals of entry for microbes. Long or broken nails can scratch skin or snag clothing.

The feet are easily infected and injured. Dirty feet, socks, or stockings harbor microbes and cause odors. Shoes and socks provide a warm, moist environment for the growth of microbes. Injuries occur from stubbing toes, stepping on sharp objects, or being stepped on. Shoes that fit poorly cause blisters. Healing is prolonged in persons with poor circulation to the feet. Diabetes mellitus and vascular disease are common causes of poor circulation. Infections or foot injuries are particularly serious for older persons and persons with circulatory disorders. Gangrene and amputation are serious complications (see Chapter 30). Trimming and clipping toenails can easily result in injuries. *Therefore assistive personnel do not cut or trim toenails.*

> **Focus On... HOME CARE**
>
> Tub baths are a good time for soaking toes. If soaking is done at other times, the person can sit on the side of the tub and soak the feet. Make sure the person can step into and out of the tub. Otherwise, soak the feet in a basin.
>
> If the position is comfortable for the person, fingers can soak in the sink. Or a bowl is useful if a small basin is not available.

Cleaning and trimming fingernails are easier after soaking. Use nail clippers to cut fingernails. *Never use scissors.* Be very careful when clipping and trimming fingernails. You must not damage surrounding tissues. Also, check with the nurse about the water temperature. The feet are easily burned. Persons with decreased sensation or circulatory problems may not feel hot temperatures. *(See Focus on Home Care box.)*

Giving Nail and Foot Care

QUALITY OF LIFE

Remember to:
- Knock before entering the person's room
- Address the person by name
- Introduce yourself by name and title

Pre-Procedure

1 Explain the procedure to the person.
2 Wash your hands.
3 Collect the following:
   - Wash basin
   - Bath thermometer
   - Bath towel
   - Face towel
   - Washcloth
   - Kidney basin
   - Nail clippers
   - Orange stick
   - Emery board or nail file
   - Lotion or petroleum jelly
   - Paper towels
   - Disposable bath mat
   - Gloves (optional)
4 Arrange items on the overbed table.
5 Identify the person. Check the ID bracelet against the assignment sheet.
6 Provide for privacy.

Procedure

7 Help the person to a bedside chair. Place the signal light within reach.
8 Place the bath mat under the feet.
9 Fill the wash basin. Water temperature should be 105° F (40.5° C) unless otherwise instructed by the nurse.
10 Place the basin on the bath mat. Help the person put the feet into the basin.
11 Position the overbed table in front of the person. It should be low and close to the person.
12 Fill the kidney basin. Water temperature should be 105° F (40.5° C).
13 Place the basin on the overbed table on top of the paper towels.
14 Place the person's fingers into the basin. Position the arms for comfort (Fig. 15-6).
15 Let the feet and fingernails soak for 10 to 20 minutes. Rewarm the water as needed.
16 Clean under the fingernails with the orange stick.
17 Remove the kidney basin, and dry the fingers thoroughly.
18 Clip fingernails straight across with the nail clippers (Fig. 15-7).
19 Shape nails with an emery board or nail file.
20 Push cuticles back with the orange stick or a washcloth (Fig. 15-8).
21 Move the overbed table to the side.
22 Scrub calloused areas of the feet with a washcloth.
23 Remove the feet from the basin. Dry thoroughly.
24 Apply lotion or petroleum jelly to the feet.

Post-Procedure

25 Assist the person back to bed and to a comfortable position. Place the signal light within reach.
26 Raise or lower bed rails. Follow the care plan.
27 Clean and return equipment and supplies to the proper place. Discard disposable items.
28 Unscreen the person.
29 Follow agency policy for dirty linen.
30 Wash your hands.
31 Report your observations to the nurse:
   - Reddened, irritated, or calloused areas
   - Breaks in the skin
   - Changes in color of the skin and nails
   - Hot or cold hands and feet

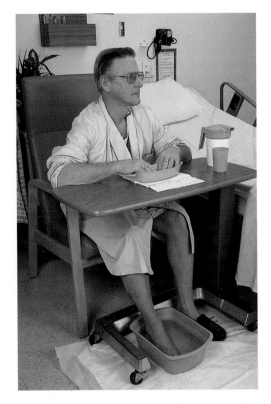

Fig. 15-6 Nail and foot care. The feet soak in a foot basin, and the fingers soak in a kidney basin.

Fig. 15-7 Clip fingernails straight across. Use a nail clipper.

Fig. 15-8 Push the cuticle back with an orange stick.

CHANGING HOSPITAL GOWNS AND CLOTHING

Hospital gowns or pajamas are changed after the bath and when wet or soiled. Persons who wear street clothing during the day change into a gown or pajamas for bed. Then they dress in the morning. Incontinent persons may change more often. Patients and residents may need help with these activities. The following rules are followed:

- Provide for privacy. Do not expose the person.
- Encourage the person to do as much as possible.
- Allow the person to choose what to wear. Make sure the person chooses the right undergarments.
- Remove clothing from the strong or "good" side first.
- Put clothing on the weak side first.
- Support the arm or leg when removing or putting on a garment.

► CHANGING HOSPITAL GOWNS

Special measures are needed for arm injuries, paralysis, or IV infusions. If there is injury or paralysis, the gown is removed from the good arm first. Support the weak arm while removing the gown. Put the clean gown on the weak arm first and then on the good arm.

Some agencies have special gowns for persons receiving IV infusions. The gowns open along the entire sleeve and close with ties, snaps, or Velcro. Standard hospital gowns may be used for persons with IV infusions.

Fig. 15-9 Changing a hospital gown. **A,** The gown is removed from the good arm. The sleeve on the arm with the IV is gathered up, slipped over the IV site and tubing, and removed from the arm and hand. **B,** The gathered sleeve is slipped along the IV tubing to the bag. **C,** The IV bag is removed from the pole and passed through the sleeve. **D,** The gathered sleeve of the clean gown is slipped over the IV bag at the shoulder part of the gown.

Changing the Gown of a Person With an IV

QUALITY OF LIFE

Remember to:
- Knock before entering the person's room
- Address the person by name
- Introduce yourself by name and title

Pre-Procedure

1. Explain the procedure to the person.
2. Wash your hands.
3. Get a clean gown.
4. Identify the person. Check the ID bracelet, and call the person by name.
5. Provide for privacy.
6. Raise the bed to a level for good body mechanics. Make sure both bed rails are up.

Procedure

7. Lower the bed rail near you.
8. Untie the gown. Free parts of the gown that the person is lying on.
9. Remove the gown from the arm with no IV.
10. Gather up the sleeve of the arm with the IV. Slide it over the IV site and tubing. Remove the arm and hand from the sleeve (Fig. 15-9, A).
11. Keep the sleeve gathered. Slide your arm along the tubing to the bag (Fig. 15-9, B).
12. Remove the bag from the pole. Slide the bag and tubing through the sleeve (Fig. 15-9, C). Do not pull on the tubing. Keep the bag above the person's arm.
13. Hang the IV bag on the pole.
14. Gather the sleeve of the clean gown that will go on the arm with the IV infusion.
15. Remove the bag from the pole. Quickly slip the gathered sleeve over the bag at the shoulder part of the gown (Fig. 15-9, D). Hang the bag on the pole.
16. Slide the gathered sleeve over the tubing, hand, arm, and IV site. Then slide the sleeve onto the person's shoulder.
17. Put the other side of the gown on the person.
18. Fasten the gown.

Post-Procedure

19. Provide for comfort.
20. Place the signal light within reach.
21. Lower the bed to its lowest position.
22. Raise or lower bed rails. Follow the care plan.
23. Unscreen the person.
24. Follow agency policy for dirty linen.
25. Wash your hands.
26. Ask the nurse to check the IV flow rate.

► DRESSING AND UNDRESSING

Clothing changes are usually necessary on admission and discharge. Some people enter and leave the agency in a gown or pajamas. Most wear street clothes. The rules listed on p. 364 are followed when dressing or undressing individuals. *(See Focus on Long-Term Care box and Focus on Home Care box.)*

Focus On... LONG-TERM CARE

Most residents wear street clothes during the day. Some dress and undress themselves. Others need help. Remember, personal choice is a resident right. Allow the person to choose what to wear.

Focus On... HOME CARE

Patients often wear street clothes during the day. Some wear nightgowns and pajamas and robes. The procedures that follow apply to nightgowns, pajamas, and robes as well as street clothes.

► Undressing a Person

QUALITY OF LIFE

Remember to:
- Knock before entering the person's room
- Address the person by name
- Introduce yourself by name and title

Pre-Procedure

1 Explain the procedure to the person.

2 Wash your hands.

3 Get a bath blanket.

4 Identify the person. Check the ID bracelet, and call the person by name.

5 Provide for privacy.

6 Raise the bed to the best level for good body mechanics. Make sure bed rails are up.

7 Lower the bed rail on the person's weak side.

8 Position him or her supine.

9 Cover the person with the bath blanket. Fanfold linens to the foot of the bed. Do not expose the person during the procedure.

Procedure

10 Remove garments that open in the back:

  a Raise the person's head and shoulders. Or turn him or her onto the side away from you.

  b Undo buttons, zippers, ties, or snaps.

  c Bring the sides of the garment to the sides of the person (Fig. 15-10, p. 368).

Do the following if he or she is in a side-lying position:

  (1) Tuck the far side under the person.

  (2) Fold the near side onto the chest (Fig. 15-11, p. 368).

  d Position the person supine.

Undressing a Person—cont'd

Procedure—cont'd

e Slide the garment off the shoulder on the strong side. Remove it from the arm (Fig. 15-12, p. 368).

f Repeat step 10e for the weak side.

11 Remove garments that open in the front.

　a Undo buttons, zippers, snaps, or ties.

　b Slide the garment off the shoulder and arm on the strong side.

　c Raise the head and shoulders. Bring the garment over to the weak side (Fig. 15-13, p. 369). Lower the head and shoulders.

　d Remove the garment from the weak side.

　e Do the following if you cannot raise the person's head and shoulders:

　　(1) Turn the person toward you. Tuck the removed part of the garment under the person.

　　(2) Turn him or her onto the side away from you.

　　(3) Pull the side of the garment out from under the person. Make sure he or she will not lie on it when supine.

　　(4) Return the person to the supine position.

　　(5) Remove the garment from the weak side.

12 Remove pullover garments:

　a Undo any buttons, zippers, ties, or snaps.

　b Remove the garment from the strong side.

　c Raise the head and shoulders. You may need to turn the person onto the side away from you. Bring the garment up to the person's neck (Fig. 15-14, p. 369).

　d Remove the garment from the weak side.

　e Bring the garment over the person's head.

　f Position him or her in the supine position.

13 Remove pants or slacks:

　a Remove shoes or slippers.

　b Position the person supine.

　c Undo buttons, zippers, ties, snaps, or buckles.

　d Remove the belt if one is worn.

　e Ask the person to lift the buttocks off the bed. Slide the pants down over the hips and buttocks (Fig. 15-15, p. 369). Have the person lower the hips and buttocks.

　f Do the following if the person cannot raise the hips off the bed:

　　(1) Turn the person toward you.

　　(2) Slide the pants off the hip and buttock on the strong side (Fig. 15-16, p. 370).

　　(3) Turn the person away from you.

　　(4) Slide the pants off the hip and buttock on the weak side (Fig. 15-17, p. 370).

　g Slide the pants down the legs and over the feet.

14 Dress or put a clean gown or pajamas on the person.

15 Help the person get out of bed if he or she is to be up. Cover the person and remove the bath blanket if the person will not be up.

Post-Procedure

16 Lower the bed to its lowest position.

17 Raise or lower bed rails. Follow the care plan.

18 Place the signal light within reach.

19 Unscreen the person.

20 Follow agency policy for soiled clothing.

21 Report your observations to the nurse.

Fig. 15-10 The sides of the garment are brought from the back to the sides of the person.

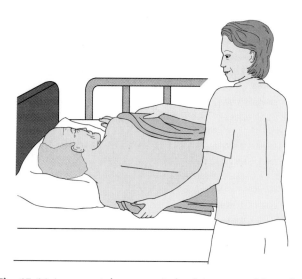

Fig. 15-11 A garment that opens in back is removed from the person in the side-lying position. The far side of the garment is tucked under the person. The near side is folded onto the person's chest.

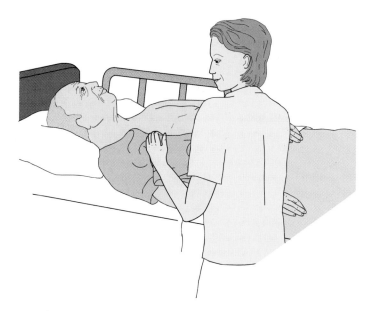

Fig. 15-12 The garment is removed from the strong side first.

Fig. 15-13 A front-opening garment is removed with the person's head and shoulders raised. The garment is removed from the strong side first. Then it is brought around the back to the weak side.

Fig. 15-14 A pullover garment is removed from the strong side first. Then the garment is brought up to the person's neck so that it can be removed from the weak side.

Fig. 15-15 The person lifts the hips and buttocks for removing the pants. The pants are slid down over the hips and buttocks.

Fig. 15-16 Pants are removed in the side-lying position. They are removed from the strong side first. They are slid over the hips and buttocks.

Fig. 15-17 The person is turned onto the other side. The pants are removed from the weak side.

Dressing the Person

NNAAP™

QUALITY OF LIFE

Remember to:
- Knock before entering the person's room
- Address the person by name
- Introduce yourself by name and title

Pre-Procedure

1 Explain the procedure to the person.
2 Wash your hands.
3 Get a bath blanket and necessary clothing.
4 Identify the person. Check the ID bracelet, and call the person by name.
5 Provide for privacy.
6 Raise the bed to a level for good body mechanics. Make sure bed rails are up.
7 Undress the person (see *Undressing the Person*, p. 366).
8 Lower the bed rail on the person's strong side. Make sure the other bed rail is up.
9 Position the person supine.

Procedure

10 Cover the person with the bath blanket. Fanfold linens to the foot of the bed. Do not expose the person during the procedure.
11 Put on garments that open in the back:
  a Slide the garment onto the arm and shoulder of the weak side.
  b Slide the garment onto the arm and shoulder of the strong side.
  c Raise the person's head and shoulders.
  d Bring the sides to the back if he or she is in a semisitting position.
  e Do the following if the person is in a side-lying position:
    (1) Turn the person toward you.
    (2) Bring one side of the garment to the person's back (Fig. 15-18, A, p. 372).
    (3) Turn the person away from you.
    (4) Bring the other side to the person's back (Fig. 15-18, *B*, p. 372).
  f Fasten buttons, snaps, ties, or zippers.
  g Position the person in the supine position.
12 Put on garments that open in the front:
  a Slide the garment onto the arm and shoulder on the weak side.
  b Raise the person's head and shoulders. Bring the other side of the garment around to the back. Lower the person to the supine position. Slide the garment onto the arm and shoulder of the strong arm.

  c Do the following if the person cannot raise the head and shoulders:
    (1) Turn the person toward you.
    (2) Tuck the garment under him or her.
    (3) Turn the person away from you.
    (4) Pull the garment out from under him or her.
    (5) Turn the person back to the supine position.
    (6) Slide the garment over the arm and shoulder of the strong arm.
  d Fasten buttons, snaps, ties, or zippers.
13 Put on pullover garments:
  a Position the person supine.
  b Bring the neck of the garment over the head.
  c Slide the arm and shoulder of the garment onto the person's weak side.
  d Raise the person's head and shoulders.
  e Bring the garment down.
  f Slide the arm and shoulder of the garment onto the person's strong side.
  g Do the following if the person cannot assume a semisitting position:
    (1) Turn the person toward you.
    (2) Tuck the garment under him or her.
    (3) Turn the person away from you.
    (4) Pull the garment out from under him or her.

Continued

Dressing the Person—cont'd

NNAAP™

Procedure—cont'd

(5) Return the person to the supine position.

(6) Slide the arm and shoulder of the garment onto the strong side.

h Fasten buttons, snaps, ties, or zippers.

14 Put on pants or slacks:

  a Slide the pants over the feet and up the legs.

  b Ask him or her to raise the hips and buttocks off the bed.

  c Bring the pants up over the buttocks and hips.

  d Ask the person to lower the hips and buttocks.

  e Do the following if the person cannot raise the hips and buttocks:

    (1) Turn person onto the strong side.

    (2) Pull the pants over the buttock and hip on the weak side.

    (3) Turn the person onto the weak side.

    (4) Pull the pants over the buttock and hip on the strong side.

    (5) Return the person to the supine position.

  f Fasten buttons, ties, snaps, zipper, and belt buckle.

15 Put socks and shoes or slippers on the person.

16 Help the person to the chair if he or she can be up. Otherwise, help the person assume a comfortable position in bed.

17 Cover the person, and remove the bath blanket.

Post-Procedure

18 Lower the bed to its lowest position.

19 Raise or lower bed rails. Follow the care plan.

20 Make sure the signal light is within reach.

21 Unscreen the person.

22 Follow agency policy for soiled clothing.

23 Report your observations to the nurse.

A   **B**

Fig. 15-18 Dressing a person. **A,** The side-lying position can be used to put on garments that open in the back. Turn the person toward you after the garment is put on the arms. The side of the garment is brought to the person's back. **B,** Then turn the person away from you. The other side of the garment is brought to the back and fastened.

Circle the BEST answer.

1. You read the word *alopecia* in Mr. Lee's medical record. The term means
   A. Excessive body hair
   B. Dry, white flakes from the scalp
   C. An infestation of lice
   D. Hair loss

2. You are going to brush a woman's hair. The hair is not matted or tangled. When brushing the hair, start at
   A. The forehead
   B. The hair ends
   C. The scalp
   D. The back of the neck

3. Brushing is important to keep the hair
   A. Soft and shiny
   B. Clean
   C. Free from pediculosis
   D. Long

4. Mr. Lee wants his hair washed. You should
   A. Wash his hair during his shower
   B. Wash his hair at the sink
   C. Shampoo him in bed
   D. Follow the nurse's instructions

5. When shaving Mr. Lee, you need to do the following *except*
   A. Practice Standard Precautions
   B. Follow the Bloodborne Pathogen Standard
   C. Shave in the opposite direction of hair growth
   D. Make sure the skin is soft before shaving

6. Mr. Lee is nicked during shaving. Your first action is to
   A. Wash your hands
   B. Apply direct pressure
   C. Report the nick to the nurse immediately
   D. Switch to an electric razor

7. You are going to cut a person's fingernails. You should use
   A. Toenail clippers
   B. Scissors
   C. An emery board
   D. Nail clippers

8. Fingernails are trimmed
   A. Before they are soaked
   B. After they are soaked
   C. Before the toenails are trimmed
   D. After the toenails are trimmed

Circle T if the answer is true and F if it is false.

9. T F Mr. Lee has a mustache and beard. You think he would be more comfortable without facial hair. You can shave his beard and mustache.

10. T F You can cut and trim toenails.

11. T F Clothing is removed from the strong side first.

12. T F The person is allowed to choose what to wear.

The answers to these questions are on p. 836.

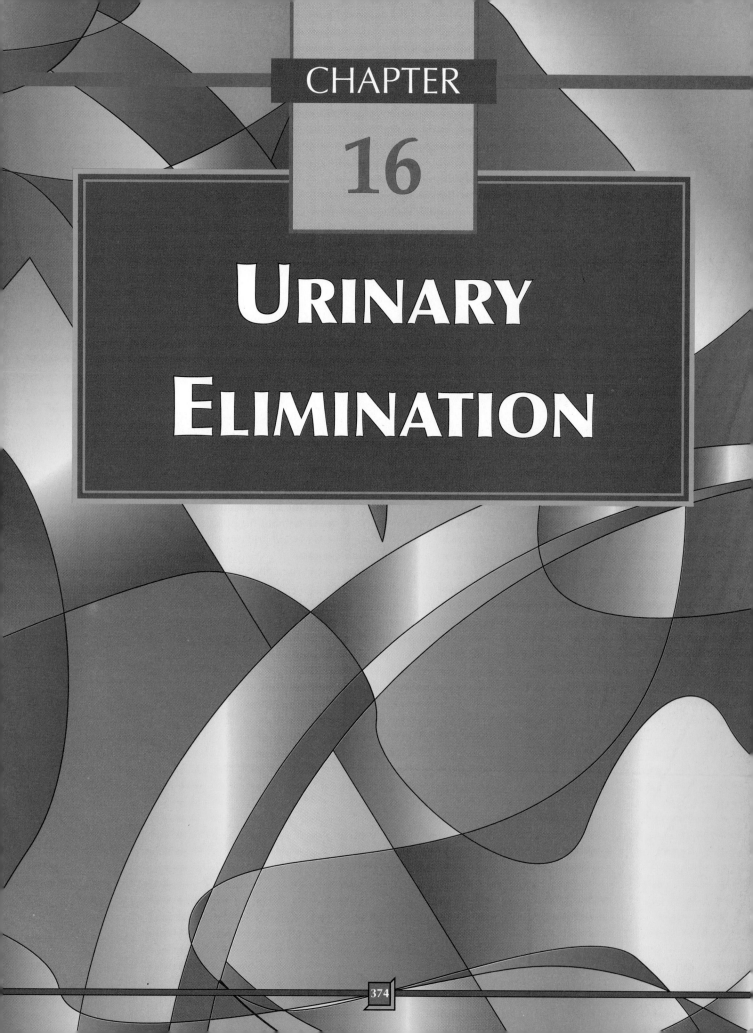

CHAPTER

16

URINARY ELIMINATION

OBJECTIVES

Define the key terms listed in this chapter
Identify the characteristics of normal urine
Describe the rules for maintaining normal urinary elimination
List the observations to make about urine
Describe urinary incontinence and the care required
Explain why catheters are used
Describe the rules for caring for persons with catheters
Explain the differences between straight, indwelling, and condom catheters
Describe two methods of bladder training
Describe the rules for collecting urine specimens
Perform the procedures described in this chapter

KEY TERMS

acetone Ketone bodies that appear in the urine because of the rapid breakdown of fat for energy

catheter A tube used to drain or inject fluid through a body opening

catheterization The process of inserting a catheter

dysuria Painful or difficult *(dys)* urination *(uria)*

Foley catheter A catheter that is left in place in the urinary bladder so urine drains constantly into a drainage bag; an indwelling or retention catheter

functional incontinence The involuntary, unpredicted loss of urine from the bladder

glucosuria Sugar *(glucos)* in the urine *(uria)*; glycosuria

glycosuria Sugar *(glycos)* in the urine *(uria)*; glucosuria

hematuria Blood *(hemat)* in the urine *(uria)*

indwelling catheter A retention or Foley catheter

ketones Ketone bodies, acetone

ketone body Acetone

micturition The process of emptying urine from the bladder; urination or voiding

mixed incontinence A combination of urge and stress incontinence

nocturia Frequent urination *(uria)* at night *(noct)*

oliguria Scant amount *(olig)* of urine *(uria)*; usually less than 500 ml in 24 hours

overflow incontinence The loss of urine when the bladder is too full

polyuria The production of abnormally large amounts *(poly)* of urine *(uria)*

reflex incontinence The loss of urine at predictable intervals; unconscious incontinence

retention catheter A Foley or indwelling catheter

straight catheter A catheter that drains the bladder and is removed

stress incontinence The loss of small amounts of urine with exercise and certain movements

unconscious incontinence Reflex incontinence

urge incontinence The involuntary loss of urine after feeling a strong need to void

urinary frequency Voiding at frequent intervals

urinary incontinence The inability to control the loss of urine from the bladder

urinary urgency The need to void immediately

urination The process of emptying urine from the bladder; micturition or voiding

voiding Urination or micturition

Eliminating waste is a physical need. The respiratory, digestive, integumentary, and urinary systems all remove body wastes. The digestive system rids the body of solid wastes. The lungs rid the body of carbon dioxide. Sweat contains water and other substances. Blood contains waste products from body cells burning food for energy. The urinary system removes waste products from the blood and maintains the body's water balance Box 16-1 contains a review of the structure and function of the urinary system. See Chapter 6 for more detailed information.

NORMAL URINATION

The healthy adult excretes about 1500 ml (milliliters) (3 pints) of urine a day. Many factors affect urine production. They include age, disease, the amount and kinds of fluid ingested, dietary salt, and drugs. Some substances increase urine production. Examples are coffee, tea, alcohol, and some drugs. A diet high in salt causes the body to retain water. When water is retained, less urine is produced.

Urination, micturition, and voiding mean the process of emptying urine from the bladder. Urination patterns depend on many factors. The amount of fluid intake, personal habits, and available toilet facilities affect frequency. So do activity, work, and illness. People usually urinate at bedtime, after getting up, and before meals. Some people urinate every 2 to 3 hours. The need to urinate at night disturbs sleep.

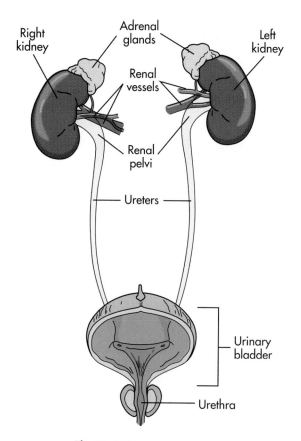

Fig. 16-1 The urinary system.

Box 16-1	The Urinary System: Review of Body Structure and Function

The kidneys, ureters, urinary bladder, and urethra are the major urinary tract structures (Fig. 16-1). The two kidneys lie in the upper abdomen against the muscles of the back on each side of the spine. Blood passes through the two kidneys, where urine is formed. Urine consists of wastes and excess fluids filtered out of the blood. Urine flows through the two ureters to the urinary bladder, where it is stored until urination. The urethra is the tube that connects the urinary bladder to the outside of the body. Urine is eliminated from the body through the urethra. **Urination, micturition,** and **voiding** all mean the process of emptying the bladder.

MAINTAINING NORMAL URINATION

Some persons need help getting to the bathroom. Others use bedpans, urinals, or commodes. Follow the rules listed in Box 16-2 to help maintain normal elimination.

OBSERVATIONS

Urine is normally pale yellow, straw colored, or amber. It is clear with no particles. A faint odor is normal. Observe urine for color, clarity, odor, amount, and particles. Some foods normally affect urine color. Red food dyes, beets, blackberries, and rhubarb cause red-colored urine. Carrots and sweet potatoes cause bright yellow urine. Certain drugs cause changes in urine color. Asparagus causes a urine odor.

Ask the nurse to observe any urine that looks or smells abnormal. Report complaints of urgency, burning on urination, or dysuria. **Dysuria** means painful or difficult (*dys*) urination (*uria*). Also report the problems described in Table 16-1. The RN uses the information for the nursing process.

Box 16-2	Rules for Maintaining Normal Elimination

- Practice medical asepsis and Standard Precautions. Also follow the Bloodborne Pathogen Standard.
- Provide fluids as instructed by the nurse.
- Follow the person's normal voiding routines and habits. Check with the nurse and the nursing care plan.
- Help the person to the bathroom when the request is made. Or provide the commode, bedpan, or urinal. The need to void may be urgent.
- Help the person assume a normal position for voiding if possible. Women sit or squat; men stand.
- Warm the bedpan or urinal.
- Cover the person for warmth and privacy.
- Provide for privacy. Pull the curtain around the bed, close room and bathroom doors, and pull drapes or window shades. Leave the room if the person can be alone.
- Tell the person that running water, flushing the toilet, or playing music can mask urination sounds. Some persons are embarrassed about voiding with others close by.

- Remain nearby if the person is weak or unsteady.
- Place the signal light and toilet tissue within reach.
- Allow the person enough time to void. Do not rush the person.
- Promote relaxation. Some people like to read when eliminating.
- Run water in a nearby sink if the person has difficulty starting the stream. Or place the person's fingers in some warm water.
- Provide perineal care as needed.
- Have the person wash his or her hands after voiding. Provide a wash basin, soap, washcloth, and towel. Assist as necessary.
- Assist the person to the bathroom or offer the bedpan, urinal, or commode at regular times. Some people are embarrassed or are too weak to ask.

Table 16-1	Common Urinary Elimination Problems

	Definition	Causes
dysuria	Painful or difficult *(dys)* urination *(uria)*	Urinary tract infection, trauma, urinary tract obstruction
hematuria	Blood *(hemat)* in the urine *(uria)*	Kidney disease, urinary tract infection, trauma
nocturia	Frequent urination *(uria)* at night *(noct)*	Excessive fluid intake, kidney disease, disease of the prostate
oliguria	Scant amount *(olig)* of urine *(uria)*, usually less than 500 ml in 24 hours	Inadequate fluid intake, shock, burns, kidney disease, heart failure
polyuria	The production of abnormally large amounts *(poly)* of urine *(uria)*	Drugs, excessive fluid intake, diabetes mellitus, hormone imbalance
urinary frequency	Voiding at frequent intervals	Excessive fluid intake, bladder infections, pressure on the bladder, drugs
urinary incontinence	Inability to control the loss of urine from the bladder	Trauma, disease, urinary tract infections, reproductive or urinary tract surgeries, aging, fecal impaction, constipation, not getting to the bathroom
urinary urgency	The need to void immediately	Urinary tract infection, fear of incontinence, full bladder, stress

▶ BEDPANS

Bedpans are used when persons cannot be out of bed. Women use bedpans for voiding and bowel movements. Men use them only for bowel movements. Bedpans are made of plastic or stainless steel. Stainless steel bedpans are often cold. They are warmed with water and dried before use.

A *fracture pan* has a thinner rim and is only about ½-inch deep at one end (Fig. 16-2). The smaller end is placed under the buttocks (Fig. 16-3). Fracture pans are used for persons with casts or those in traction. *(See Focus on Older Persons box.)*

Follow medical asepsis, Standard Precautions, and the Bloodborne Pathogen Standard when handling bedpans and their contents.

Text continued on p. 382

Focus On... OLDER PERSONS

Regular bedpans are uncomfortable for some older persons. They may have fragile bones from osteoporosis, painful joints from arthritis, or a hip replacement (see Chapter 30). Fracture pans are often more comfortable for these people.

Fig. 16-2 The regular bedpan and the fracture pan.

Fig. 16-3 A person positioned on a fracture pan. The smaller end is placed under the buttocks.

Giving the Bedpan

NNAAP™

QUALITY OF LIFE

Remember to:
- Knock before entering the person's room
- Address the person by name
- Introduce yourself by name and title

Pre-Procedure

1 Provide for privacy.
2 Put on gloves.
3 Collect the following:
   - Bedpan
   - Bedpan cover
   - Toilet tissue
4 Arrange equipment on the chair or bed.
5 Explain the procedure to the person.
6 Raise the bed to the best level for good body mechanics. Make sure bed rails are up.

Procedure

7 Warm and dry the bedpan if necessary.
8 Lower the bed rail near you.
9 Position the person supine. Raise the head of the bed slightly.
10 Fold the top linens and gown out of the way. Keep the lower body covered.
11 Ask the person to flex the knees and raise the buttocks by pushing against the mattress with his or her feet.
12 Slide your hand under the lower back, and help him or her raise the buttocks.
13 Slide the bedpan under the person (Fig. 16-4, p. 380).
14 Do the following if the person cannot assist in getting on the bedpan:
   a Turn the person onto the side away from you.
   b Place the bedpan firmly against the buttocks (Fig. 16-5, *A*, p. 381).
   c Push the bedpan down and toward the person (Fig. 16-5, *B*, p. 381).
   d Hold the bedpan securely. Turn the person onto the back. Make sure the bedpan is centered under the person.
15 Return top linens to their proper position.
16 Raise the head of the bed so the person is in a sitting position.
17 Make sure the person is correctly positioned on the bedpan (Fig. 16-6, p. 381).
18 Raise the bed rail.
19 Place the toilet tissue and signal light within reach.
20 Ask the person to signal when done or when help is needed.
21 Remove the gloves, and wash your hands.
22 Leave the room, and close the door.
23 Return when the person signals. Knock before entering.
24 Lower the bed rail and the head of the bed.
25 Put on gloves.
26 Ask the person to raise the buttocks. Remove the bedpan. Or hold the bedpan securely and turn him or her onto the side away from you.
27 Clean the genital area if the person cannot do so. Clean from front to back with toilet tissue. Use fresh tissue for each wipe. Provide perineal care if necessary.
28 Cover the bedpan. Take it to the bathroom or dirty utility room. Raise the bed rail before leaving the bedside.
29 Note the color, amount, and character of urine or feces.
30 Empty and rinse the bedpan. Clean it with a disinfectant.
31 Remove soiled gloves. Wash your hands, and put on clean gloves.
32 Return the bedpan and clean cover to the bedside stand.
33 Help the person wash the hands.
34 Remove the gloves.

Continued

Giving the Bedpan—cont'd

NNAAP™

Post-Procedure

35 Provide for comfort.

36 Place the signal light within reach.

37 Raise or lower bed rails. Follow the care plan.

38 Lower the bed to its lowest position.

39 Unscreen the person.

40 Follow agency policy for soiled linen.

41 Wash your hands.

42 Report your observations to the nurse.

Fig. 16-4 The person raises the buttocks off the bed with help. The bedpan is slid under the person.

Fig. 16-5 Giving a bedpan. **A,** Position the person on one side, and place the bedpan firmly against the buttocks. **B,** Push downward on the bedpan and toward the person.

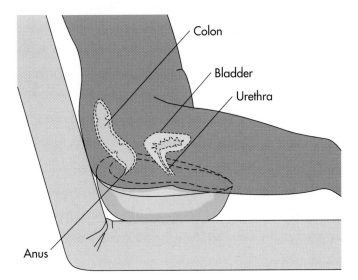

Fig. 16-6 The person is positioned on the bedpan so the urethra and anus are directly over the opening.

▶ URINALS

Men use urinals to void (Fig. 16-7). Plastic urinals have caps at the top and hook-type handles. The urinal hooks to the bed rail within the man's reach. The man stands to use the urinal if possible. Otherwise he sits on the side of the bed or lies in bed. Some men stand with the support of 1 or 2 people. You may have to place and hold the urinal for some men.

Remind men to hang urinals on bed rails and to signal when urinals need emptying. Remind them not to place urinals on overbed tables and bedside stands. The overbed table is used for eating and as a work surface. Bedside stands are used for supplies. For these reasons, table surfaces must not be contaminated with urine.

Follow medical asepsis, Standard Precautions, and the Bloodborne Pathogen Standard when handling urinals and their contents. Empty urinals promptly to prevent odors and the spread of microbes. A filled urinal spills easily, causing safety hazards. Also, it is an unpleasant site and a source of odor. Urinals are cleaned like bedpans.

A

B

Fig. 16-7 **A,** Male urinal. **B,** The urinal hangs from the bed rail.

Giving the Urinal

QUALITY OF LIFE

Remember to: • Knock before entering the person's room
• Address the person by name
• Introduce yourself by name and title

Procedure

1   Provide for privacy.
2   Determine if the man will stand or stay in bed.
3   Put on gloves.
4   Give him the urinal if he is in bed. Remind him to tilt the bottom down to prevent spills.
5   Do the following if he is going to stand:
  a   Help him sit on the side of the bed.
  b   Put shoes or nonskid slippers on him.
  c   Assist him to a standing position.
  d   Provide support if he is unsteady.
  e   Give him the urinal.
6   Position the urinal between his legs if necessary. Position his penis in the urinal if he cannot hold the urinal.
7   Cover him to provide for privacy.
8   Place the signal light within reach. Ask him to signal when done or when he needs help.
9   Remove the gloves, and wash your hands.
10   Leave the room, and close the door.
11   Return when he signals for you. Knock before entering.
12   Put on gloves.
13   Cover the urinal. Take it to the bathroom or dirty utility room.
14   Note the color, amount, and character of the urine.
15   Empty the urinal, and rinse it with cold water. Clean it with a disinfectant.
16   Return the urinal to its proper place.
17   Remove soiled gloves. Wash your hands, and put on clean gloves.
18   Help the person wash his hands.
19   Remove the gloves.

Post-Procedure

20   Provide for comfort.
21   Place the signal light within reach.
22   Raise or lower bed rails. Follow the care plan.
23   Unscreen him.
24   Follow agency policy for soiled linen.
25   Wash your hands.
26   Report your observations to the nurse.

► COMMODES

A bedside commode is a portable chair or wheelchair with an opening for a bedpan or container (Fig. 16-8). Persons unable to walk to the bathroom often use commodes. The commode allows a normal position for elimination. The bedpan or container is cleaned after use like the regular bedpan.

Some commodes are wheeled into the bathroom and placed over the toilet. The container is removed if the commode is used with the toilet. Make sure the commode wheels are locked and that the commode is positioned over the toilet.

Fig. 16-8 The bedside commode has a toilet seat with a container. The container slides out from under the toilet seat for emptying.

Helping the Person to the Commode

QUALITY OF LIFE

Remember to:
- Knock before entering the person's room
- Address the person by name
- Introduce yourself by name and title

Pre-Procedure

1 Explain the procedure to the person.
2 Provide for privacy.
3 Put on gloves.

4 Collect the following:
- Commode
- Toilet tissue
- Bath blanket

Procedure

5 Bring the commode next to the bed. Remove the chair seat and lid from the container.
6 Help the person sit on the side of the bed.
7 Help him or her put on a robe and shoes or nonskid slippers.
8 Assist the person to the commode.
9 Place a bath blanket over his or her lap for warmth.
10 Place the toilet tissue and signal light within reach.
11 Ask him or her to signal when done or when help is needed.
12 Remove the gloves, and wash your hands.
13 Leave the room, and close the door. (Stay in the room if it is not safe to leave the person alone. Allow as much privacy as possible.)
14 Return when the person signals. Knock before entering.
15 Put on the gloves.

16 Help the person clean the genital area if indicated. Remove the gloves.
17 Help the person back to bed. Remove the robe and slippers. Raise the bed according to the care plan.
18 Put on clean gloves. Cover and remove the container from the commode. Clean the commode if necessary.
19 Take the container to the bathroom or dirty utility room.
20 Check urine and feces for color, amount, and character.
21 Clean and disinfect the container.
22 Return the container to the commode. Return other supplies to their proper place.
23 Return the commode to its proper place.
24 Remove soiled gloves. Wash your hands, and put on clean gloves.
25 Help the person wash the hands.
26 Remove the gloves.

Post-Procedure

27 Provide for comfort.
28 Place the signal light within reach.
29 Raise or lower bed rails. Follow the care plan.
30 Unscreen the person.
31 Follow agency policy for soiled linen.
32 Wash your hands.
33 Report your observations to the nurse.

URINARY INCONTINENCE

Urinary incontinence is the involuntary loss of urine from the bladder. It may be temporary or permanent. There are different types of incontinence:

- **Urge incontinence** is the involuntary loss of urine after feeling a strong need to void. The person cannot stop urinating and cannot get to the bathroom in time. Urinary frequency, urinary urgency, and nighttime voidings are common. Urinary tract infections, decreased bladder capacity, alcohol and caffeine intake, and increased fluid intake are causes.
- **Stress incontinence** is the loss of small amounts of urine with exercise and certain movements. Urine loss is usually small (less than 50 ml). Often called *dribbling*, stress incontinence occurs with laughing, sneezing, coughing, lifting, or other activities. Late pregnancy and obesity are other causes. The problem is common in women. Pelvic muscles weaken after multiple pregnancies and with aging.
- **Mixed incontinence** is a combination of urge and stress incontinence. This type is more common in older women.
- **Overflow incontinence** is the loss of urine when the bladder is too full. The person feels like the bladder is never completely empty. Much time is spent trying to void. However, the person only dribbles or has a weak stream of urine. Small amounts of urine are lost during the day and night. Nocturia is common. Fecal impaction, diabetes, and spinal cord injury are causes. Prostate enlargement is a common cause in men.
- **Functional incontinence** is the involuntary, unpredictable loss of urine. The person does not have nervous system or urinary system injuries. The person cannot use the bathroom, bedpan, urinal, or commode in time. Immobility, restraints, unanswered signal lights, not having a signal light within reach, and not knowing where to find the bathroom also are causes. So is difficulty removing clothes. Confusion and disorientation are other causes.
- **Unconscious or reflex incontinence** is the loss of urine at predictable intervals. Urine is lost when the bladder is full. The person does not know the bladder is full and has no urge to void. Central nervous system disorders and injuries are common causes.

Incontinence is embarrassing. Clothing gets wet, odors develop, and the person is uncomfortable. Skin irritation, infection, and pressure ulcers can occur. Falling is a risk as the person tries to get to the bathroom quickly. The person's pride, dignity, and self-esteem are affected.

The RN uses the nursing process to meet the person's needs. Follow the nurse's instructions and the nursing care plan. Nursing measures depend on the type of incontinence. The person's care plan may include some of the nursing measures listed in Box 16-3. *Good skin care and dry clothing and linens are always essential.* Following the rules for maintaining normal urinary elimination prevents incontinence in some people. Others need bladder training programs. Sometimes catheters are ordered. Some people wear garment protectors or incontinence pads (Fig. 16-9). Incontinence drawsheets help keep the person dry. The drawsheet has two layers and a waterproof back. Fluid passes through the first layer and is absorbed by the lower layer. A variety of incontinence products are available. The nurse selects products best suited to the person's needs.

Incontinence is a link to abuse, mistreatment, and neglect. Caring for these persons is stressful. They need frequent care and may wet again just after you changed wet garments and linens and gave skin care. Do not lose patience. Their needs are great, and your role is to meet their needs. If you find yourself short tempered and impatient, discuss the problem with the nurse immediately. Remember, the person has the right to be free from abuse, mistreatment, or neglect. The incontinence is beyond the person's control. It is not something he or she chooses to let happen. Kindness, empathy, understanding, and patience are very important. *(See Focus on Older Persons box and Focus on Home Care box.)*

Fig. 16-9 Garment protector. **A,** Complete incontinence brief. **B,** Pant liner and undergarment.

Box 16-3 Nursing Measures for Persons With Urinary Incontinence

- Keep records of the person's voidings. This includes incontinent episodes and successful use of the toilet, commode, bedpan, or urinal.
- Answer signal lights promptly. The person may have an urgent need to void.
- Promote normal urinary elimination (see Box 16-2).
- Promote normal bowel elimination (see Chapter 17).
- Encourage urination at scheduled intervals.
- Follow the person's bladder training program.
- Encourage the person to wear clothing that is easy to remove. Incontinence can occur as the person is trying to deal with buttons, zippers, and undergarments.
- Encourage the person to do pelvic muscle exercises as instructed by the nurse.
- Encourage fluid intake as directed by the nurse.
- Decrease fluid intake before bedtime.
- Provide good skin care.
- Keep the perineal area clean and dry.
- Provide dry gowns and linens.
- Observe the skin for signs of breakdown.
- Use incontinence products as directed by the nurse.

Focus On... OLDER PERSONS

Urinary incontinence is a common problem among older persons. They are at greater risk for the disorders and physical problems that cause incontinence. These include disorders of the nervous, endocrine, and reproductive systems. Dementia, tumors, and poor mobility are other causes. Complications from incontinence pose serious health risks for older persons. These include falls, pressure ulcers, and urinary tract infections. Prolonged hospital care or long-term care is often necessary. The resulting health care costs are high.

Persons with dementia present other problems. They may urinate in inappropriate places (trash cans, planters, heating vents, closets, and other places). Some persons flush wet undergarments or incontinence products down the toilet. Others resist staff efforts to keep them clean and dry. Check with the nurse and the care plan for the special measures needed to help the person.

Focus On... HOME CARE

Incontinence is stressful for the family. Family caregivers often cannot cope with the person's incontinence. It is a common reason for seeking long-term care.

CATHETERS

A **catheter** is a rubber or plastic tube used to drain or inject fluid through a body opening. Inserted through the urethra into the bladder, a urinary catheter drains urine. A **straight catheter** drains the bladder and is removed. An **indwelling catheter** (**retention** or **Foley catheter**) is left in the bladder so urine drains constantly into a drainage bag. A balloon near the tip is inflated after the catheter is inserted. The balloon prevents the catheter from slipping out of the bladder (Fig. 16-10). Tubing connects the catheter to the collection bag. Catheter insertion (**catheterization**) is done by a nurse or doctor. With the proper education and supervision, some states and agencies allow assistive personnel to perform catheterizations.

Catheters often are used before, during, and after surgery to keep the bladder empty. This reduces the risk of accidental bladder injury during surgery. After surgery, a full bladder causes pressure on nearby organs.

Catheters also allow hourly urinary output measurements in critically ill persons. Catheters are a last resort for incontinence. Catheters do not treat the cause of incontinence, and the risk of infection is high. However, some persons have wounds and pressure ulcers that need protection from urine. Catheters can protect the wounds and pressure ulcers from contamination with urine.

Some people are too weak or disabled to use the bedpan, commode, or toilet. Dying persons are an example. For them, catheters can promote comfort. Also, the person is protected from incontinence.

Catheters are inserted for diagnostic purposes. They are used to collect sterile urine specimens. Another test involves inserting a catheter to see how much urine is left in the bladder *(residual urine)*. The catheter is inserted after the person voids.

You will care for persons with indwelling catheters. The rules listed in Box 16-4 promote their comfort and safety.

Text continued on p. 392

Fig. 16-10 A, Indwelling catheter in the female bladder. The inflated balloon at the top prevents the catheter from slipping out through the urethra. **B,** Indwelling catheter with the balloon inflated in the male bladder.

Box 16-4   Caring for Persons With Indwelling Catheters

- Follow the rules of medical asepsis, Standard Precautions, and the Bloodborne Pathogen Standard.
- Make sure urine flows freely through the catheter or tubing. Tubing should not have kinks. The person should not lie on the tubing.
- Make sure the catheter is connected to the drainage tubing. Follow the measures on p. 392 if the catheter and drainage tube are disconnected.
- Keep the drainage bag below the bladder. This prevents urine from flowing backward into the bladder.
- Attach the drainage bag to the bed frame. *Never attach the drainage bag to the bed rail.* Otherwise the drainage bag is higher than the bladder when the bed rail is raised. If the person is in a wheelchair, attached the drainage bag to the back of the chair. If the person is ambulatory, attach the drainage bag to the lower part of an IV pole.
- Do not let the drainage bag rest on the floor. This can contaminate the system.
- Coil the drainage tubing on the bed, and secure it to the bottom linen (Fig. 16-11). Use a clip, tape, or a safety pin following agency policy. Tubing must not loop below the drainage bag.
- Secure the catheter to the inner thigh as in Figure 16-11. Or secure it to the man's abdomen. This prevents excessive movement of the catheter and reduces friction at the insertion site. Secure the catheter with tape or elastic strap as ordered by the nurse.
- Check for leaks. Check the site where the catheter connects to the drainage bag. Report any leaks to the nurse immediately.
- Provide catheter care if ordered. Catheter care is done daily or twice a day (see *Giving Catheter Care*). Some agencies consider perineal care to be sufficient. Catheter care is sometimes needed after bowel movements and when there is vaginal drainage.
- Provide perineal care daily and after bowel movements.
- Empty the drainage bag at the end of the shift or at time intervals as directed by the nurse. Measure and record the amount of urine (see *Emptying a Urinary Drainage Bag*). Report increases or decreases in the amount of urine.
- Use a separate measuring container for each person. This prevents the spread of microbes from one person to another.
- Do not the let the drain on the drainage bag touch any surface.
- Report complaints to the nurse immediately. These include complaints of pain, burning, the need to urinate, or irritation. Also report the color, clarity, and odor of urine and the presence of particles.
- Encourage fluid intake as instructed by the nurse.

Fig. 16-11 Securing catheters. **A,** The drainage tubing is coiled on the bed and secured to the bottom linens so urine flows freely. The catheter is taped to the inner thigh. Enough slack is left on the catheter to prevent friction at the urethra. **B,** The catheter is secured to the man's abdomen.

Giving Catheter Care

NNAAP™

QUALITY OF LIFE

Remember to:
- Knock before entering the person's room
- Address the person by name
- Introduce yourself by name and title

Pre-Procedure

1 Explain the procedure to the person.

2 Wash your hands.

3 Collect the following:
- Equipment for perineal care
- Gloves
- Bed protector
- Bath blanket

4 Identify the person. Check the ID bracelet against the assignment sheet.

5 Provide for privacy.

6 Raise the bed to the best level for good body mechanics. Make sure bed rails are up.

Procedure

7 Lower the bed rail near you.

8 Put on the gloves.

9 Cover the person with a bath blanket. Fanfold top linens to the foot of the bed.

10 Drape the person for perineal care (see Fig. 14-28).

11 Fold back the bath blanket between the legs to expose the genital area.

12 Place the bed protector under the buttocks. Ask the person to flex the knees and raise the buttocks off the bed by pushing against the mattress with the feet.

13 Perform perineal care (see *Female Perineal Care,* p. 345 or *Male Perineal Care,* p. 348).

14 Separate the labia (female), or retract the foreskin (uncircumcised male) as in Figure 16-12. Check for crusts, abnormal drainage, or secretions.

15 Clean the catheter from the meatus down the catheter about 4 inches (Fig. 16-13). Use soap and water and a clean washcloth. Avoid tugging or pulling on the catheter. Repeat if necessary with a clean washcloth.

16 Make sure the catheter is secured properly. Coil and secure tubing (see Fig. 16-11).

17 Remove the bed protector.

18 Cover the person, and remove the bath blanket.

19 Remove the gloves.

Post-Procedure

20 Provide for comfort.

21 Raise or lower bed rails. Follow the care plan.

22 Lower the bed to its lowest position.

23 Clean and return equipment to its proper place. Discard disposable items. (Wear gloves for this step.)

24 Unscreen the person.

25 Follow agency policy for soiled linen.

26 Wash your hands.

27 Report your observations to the nurse.

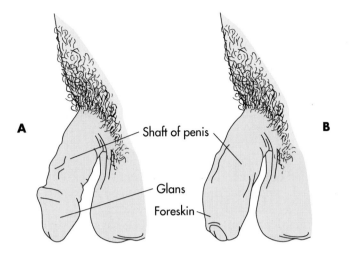

Fig. 16-12 A, Circumcised male. **B,** Uncircumcised male.

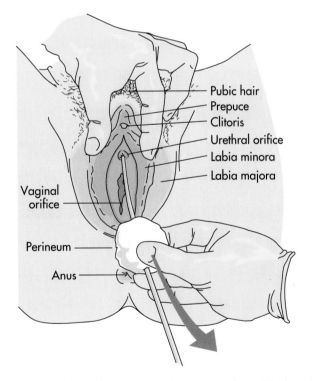

Fig. 16-13 The catheter is cleaned beginning at the meatus. About 4 inches of the catheter is cleaned.

▶ DRAINAGE SYSTEMS

A closed drainage system is used for indwelling catheters. That means that nothing can enter the system from the catheter to the drainage bag. Remember, the urinary system is sterile. Infection can occur if microbes enter the drainage system and travel up the tubing or catheter into the bladder and kidneys. Such an infection can seriously threaten the person's health and life.

The drainage system consists of a tubing and a drainage bag. The tubing is attached at one end to the catheter. At the other end, it is attached to the drainage bag.

The bag hangs from the bed frame, chair, or wheelchair. It must not touch the floor. The bag must always be lower than the level of the person's bladder (see Fig. 16-11). Some people wear leg bags when up. The bag is attached to the thigh or calf.

Urine provides an environment for the growth of microbes. If the bag is higher than the bladder, urine can flow back into the bladder. An infection can develop. Therefore do not hang the drainage bag on a bed rail. When the bed rail is raised, the bag is higher than bladder level. When the person ambulates, the bag is held lower than the bladder.

Sometimes catheters are disconnected accidentally. If that happens, tell the nurse immediately. Do not touch the ends of the catheter or tubing. Do the following:

- Wipe the end of the tube and the end of the catheter with antiseptic wipes. Use a separate wipe for the tube end and catheter end.
- Do not put the ends down. Do not touch the ends after you clean them.
- Connect the tubing to the catheter.
- Discard the wipes into a biohazard plastic bag.

Leg bags are switched to drainage bags when the person is in bed. This is so that the drainage bag is kept lower than bladder level. This means that you will have to open the closed drainage system. You must take measures to prevent microbes from entering the system.

Drainage bags are emptied at the end of every shift. They also are emptied when changing from a leg bag to a drainage bag or from a drainage bag to a leg bag. Always measure the contents of the leg bag or drainage bag. Also note the observations listed in Box 16-4.

Text continued on p. 396

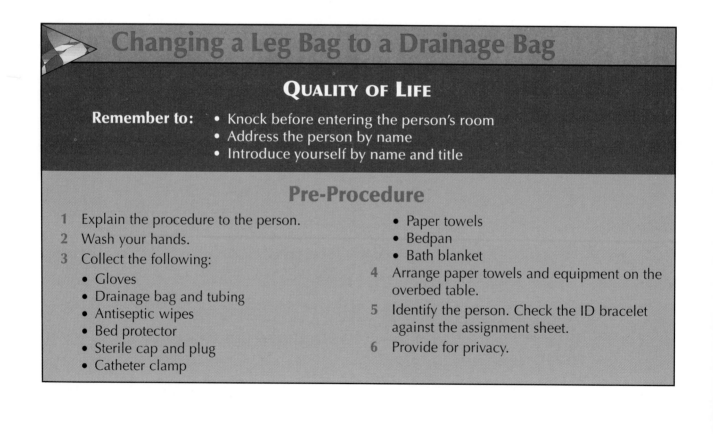

Changing a Leg Bag to a Drainage Bag

QUALITY OF LIFE

Remember to:
- Knock before entering the person's room
- Address the person by name
- Introduce yourself by name and title

Pre-Procedure

1 Explain the procedure to the person.
2 Wash your hands.
3 Collect the following:
- Gloves
- Drainage bag and tubing
- Antiseptic wipes
- Bed protector
- Sterile cap and plug
- Catheter clamp
- Paper towels
- Bedpan
- Bath blanket

4 Arrange paper towels and equipment on the overbed table.
5 Identify the person. Check the ID bracelet against the assignment sheet.
6 Provide for privacy.

Changing a Leg Bag to a Drainage Bag—cont'd

Procedure

7   Have the person sit on the side of the bed.

8   Put on the gloves

9   Expose the catheter and leg bag. Make sure the person is not exposed unnecessarily.

10 Clamp the catheter (Fig. 16-14, p. 394). This prevents urine from draining from the catheter into the drainage tubing.

11 Let urine drain from below the clamp site into the drainage tubing. This empties the lower end of the catheter.

12 Help the person lie down in bed.

13 Raise the bed rails. Then raise the bed to a level for good body mechanics.

14 Lower the bed rail near you.

15 Cover the person with a bath blanket. Expose the catheter and leg bag.

16 Place the bed protector under the person's leg.

17 Open the alcohol wipes. Set them on the paper towels.

18 Open the package with the sterile cap and plug. Set the package on the paper towels. Do not let anything touch the sterile cap or plug (Fig. 16-15, p. 394).

19 Open the package with the drainage bag and tubing.

20 Attach the drainage bag to the bed frame.

21 Disconnect the catheter from the drainage tubing. Do not let anything touch the ends.

22 Insert the sterile plug into the catheter end (Fig. 16-16, p. 394). Touch only the end of the plug. Do not touch the part that goes inside the catheter. (Wipe the catheter end with an antiseptic wipe if you accidentally contaminate the end of the catheter. Wipe the end before you insert the sterile plug.)

23 Place the sterile cap on the end of the leg bag drainage tube (see Fig. 16-16). (Wipe the tubing end with an antiseptic wipe if you accidentally contaminate the end of the catheter. Wipe the end before you insert the sterile plug.)

24 Remove the cap from the new drainage tubing.

25 Remove the sterile plug from the catheter.

26 Insert the end for the drainage tubing into the catheter.

27 Remove the clamp from the catheter.

28 Loop drainage tubing on the bed. Secure the tubing to the mattress.

29 Remove the leg bag. Place it in the bedpan.

30 Remove and discard the bed protector.

31 Cover the person, and remove the bath blanket. Raise the bed rails.

32 Take the bedpan to the bathroom.

33 Remove the gloves. Wash your hands.

Post-Procedure

34 Provide for comfort.

35 Place the signal light within reach.

36 Raise or lower bed rails. Follow the care plan.

37 Lower the bed to its lowest position.

38 Unscreen the person.

39 Put on clean gloves. Discard disposable supplies.

40 Empty the drainage bag (see *Emptying a Urinary Drainage Bag,* p. 395).

41 Discard the drainage tubing and bag following agency policy. If reusable, clean the bag following agency policy.

42 Clean the bedpan. Place it in a clean cover.

43 Remove the gloves, and wash your hands.

44 Return the bedpan and other supplies to their proper place.

45 Report your observations to the nurse.

46 Reverse the procedure to attach a leg bag to the catheter.

Fig. 16-14 The catheter is clamped.

Fig. 16-15 Sterile cap and catheter plug. The inside of the cap is sterile. It is inserted into the catheter. Touch only the end of the plug.

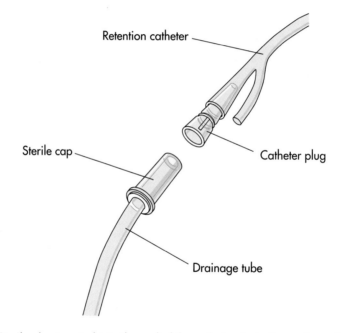

Fig. 16-16 Sterile plug inserted into the end of the catheter. A sterile cap is on the end of the drainage tube.

Emptying a Urinary Drainage Bag

QUALITY OF LIFE

Remember to:
- Knock before entering the person's room
- Address the person by name
- Introduce yourself by name and title

Pre-Procedure

1. Collect equipment:
   - Graduate (measuring container)
   - Gloves
   - Paper towels
2. Wash your hands.
3. Explain the procedure to the person.
4. Identify the person. Check the ID bracelet against the assignment sheet.
5. Provide for privacy.

Procedure

6. Put on the gloves.
7. Place a paper towel on the floor. Place the measuring container on top of the paper towel.
8. Place the measuring container (graduate) so urine is collected when you open the drain.
9. Open the clamp on the bottom of the drainage bag.
10. Let all urine drain into the graduate. Do not let the drain touch the graduate (Fig. 16-17).
11. Close the clamp. Replace the clamped drain in the holder on the bag (see Fig. 16-11).
12. Measure urine.
13. Remove and discard the paper towel.
14. Rinse the graduate, and return it to its proper place.
15. Remove the gloves, and wash your hands.
16. Record the time and amount on the I&O record (see Chapter 18).

Post-Procedure

17. Unscreen the person.
18. Report the amount and other observations to the nurse (Fig. 16-18).

Fig. 16-17 The clamp on the drainage bag is opened, and the drain is directed into the measuring container. The drain must not touch the inside of the container.

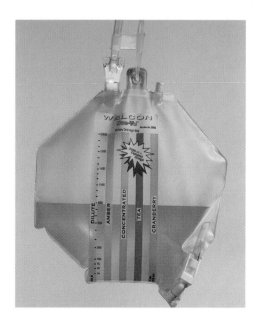

Fig. 16-18 This urinary drainage bag has a comparison chart for the color of urine. (*Courtesy of Welcon, Inc. Fort Worth, Tex.*)

THE CONDOM CATHETER

Condom catheters (external catheter, urinary sheath) are often used for incontinent men. A condom catheter is a soft, rubber sheath that slides over the penis. Tubing connects the condom catheter and the drainage bag. Many men prefer leg bags (Fig. 16-19).

A new condom catheter is applied daily. The manufacturer's instructions are followed. The penis is thoroughly washed with soap and water and dried before applying a new catheter. Elastic tape secures the catheter in place. Elastic tape expands when the penis changes size. This allows blood flow to the penis. *Never use adhesive tape to secure catheters. It does not expand. Blood flow to the penis is cut off, injuring the penis.* Medical asepsis, Standard Precautions, and the Bloodborne Pathogen Standard are followed when removing or applying condom catheters.

Fig. 16-19 A condom catheter attached to a leg bag.

Fig. 16-20 A condom catheter applied to the penis. There is a 1-inch space between the penis and the end of the catheter.

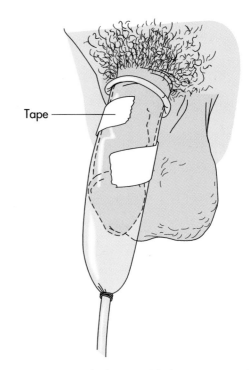

Fig. 16-21 Tape is applied in spiral fashion to secure the condom catheter to the penis.

Applying a Condom Catheter

QUALITY OF LIFE

Remember to:
- Knock before entering the person's room
- Address the person by name
- Introduce yourself by name and title

Pre-Procedure

1 Explain the procedure to the man.
2 Wash your hands.
3 Collect the following:
- Condom catheter
- Elastic tape
- Drainage bag or leg bag
- Cap for the drainage bag
- Basin of warm water
- Soap
- Towel and washcloths
- Bath blanket
- Gloves
- Bed protector
- Paper towels

4 Arrange paper towels and equipment on the overbed table.
5 Provide for privacy.
6 Identify the person. Check the ID bracelet against the assignment sheet.
7 Raise the bed to the best level for good body mechanics. Make sure bed rails are up.

Procedure

8 Lower the bed rail near you.
9 Cover the person with a bath blanket. Lower top linens to the knees.
10 Ask the person to raise his buttocks off the bed. Or turn him onto his side away from you.
11 Slide the bed protector under his buttocks.
12 Have the person lower his buttocks, or turn him onto his back.
13 Secure the drainage bag to the bed frame, or have a leg bag ready. Close the drain.
14 Expose the genital area.
15 Put on the gloves.
16 Remove the condom catheter:
  a Remove the tape and roll the sheath off the penis.
  b Disconnect the drainage tubing from the condom. Cap the drainage tube.
  c Discard the tape and condom.

17 Provide perineal care (see *Giving Male Perineal Care*, p. 348). Observe the penis for skin breakdown or irritation.
18 Remove the protective backing from the condom. This exposes the adhesive strip.
19 Hold the penis firmly. Roll the condom onto the penis. Leave a 1-inch space between the penis and the end of the catheter (Fig. 16-20).
20 Secure the condom with elastic tape. Apply tape in a spiral (Fig. 16-21). Do not apply tape completely around the penis.
21 Connect the condom to the drainage tubing. Coil excess tubing on the bed as shown in Figure 16-11, or attach a leg bag.
22 Remove the bed protector and gloves.
23 Return top linens, and remove the bath blanket.

Post-Procedure

24 Provide for comfort.
25 Place the signal light within reach.
26 Raise or lower bed rails. Follow the care plan.
27 Lower the bed to its lowest position.
28 Unscreen the person.
29 Wash your hands. Put on clean gloves.
30 Measure and record the amount of urine in the bag. Discard the collection bag and disposable items.
31 Clean and return the wash basin and other equipment. Return items to their proper place.
32 Remove the gloves, and wash your hands.
33 Report your observations to the nurse.

BLADDER TRAINING

Bladder training programs are developed for persons with urinary incontinence. Some persons need bladder training after indwelling catheter removal. Voluntary control of urination is the goal. The bladder training program is part of the nursing care plan. You assist with bladder training as directed by the nurse.

There are two basic methods for bladder training. With one, the person uses the toilet, commode, bedpan, or urinal at scheduled times. The person is given 15 or 20 minutes to start voiding. The rules for maintaining normal urination are followed. The normal position for urination is assumed if possible. Privacy is important.

The second method is used with catheters. Clamping the catheter prevents urine from draining out of the bladder. Usually the catheter is clamped for 1 hour at first. Eventually it is clamped for 3 to 4 hours at a time. Urine drains from the bladder when the catheter is unclamped. When the catheter is removed, urination is encouraged every 3 to 4 hours.

COLLECTING URINE SPECIMENS

Urine specimens (samples) are collected for urine tests. Doctors use test results to make a diagnosis or evaluate treatment. Each specimen sent to the laboratory needs a requisition slip. The slip has the person's identifying information and the required test. Box 16-5 lists the rules to follow when collecting specimens. (See Focus on Children box.)

Box 16-5	Rules for Collecting Urine Specimens

- Follow the rules of medical asepsis, Standard Precautions, and the Bloodborne Pathogen Standard.
- Use a clean container for each specimen.
- Use a container appropriate for the specimen.
- Label the container accurately. Write the person's full name, room and bed number, date, and time the specimen was collected.
- Do not touch the inside of the container or lid.
- Collect the specimen at the time specified.
- Ask the person not to have a bowel movement during specimen collection. The specimen must not contain feces.
- Ask the person to put toilet tissue in the toilet or wastebasket. The specimen must not contain tissue.
- Take the specimen and requisition slip to the laboratory or storage place. The specimen container should be in a plastic bag.

Focus On... CHILDREN

For infants and toddlers who are not toilet trained, a collection bag is applied to the genital area, see p. 405. Toilet-trained toddlers and young children have difficulty urinating into a collecting receptacle. Potty chairs and specimen pans are useful.

Urine specimens may embarrass older children and adolescents. They do not like clear specimen containers that show urine. Placing the urine specimen in a paper bag is often helpful.

▶ THE RANDOM URINE SPECIMEN

The random urine specimen is collected for a urin-alysis. No special measures are needed. It is collected at any time. Many people can collect the specimen themselves. Weak and very ill persons need assistance.

Fig. 16-22 The specimen pan is placed on the rim of the toilet. It has a color chart for urine. *(Courtesy Welcon, Inc., Fort Worth, Tex.)*

Collecting a Random Urine Specimen

QUALITY OF LIFE

Remember to:
- Knock before entering the person's room
- Address the person by name
- Introduce yourself by name and title

Pre-Procedure

1 Explain the procedure to the person.
2 Wash your hands.
3 Collect the following:
- Bedpan and cover, urinal, or specimen pan (Fig. 16-22)
- Specimen container and lid
- Label
- Gloves
- Plastic bag

Procedure

4 Fill out the label. Put it on the container.
5 Put the container and lid in the bathroom.
6 Identify the person. Check the ID bracelet against the requisition slip.
7 Provide for privacy.
8 Put on the gloves.
9 Ask the person to urinate in the receptacle. Remind him or her to put toilet tissue into the wastebasket or toilet, not in the bedpan or specimen pan.
10 Take the receptacle to the bathroom.
11 Measure urine if I&O is ordered.
12 Pour about 120 ml (4 oz) of urine into the specimen container. Dispose of excess urine.
13 Place the lid on the specimen container. Put the container in the plastic bag.
14 Clean and return the receptacle to its proper place.
15 Help the person wash the hands.
16 Remove the gloves.

Post-Procedure

17 Provide for comfort.
18 Place the signal light within reach.
19 Raise or lower bed rails. Follow the care plan.
20 Unscreen the person.
21 Wash your hands.
22 Report your observations to the nurse.
23 Take the specimen and the requisition slip to the storage area or laboratory.

▶ THE MIDSTREAM SPECIMEN

The midstream specimen is also called a *clean-voided specimen* or a *clean-catch specimen*. The perineal area is cleaned before collecting the specimen. This reduces the number of microbes in the urethral area during specimen collection. The person starts to void into the toilet, bedpan, urinal, or commode. Then the stream is stopped and a sterile specimen container positioned. The person voids into the container until the specimen is obtained.

Stopping the stream of urine is hard for many people. You may need to position and hold the specimen container in place after the person starts to void.

Fig. 16-23 The labia are separated to collect a midstream specimen.

▶ Collecting a Midstream Specimen

QUALITY OF LIFE

Remember to:
- Knock before entering the person's room
- Address the person by name
- Introduce yourself by name and title

Pre-Procedure

1. Explain the procedure to the person.
2. Wash your hands.
3. Collect the following:
   - Clean-voided specimen kit with sterile specimen container
   - Label
   - Antiseptic solution
   - Disposable gloves
   - Sterile gloves (if not part of the kit)
   - Bedpan, urinal, or commode if the person cannot use the bathroom
   - Plastic bag
   - Supplies for perineal care
4. Label the container with the requested information.
5. Identify the person. Check the ID bracelet against the requisition slip.
6. Provide for privacy.

Collecting a Midstream Specimen—cont'd

Procedure

7 Let the person complete perineal care if able. Place the signal light within reach.

8 Provide perineal care if the person cannot.

9 Open the sterile kit using sterile technique.

10 Put on the sterile gloves.

11 Pour the antiseptic solution over the cotton balls.

12 Open the sterile specimen container. Do not touch the inside of the container or lid. Set the lid down so the inside is up.

13 Clean the perineum with cotton balls if the person cannot:

   a *Female:*

   (1) Spread the labia with your thumb and index finger. Use your nondominant hand. (This hand is now contaminated and must not touch anything sterile.)

   (2) Clean down the urethral area from front to back. Use a clean cotton ball for each stroke.

   (3) Keep the labia separated to collect the urine specimen (steps 15 and 16).

   b *Male:*

   (1) Hold the penis with your nondominant hand.

   (2) Clean the penis starting at the meatus. Use a cotton ball, and clean in a circular motion. Start at the center, and work outward.

   (3) Keep holding the penis until the specimen is collected (steps 15 and 16).

14 Ask the person to start urinating into the toilet, bedpan, commode, or urinal.

15 Pass the specimen container into the stream of urine. Keep the labia separated (Fig. 16-23).

16 Collect about 30 to 60 ml of urine (1 to 2 oz).

17 Remove the specimen container before the person stops urinating.

18 Release the labia or penis.

19 Let the person finish urinating into the toilet, bedpan, commode, or urinal.

20 Put the lid on the specimen container. Touch only the outside of the container or lid.

21 Wipe the outside of the container.

22 Place the container in a plastic bag.

23 Provide toilet tissue after the person finishes urinating.

24 Remove and empty the bedpan, commode container, or urinal.

25 Clean the bedpan, urinal, or commode container and other equipment. Return equipment to its proper place.

26 Remove soiled gloves. Put on clean gloves.

27 Let the person wash his or her hands.

28 Remove the gloves.

Post-Procedure

29 Follow Steps 17-23 in *Collecting a Random Urine Specimen.*

THE 24-HOUR URINE SPECIMEN

All urine voided during a 24-hour period is collected for a 24-hour urine specimen. Urine is chilled on ice or refrigerated during the collection period. This prevents the growth of microbes. A preservative is added to the collection container for some tests.

The person voids to begin the test; this voiding is discarded. *All* voidings during the next 24 hours are collected. The person and nursing staff must clearly understand the procedure and test period. The rules for collecting urine specimens are followed.

Collecting a 24-Hour Urine Specimen

QUALITY OF LIFE

Remember to:
- Knock before entering the person's room
- Address the person by name
- Introduce yourself by name and title

Pre-Procedure

1 Review the procedure with the nurse.
2 Explain the procedure to the person.
3 Wash your hands.
4 Collect the following:
- Urine container for a 24-hour collection
- Preservative from the laboratory if needed
- Bucket with ice if needed
- Two 24-hour urine specimen labels
- Funnel
- Bedpan, urinal, commode, or specimen pan
- Gloves
- Measuring containers

Collecting a 24-Hour Urine Specimen—cont'd

Procedure

5 Label the specimen container.

6 Identify the person. Check the ID bracelet against the requisition slip.

7 Arrange equipment in the person's bathroom or dirty utility room.

8 Place one 24-hour specimen label in the bathroom or dirty utility room. Place the other near the bed.

9 Put on the gloves.

10 Offer the bedpan or urinal, or assist the person to the bathroom or bedside commode.

11 Ask the person to void.

12 Discard the specimen, and note the time. This starts the 24-hour collection period.

13 Clean the bedpan, urinal, commode, or specimen pan.

14 Remove the gloves.

15 Mark the time the test began and the time it ends on the room and bathroom labels. Also mark the specimen container.

16 Ask the person to use the bedpan, urinal, commode, or specimen pan when voiding during the next 24 hours. Tell the person to signal after voiding. Remind him or her not to have a bowel movement at the same time and not to put toilet tissue in the receptacle.

17 Put on the gloves.

18 Measure all urine if I&O is ordered.

19 Pour urine into the specimen container, using the funnel. Do not spill any urine. Restart the test if you spill or discard urine.

20 Clean the bedpan, urinal, commode, or specimen pan. Remove the gloves.

21 Add ice to the bucket as necessary.

22 Ask the person to void at the end of the 24-hour period. Pour the urine into the specimen container.

23 Thank the person for cooperating.

Post-Procedure

24 Provide for comfort.

25 Place the signal light within reach.

26 Raise or lower bed rails. Follow the care plan.

27 Remove the labels from the room and bathroom. Clean and return equipment to its proper place. Discard disposable items.

28 Wash your hands.

29 Report your observations to the nurse.

30 Take the specimen and requisition slip to the laboratory.

▶ THE DOUBLE-VOIDED SPECIMEN

Fresh-fractional urine specimen is another term for a double-voided specimen. The person voids twice. The first time the bladder is emptied of "stale" urine. "Fresh" urine collects in the bladder after the first voiding. In 30 minutes the person voids again. The second voiding is usually a very small or "fractional" amount of urine.

Fresh-fractional specimens are used to test urine for glucose and ketones.

▶ Collecting a Double-Voided Specimen

QUALITY OF LIFE

Remember to:
- Knock before entering the person's room
- Address the person by name
- Introduce yourself by name and title

Pre-Procedure

1   Explain the procedure to the person.
2   Wash your hands.
3   Collect the following:
- Bedpan, urinal, commode, or disposable specimen pan
- Two specimen containers
- Urine testing equipment
- Gloves

4   Identify the person. Check the ID bracelet against the assignment sheet.
5   Provide for privacy.

Procedure

6   Put on the gloves.
7   Ask the person to urinate in the receptacle. Remind him or her to put toilet tissue into the wastebasket or toilet, not in the bedpan or specimen pan.
8   Take the receptacle to the bathroom.
9   Measure urine if I&O is ordered. Pour some urine into the specimen container.
10 Test the specimen in case you cannot obtain a second specimen. Discard the urine.
11 Clean the receptacle. Remove the gloves.
12 Return the receptacle to its proper place.
13 Help the person wash the hands.
14 Ask the person to drink an 8-ounce glass of water.
15 Provide for comfort. Raise the bed rails if needed. Place the signal light within reach, and unscreen the person.
16 Wash your hands.
17 Return to the room in 20 to 30 minutes.
18 Repeat steps 5 through 17.
19 Report the results of the second test and any other observations to the RN.

COLLECTING A SPECIMEN FROM AN INFANT OR CHILD

Sometimes specimens are needed from infants and children who are not toilet trained. A collection bag is applied over the urethra. A parent or another staff member assists if the child is agitated.

Collecting a Urine Specimen From an Infant or Child

QUALITY OF LIFE

Remember to:
- Knock before entering the person's room
- Address the person by name
- Introduce yourself by name and title

Pre-Procedure

1 Explain the procedure to the child and parents.
2 Wash your hands.
3 Collect the following:
   - Collection bag
   - Wash basin
   - Cotton balls
   - Bath towel
   - Two diapers
   - Specimen container
   - Gloves
   - Plastic bag
   - Scissors
4 Identify the child. Check the ID bracelet against the requisition slip.
5 Provide for privacy.

Procedure

6 Put on the gloves.
7 Remove and dispose of the diaper.
8 Clean the perineal area. Use a new cotton ball for each stroke. Rinse and dry the area.
9 Put on clean gloves.
10 Position the child on the back. Flex the child's knees, and separate the legs.
11 Remove the adhesive backing from the collection bag.
12 Apply the bag to the perineum. Do not cover the anus (Fig. 16-24, p. 406).
13 Cut a slit in the bottom of a new diaper.
14 Diaper the child.
15 Pull the collection bag through the slit in the bottom of the diaper.
16 Remove the gloves.
17 Raise the head of the crib if allowed. This helps urine to collect in the bottom of the bag.
18 Raise the crib rail and unscreen the child.
19 Return to the room periodically. Check the bag to see if the child has urinated. (Wear gloves, and provide for privacy.)
20 Provide privacy if the child has urinated.
21 Lower the crib rail.
22 Remove the diaper.
23 Remove the collection bag gently.
24 Press the adhesive surfaces of the bag together. Or transfer urine to the specimen container through the drainage tab.
25 Clean the perineal area, rinse, and dry well.
26 Diaper the child.
27 Remove the gloves, and wash your hands.

Continued

Collecting a Urine Specimen From an Infant or Child—cont'd

Post-Procedure

28 Provide for comfort. Raise the bed rail.

29 Unscreen the child.

30 Write the requested information on the specimen container. Place the container in the plastic bag.

31 Clean and return equipment to its proper place. Discard disposable items. (Wear gloves for this step.)

32 Wash your hands.

33 Report your observations to the nurse.

34 Take the requisition slip and the specimen to the storage area or laboratory.

Fig. 16-24 A disposable collection bag is applied to the perineal area of the infant. Urine collects in the bag for a specimen.

TESTING URINE

The nurse may ask you to do simple urine tests. You can test for pH, glucose, ketones, blood, and specific gravity using reagent strips. Straining urine for stones is another simple test. You must be accurate when testing urine. Promptly report the results to the nurse.

- *Testing for pH*—Urine pH measures if urine is acidic or alkaline. Changes in normal pH (4.6 to 8.0) occur from illness, foods, and drugs. Use reagent strips to test for urine pH. A routine urine specimen is needed.

- *Testing for glucose and ketones*—*Diabetes mellitus* is a chronic disease in which the pancreas fails to secrete enough insulin (see Chapter 30). The body needs insulin to use sugar for energy. Sugar builds up in the blood if it cannot be used. Some sugar appears in the urine. **Glucosuria** or **glycosuria** means sugar *(glucos, glycos)* in the urine *(uria)*. The diabetic person may also have **acetone (ketone bodies, ketones)** in the urine. These appear in urine because of the rapid breakdown of fat for energy. The body uses fat for energy if it cannot use sugar. Urine is also tested for ketones. The doctor orders the type and frequency of urine tests. They are usually done four times a day: 30 minutes before each meal (ac) and at bedtime (HS). The doctor uses the test results to regulate the person's medication and diet. Double-voided specimens are best for testing urine for sugar and ketones. Reagent strips are used for testing.

- *Testing for blood*—Normal urine is free of blood. Injury and disease can cause blood *(hemat)* to appear in the urine *(uria)*. This is called **hematuria.** Sometimes blood is seen in the urine. At other times it is unseen *(occult).* You use reagent strips to test for occult blood. A routine urine specimen is needed.

► USING REAGENT STRIPS

Reagent strips have different sections that change color when they react with urine. To use a reagent strip, dip the strip into urine. Then compare the strip with the color chart on the bottle (Fig. 16-25). The nurse gives you specific instructions for the urine test ordered. You must read the manufacturer's instructions before you begin.

Fig. 16-25 Reagent strip for sugar and ketones.

Testing Urine With Reagent Strips

QUALITY OF LIFE

Remember to:
- Knock before entering the person's room
- Address the person by name
- Introduce yourself by name and title

Pre-Procedure

1 Explain the procedure to the person.

2 Wash your hands.

3 Identify the person. Check the ID bracelet against the assignment sheet.

Procedure

4 Put on the gloves.

5 Collect the following:
- Urine specimen (routine specimen for pH, occult blood, and specific gravity; double-voided specimen for sugar and ketones)
- Reagent strip as ordered
- Gloves

6 Remove a strip from the bottle. Put the cap on the bottle immediately. Make sure it is tight.

7 Dip the strip test areas into the specimen.

8 Remove the strip after the correct amount of time (see the manufacturer's instructions).

9 Tap the strip gently against the container to remove excess urine.

10 Wait the required amount of time (see the manufacturer's instructions).

11 Compare the strip with the color chart on the bottle. Read the results.

12 Discard disposable items and the specimen.

Post-Procedure

13 Clean and return equipment to its proper place.

14 Remove the gloves, and wash your hands.

15 Report the results and other observations to the nurse.

▶ STRAINING URINE

Stones (calculi) can develop in the kidneys, ureters, or bladder. Stones vary in size. Some are pinhead size; others are the size of an orange. Stones causing severe pain and damage to the urinary system may require surgical removal. Some stones exit the body through urine. Therefore all of the person's urine is strained. Passed stones are sent to the laboratory for examination.

Fig. 16-26 A disposable strainer is placed in a specimen container. Urine is poured through the strainer into the specimen container.

Straining Urine

QUALITY OF LIFE

Remember to:
- Knock before entering the person's room
- Address the person by name
- Introduce yourself by name and title

Pre-Procedure

1. Explain the procedure to the person. Also explain that the urinal, bedpan, commode, or specimen pan is used for voiding.
2. Wash your hands.
3. Collect the following:
   - Strainer or 4 × 4 gauze
   - Specimen container
   - Urinal, bedpan, commode, or specimen pan
   - Two labels stating that all urine is strained
   - Gloves
   - Plastic bag
4. Identify the person. Check the ID bracelet against the assignment sheet.

Procedure

5. Arrange items in the person's bathroom.
6. Place one label in the bathroom. Place the other near the bed.
7. Put on the gloves.
8. Offer the bedpan or urinal. Or assist the person to the bedside commode or bathroom.
9. Provide for privacy.
10. Tell the person to signal after voiding.
11. Remove the gloves, and wash your hands.
12. Return when the person signals for you. Knock before entering the room.
13. Put on gloves.
14. Place the strainer or gauze into the specimen container.
15. Pour urine into the specimen container. Urine passes through the strainer or gauze (Fig. 16-26).
16. Discard the urine.
17. Place the strainer or gauze in the container if any crystals, stones, or particles appear.
18. Help the person clean the perineal area if necessary.
19. Clean and return equipment to its proper place.
20. Remove soiled gloves. Wash your hands, and put on clean gloves.
21. Help the person wash the hands.
22. Remove the gloves.

Post-Procedure

23. Provide for comfort.
24. Place the signal light within reach.
25. Raise or lower bed rails. Follow the care plan.
26. Unscreen the person.
27. Label the specimen container with the requested information. Put the container in the plastic bag. (Wear gloves for this step.)
28. Wash your hands.
29. Report your observations to the nurse.
30. Take the specimen and requisition slip to the laboratory.

Circle the BEST answer.

1. Which is *false?*
   A. Urine is normally clear and yellow or amber in color.
   B. Urine normally has an ammonia odor.
   C. Micturition usually occurs before going to bed and on rising.
   D. A person normally voids about 1500 ml a day.

2. Which is *not* a rule for maintaining normal elimination?
   A. Help the person assume a normal position for urination.
   B. Provide for privacy.
   C. Help the person to the bathroom or commode, or provide the bedpan or urinal as soon as requested.
   D. Always stay with the person who is on a bedpan.

3. The best position for using a bedpan is
   A. Fowler's position
   B. The supine position
   C. The prone position
   D. The side-lying position

4. After a man uses the urinal, he should
   A. Put the urinal on the bedside stand
   B. Use the signal light
   C. Put the urinal on the overbed table
   D. Empty the urinal

5. Urinary incontinence
   A. Is always permanent
   B. Requires good skin care
   C. Is treated with an indwelling catheter
   D. Requires tests for sugar and ketones

6. A person has an indwelling catheter. Which is *incorrect?*
   A. Keep the drainage bag above the level of the bladder.
   B. Make sure the drainage tubing is free of kinks.
   C. Coil the drainage tubing on the bed.
   D. Tape the catheter to the inner thigh.

7. A person has an indwelling catheter. Which is *incorrect?*
   A. Tape any leaks at the connection site.
   B. Follow the rules of medical asepsis and Standard Precautions.
   C. Empty the drainage bag at the end of each shift.
   D. Report complaints of pain, burning, the need to urinate, or irritation immediately.

8. Mr. Powers has a condom catheter. You apply elastic tape
   A. Completely around the penis
   B. To the inner thigh
   C. To the abdomen
   D. In a spiral fashion

9. The goal of bladder training is to
   A. Remove the catheter
   B. Allow the person to walk to the bathroom
   C. Gain voluntary control of urination
   D. All of the above

10. When collecting a urine specimen, you should do the following *except*
    A. Label the container with the requested information
    B. Use the correct container
    C. Collect the specimen at the time specified
    D. Use sterile supplies

11. The perineum is cleaned immediately before collecting a
    A. Random specimen
    B. Midstream specimen
    C. 24-hour urine specimen
    D. Double-voided specimen

12. A 24-hour urine specimen involves
    A. Collecting all urine voided by a person during a 24-hour period
    B. Collecting a random specimen every hour for 24 hours
    C. A catheterization
    D. Testing the urine for sugar and acetone

13. Urine is tested for sugar and ketones
    A. At bedtime
    B. 30 minutes after meals and at bedtime
    C. 30 minutes before meals and at bedtime
    D. Before breakfast

14. Which specimen is best for sugar and ketone testing?
    A. A random specimen
    B. A clean-voided specimen
    C. A 24-hour urine specimen
    D. A double-voided specimen

15. You are instructed to strain Mr. Powers' urine. You know that straining urine is done to find
    A. Hematuria
    B. Stones
    C. Nocturia
    D. Urgency

Answers to these questions are on p. 836.

CHAPTER 17

BOWEL ELIMINATION

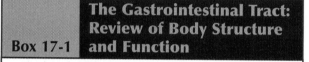Like urinary elimination, bowel elimination is a basic physical need. Many factors affect bowel elimination. They include privacy, personal habits, age, diet, exercise and activity, fluids, and drugs. Problems easily occur. Promoting normal bowel elimination is important. You will assist patients and residents in meeting their elimination needs. See Box 17-1 for a review of the gastrointestinal tract.

NORMAL BOWEL MOVEMENTS

The frequency of bowel movements varies from person to person. Some have a bowel movement every day. Others have one every 2 to 3 days. Some people have 2 or 3 bowel movements a day. The elimination pattern also involves the time of day. Many people defecate after breakfast, others in the evening.

Stools are normally brown in color. Bleeding in the stomach and small intestine causes black or tarry stools. Bleeding in the lower colon and rectum causes red-colored stools. So do beets. A diet high in green vegetables can cause green stools. Diseases and infection can also cause clay-colored or white, pale, orange-colored, or green-colored stools.

Stools are normally soft, formed, moist, and shaped like the rectum. They have a characteristic odor. The odor is from bacterial action in the intestines. Certain foods and drugs also cause odors.

OBSERVATIONS

The RN uses your observations for the nursing process. Therefore stools are carefully observed before disposal. Ask the nurse to observe abnormal stools. You need to observe stools and report the following to the nurse: color, amount, consistency, odor, shape, size, frequency of defecation, and any complaints of pain.

Box 17-1	The Gastrointestinal Tract: Review of Body Structure and Function

The gastrointestinal (GI) tract is part of the digestive system (see Chapter 6). Bowel elimination is the excretion of wastes from the GI tract. Foods and fluids are normally taken in through the mouth and are partially digested in the stomach. The partially digested foods and fluids are called *chyme*. Chyme passes from the stomach into the small intestine. Further digestion and absorption of nutrients occur as the chyme passes through the small bowel. Chyme eventually enters the large intestine (large bowel or colon), where fluid is absorbed. There the chyme becomes less fluid and more solid in consistency. **Feces** refers to the semisolid mass of waste products in the colon.

Feces move through the intestines by peristalsis. **Peristalsis** is the alternating contraction and relaxation of intestinal muscles. The feces move through the large intestine to the rectum. Feces are stored in the rectum until excreted from the body (Fig. 17-1). **Defecation** (bowel movement) is the process of excreting feces from the rectum through the anus. The term **stool** refers to feces that have been excreted.

See Chapter 6 for more detailed information.

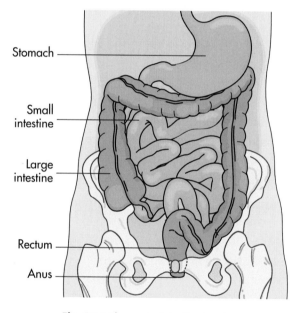

Fig. 17-1 The gastrointestinal system.

FACTORS AFFECTING BOWEL ELIMINATION

Normal, regular defecation is affected by many factors. The following factors affect the frequency, consistency, color, and odor of stools. The RN considers these factors when using the nursing process to meet the person's elimination needs. Normal, regular elimination is the goal:

- *Privacy*—Like voiding, bowel elimination is a private act. Lack of privacy prevents many people from defecating despite having the urge. Bowel movement odors and sounds are embarrassing. Ignoring the urge to defecate can lead to constipation.
- *Personal habits*—Many people routinely have a bowel movement after breakfast. Some drink a hot beverage, read a book or newspaper, or take a walk. These activities relax the person. Defecation is easier when a person is relaxed rather than tense.
- *Diet*—A well-balanced diet and bulk are needed. High-fiber foods leave a residue that provides needed bulk. Fruits, vegetables, and whole grain cereals and breads are high in fiber. Certain foods can cause diarrhea or constipation. Milk causes constipation in some people and diarrhea in others. Other milk products and chocolate can cause similar reactions. Spicy foods can irritate the intestines. Frequent stools or diarrhea can result. Gas-forming foods stimulate peristalsis. Increased peristalsis results in defecation. Gas-forming foods include onions, beans, cabbage, cauliflower, radishes, and cucumbers.
- *Fluids*—Feces contain water. Stool consistency depends on the amount of water absorbed in the large intestine. The amount of fluid ingested, urine output, and vomiting are factors. Feces become hard and dry when large amounts of water are absorbed or when fluid intake is poor. Hard, dry feces move through the intestines at a slower rate. Constipation can occur. Drinking 6 to 8 glasses of water every day promotes normal bowel elimination. Warm fluids—coffee, tea, hot cider, and warm water—increase peristalsis.
- *Activity*—Exercise and activity maintain muscle tone and stimulate peristalsis. Irregular elimination and constipation often occur from inactivity and bedrest. Inactivity may result from disease, surgery, injury, and aging.

Focus On... CHILDREN

Infants and toddlers do not have voluntary control of bowel movements. Defecation occurs whenever feces enter the rectum. Bowel training is learned between 2 and 3 years of age.

Focus On... OLDER PERSONS

Aging causes changes in the gastrointestinal system. Feces pass through the intestine at a slower rate. Constipation is a risk. Body changes from aging cause some older persons to lose control over defecation. Older persons are also at risk for intestinal tumors and disorders.

Older persons do not always completely empty the rectum. They often need to use the bathroom, commode, or bedpan again. This usually occurs about 30 to 45 minutes after the first bowel movement.

Many older persons expect to have a bowel movement every day. The slightest irregularity concerns them. The nurse provides teaching about normal elimination.

- *Medications*—Drugs can prevent constipation or control diarrhea. Other drugs have diarrhea or constipation as side effects. Drugs for pain relief often cause constipation. Antibiotics, used to fight or prevent infection, often cause diarrhea. Diarrhea occurs when the antibiotics kill normal flora in the large intestine. Normal flora is necessary in forming stools.
- *Age*—Age affects bowel elimination. (*See Focus on Children box and Focus on Older Persons box.*)

COMMON PROBLEMS

Many factors affect normal bowel elimination. Common problems include constipation, fecal impaction, diarrhea, anal incontinence, and flatulence.

CONSTIPATION

Constipation is the passage of a hard, dry stool. The person usually strains to have a bowel movement. Stools are large or marble-size. Large stools cause pain as they pass through the anus. Constipation occurs when feces move through the intestine slowly. This allows more time for water absorption. Common causes include a low-fiber diet, ignoring the urge to defecate, decreased fluid intake, inactivity, drugs, aging, and certain diseases. Dietary changes, fluids, activity, enemas, and medications prevent or relieve constipation.

▶ FECAL IMPACTION

A **fecal impaction** is the prolonged retention and accumulation of feces in the rectum. Feces are hard or puttylike in consistency. Fecal impaction results if constipation is not relieved. The person cannot defecate. More water is absorbed from the already hardened feces. Liquid seeping from the anus is a sign of fecal impaction. Liquid feces pass around the hardened fecal mass in the rectum.

The person tries many times to have a bowel movement. Abdominal discomfort, cramping, and rectal pain are common. A digital examination is done to check for an impaction. (Digital refers to a finger.) This is done by inserting a gloved finger into the rectum and feeling for a hard mass (Fig. 17-2). The mass is felt in the lower rectum. Sometimes it is higher in the colon and out of reach. The digital examination often produces the urge to defecate. The doctor may order drugs and enemas to remove the impaction.

Often it is necessary to remove the fecal mass with a lubricated, gloved finger. This is called *digital removal of an impaction*. A doctor's order is required. A finger is inserted into the rectum and the finger hooked around a piece of feces. Then the finger and stool are removed. The stool is dropped into the bedpan. The process is repeated until the impaction is removed. The procedure is uncomfortable and embarrassing for most people.

Checking for and removing impactions are very dangerous. The vagus nerve in the rectum can be stimulated. This nerve also affects the heart. Stimulation of the vagus nerve slows the heart rate. The heart rate can slow to dangerous levels in some persons. In some agencies, assistive personnel check for and remove impactions. Before you perform these procedures make sure that:

- Your state allows you to perform them
- They are in your job description
- You have the necessary education and training
- You review the procedure with a nurse
- A nurse is available to answer questions and to supervise you

You must be very careful and gentle. Rectal bleeding can occur with both procedures. You must follow Standard Precautions and the Bloodborne Pathogen Standard.

Fig. 17-2 An index finger is used to check for a fecal impaction.

Checking for a Fecal Impaction

QUALITY OF LIFE

Remember to:
- Knock before entering the person's room
- Address the person by name
- Introduce yourself by name and title

Pre-Procedure

1. Explain the procedure to the person.
2. Wash your hands.
3. Collect the following:
   - Bedpan and bedpan cover
   - Bath blanket
   - Toilet tissue
   - Gloves
   - Lubricant
   - Waterproof pad
   - Basin of warm water
   - Soap
   - Washcloth
   - Bath towel
4. Identify the person. Check the ID bracelet against the assignment sheet.
5. Provide for privacy.
6. Raise the bed to the best level for body mechanics. Make sure bed rails are up.

Procedure

7. Lower the bed rail near you.
8. Cover the person with a bath blanket. Fan-fold top linens to the foot of the bed.
9. Position the person in the Sims' position, or in a left side-lying position.
10. Place the waterproof pad under the buttocks.
11. Put on the gloves.
12. Expose the anal area.
13. Lubricate your gloved index finger.
14. Ask the person to take a deep breath through his or her mouth.
15. Insert the gloved finger while the person is taking a deep breath.
16. Check for a fecal mass.
17. Withdraw your finger.
18. Help the person onto the bedpan or to the bathroom or commode if needed. Provide for privacy. See *Giving the Bedpan*, p. 379 or *Helping the Person to the Commode*, p. 385.
19. Remove and discard the gloves. Wash your hands.
20. Put on clean gloves.
21. Wash the person's anal area with soap and water. Pat dry.
22. Remove the waterproof pad.
23. Provide for comfort.

Post-Procedure

24. Return top linens, and remove the bath blanket.
25. Place the signal light within the person's reach.
26. Lower the bed to its lowest position.
27. Raise or lower bed rails. Follow the care plan.
28. Unscreen the person.
29. Clean and return equipment to its proper place. Discard disposable items.
30. Follow agency policy for soiled linen.
31. Remove the gloves, and wash your hands.
32. Report your observations to the nurse.

Removing a Fecal Impaction

QUALITY OF LIFE

Remember to:
- Knock before entering the person's room
- Address the person by name
- Introduce yourself by name and title

Procedure

1 Follow steps 1 through 13 in *Checking for a Fecal Impaction,* p. 417.

2 Check the person's pulse. Note the rate and rhythm.

3 Ask the person to take a deep breath through the mouth.

4 Insert your lubricated, gloved index finger.

5 Hook your index finger around a small piece of feces.

6 Remove your finger and the feces.

7 Drop the stool into the bedpan.

8 Clean your finger with toilet tissue. Reapply lubricant as needed.

9 Repeat steps 2 through 7 until you no longer feel feces. Check the person's pulse at intervals using your clean gloved hand. Note the rate and rhythm. Stop the procedure and call for the nurse if the pulse rate has slowed or if the rhythm is irregular.

10 Wipe the anal area with toilet tissue.

11 Cover the person with the bath blanket.

12 Cover the bedpan.

13 Remove and discard the gloves. Put on clean gloves.

14 Raise the bed rail. Take the bedpan to the bathroom.

15 Empty, clean, and disinfect the bedpan.

16 Return the bedpan to the bedside stand.

17 Remove and discard the gloves. Wash your hands.

18 Fill the wash basin with warm water.

19 Return to the bedside, and lower the bed rail near you.

20 Put on clean gloves.

21 Wash the buttocks, and give perineal care.

22 Remove the waterproof pad. Also remove your gloves.

Post-Procedure

23 Provide for comfort.

24 Return top linens, and remove the bath blanket.

25 Place the signal light within the person's reach.

26 Lower the bed to its lowest position.

27 Raise or lower bed rails. Follow the care plan.

28 Unscreen the person.

29 Clean and return equipment to its proper place. Discard disposable items. Wear gloves for this step.

30 Follow agency policy for soiled linen.

31 Remove the gloves, and wash your hands.

32 Report your observations to the nurse.

DIARRHEA

Diarrhea is the frequent passage of liquid stools. Feces move through the intestines rapidly. This reduces the time for fluid absorption. The need to defecate is urgent. Some people cannot get to a bathroom in time. Abdominal cramping, nausea, and vomiting may also occur.

Causes of diarrhea include infections, certain drugs, irritating foods, and microbes in food and water. Diet and drugs reduce peristalsis. Nursing measures include promptly assisting the person to the bathroom or providing the commode or bedpan. Stools require prompt disposal to reduce odors and prevent the spread of microbes. Good skin care is essential. Liquid feces are very irritating to the skin. So is frequent wiping of the anal area with toilet tissue. Skin breakdown and pressure ulcers are risks if cleanliness and good skin care are not practiced.

Fluid lost through diarrhea is replaced. Otherwise dehydration occurs. **Dehydration** is the excessive loss of water from tissues. Signs and symptoms include pale or flushed skin, dry skin, coated tongue, oliguria (scant amount of urine), thirst, weakness, dizziness, and confusion. Falling blood pressure and increased pulse and respirations are serious signs. The RN uses the nursing process to meet the person's fluid needs. The doctor orders intravenous fluids in severe cases.

Microbes often cause diarrhea. Preventing the spread of infection is important. Always practice Standard Precautions when in contact with stools.

(See Focus on Children and Focus on Older Persons boxes below.)

FECAL INCONTINENCE

Fecal incontinence (anal incontinence) is the inability to control the passage of feces and gas through the anus. Causes include intestinal diseases and nervous system diseases and injuries. Fecal impaction, diarrhea, and some drugs are other causes. Persons with mental health problems or cognitive disorders (Chapters 31 and 32) may not recognize the need or act of defecating. Fecal incontinence also can result from unanswered signal lights when the person needs to use the bathroom, commode, or bedpan. When in a new setting, it is hard for some people to find the bathroom in time.

Good skin care is required. A bowel training program may be developed. Providing the bedpan or commode after meals or every 2 to 3 hours may be helpful. Waterproof pads or incontinence products keep linens and clothes clean. Fecal incontinence affects the person emotionally. Frustration, embarrassment, anger, and humiliation are common emotions. *(See Focus on Children and Focus on Older Persons boxes below.)*

Focus On... CHILDREN

Infants and toddlers normally have fecal incontinence until toilet trained.

Focus On... OLDER PERSONS

Some older persons suffer from dementia. They may smear feces on themselves, furniture, and walls. Some do not know when they are having bowel movements. Resisting care is a common problem. It may be hard to keep the person clean. Follow the person's care plan. Also talk to the nurse if you have problems keeping the person clean.

Focus On... CHILDREN

The bodies of infants and young children contain large amounts of water. They are at risk for dehydration. Death can occur quickly. Report any liquid or watery stool to the nurse immediately. Ask the nurse to observe the stool. Also note the number of wet diapers. Infants wet less when dehydrated.

Focus On... OLDER PERSONS

Older persons also are at risk for dehydration. The amount of body water decreases with aging. Many diseases common in older persons also affect body fluids. So do many drugs. Report any signs of diarrhea to the nurse immediately. Ask the nurse to observe the stool. Death is a risk from unrecognized and untreated dehydration.

FLATULENCE

Gas and air are normally found in the stomach and intestines. They are expelled through the mouth (belching, eructating) and anus. Gas and air passed through the anus is called **flatus**. **Flatulence** is the excessive formation of gas or air in the stomach and intestines. Common causes are:

- Swallowing air while eating and drinking (This includes chewing gum, eating fast, drinking through a straw, and drinking carbonated beverages. Tense or anxious people may swallow large amounts of air when drinking.)
- Bacterial action in the intestines
- Gas-forming foods (onions, beans, cabbage, cauliflower, radishes, cucumbers)
- Constipation
- Bowel and abdominal surgeries
- Drugs that decrease peristalsis

If flatus is not expelled, the intestines distend. That is, they swell or enlarge from the pressure of the gases. Abdominal cramping or pain, shortness of breath, and a swollen abdomen occur. "Bloating" is a common complaint. Walking and the left side-lying position often produce flatus. Doctors may order enemas, medications, or rectal tubes to relieve flatulence.

COMFORT AND SAFETY DURING ELIMINATION

Certain measures help promote normal bowel elimination. The RN uses the nursing process to meet the person's elimination needs. The nursing care plan may include measures that involve diet, fluids, and exercise. The actions listed in Box 17-2 are routinely practiced to promote comfort and safety during bowel elimination.

BOWEL TRAINING

Bowel training has two goals. One is to gain control of bowel movements. The other is to develop a regular pattern of elimination. Fecal impaction, constipation, and fecal incontinence are prevented.

The urge to defecate is usually felt after a meal, usually breakfast. Toilet, commode, or bedpan use is encouraged at this time. Other factors that promote elimination are included in the nursing care plan and bowel training program. These include a high-fiber diet, increased fluids, warm fluids, activity, and privacy. The nurse tells you about a person's bowel training program.

Box 17-2	Comfort and Safety During Bowel Elimination

- Help the person to the toilet or commode or provide the bedpan as soon as requested. If the person cannot walk, the nurse may have you wheel the person into the bathroom on the commode. The commode is placed over the toilet. This provides the person with privacy.
- Provide for privacy. Ask visitors to leave the room. Close doors, pull curtains around the bed, and pull window curtains or shades. Remember, defecation is a private act. Leave the room if the person can be alone.
- Make sure the bedpan is warm.
- Position the person in a normal sitting or squatting position.
- Cover the person for warmth and privacy.
- Allow enough time for defecation.
- Place the signal light and toilet tissue within the person's reach.
- Stay nearby if the person is weak or unsteady.
- Provide perineal care.
- Dispose of feces promptly. This reduces odors and prevents the spread of microbes.
- Let the person wash the hands after defecating and wiping with toilet tissue.
- Assist the person to the bathroom or commode or offer the bedpan after meals if the person has the problem of incontinence.
- Practice Standard Precautions, and follow the Bloodborne Pathogen Standard.

The doctor may order a suppository to stimulate defecation. A **suppository** is a cone-shaped, solid medication that is inserted into a body opening. It melts at body temperature. The rectal suppository is inserted into the rectum by a nurse (Fig. 17-3). A bowel movement occurs about 30 minutes later. Enemas are sometimes ordered.

ENEMAS

An **enema** is the introduction of fluid into the rectum and lower colon. Enemas are ordered by doctors. They are given to remove feces and to relieve constipation or fecal impaction. They also are ordered to clean the bowel of feces before certain surgeries, x-ray procedures, or childbirth. Sometimes enemas are ordered to relieve flatulence and intestinal distention. Bowel training programs can involve enemas.

Enemas are usually safe procedures. Many people give themselves enemas at home. However, enemas are dangerous for older persons and those with certain heart and kidney diseases. Comfort and safety measures are practiced when giving an enema. The rules in Box 17-3 also are followed.

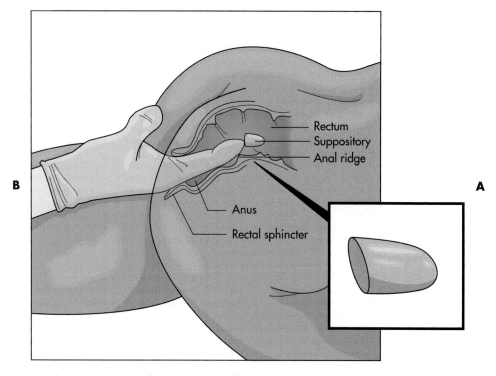

Fig. 17-3 A, A rectal suppository, **B,** The suppository is inserted into the rectum.

Box 17-3	**Comfort and Safety Measures for Giving Enemas**

- Solution temperature for adults is 105° F (40.5° C). The temperature should be 98.6° F (37° C) for children. Measure the temperature with a bath thermometer. Ask the nurse what the temperature should be for the person.
- The amount of solution given depends on the enema's purpose and the person's age. Adults generally receive 500 to 1000 ml. The doctor orders the amount of solution to be given. *(See Focus on Children box, p. 422.)*
- The Sims' position or a comfortable left side-lying position is preferred.
- For adults, the enema bag is raised 12 inches above the anus. For infants, the bag is raised no more than 3 inches above the anus. Ask the nurse how high to raise the bag for the person.
- The nurse and agency manual tell you how far to insert the enema tubing. In the adult, the tubing is usually inserted 3 to 4 inches but never more than 6 inches. *(See Focus on Children box, p. 422.)* Enema tubing can injure the intestine. Stop inserting the tube if you feel resistance, the person complains of pain, or bleeding occurs.

- The solution is given slowly. Usually it takes 10 to 15 minutes to give 750 to 1000 ml.
- The solution should be retained in the bowel for a certain length of time. The length of time depends on the amount and type of solution. Ask the nurse how long the person should retain the enema solution.
- The enema tube is held in place while giving the solution.
- The bathroom must be vacant when the person has the urge to defecate. Make sure that the bathroom will not be used by another person.
- The nurse observes the enema results.
- Standard Precautions and the Bloodborne Patho-gen Standard are followed.

Some states allow assistive personnel to give enemas. Others do not. Before giving an enema, make sure that:

- Your state allows you to perform the procedure
- The procedure is in your job description
- You have the necessary education and training
- You review the procedure with a nurse
- A nurse is available to answer questions and to supervise you

ENEMA SOLUTIONS

The enema solution is ordered by the doctor. The kind of solution ordered depends on the purpose of the enema:

- *Tap-water enema*—obtained from a faucet.
- *Soapsuds enema (SSE)*—add 5 ml of castile soap to 1000 ml of tap water.
- *Saline enema*—add 2 teaspoons of table salt to 1000 ml of tap water.
- *Oil-retention enema*—mineral oil or a commercial oil-retention enema is used.
- *Commercial enema*—contains about 120 ml (4 ounces) of solution.

Other enema solutions may be ordered. Consult with the nurse and use the agency procedure manual to safely prepare and give uncommon enemas. Do not administer enemas that contain drugs. Nurses give these enemas.

▶ THE CLEANSING ENEMA

Cleansing enemas clean the bowel of feces and flatus. They are sometimes given before surgery, x-ray procedures, and childbirth. The doctor orders a soapsuds, tap-water, or saline enema. The doctor may order *enemas until clear*. This means that enemas are given until the return solution is clear and free of fecal material. Ask the nurse how many enemas to give. Agency policy may allow repeating cleansing enemas only 2 or 3 times.

Tap-water enemas can be dangerous. The large intestine may absorb some of the water into the bloodstream. This creates a fluid imbalance in the body. Only one tap-water enema is given. Do not repeat the enema. Repeated enemas increase the risk of excessive fluid absorption.

Soapsuds enemas are very irritating to the bowel's mucous lining. Repeated enemas can damage the bowel. Using more than 5 ml (1 teaspoon) of castile soap or using stronger soaps also can damage the bowel.

The saline enema solution is similar to body fluid. However, some of the salt solution may be absorbed. This too can cause a fluid imbalance. When there is excess salt in the body, the body retains water. (*See Focus on Children box.*)

Text continued on p. 426

Focus On... CHILDREN

Only saline enemas are used for children. The amount of enema solution varies for infants and children. Always check with the nurse for the amount of solution to give. The following are guidelines:

- Infants—50 to 250 ml
- Toddlers—200 to 300 ml
- School-age children—300 to 500 ml
- Adolescents—500 to 1000 ml

Ask the nurse about tube size. The following are size guidelines:

- Infants—#10 to #12 (10 to 12 Fr)
- Toddlers—#14 to #16 (14 to 16 Fr)
- School-age children—#16 to #18 (16 to 18 Fr)

In children, enema solutions are given at body temperature (98.6° F, 37° C). In infants, the tube is inserted 1 inch. In toddlers, the tube is inserted 2 inches. Also ask the nurse how high to raise the enema bag. In infants, the bag should be only 3 inches above the anus.

Giving a Cleansing Enema

QUALITY OF LIFE

Remember to:
- Knock before entering the person's room
- Address the person by name
- Introduce yourself by name and title

Pre-Procedure

1. Explain the procedure to the person.
2. Wash your hands.
3. Collect the following:
   - Bedpan or commode
   - Disposable enema kit (enema bag, tube, clamp, and waterproof pad); for adults, the tube size is #22 to #30 (22 to 30 Fr)
   - Bath thermometer
   - Waterproof pad
   - Water-soluble lubricant
   - Gloves
   - Material for enema solution: 5 ml (1 teaspoon) castile soap or 2 teaspoons of salt
   - Toilet tissue
   - Bath blanket
   - IV pole
   - Robe and shoes or nonskid slippers
   - Specimen container if needed
   - Paper towels
4. Identify the person. Check the ID bracelet against the assignment sheet.
5. Provide for privacy.
6. Raise the bed to the best level for good body mechanics. Make sure bed rails are up.

Procedure

7. Lower the bed rail near you.
8. Cover the person with a bath blanket. Fanfold top linens to the foot of the bed.
9. Position the IV pole so the enema bag is above the anus:
   a. Adults—12 inches above the anus
   b. Infants—3 inches above the anus
10. Raise the bed rail.
11. Prepare the enema:
    a. Close the clamp on the tube.
    b. Adjust water flow until it is lukewarm.
    c. Fill the enema bag to the 1000-ml mark or as otherwise ordered.
    d. Measure water temperature. For adults it should be 105° F (40.5° C).
    e. Prepare the enema solution:
       (1) Saline enema: add 2 teaspoons of salt
       (2) Soapsuds enema: add 5 ml (1 teaspoon) of castile soap
       (3) Tap-water enema: add nothing to the water
    f. Stir the solution with the bath thermometer. Scoop off any suds (SSE).
    g. Seal the top of the bag.
    h. Hang the bag on the IV pole.
12. Lower the bed rail near you.
13. Position the person in the Sims' position or in a comfortable left side-lying position.
14. Place a waterproof pad under the buttocks.
15. Put on the gloves.
16. Expose the anal area.
17. Place the bedpan behind the person.
18. Position the enema tube in the bedpan. Open the clamp. Let solution flow through the tube to remove air. Clamp the tube.
19. Lubricate the tube with the lubricant. For adults, lubricate 3 to 4 inches from the tip or as directed by the nurse.
20. Separate the buttocks to see the anus.
21. Ask the person to take a deep breath through the mouth.
22. Insert the tube gently 3 to 4 inches into the adult rectum or to a distance directed by the nurse when the person is exhaling (Fig. 17-4, p. 425). Stop and call for the nurse if the person complains of pain, if you feel resistance, or if bleeding occurs.

Continued

Giving a Cleansing Enema—cont'd

Procedure—cont'd

23 Check how much solution is in the enema bag.

24 Unclamp the tube, and administer the solution slowly (Fig. 17-5, p. 425).

25 Ask the person to take slow, deep breaths. This helps the person relax while the enema is given.

26 Clamp the tube if the person needs to defecate, has abdominal cramping, or starts to expel solution. Unclamp when symptoms subside.

27 Give the amount of solution ordered. Stop if the person cannot tolerate the procedure.

28 Clamp the tube before it is empty. This prevents air from entering the bowel.

29 Hold several thicknesses of toilet tissue around the tube and against the anus. Remove the tube.

30 Discard the soiled toilet tissue into the bedpan.

31 Wrap the tubing tip with paper towels, and place it inside the enema bag.

32 Help the person onto the bedpan. Raise the head of the bed. Raise or lower the bed rails according to the care plan. Or assist the person to the bathroom or commode. The person wears a robe and shoes or nonskid slippers when up. The bed is in the lowest position.

33 Place the signal light and toilet tissue within reach. Remind the person not to flush the toilet.

34 Discard disposable items.

35 Remove the gloves, and wash your hands.

36 Leave the room if the person can be left alone.

37 Return when the person signals. Knock before entering. Lower the bed rail.

38 Observe enema results for amount, color, consistency, and odor.

39 Put on the gloves.

40 Obtain a stool specimen if ordered.

41 Provide perineal care as needed.

42 Remove the bed protector.

43 Empty, clean, and disinfect the bedpan or commode. Flush the toilet after the nurse observes the results. Return items to their proper place. Remove the gloves, and wash your hands.

44 Help the person wash the hands. Wear gloves for this step if necessary.

45 Return top linens, and remove the bath blanket.

Post-Procedure

46 Provide for comfort.

47 Place the signal light within reach.

48 Lower the bed to its lowest position.

49 Raise or lower bed rails. Follow the care plan.

50 Unscreen the person.

51 Follow agency policy for soiled linen and used supplies.

52 Wash your hands.

53 Report your observations.

Colon

Rectum

Anus

Tubing

Fig. 17-4 The enema tubing inserted into the adult.

Fig. 17-5 An enema is given in the Sims' position. The IV pole is positioned so that the enema bag is 12 inches above the anus and 18 inches above the mattress.

► THE COMMERCIAL ENEMA

Commercial enemas irritate and distend the rectum. This causes defecation. They are often ordered for constipation or when complete cleansing of the bowel is not needed.

Manufacturers prepare and package the commercial enema. It is ready to give. The solution is usually given at room temperature. However, the nurse may have you warm the enema in a basin of warm water.

To give the enema, squeeze and roll up the plastic bottle from the bottom. Do not release pressure on the bottle. Otherwise solution is drawn from the rectum back into the bottle. Encourage the person to retain the solution until feeling the urge to defecate. Remaining in the Sims' or left side-lying position helps retain the enema longer.

Fig. 17-6 The tip of the commercial enema is inserted 2 inches into the rectum.

Giving a Commercial Enema

QUALITY OF LIFE

Remember to:
- Knock before entering the person's room
- Address the person by name
- Introduce yourself by name and title

Pre-Procedure

1 Explain the procedure to the person.
2 Wash your hands.
3 Collect the following:
- Commercial enema
- Bedpan or commode
- Waterproof pad
- Toilet tissue
- Gloves
- Bath blanket

4 Identify the person. Check the ID bracelet against the assignment sheet.
5 Provide for privacy.
6 Raise the bed to the best level for good body mechanics. Make sure bed rails are raised.

Procedure

7 Lower the bed rail near you.
8 Cover the person with a bath blanket. Fan-fold top linens to the foot of the bed.
9 Position the person in the Sims' or a comfortable left side-lying position.
10 Place the waterproof pad under the buttocks.
11 Put on the gloves.
12 Expose the anal area.
13 Position the bedpan near the person.
14 Remove the cap from the enema tip.
15 Separate the buttocks to see the anus.
16 Ask the person to take a deep breath through the mouth.
17 Insert the enema tip 2 inches into the rectum when the person is exhaling (Fig. 17-6).
18 Squeeze and roll the bottle gently. Release pressure on the bottle *after* you remove the tip from the rectum.
19 Put the bottle into the box, tip first.
20 Help the person onto the bedpan; raise the head of the bed. Raise or lower bed rails according to the care plan. Or assist the person to the bathroom or commode. The person wears a robe and shoes or nonskid slippers when up, and the bed is in the lowest position.
21 Place the signal light and toilet tissue within reach. Remind the person not to flush the toilet.
22 Discard used disposable items. Remove the gloves, and wash your hands.
23 Leave the room if the person can be left alone.
24 Return when the person signals. Knock before entering. Lower the bed rail.
25 Observe enema results for amount, color, consistency, and odor.
26 Put on gloves.
27 Help the person clean the perineal area if indicated.
28 Remove the bed protector.
29 Empty, clean, and disinfect the bedpan or commode. Flush the toilet after the nurse observes the results. Return equipment to its proper place. Remove the gloves, and wash your hands.
30 Help the person wash the hands. Wear gloves for this step if necessary.

Post-Procedure

31 Follow steps 46 through 53 in *Giving a Cleansing Enema.*

▶ THE OIL-RETENTION ENEMA

Oil-retention enemas are given for constipation or fecal impactions. The oil is retained for 30 to 60 minutes to soften feces and lubricate the rectum. This allows feces to pass with ease. Most oil-retention enemas are commercially prepared.

Giving an Oil-Retention Enema

QUALITY OF LIFE

Remember to:
- Knock before entering the person's room
- Address the person by name
- Introduce yourself by name and title

Pre-Procedure

1 Explain the procedure to the person.
2 Wash your hands.
3 Collect the following:
   - Commercial oil-retention enema
   - Waterproof pad
   - Gloves
   - Bath blanket

4 Identify the person. Check the ID bracelet against the assignment sheet.
5 Provide for privacy.
6 Raise the bed to the best level for good body mechanics. Make sure bed rails are up.

Procedure

7 Lower the bed rail near you.
8 Cover the person with a bath blanket. Fanfold top linens to the foot of the bed.
9 Position the person in the Sims' or left side-lying position.
10 Place a waterproof pad under the buttocks.
11 Put on the gloves.
12 Expose the anal area.
13 Remove the cap from the enema tip.
14 Separate the buttocks to see the anus.
15 Ask the person to take a deep breath through the mouth.
16 Insert the tip 2 inches into the rectum when the person is exhaling. Insert the tip gently.
17 Squeeze and roll the bottle slowly and gently. Release pressure on the bottle *after* you remove the tip from the rectum.
18 Put the bottle in the box, tip first.

19 Cover the person. Leave him or her in the Sims' or side-lying position.
20 Encourage him or her to retain the enema for the time ordered.
21 Place additional waterproof pads on the bed if needed.
22 Remove the gloves.
23 Lower the bed to its lowest position.
24 Raise or lower bed rails. Follow the care plan.
25 Provide for comfort. Place the signal light within reach.
26 Unscreen the person.
27 Follow agency policy for soiled linen and used supplies.
28 Wash your hands.
29 Report your observations.
30 Check the person often.

RECTAL TUBES

A rectal tube is inserted into the rectum to relieve flatulence and intestinal distention. Flatus passes from the body without effort or straining. The rectal tube is inserted 6 inches into the adult rectum. It is left in place for 20 to 30 minutes. This helps prevent rectal irritation. It can be reinserted every 2 to 3 hours. The nurse tells you when to insert the tube and how long to leave it in place. *Rectal tubes are not used after rectal surgery.*

Size #22 to #30 (22 to 30 Fr) tubes are used for adults. (Tubes are sized in the French scale. The abbreviation "Fr" means French. Either *Fr* follows the number or the # sign is before the number.) *(See Focus on Children box.)*

Often the tube is connected to a flatus bag or to a container with water (Fig. 17-7). The bag inflates as gas passes into it. If the tube is connected to a container with water, the water bubbles as gas passes through the tube into the water. For this system, the rectal tube is attached to connecting tubing. The connecting tubing attaches to the water container.

Feces may be expelled along with flatus. If a flatus bag is not used, place the open end of the tube in a folded waterproof pad.

Focus On... CHILDREN

Smaller rectal tubes are used for children. Sizes range from #10 to #18 (10 to 18 Fr). The tube is inserted 2 to 4 inches into the child's rectum. The nurse tells you what size to use and how far to insert the tube.

Fig. 17-7 The tube is inserted 6 inches into the adult rectum. The rectal tube is taped to the buttocks. The flatus bag rests on the bed.

Inserting a Rectal Tube

QUALITY OF LIFE

Remember to:
- Knock before entering the person's room
- Address the person by name
- Introduce yourself by name and title

Pre-Procedure

1 Explain the procedure to the person.
2 Wash your hands.
3 Collect the following:
   - Disposable rectal tube with flatus bag
   - Water-soluble lubricant
   - Tape
   - Gloves
   - Waterproof pad
4 Identify the person. Check the ID bracelet against the assignment sheet.
5 Provide for privacy.
6 Raise the bed to the best level for good body mechanics. Make sure bed rails are up.

Procedure

7 Lower the bed rail near you.
8 Position the person in the Sims' or left side-lying position.
9 Place the waterproof pad under the buttocks.
10 Put on the gloves.
11 Expose the anal area.
12 Lubricate the tip of the tube. For adults, lubricate 6 inches.
13 Separate the buttocks to see the anus.
14 Ask the person to take a deep breath through the mouth.
15 Insert the tube 6 inches into the adult rectum when the person is exhaling. Stop if person complains of pain or if you feel resistance. Insert the tube gently.
16 Tape the rectal tube to the buttocks.
17 Position the flatus bag so it rests on the bed protector (see Fig. 17-7).
18 Cover the person.
19 Leave the tube in place no longer than 30 minutes.
20 Lower the bed to its lowest position. Place the signal light within reach. Raise or lower bed rails according to the care plan.
21 Remove the gloves, and wash your hands.
22 Leave the room. Check the person often.
23 Return to the room in 30 minutes. Knock before entering the room.
24 Put on gloves, and remove the tube. Wipe the rectal area.
25 Wrap the rectal tube and flatus bag in the bed protector. Remove the bed protector and your gloves.
26 Ask the person about the amount of gas expelled.

Post-Procedure

27 Provide for comfort.
28 Place the signal light within reach.
29 Unscreen the person.
30 Discard disposable items. Follow agency policy for soiled linen. Wear gloves for this step.
31 Remove the gloves, and wash your hands.
32 Report your observations to the nurse.

THE PERSON WITH AN OSTOMY

Sometimes surgical removal of part of the intestines is necessary. Cancer, diseases of the bowel, and trauma (such as stab or bullet wounds) are common reasons for intestinal surgery. An ostomy is sometimes necessary. An **ostomy** is the surgical creation of an artificial opening. The opening is called a **stoma.** The person wears a pouch over the stoma to collect feces and flatus. Stomas do not have nerve endings and are not painful. You will not hurt the person when touching the stoma.

You may assist the nurse with the person's postoperative care. Some states let assistive personnel change ostomy pouches. Before changing an ostomy pouch, make sure that:

- Your state allows you to perform the procedure
- The procedure is in your job description
- You have the necessary education and training
- You review the procedure with a nurse
- A nurse is available to answer questions and to supervise you

COLOSTOMY

A **colostomy** is the surgical creation of an artificial opening *(stomy)* between the colon *(colo)* and abdominal wall. Part of the colon is brought out onto the abdominal wall and a stoma made. Feces and flatus pass through the stoma rather than the anus. Colostomies are permanent or temporary. If the colostomy is permanent, the diseased part of the colon is removed. A temporary colostomy gives the diseased or injured bowel time to heal. After healing, surgery is done to reconnect the bowel.

The colostomy site depends on the site of colon disease or injury. Figure 17-8 shows common colostomy sites. Stools consistency ranges from liquid to formed. The more colon remaining to absorb water, the more solid and formed the stool. If the colostomy is near the beginning of the colon, stools are liquid. A colostomy near the end of the large intestine results in formed stools.

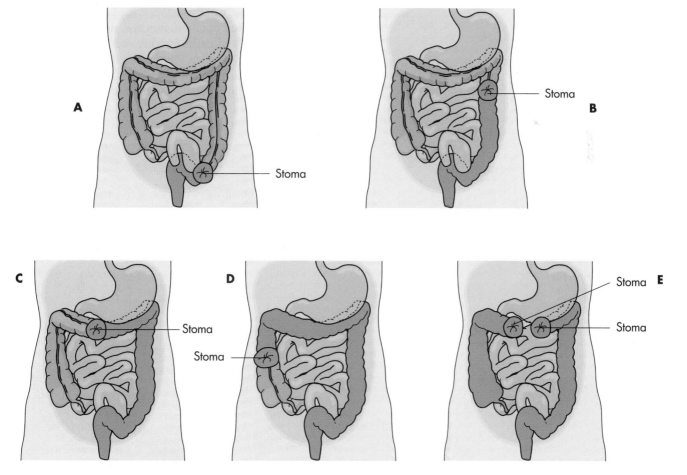

Fig. 17-8 Colostomy sites. *Shading* shows the part of the bowel that was surgically removed. **A,** Sigmoid colostomy. **B,** Descending colostomy. **C,** Transverse colostomy. **D,** Ascending colostomy. **E,** Double-barrel colostomy. Two stomas are created: one allows for the excretion of fecal material. The other is for the introduction of medicine to help the bowel heal. This type of colostomy is usually temporary.

Feces irritate the skin. Skin care prevents skin breakdown around the stoma. The skin is washed and dried when the pouch is removed. Then a skin barrier is applied around the stoma. The skin barrier prevents feces from coming in contact with the skin. The skin barrier may be part of the pouch or a separate device.

ILEOSTOMY

An **ileostomy** is the surgical creation of an artificial opening (stomy) between the ileum (small intestine [ileo]) and the abdominal wall. Part of the ileum is brought out onto the abdominal wall and a stoma made. The entire large intestine is removed (Fig. 17-9). Liquid feces drain constantly from an ileostomy. Water is not absorbed because the colon was removed. Feces in the small intestine contain digestive juices that are very irritating to the skin. The ileostomy pouch must fit well so feces do not touch the skin. Good skin care is essential.

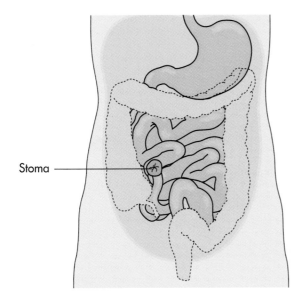

Fig. 17-9 An ileostomy. The entire large intestine is surgically removed.

 Ostomy Pouches. The pouch has an adhesive backing that is applied to the skin. Sometimes pouches are secured to ostomy belts (Fig. 17-10). Many pouches have a drain at the bottom that is closed with clips, clamps, or wire closures. The drain is opened to empty the pouch of feces (see Fig. 17-10). The pouch is emptied when $\frac{1}{3}$ to $\frac{1}{2}$ full. It is also opened when it balloons or bulges with flatus. The drain is wiped with toilet tissue before it is closed.

The pouch is changed every 3 to 7 days. Some people change the pouch whenever soiling occurs. Many people manage their colostomies without help.

Odors are prevented. Good hygiene is essential. The pouch is emptied when feces are present. Avoiding gas-forming foods also control odors. Special deodorants can be put into the pouch. The nurse tells you what to use.

The person can wear normal clothes with an ostomy pouch. However, tight undergarments can interfere with feces being expelled into the pouch. Also, bulging from feces and flatus can be seen with tight clothes.

Peristalsis increases after eating. Therefore stomas are usually quieter before breakfast. That is, expelling feces is less likely at this time. If the person showers or bathes with the pouch off, it is best done before breakfast. Showers and baths are delayed 1 or 2 hours after applying a new pouch. This gives the adhesive backing on the pouch time to stick to the skin.

Do not flush pouches down the toilet. Follow agency policy for disposing of used pouches. *(See Focus on Children box.)*

Focus On... CHILDREN

Children of all ages can have ostomies, even premature infants. If changing a child's ostomy pouch is delegated to you, the nurse will give you the necessary instructions.

Fig. 17-10 The ostomy pouch is secured to an ostomy belt. The pouch is emptied by directing it into the toilet and unclamping the end.

Changing an Ostomy Pouch

Pre-Procedure

1. Explain the procedure to the person.
2. Wash your hands.
3. Collect the following:
   - Clean pouch with skin barrier
   - Skin barrier (if not part of the pouch)
   - Pouch clamp, clip, or wire closure
   - Clean ostomy belt (if used)
   - Skin barrier as ordered
   - Gauze squares or wash cloths
   - Adhesive remover
   - Cotton balls
   - Bedpan with cover
   - Waterproof pad
   - Bath blanket
   - Toilet tissue
   - Wash basin
   - Bath thermometer
   - Prescribed soap or cleansing agent
   - Pouch deodorant
   - Paper towels
   - Gloves
   - Disposable bag
4. Arrange your work area.
5. Identify the person. Check the ID bracelet against the assignment sheet.
6. Provide for privacy.
7. Raise the bed to the best level for good body mechanics. Make sure bed rails are up.

Procedure

8. Lower the bed rail near you.
9. Cover the person with a bath blanket. Fan-fold linens to the foot of the bed.
10. Place the waterproof pad under the buttocks.
11. Put on the gloves.
12. Disconnect the pouch from the belt if one is worn. Remove the belt.
13. Remove the pouch gently. Gently push the skin down and away from the skin barrier. Place the pouch in the bedpan.
14. Wipe around the stoma with toilet tissue or a gauze square. This removes mucus and feces. Place soiled tissue or gauze in the bedpan.
15. Moisten a cotton ball with adhesive remover. Clean around the stoma to remove any remaining skin barrier. Clean from the stoma outward.
16. Cover the bedpan, and take it to the bathroom. (Raise the bed rail before you leave the bedside.)
17. Measure feces as directed by the nurse. Ask the nurse to observe abnormal feces. Then empty the pouch and bedpan into the toilet. Note the color, amount, consistency, and odor of feces. Put the pouch in the disposable bag.
18. Remove the gloves, and wash your hands. Put on clean gloves.
19. Fill the wash basin with warm water. Place the basin on the overbed table on top of the paper towels. Lower the bed rail near you.
20. Clean the skin around the stoma with water. Rinse and pat dry. Use soap or other cleansing agent as directed by the nurse.
21. Apply the skin barrier if it is a separate device.
22. Put a clean ostomy belt on the person if a belt is worn.
23. Add deodorant to the new pouch.
24. Remove adhesive backing on the pouch.

Continued

Changing an Ostomy Pouch—cont'd

Procedure—cont'd

25 Center the pouch over the stoma. Make sure the drain points downward.

26 Press around the skin barrier so the pouch seals to the skin. Apply gentle pressure from the stoma outward.

27 Maintain pressure for 1 to 2 minutes.

28 Connect the belt to the pouch (if a belt is worn).

29 Remove the waterproof pad.

30 Remove the gloves.

31 Cover the person. Remove the bath blanket.

Post-Procedure

32 Provide for comfort.

33 Raise or lower bed rails. Follow the care plan.

34 Lower the bed to its lowest position.

35 Place the signal light within reach.

36 Unscreen the person.

37 Clean the bedpan, wash basin, and other equipment. Wear gloves for this step.

38 Return equipment to its proper place.

39 Discard the disposable bag according to agency policy. Follow agency policy for soiled linen.

40 Remove the gloves, and wash your hands.

41 Report your observations to the nurse. Normally the stoma is red like mucous membranes.

► STOOL SPECIMENS

When internal bleeding is suspected, feces are checked for blood. Stools are also studied for fat, microbes, worms, and other abnormal contents. The rules for collecting urine specimens (see Chapter 16) apply when collecting stool specimens. Standard Precautions and the Bloodborne Pathogen Standard are followed.

The stool specimen must not be contaminated with urine. Some tests require a warm stool. The specimen is taken to the laboratory immediately if a warm stool is needed.

► Collecting a Stool Specimen

QUALITY OF LIFE

Remember to:
- Knock before entering the person's room
- Address the person by name
- Introduce yourself by name and title

Pre-Procedure

1. Explain the procedure to the person.
2. Wash your hands.
3. Collect the following:
   - Bedpan and cover (two bedpans if the person needs to urinate) or bedside commode
   - Urinal
   - Specimen pan for the toilet or commode
   - Specimen container and lid
   - Tongue blade
   - Disposable bag
   - Gloves
   - Toilet tissue
   - Laboratory requisition slip
   - Plastic bag

Procedure

4. Label the container with the requested information.
5. Identify the person. Check the ID bracelet against the requisition slip.
6. Provide for privacy.
7. Offer the bedpan or urinal for voiding.
8. Assist the person onto the bedpan or to the toilet or commode. Place the specimen pan under the toilet seat (Fig. 17-11, p. 436). The person wears a robe and shoes or non-skid slippers when up.
9. Ask the person not to put toilet tissue in the bedpan, commode, or specimen pan. Provide a disposable bag for toilet tissue.
10. Place the signal light and toilet tissue within reach. Raise or lower bed rails according to the care plan.
11. Wash your hands, and leave the room.
12. Return when the person signals. Knock before entering.
13. Lower the bed rail near you.
14. Put on the gloves. Provide perineal care if necessary.
15. Use a tongue blade to take about 2 tablespoons of feces from the bedpan, commode, or specimen pan to the specimen container (Fig. 17-12, p. 436).
16. Put the lid on the specimen container. Do not touch the inside of the lid or container. Place the container in the plastic bag.
17. Place the tongue blade in the disposable bag.
18. Empty, clean, and disinfect the bedpan, commode container, or specimen pan. Remove the gloves, and wash your hands.
19. Return equipment to its proper place.
20. Help the person wash the hands. Wear gloves for this step if necessary.

Continued

Collecting a Stool Specimen—cont'd

Post-Procedure

21 Provide for comfort.
22 Place the signal light within reach.
23 Lower the bed to its lowest position.
24 Raise or lower bed rails. Follow the care plan.
25 Unscreen the person.
26 Take the specimen and requisition slip to the laboratory.
27 Wash your hands.
28 Report your observations to the nurse.

Fig. 17-11 A specimen pan is placed in the toilet for a stool specimen.

Fig. 17-12 A tongue blade is used to transfer a small amount of stool from the bedpan to the specimen container.

TESTING STOOLS FOR BLOOD

Blood can appear in stools for many reasons. Ulcers, colon cancer, and hemorrhoids are common causes. Often blood is visible. Blood can usually be seen if bleeding is low in the gastrointestinal tract. Stools are black and tarry if there is bleeding in the stomach or upper GI tract. **Melena** is a black, tarry stool.

Sometimes bleeding occurs in very small amounts. It is difficult to detect such bleeding by just observing the stools. Therefore stools are often tested for the presence of *occult blood*. Occult means *hidden* or *unseen*. The test is commonly done to screen for colon cancer.

There are many types of tests. You must follow the manufacturer's instructions for the test ordered. Also follow Standard Precautions and the Bloodborne Pathogen Standard. The nurse tells you when to collect the specimen. Many factors can affect the test results. One is eating red meat. Therefore the person cannot eat red meat for 3 days before the test. Bleeding from hemorrhoids and menstrual periods also affect the test results.

Testing a Stool Specimen for Blood

QUALITY OF LIFE

Remember to:
- Knock before entering the person's room
- Address the person by name
- Introduce yourself by name and title

Pre-Procedure

1 Explain the procedure to the person.

2 Wash your hands.

Procedure

3 Collect a stool specimen (see *Collecting a Stool Specimen,* p. 435).

4 Collect the following:
- Paper towel
- Hemoccult test kit (includes developer)
- Tongue blades
- Gloves

5 Put on the gloves.

6 Open the test kit.

7 Use a tongue blade to obtain a small amount of stool.

8 Apply a thin smear of stool on box **A** on the test paper (Fig. 17-13, *A*, p. 438).

9 Use another tongue blade to obtain some feces from another part of the specimen.

10 Apply a thin smear of stool on box **B** on the test paper (Fig. 17-13, *B*, p. 438).

11 Close the test packet.

12 Turn the test packet to the other side. Open the flap. Apply developer to boxes **A** and **B**. Follow the manufacturer's instructions (Fig. 17-13, *C*, p. 438).

13 Wait the amount of time noted in the manufacturer's instructions. Time can vary from 10 to 60 seconds.

14 Note and record the color changes (Fig. 17-13, *D*, p. 438). Follow the manufacturer's instructions.

15 Dispose of the test packet.

16 Discard the tongue blade.

17 Dispose of the specimen.

18 Remove the gloves, and wash your hands.

19 Report the test results and your observations to the nurse.

Fig. 17-13 Testing for occult blood. **A,** Stool is smeared on box A. **B,** Stool is smeared on box B. **C,** Developer is applied to boxes A and B. **D,** Color changes are noted.

Circle the BEST answer.

1. Which is *false?*
   A. A person must have a bowel movement every day.
   B. Stools are normally brown, soft, and formed.
   C. Diarrhea occurs when feces move through the intestines rapidly.
   D. Constipation results when feces move through the large intestine slowly.

2. The prolonged retention and accumulation of feces in the rectum is called
   A. Constipation
   B. Fecal impaction
   C. Diarrhea
   D. Anal incontinence

3. Which will *not* promote comfort and safety in relation to bowel elimination?
   A. Asking visitors to leave the room
   B. Helping the person assume a sitting position
   C. Offering the bedpan after meals
   D. Telling the person that you will return very soon

4. Bowel training is aimed at
   A. Gaining control of bowel movements and developing a regular elimination pattern
   B. Ostomy control
   C. Preventing fecal impaction, constipation, and anal incontinence
   D. All of the above

5. Which is *not* used for a cleansing enema?
   A. Soap suds
   B. Saline
   C. Oil
   D. Tap water

6. Which is *false?*
   A. Enema solutions should be 105° F (40.5° C).
   B. The Sims' position is used for an enema.
   C. The enema bag is held 12 inches above the anus.
   D. The enema solution is administered rapidly.

7. In adults, the enema tube is inserted
   A. 2 inches
   B. 4 inches
   C. 6 inches
   D. 8 inches

8. The oil-retention enema is retained for
   A. 10 to 15 minutes
   B. 15 to 30 minutes
   C. 30 to 60 minutes
   D. 60 to 90 minutes

9. Rectal tubes are left in place no longer than
   A. 60 minutes
   B. 30 minutes
   C. 20 minutes
   D. 10 minutes

10. Which statement about ostomies is *false?*
    A. Good skin care around the stoma is essential.
    B. Deodorants can control odors.
    C. The person wears a pouch.
    D. Fecal material is always liquid.

11. A person wears an ostomy pouch. It is usually emptied
    A. Every 4 to 6 hours
    B. Every morning
    C. Every 3 to 7 days
    D. When $\frac{1}{3}$ to $\frac{1}{2}$ full

12. You note a black, tarry stool. This is called
    A. Melena
    B. Feces
    C. Hemostool
    D. Occult blood

Answers to these questions are on p. 836.

CHAPTER

18

NUTRITION AND FLUIDS

440

Define the key terms listed in this chapter

Explain the purpose and use of the Food Guide Pyramid

Describe the functions and major sources of protein, carbohydrates, fats, vitamins, and minerals

Explain how to use food labels

Describe factors that affect eating and nutrition

Describe the special diets and between-meal nourishments

Explain how to assist with calorie counts

Explain the purpose of enteral nutrition and necessary comfort measures

Explain how to prevent aspiration and regurgitation

Identify the signs and symptoms of aspiration

Describe normal adult fluid requirements and the common causes of dehydration

Explain your responsibilities when the person has special fluid orders

Explain the purpose of intake and output records

Identify foods that are counted as fluid intake

Identify the solutions, equipment, and complications involved in IV therapy

Explain the safety measures necessary for IV therapy and your role in maintaining the flow rate

Perform the procedures described in this chapter

KEY TERMS

anorexia The loss of appetite

aspiration Breathing of fluid or an object into the lungs

calorie The amount of energy produced from the burning of food by the body

Daily Reference Values (DRVs) The maximum daily intake values for total fat, saturated fat, cholesterol, sodium, carbohydrate, and dietary fiber

Daily Value (DV) How a serving fits into the daily diet; it is expressed in a percent based on a daily diet of 2000 calories

dehydration A decrease in the amount of water in body tissues

dysphagia Difficulty or discomfort *(dys)* in swallowing *(phagia)*

edema Swelling of body tissues with water

enteral nutrition Giving nutrients through the gastrointestinal tract *(enteral)*

flow rate The number of drops per minutes (gtt/min)

gastrostomy A surgically created opening *(stomy)* in the stomach *(gastro)*

gavage Tube feeding

graduate A calibrated container used to measure fluid

hyperalimentation The intravenous administration of a solution highly concentrated with proteins, carbohydrates, vitamins, and minerals; fat also may be added

intake The amount of fluids taken in by the body

intravenous therapy Administration of fluids into a vein; IV, IV therapy, and IV infusion

jejunostomy A surgically created opening *(stomy)* into the middle part of the small intestine *(jejunum)*

nasogastric (NG) tube A tube inserted through the nose *(naso)* into the stomach *(gastro)*

nasointestinal tube A tube inserted through the nose into the duodenum or jejunum of the small intestine

nutrient A substance that is ingested, digested, absorbed, and used by the body

nutrition The many processes involved in the ingestion, digestion, absorption, and use of foods and fluids by the body

output The amount of fluid lost by the body

percutaneous endoscopic gastrostomy (PEG) tube A tube inserted into the stomach *(gastro)* through a stab or puncture wound *(stomy)* made through *(per)* the skin *(cutaneous)*; a lighted instrument *(scope)* allows the doctor to see inside a body cavity or organ *(endo)*

regurgitation The backward flow of food from the stomach into the mouth

---

Caring About Culture

MEALTIME PRACTICES

Unlike Americans, many cultural groups have their main meal at midday. For example, the Austrians have their main meal at midday and eat light meals in the early evening and at the end of the day. Persons from Brazil also eat their main meal at noon. They have a light meal around 8 PM. A main meal at noon also is common in Finland, France, Germany, Greece, and Iran. In South Korea, breakfast is the main meal.

Remember, individuals may not follow every belief and practice of their culture and religion. Each person is unique. Do not judge the person by your own standards.

Modified from Geissler EM: *Pocket guide to cultural assessment,* ed 2, St Louis, 1998, Mosby.

The need for food and water is a basic physical need necessary for life and health. The amount and quality of foods in the diet are important. They affect a person's current and future well-being. A poor diet and poor eating habits increase a person's risk for infection and acute and chronic diseases. Healing problems and abnormal physical and mental function also are related to poor diet and eating habits. Poor physical and mental functioning increase the risk for accidents and injuries.

Eating and drinking also provide pleasure. They are part of social activity with family and friends. Many people need a friendly, social setting for meals. Otherwise they eat poorly.

Many factors affect dietary practices. They include culture, finances, and personal choice. *(See Caring About Culture [Mealtime Practices] box.)* Dietary practices also include selecting, preparing, and serving food. The RN considers these factors when using the nursing process to meet the person's nutritional needs. The dietitian also is involved in developing the care plan.

See Box 18-1 for a review of the structure and function of the digestive system.

BASIC NUTRITION

Nutrition is the many processes involved in the ingestion, digestion, absorption, and use of foods and fluids by the body. Good nutrition is needed for growth, healing, and maintaining body functions. Selected foods must provide a well-balanced diet and correct calorie intake. A diet high in fat and calories causes weight gain and obesity. Weight loss occurs when the person consumes fewer calories than needed.

Foods and fluids contain nutrients. A **nutrient** is a substance that is ingested, digested, absorbed, and used by the body. Many nutrients are needed for body functions. Nutrients are grouped into fats, proteins, carbohydrates, vitamins, and minerals.

Fats, proteins, and carbohydrates give the body fuel for energy. The amount of energy provided by a nutrient is measured in calories. A **calorie** is the amount of energy produced from the burning of food by the body:

- 1 gram of fat supplies the body with 9 calories
- 1 gram of protein supplies 4 calories
- 1 gram of carbohydrate supplies 4 calories

The digestive system breaks down food physically and chemically so it can be absorbed for use by the cells. This process is called *digestion.* The digestive system is also called the *gastrointestinal system (GI system).* The digestive system consists of the *alimentary canal (GI tract)* and the accessory organs of digestion (Fig. 18-1). The alimentary canal is a long tube extending from the mouth to the anus. Its major parts are the mouth, pharynx, esophagus, stomach, small intestine, and large intestine. The accessory organs of digestion are the teeth, tongue, salivary glands, liver, gallbladder, and pancreas.

Digestion begins in the *mouth (oral cavity).* The oral cavity receives food and prepares it for digestion. Using chewing motions, the *teeth* cut, chop, and grind food into smaller particles for digestion and swallowing. The *tongue* aids in chewing and swallowing. *Taste buds* on the tongue contain nerve endings. Taste buds allow sensing of sweet, sour, bitter, and salty tastes. *Salivary glands* in the mouth secrete *saliva.* Saliva moistens food particles for easier swallowing and begins the digestion of food. During swallowing, the tongue pushes food into the pharynx.

The *pharynx* (throat) is a muscular tube. The act of swallowing is continued as the pharynx contracts. Contraction of the pharynx pushes food into the *esophagus.* The esophagus is a muscular tube about 10 inches long. It extends from the pharynx to the stomach. Involuntary muscle contractions called *peristalsis* move food down the esophagus into the stomach.

The *stomach* is a muscular, pouchlike sac in the upper left portion of the abdominal cavity. Strong stomach muscles stir and churn food to break it up into even smaller particles. The stomach is lined with a mucous membrane containing glands that secrete *gastric juices.* Food is mixed and churned with the gastric juices to form a semiliquid substance called *chyme.* Through peristalsis, the chyme is pushed from the stomach into the small intestine.

The *small intestine* is about 20 feet long and has three parts. The first part is the *duodenum.* In the duodenum, more digestive juices are added to the chyme. One is called *bile.* Bile is a greenish liquid produced by the *liver* and stored in the *gallbladder.* Juices from the *pancreas* and small intestine are also added to the chyme. The digestive juices chemically break down food so it can be absorbed.

Peristalsis moves the chyme through the two remaining portions of the small intestine: the *jejunum* and the *ileum.* Tiny projections called *villi* line the small intestine. Villi absorb the digested food into the capillaries. Most of the absorption of food takes place in the jejunum and ileum. Chyme eventually enters the large intestine. More fluid is absorbed. The solid waste that remains is eventually eliminated through the anus.

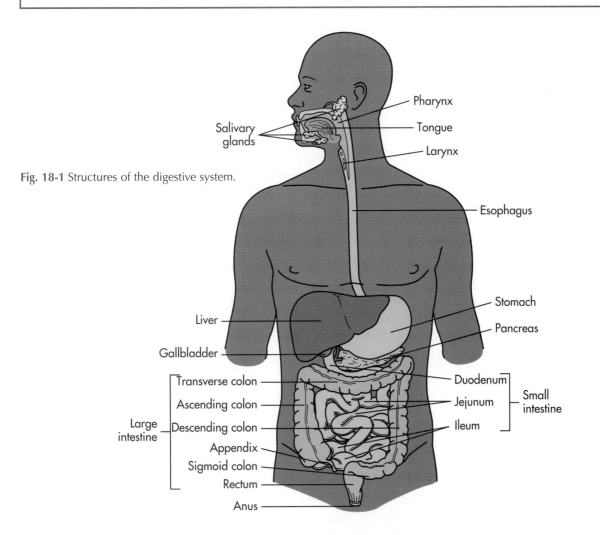

Fig. 18-1 Structures of the digestive system.

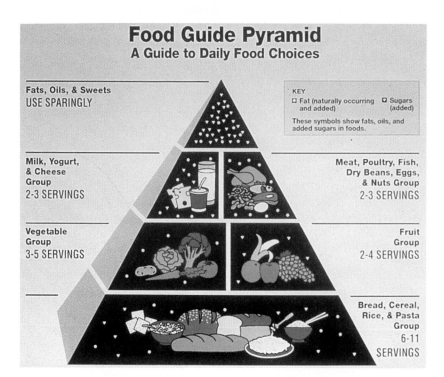

Fig. 18-2 Food Guide Pyramid. *(Courtesy U.S. Dept. of Agriculture, Washington, D.C.)*

FOOD GUIDE PYRAMID

In 1992 the U.S. Dept. of Agriculture (USDA) released its *Food Guide Pyramid*. The Food Guide Pyramid promotes wise food choices (Fig. 18-2). The pyramid has 6 food groups:

- Bread, cereal, rice, and pasta
- Vegetables
- Fruits
- Milk, yogurt, and cheese
- Meat, poultry, fish, dry beans, eggs, and nuts
- Fats, oils, and sweets

The pyramid suggests eating more foods at the bottom level (level 1) and lesser amounts at each level moving to the top (level 4). The Food Guide Pyramid encourages a low-fat diet. More bread, cereal, rice, and pasta (level 1) and more vegetables and fruits (level 2) are eaten. Food from the milk, yogurt, and cheese group are eaten in moderate amounts. So are foods from the meat, poultry, fish, beans, eggs, and nut group (level 3). Fats, oils, and sweets (level 4) are used sparingly.

Foods from the 5 food groups in levels 1, 2, and 3 are needed daily. Those foods contain varying amounts of the essential nutrients. No one food or food group contains every nutrient needed by the body.

Note the small circles and triangles in the pyramid (see Fig. 18-2). The circles are for fat and the triangles for sugar. Some sugar and fat naturally occur in all

Box 18-2	**Dietary Guidelines for Americans**

- Eat a variety of foods.
- Maintain a healthy weight.
- Choose a diet low in fat, saturated fat, and cholesterol.
- Choose a diet with plenty of vegetables, fruits, and grain products.
- Use sugars only in moderation.
- Use salt and sodium only in moderation.
- If you drink alcoholic beverages, do so in moderation.

foods. They appear in all levels of the pyramid. There are fewer fats and sugars at levels 1 and 2. More servings are allowed from these groups than the others. The result is a low-fat diet. Level 4 foods contain more fat and calories than do foods at level 1. As you move up the Food Guide Pyramid, fat and calorie amounts increase.

The pyramid is for everyone older than 2 years. Better health is the goal. Many diseases are related to diet and the kinds of food eaten. They include heart disease, high blood pressure, stroke, diabetes, and certain cancers. Following the Dietary Guidelines for Americans reduces the risk for such diseases. Box 18-2 lists the guidelines developed by the U.S. Dept. of Agriculture and the U.S. Dept. of Health and Human Services.

Box 18-3	Food Guide Pyramid Serving Sizes

Bread, Cereals, Rice, and Pasta Group
  1 slice of bread = 1 serving
  1 ounce of ready-to-eat cereal = 1 serving
  $1/2$ cup of cooked cereal, rice, or pasta = 1 serving
Vegetable Group
  1 cup raw leafy vegetables = 1 serving
  $1/2$ cup other cooked or chopped raw vegetables = 1 serving
  $3/4$ cup vegetable juice = 1 serving
Fruit Group
  1 medium apple, orange, or banana = 1 serving
  $1/2$ cup chopped, cooked, or canned fruit = 1 serving
  $3/4$ cup fruit juice = 1 serving

Milk, Cheese, and Yogurt Group
  1 cup of milk or yogurt = 1 serving
  $1/2$ to 1 ounce cheese = 1 serving
  2 ounces process cheese = 1 serving
Meat, Poultry, Fish, Dry Beans, Eggs, and Nuts Group
  2 to 3 ounces cooked lean meat, poultry, or fish = 1 serving
  $1/2$ cup cooked dry beans = 1 serving
  1 egg = 1 serving
  2 tablespoons peanut butter = 1 serving
Fats, Oils, and Sweets Group
  Use sparingly

Breads, Cereals, Rice, and Pasta Group. This group forms the base of the pyramid. More servings are allowed from this group than any other group. The USDA recommends 6 to 11 servings a day (Box 18-3). All foods in the group come from grain (e.g., wheat, oats, rice). Protein, carbohydrates, iron, thiamin, niacin, and riboflavin are the main nutrients in this group. There are small amounts of fats and sugars.

Foods such as pie, cake, cookies, pastries, doughnuts, and muffins are made from grains. However, they are also made with fats and sugars. They are high-fat food choices depending on the amount of fat and sugar added.

Vegetable Group. The USDA recommends 3 to 5 servings a day from this group (see Box 18-3). Vegetables provide fiber, vitamins A and C, carbohydrates, and minerals. They are naturally low in fat. A variety of vegetables are eaten: dark green and yellow vegetables, tomatoes, potatoes, and vegetable juices.

Vegetables can become high in fat from food preparation. French fries are very high in fat compared with a baked or boiled potato. Butter, oil, mayonnaise, salad dressing, sour cream, and sauces are often added to vegetables. These toppings are high in fat. Small amounts of low-fat toppings help keep vegetables low in fat.

Fruit Group. Fruits naturally contain some sugar and are low in fat. The USDA recommends 2 to 4 servings of fruit daily (see Box 18-3). Fruits provide carbohydrates, vitamins A and C, potassium, and other minerals. This group includes all fruits and fruit juices. Fresh fruits and juices are best. Frozen or canned fruits should be unsweetened. Often they are sweetened or syrupy and therefore higher in sugar and calories.

Milk, Yogurt, and Cheese Group. Milk and milk products are high in protein, carbohydrates, fat, calcium, and riboflavin. The USDA recommends 2 to 3 daily servings from the milk group—milk, cheese, and yogurt (see Box 18-3). Children and breast-feeding mothers need 3 servings a day.

Skim milk has less fat than whole milk. One cup of skim milk has only a trace of fat (86 calories); 1 cup of whole milk has 8 grams of fat. One cup of whole milk has about 150 calories—72 of the calories come from fat. Other low-fat foods in this group include cheeses made with skim milk, low-fat or nonfat yogurt, and ice milk rather than ice cream.

Meat, Poultry, Fish, Dry Beans, Eggs, and Nuts Group. This food group is higher in fat than the milk, fruit, vegetable, and bread groups. The USDA recommends 2 to 3 servings a day (see Box 18-3). Protein, fat, iron, and thiamin are the main nutrients found in this group.

Serving size is very important for a well-balanced diet. This is very important for meat, poultry, and fish because they contain many calories. Culture, appetite, personal choice, and the recipe used are some factors affecting serving size. A quarter-pound hamburger, a 12-ounce steak, a 10-ounce lobster tail, and a quarter of a chicken are servings offered by restaurants. *One serving* in this group is 2 to 3 ounces of boned meat, fish, or poultry. A 12-ounce steak is 4 to 6 servings from this group!

Remember, foods in this group are high in fat. The more fat, the more calories. Wise food choices lower fat intake from this group. Fish and shellfish are low in fat. Chicken and turkey have less fat than veal, beef, pork, and lamb. Skinless chicken and turkey are even lower in fat. Veal is lower in fat than beef. Lean cuts of beef and pork should be used. Egg yolks have more

Fig. 18-3 Two tablespoons of peanut butter (1 serving) equals this 3-ounce chicken breast (1 serving).

fat than egg whites. Low-fat egg substitutes can be used for cooking and baking.

Food preparation is also important. Trim fat from meat and poultry. Remove skin from poultry. Roasting, broiling, and baking are better than frying. Gravies and sauces also add fat.

Nuts and peanut butter have the most fat in this group. Use them wisely. As shown in Figure 18-3, 1 serving of peanut butter (2 tablespoons) equals 1 meat serving (2 to 3 ounces)! Peas and cooked dry beans are very low in fat. Use them often.

Fats, Oils, and Sweets Group. This group is at the top of the pyramid. The USDA recommends that it be used sparingly and as little as possible. Fats, oils, and sweets (foods with added sugar) have little nutritional value. However, they are very high in calories. Foods in this group include cooking oils, shortening, butter, margarine, salad dressing, soft drinks, sour cream, cream cheese, and frosting. They also include all candy, many desserts (cookies, cake, pie, ice cream), jelly and jam, syrup, and alcohol.

You can buy many low-fat foods. Use food labels to determine fat content.

NUTRIENTS

No one food or food group has every essential nutrient. A well-balanced diet has servings from the five food groups in levels 1, 2, and 3 of the Food Guide Pyramid. It ensures an adequate intake of the essential nutrients:

- *Protein*—the most important nutrient, it is needed for tissue growth and repair. Protein sources include meat, fish, poultry, eggs, milk and milk products, cereals, beans, peas, and nuts.
- *Carbohydrates*—provide energy and fiber for bowel elimination. They are found in fruits, vegetables, breads, cereals, and sugar. Carbohydrates are broken down into sugars during digestion. The sugars are then absorbed into the bloodstream. The fiber is not digested. It provides the bulky part of chyme for elimination.
- *Fats*—provide energy and add flavor to food and help the body use certain vitamins. Fat sources include the fat in meats, lard, butter, shortening, salad and vegetable oils, milk, cheese, egg yolks, and nuts. Dietary fat not needed by the body is stored as body fat (adipose tissue).
- *Vitamins*—do not provide calories but are essential nutrients. The body stores vitamins A, D, E, and K. Vitamin C and the B complex vitamins are not stored. They must be ingested daily. Each vitamin is needed for certain body functions. The lack of a specific vitamin results in signs and symptoms of an illness. Table 18-1 lists the sources and major functions of common vitamins.
- *Minerals*—are used for many body processes. They are needed for bone and tooth formation, nerve and muscle function, fluid balance, and other body processes. Table 18-2 lists the major functions and dietary sources of common minerals.

FOOD LABELS

The Nutrition Labeling and Education Act of 1990 (NLEA) requires food labeling for almost all foods (Fig. 18-4, p. 448). Food labels are useful for planning a healthy diet and for following special diets ordered by the doctor. The food label (Fig. 18-5, p. 448) has information about:

- Serving size and how the serving fits into the daily diet
- Total number of calories per serving and the number of calories from fat
- The total amount of fat and the amount of saturated fat
- Amount of cholesterol, sodium, and protein
- Total amount of carbohydrates and the amount of dietary fiber and sugars
- Amount of Vitamins A and C
- Amount of calcium and iron

Table 18-1	Functions and Sources of Common Vitamins	
Vitamin	**Major Functions**	**Sources**
Vitamin A	Growth; vision; healthy hair, skin, and mucous membranes; resistance to infection	Liver, spinach, green leafy and yellow vegetables, yellow fruits, fish liver oils, egg yolk, butter, cream, whole milk
Vitamin B_1 (thiamin)	Muscle tone; nerve function; digestion; appetite; normal elimination; carbohydrate use	Pork, fish, poultry, eggs, liver, breads, pastas, cereals, oatmeal, potatoes, peas, beans, soybeans, peanuts
Vitamin B_2 (riboflavin)	Growth; healthy eyes; protein and carbohydrate metabolism; healthy skin and mucous membranes	Milk and milk products, liver, green leafy vegetables, eggs, breads, cereals
Vitamin B_3 (niacin)	Protein, fat, and carbohydrate metabolism; nervous system function; appetite; digestive system function	Meat, pork, liver, fish, peanuts, breads and cereals, green vegetables, dairy products
Vitamin B_{12}	Formation of red blood cells; protein metabolism; nervous system functioning	Liver, meats, poultry, fish, eggs, milk, cheese
Folic acid	Formation of red blood cells; functioning of the intestines; protein metabolism	Liver, meats, fish, poultry, green leafy vegetables, whole grains
Vitamin C (ascorbic acid)	Formation of substances that hold tissues together; healthy blood vessels, skin, gums, bones, and teeth; wound healing; prevention of bleeding; resistance to infection	Citrus fruits, tomatoes, potatoes, cabbage, strawberries, green vegetables, melons
Vitamin D	Absorption and metabolism of calcium and phosphorus; healthy bones	Fish liver oils, milk, butter, liver, exposure to sunlight
Vitamin E	Normal reproduction; formation of red blood cells; muscle function	Vegetable oils, milk, eggs, meats, cereals, green leafy vegetables
Vitamin K	Blood clotting	Liver, green leafy vegetables, egg yolk, cheese

Table 18-2	Functions and Sources of Common Minerals	
Mineral	**Major Functions**	**Sources**
Calcium	Formation of teeth and bones; blood clotting; muscle contraction; heart function; nerve function	Milk and milk products, green leafy vegetables, whole grains, egg yolks, dried peas and beans, nuts
Phosphorus	Formation of bones and teeth; use of proteins, fats, and carbohydrates; nerve and muscle function	Meat, fish, poultry, milk and milk products, nuts, egg yolks, dried peas and beans
Iron	Allows red blood cells to carry oxygen	Liver, meat, eggs, green leafy vegetables, breads and cereals, dried peas and beans, nuts
Iodine	Thyroid gland function; growth; and metabolism	Iodized salt, seafood, and shellfish
Sodium	Fluid balance; nerve and muscle function	Almost all foods
Potassium	Nerve function; muscle contraction; heart function	Fruits, vegetables, cereals, meats, dried peas and beans

How a serving fits into the daily diet is called the **Daily Value (DV)**. The Daily Value is expressed in a percent (%). The percent is based on a daily diet of 2000 calories. Some food labels show the maximum daily intake values for total fat, saturated fat, cholesterol, sodium, carbohydrate, and dietary fiber. These are **Daily Reference Values (DRVs)**. The DV and DRVs are used as follows:

- No more than 30% of the calories in the daily diet should come from fat.
- Based on a 2000-calorie diet, the diet should have no more than 65 grams of fat.
- The food label in Figure 18-5 shows that one serving has 13 grams of fat or 20% of the Daily Value.
- The person can have 52 more grams of fat (80%) that day.

Fig. 18-4 Food labels are required on most foods.

Nutrition Facts

Serving Size 1 cup (228g)
Servings Per Container 2

Amount Per Serving

Calories 260   Calories from Fat 120

	% Daily Value*
Total Fat 13g	**20%**
Saturated Fat 5g	**25%**
Cholesterol 30mg	**10%**
Sodium 660mg	**28%**
Total Carbohydrate 31g	**10%**
Dietary Fiber 0g	**0%**
Sugars 5g	
Protein 5g	

Vitamin A 4%	•	Vitamin C 2%
Calcium 15%	•	Iron 4%

* Percent Daily Values are based on a 2,000 calorie diet. Your daily values may be higher or lower depending on your calorie needs:

	Calories:	2,000	2,500
Total Fat	Less than	65g	80g
Sat Fat	Less than	20g	25g
Cholesterol	Less than	300mg	300mg
Sodium	Less than	2,400mg	2,400mg
Total Carbohydrate		300g	375g
Dietary Fiber		25g	30g

Calories per gram:
Fat 9 • Carbohydrate 4 • Protein 4

Fig. 18-5 Information contained on a food label. *(From U.S. Food and Drug Administration: FDA consumer: an FDA consumer special report, May 1993).*

Caring About Culture

FOOD PRACTICES

Food practices vary among cultural groups. Rice and beans are protein sources in *Mexico*. Rice also is common in the *Philippines*. It is preferred with every meal. A diet high in starch and fat is common in *Poland*. Potatoes, rye, and wheat are common. A low-fat diet is common in *China*, but high in sodium. The sodium content is from the use of soy sauce and dried and preserved foods.

Whereas eating beef is common in the *United States*, beef is not eaten in India. Organ meats are common in *England*.

Remember, individuals may not follow every belief and practice of their culture and religion. Each person is unique. Do not judge the person by your own standards.

Modified from Geissler EM: *Pocket guide to cultural assessment*, ed 2, St Louis, 1998, Mosby.

FACTORS THAT AFFECT EATING AND NUTRITION

Many factors affect nutrition and eating habits. Some begin during infancy and continue throughout life. Others develop later.

- *Culture*—Culture influences dietary practices, food choices, and food preparation. *(See Caring About Culture [Food Practices] box.)* Frying, baking, smoking, and roasting food and eating raw food are cultural practices. The use of sauces and spices is also related to culture.
- *Religion*—Selecting, preparing, and eating food often involve religious practices (Box 18-4). Members of a religious group may follow all, some, or none of the dietary practice of their faith. You need to respect the person's religious practices.
- *Finances*—People with limited incomes often buy the cheaper carbohydrate foods. Their diets often lack protein and certain vitamins and minerals.
- *Appetite*—Appetite relates to the desire for food. When hungry, a person seeks food and eats until the appetite is satisfied. Aromas and thoughts of food can also stimulate the appetite. However, loss of appetite **(anorexia)** can occur. Illness, drugs, anxiety, pain, and depression are some causes of anorexia. So are unpleasant sights, thoughts, and smells.

Box 18-4   Religion and Dietary Practices

Adventist (Seventh Day Adventist)
- Coffee, tea, and alcohol are not allowed.
- Beverages with caffeine (colas) are not allowed.
- Some groups forbid eating meat.

Baptist
- Some groups forbid coffee, tea, and alcohol.

Christian Scientist
- Alcohol and coffee are not allowed.

Church of Jesus Christ of Latter Day Saints (Mormon)
- Alcohol and hot drinks, such as coffee and tea, are not allowed.
- Meat is not forbidden, but members are encouraged to eat meat infrequently.

Greek Orthodox Church
- Wednesdays, Fridays, and Lent are days of fasting.
- Meat and dairy products usually are avoided during days of fast.

Islam (Muslim or Moslem)
- All pork and pork products are forbidden.
- Alcohol is not allowed except for medical reasons.

Judaism (Jewish faith)
- Foods must be kosher (prepared according to Jewish law).
- Meat of kosher animals (cows, goats, and sheep) can be eaten.
- Chickens, ducks, and geese are kosher fowls.
- Kosher fish have scales and fins, such as tuna, sardines, carp, and salmon.
- Shellfish cannot be eaten.
- Milk, milk products, and eggs from kosher animals and fowl are acceptable.
- Milk and milk products cannot be eaten with or immediately after eating meat.
- Milk and milk products can be eaten 6 hours after eating meat.
- Milk and milk products can be a part of the same meal with meat—they are served separately and before the meat.
- Kosher foods are not prepared in utensils used to prepare nonkosher foods.
- Breads, cakes, cookies, noodles, and alcoholic beverages are not consumed during Passover.

Roman Catholic
- Fasting for 1 hour before receiving Holy Communion.
- Fasting from meat on Ash Wednesday, Good Friday, and all Fridays during Lent.

Focus On... HOME CARE

A home care assignment may involve shopping for groceries, planning meals, and cooking. These require knowledge of the Food Guide Pyramid, basic nutrition, and food labels. Also know the person's food preferences and eating habits. For example, some people have their large meal in the evening, others at noon. Some people eat the same thing for breakfast every day. Also review what foods are allowed on the person's diet. Special eating and digestive problems caused by illness, injury, or aging are considered when preparing and serving meals. The person's finances are another factor when planning meals. The nurse and dietitian advise you about what to prepare. A good cookbook is a helpful guide for planning and preparing meals.

Plan menus for a full week. Check recipes to make sure all ingredients are on hand or are on the shopping list. You can save money by checking newspapers for sales and using coupons. Save all grocery receipts for the person or family member.

Properly store foods when you return from the store. Refrigerate dairy products and most fresh fruits and vegetables right away. Freeze meat, poultry, fish, and frozen foods unless they are used that day. Dried, packaged, canned, and bottled foods keep well in cabinets. See Chapter 10 for how to safely handle food.

Focus On... LONG-TERM CARE

OBRA has the following requirements for food served in long-term care centers:
- The nutritional and special dietary needs of each person must be met.
- Residents must receive a well-balanced diet. The diet must be nourishing and taste good. Food must be well seasoned. It must not be too salty or too sweet.
- Food must be appetizing. It must have an appealing aroma and be attractive.
- Hot food must be served hot and cold food served cold. Centers have special food servers to keep food at the correct temperature. Food is served promptly. Otherwise, hot food will cool and cold food will warm.
- Food must be prepared to meet the person's individual needs. Some persons need food cut, ground, or chopped. Others have special diets ordered by the doctor.
- Each person must receive at least 3 meals per day and be offered a bedtime snack.
- The center must provide any special eating equipment and utensils that are needed (Fig. 18-6). Hands, wrists, and arms may be affected by disease or injury. The person may need special equipment to eat independently. You must make sure needed equipment is used by the person.

Some centers have dining areas where residents can dine with guests. The resident can have a family meal with a spouse, children, grandchildren, other relatives, or friends. They can celebrate holidays, birthdays, anniversaries, and other special events. The dietary department provides the meal, or it is brought by the family.

- *Personal choice*—The like or dislike of certain foods is a personal matter. Food likes begin in childhood. They are influenced by the way food looks, how it is prepared, its smell, or the recipe. Body reactions affect food choices. People usually avoid foods that cause allergic reactions, nausea, vomiting, diarrhea, indigestion, or headaches.
- *Illness*—Appetite usually decreases during illness and recovery from injuries. However, nutritional needs increase at these times. The body must fight infection, heal tissue, and replace lost blood cells. Nutrients lost through vomiting and diarrhea must be replaced. Illness can affect a person's ability to prepare and serve meals. *(See Focus on Home Care box.)*
- *Health*—Some diseases and drugs cause a sore mouth, which makes eating painful. Loss of teeth affects chewing, especially protein foods. Some illnesses and drugs cause loss of appetite (anorexia). Poor nutrition is common problem among persons needing long-term care. For them, good nutrition is important in correcting or preventing health problems. *(See Focus on Long-Term Care box.)*
- *Age*—Age affects nutrition. *(See Focus on Children box and Focus on Older Persons box.)*

Focus On... CHILDREN

Infants are breast fed or bottle fed (see Chapter 35. For bottle-fed babies, the doctor prescribes the formula to use. Solid foods are introduced at about 5 months of age. Usually cereal is the first solid food given. Others are added as the infant grows. The nurse tells you what foods the infant can have.

The Food Guide Pyramid applies to children 2 years of age and older. The nurse tells you about the child's special needs.

Fig. 18-6 Eating utensils for persons with special needs. **A,** The curved fork fits over the hand. The rounded plate helps keep food on the plate. Special grips and swivel handles are helpful for some persons. **B,** Plate guards help keep food on the plate. **C,** Knives with rounded blades are rocked back and forth to cut food. The person does not need a fork in one hand and a knife in the other. **D,** Glass or cup holder. *(Courtesy Sammons Preston; An AbilityOne Company, Bolingbrook, Ill.)*

Focus On... OLDER PERSONS

Many changes occur in the gastrointestinal system. Difficulty swallowing often occurs from decreases in the amount of saliva. **Dysphagia** is difficulty or discomfort (dys) in swallowing (phagia). Taste and smell dull, and appetite decreases. Secretion of digestive juices decreases. As a result, fried and fatty foods are hard to digest and may cause indigestion. Loss of teeth and ill-fitting dentures affect chewing. This results in digestion problems. Hard to chew foods, such as high-protein foods, are avoided. Decreased peristalsis results in slower emptying of the stomach and colon. Flatulence and constipation are common because of decreased peristalsis (see Chapter 17).

Dry, fried, and fatty foods are avoided. This helps swallowing and digestion problems. Good oral hygiene and denture care improve the ability to taste.

People may not have natural teeth or dentures. Their food is pureed or ground. Avoiding high-fiber foods may be necessary even though they help prevent constipation. High-fiber foods are hard to chew and can irritate the intestines. High-fiber foods include apricots, celery, and fruits and vegetables with skins and seeds. Foods providing soft bulk are often ordered for those with chewing problems or constipation. These foods include whole-grain cereals and cooked fruits and vegetables.

Older persons need fewer calories than younger persons. Energy levels and daily activity levels are lower. The diet must include foods that contain calcium to prevent musculoskeletal changes. Protein is needed for tissue growth and repair. However, the diets of some older persons may lack protein. High-protein foods are often costly.

SPECIAL DIETS

Doctors may order special diets. They are ordered because of a nutritional deficiency or a disease, to eliminate or decrease certain substances in the diet, or for weight control (Table 18-3). Special diets are common before and after surgery and for persons with diabetes. Persons with diseases of the heart, kidneys, gallbladder, liver, stomach, or intestines may receive special diets. Allergies, obesity, and other disorders also require special diets.

Table 18-3	Special Diets		
Diet	**Description**	**Use**	**Foods Allowed**
Clear liquid	Clear liquids that do not leave a residue; nonirritating and non-gas-forming	Postoperatively, acute illness, infection, and nausea and vomiting	Water, tea, and coffee (without milk or cream); carbonated beverages; gelatin; clear fruit juices (apple, grape, and cranberry); fat-free clear broth; hard candy, sugar, and Popsicles
Full liquid	Foods that are liquid at room temperature or that melt at body temperature	Advance from clear liquid diet postoperatively; for stomach irritation, fever, and nausea and vomiting	All foods allowed on a clear liquid diet; custard; eggnog; strained soups; strained fruit and vegetable juices; milk; creamed cereals; plain ice cream and sherbet
Soft	Semisolid foods that are easily digested	Advance from full liquid diet; chewing difficulties, gastrointestinal disorders, and infections	All liquids; eggs (not fried); broiled, baked, or roasted meat, fish, or poultry that is chopped or shredded; mild cheeses (American, Swiss, cheddar, cream, and cottage); strained fruit juices; refined bread (no crust) and crackers; cooked cereal; cooked or pureed vegetables; cooked or canned fruit without skin or seeds; pudding; plain cakes
Low residue	Food that leaves a small amount of residue in the colon	Diseases of the colon and diarrhea	Coffee, tea, milk, carbonated beverages, strained fruit juices; refined bread and crackers; creamed and refined cereal; rice; cottage and cream cheese; eggs (not fried); plain puddings and cakes; gelatin; custard; sherbet and ice cream; strained vegetable juices; canned or cooked fruit without skin or seeds; potatoes (not fried); strained cooked vegetables; plain pasta; *no raw fruits and vegetables*
High fiber	Foods that increase the amount of residue in the colon to stimulate peristalsis	Constipation and colon disorders	All fruits and vegetables; whole wheat bread; whole grain cereals; fried foods; whole grain rice; milk, cream, butter, and cheese; meats

Table 18-3   Special Diets—cont'd

Diet	Description	Use	Foods Allowed
Bland	Foods that are mechanically and chemically nonirritating and low in roughage; foods served at moderate temperatures; no strong spices or condiments	Ulcers, gallbladder disorders, and some intestinal disorders; postoperatively after abdominal surgery	Lean meats; white bread; creamed and refined cereals; cream or cottage cheese; gelatin, plain puddings, cakes, and cookies; eggs (not fried); butter and cream; canned fruits and vegetables without skin and seeds; strained fruit juices; potatoes (not fried); pastas and rice; strained or soft cooked carrots, peas, beets, spinach, squash, and asparagus tips; creamed soups from allowed vegetables; no fried foods
High calorie	Calorie intake is increased to about 4000; includes three full meals and between-meal snacks	Weight gain and some thyroid imbalances	Dietary increases in all foods
Low calorie	Calorie intake is reduced below the minimum daily requirements	Weight reduction	Foods low in fats and carbohydrates and lean meats; avoid butter, cream, rice, gravies, salad oils, noodles, cakes, pastries, carbonated and alcoholic beverages, candy, potato chips, and similar foods
High iron	Foods that are high in iron	Anemia; following blood loss; for women during the reproductive years	Liver and other organ meats; lean meats; egg yolks; shellfish; dried fruits; dried beans; green leafy vegetables; lima beans; peanut butter; enriched breads and cereals
Low fat (low cholesterol)	Foods low in fat and foods prepared without adding fat	Heart disease, gallbladder disease, disorders of fat digestion, and liver disease	Skim milk or buttermilk; cottage cheese (no other cheeses allowed); gelatin; sherbet; fruit; lean meat, poultry, and fish (baked, broiled, or roasted); fat-free broth; soups made with skim milk; margarine; rice, pasta, breads and cereals; vegetables; potatoes
High protein	Aid and promote tissue healing	For burns, high fever, infection, and some liver diseases	Meat, milk, eggs, cheese, fish, poultry; breads and cereals; green leafy vegetables
Sodium restricted	A certain amount of sodium is allowed; sodium restriction ranges from mild to severe	Heart disease, fluid retention, and some kidney diseases	Fruits and vegetables and unsalted butter are allowed; adding salt at the table is not allowed; highly salted foods and foods high in sodium are not allowed; the use of salt during cooking may be restricted
Consistent-carbohydrate diabetes meal plan	The amount of carbohydrates, protein, and fat are regulated	Diabetes mellitus	Determined by nutritional and energy requirements

When a special diet is ordered, the RN and dietitian work together to meet the person's nutritional needs. The plan includes the individual's personal choice, culture, religion, and food allergies. They also plan for eating problems. For example, some people have dysphagia (difficulty swallowing). They often need pureed food. That is, food is blended to a smooth texture. The thickness depends on the person's needs.

Regular diet, general diet, and house diet have no dietary limits or restrictions. The sodium-restricted diet is often ordered. Persons with diabetes mellitus need medical nutrition therapy.

The Sodium-Restricted Diet

The average amount of sodium in the daily diet is 3000 to 5000 mg. The body needs half this amount daily. Healthy people excrete excess sodium in the urine. Heart and kidney diseases cause the body to retain the extra sodium. So do some drugs and some complications of pregnancy.

Sodium causes the body to retain water. If there is too much sodium, the body retains more water. Tissues swell with water, and there are excess amounts of fluid in the blood vessels. The heart has to work harder. That is, the workload of the heart increases. The extra workload can cause serious complications or death. Restricting sodium in the diet decreases the amount of sodium in the body. The body retains less water. Less water in the tissues and blood vessels reduces the amount of work for the heart.

The doctor orders the amount of restriction for the person. Many low-salt or salt-free foods can be bought. Food labels are used to determine salt content.

- *2000-mg to 3000-mg sodium diet*—this is called the *low-salt diet* or *no added salt diet*. Sodium restriction is mild. All high-sodium foods are omitted (Box 18-5). A minimum amount of salt is used for cooking. Salt is not added to foods at the table.
- *1000-mg sodium diet*—sodium restriction is moderate. Food is cooked without salt. Foods high in sodium are omitted. Vegetables high in sodium are restricted in amount. Salt-free products, such as salt-free bread, are used. Diet planning is necessary.
- *500-mg sodium diet*—sodium restriction is severe. Restrictions for the mild and moderate sodium diets are followed. In addition, vegetables high in sodium are omitted. Milk is limited to 1 cup per day. Only 1 egg per day is allowed. Meat is limited to 4 ounces per day. Diet planning is essential.

Medical Nutrition Therapy for Diabetes Mellitus

Medical nutrition therapy (MNT) is necessary for people with diabetes mellitus. Diabetes mellitus is a chronic disease from a lack of insulin (see Chapter 30). The pancreas produces and secretes insulin. Insulin allows the body to use sugar. If there is not enough insulin, sugar builds up in the bloodstream rather than being used by cells for energy. Diabetes is usually treated with insulin or drugs, diet, and exercise.

Carbohydrates are broken down into sugar during digestion. For the person with diabetes, the amount of carbohydrates is controlled. Only the amount of carbohydrates needed is ingested. The doctor determines the amount of carbohydrate a person should have. The dietitian develops a *consistent-carbohydrate diabetes meal plan* for the person. The meal plan also specifies a certain amount of fat and protein to meet the person's needs. The person's age, gender, activity, and weight are considered.

The person ingests a consistent amount of carbohydrate each day. The amount is the same at each breakfast, each lunch, each dinner, and for each snack. The amount of carbohydrate at each meal is not the same but the amount ingested each day is the same. The person must eat only what is allowed and all that is allowed. Otherwise the person gets too many or too few carbohydrates.

Meal and snack times also are consistent from day to day. You must serve the person's meal and snacks on time. The person must eat at regular times to maintain a certain blood sugar level. Always check the tray to see what the person ate. Report to the nurse what the person did and did not eat. If all food was not eaten, a between-meal nourishment is needed. The nourishment makes up for what was not eaten at the regular meal. The amount of insulin given also depends on the person's daily food intake.

Box 18-5   High-Sodium Foods

Bread, Cereal, Rice, and Pasta Group
Saltine crackers
Baking powder biscuits
Muffins
Bisquick
Pretzels
Salted crackers
Quick breads (corn bread, nut bread)
Pancakes
Waffles
Instant cooked cereal
Processed bran cereals
Rice
Noodle mixes
Corn chips and other salted snacks
Vegetable Group
Sauerkraut
Tomato juice
V-8 juice
Vegetables in creams or sauces
Frozen vegetables processed with salt or sodium
Bloody Mary mixes
Potato chips
French fries
Instant potatoes
Pickles
Relishes
Fruit Group
No restrictions
Milk, Yogurt, and Cheese Group
Buttermilk
Cheese
Commercial dips made with sour cream
Meat, Poultry, Fish, Dry Beans, Eggs, and Nuts Group
Bacon
Ham
Sausage
Salt pork
Hot dogs

Luncheon meats
Corned or chopped beef
Organ meats
Shellfish
Sardines
Herring
Anchovies
Caviar
Kosher meats
Canned tuna
Canned salmon
Mackerel
Salted nuts and seeds
Peanut butter
Fats, Oils, and Sweets
Salad dressings
Mayonnaise
Baked desserts
Other
Mineral water
Club soda
Canned soups
Bouillon cubes
Dried soup mixes
Olives
Salted popcorn
Frozen or canned dinners
Salt
Baking powder
Baking soda
Celery, onion, garlic, and other seasoning salts
Meat tenderizers
Worcestershire sauce
Soy sauce
Mustard
Catsup
Horseradish
Sauces: chili, tomato, steak, barbecue

Modified from Lewis SM, Heitkemper MM, Dirkson SR: *Medical-surgical nursing: assessment and management of clinical problems,* ed 5, St Louis, 2000, Mosby

ASSISTING THE PERSON WITH EATING

Weakness and illness can affect a person's appetite and ability to eat. So can odors, unpleasant equipment, an uncomfortable position, the need for oral hygiene, the need to eliminate, and pain. Nursing staff can control these factors by getting the person ready for meals.

- Assist the person with oral hygiene. Be sure dentures are in place.
- Provide for elimination needs. Assist the person to the bathroom or bedside commode. Or offer the bedpan or urinal.
- Change clothing and provide clean linens for incontinent persons.
- Make sure dentures, eyeglasses, and hearing aids are in place.
- Assist the person in washing his or her hands.
- Position the person for eating:
  - For persons in bed—raise the head of the bed to a comfortable sitting position.
  - For persons in chairs—assist the person in transferring from the bed to a chair. Position the overbed table in front of the person.
- Assist persons to the dining room.

► SERVING MEAL TRAYS

In hospitals, food is usually served in the person's room. Some persons eat in a dining room, the cafeteria, or a lounge. Food is served in containers that keep hot and cold foods at the correct temperature. You serve meal trays after preparing persons for meals. You can serve trays promptly if patients and residents are ready to eat. Serving trays promptly keeps food at the right temperature. *(See Focus on Long-Term Care box.)*

Focus On... LONG-TERM CARE

Long-term care centers have special dining programs:
- *Social dining*—residents eat in a dining room. Each table has 4 to 6 residents (Fig. 18-7). Tables have tablecloths or placemats. Food is served as in a restaurant. This program is for persons who are oriented and can feed themselves.
- *Family dining*—food is placed in bowls and on platters. Residents serve themselves as they would at home.
- *Assistive dining*—the dining room has circular or horseshoe-shaped tables. Residents who need assistance with eating are seated around these tables. You sit at the center of the table and feed as many as 4 residents (Fig. 18-8).

Fig. 18-7 Residents enjoy a pleasant meal in the dining room.

Fig. 18-8 Special dining tables are used for assistive dining programs. A nursing assistant feeds 3 residents at one time. Residents are in the company of others.

Serving Meal Trays

QUALITY OF LIFE

Remember to:
- Knock before entering the person's room
- Address the person by name
- Introduce yourself by name and title

Pre-Procedure

1 Wash your hands.

2 Make sure the tray is complete. Check items on the tray against the dietary card.

3 Identify the person. Check the ID bracelet against the dietary card.

4 Have the person in a sitting position if possible.

5 Place the tray on the overbed table within the person's reach. Adjust table height as necessary.

6 Remove food covers. Open milk cartons and cereal boxes, cut meat, and butter bread if indicated (Fig. 18-9).

7 Place the napkin, clothes protector if needed, and silverware within reach.

8 Measure and record intake if ordered. Note the amount and type of foods eaten.

9 Remove the tray.

10 Assist the person with oral hygiene. (Wear gloves for this step.)

11 Clean any spills, and change soiled linen.

12 Help the person return to bed if indicated.

Post-Procedure

13 Assist the person with handwashing. Offer the person oral hygiene.

14 Provide for comfort.

15 Place the signal light within reach.

16 Raise or lower bed rails. Follow the care plan.

17 Wash your hands.

18 Report your observations to the nurse.

Fig. 18-9 Open cartons and other containers for the person.

▶ FEEDING THE PERSON

Some persons cannot feed themselves. Weakness, paralysis, casts, and other physical limits may make self-feeding impossible. These persons are fed.

Provide a relaxed mood so that the person does not feel rushed. Many people pray before eating. Provide time and privacy for a prayer. This shows caring and respect for the person. Ask the person about the order in which to offer foods and fluids. Spoons are used. They are less likely to cause injury than forks. The spoon should be only one-third full. The portion is easily chewed and swallowed. Some people need smaller portions. Follow the person's care plan.

Remember to offer fluids during the meal. Fluids help the person chew and swallow.

Persons who cannot feed themselves may be angry, humiliated, and embarrassed. They do not like depending on others. Some are depressed or resentful. Others refuse to eat. These persons should try to feed themselves as much as possible. However, they should not exceed activity limits ordered by the doctor. Be supportive and encouraging.

Visually impaired persons are often keenly aware of food aromas. Often they can identify some foods served. Always tell the person what foods and fluids are on the tray. When feeding a visually impaired person, always identify what you are offering. For persons who feed themselves, identify foods and fluids and their location on the tray. Use the numbers on a clock to identify the location of foods (Fig. 18-10).

Meals provide social contact with others. Engage the person in pleasant conversation. However, give the person enough time to chew and swallow food. Also, sit so that you face the person. Sitting is more relaxing. It shows the person that you have time to help him or her. Standing communicates nonverbally that you do not have time and that you are in a hurry. By facing the person, you can see how well the person is eating. You can also see if the person has problems swallowing.

BETWEEN-MEAL NOURISHMENTS

Many special diets involve between-meal nourishments. Commonly served nourishments are crackers, milk, juice, a milkshake, cake, wafers, a sandwich, gelatin, and custard. Serve nourishments as soon as they arrive on the nursing unit. Provide needed eating utensils, a straw, and a napkin. Follow the same considerations and procedures described for serving meal trays and feeding persons.

CALORIE COUNTS

For some people it is important to keep track of calorie intake. A flow sheet is provided for this purpose. Your role is to note what the person ate and how much. For example, a person is served a chicken breast, a baked potato, beans, a roll, pudding, and two pats of butter. You note that the person ate all the chicken, half the potato, and the roll. One pat of butter was used. The beans and pudding were not eaten. You note these on the form. A nurse or dietitian then converts these portions into calories. The nurse tells you what patients and residents require calorie counts.

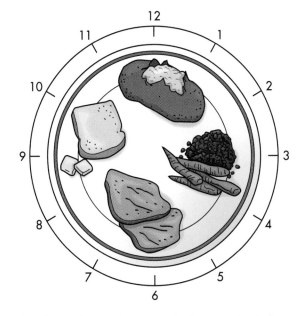

Fig. 18-10 The numbers on a clock are used to help a visually impaired person locate food on the tray.

Fig. 18-11 A spoon is used to feed the person. The spoon is no more than one-third full.

Feeding a Person

NNAAP™

QUALITY OF LIFE

Remember to:
- Knock before entering the person's room
- Address the person by name
- Introduce yourself by name and title

Pre-Procedure

1 Explain the procedure to the person.
2 Wash your hands.
3 Position the person in a comfortable sitting position.
4 Bring the tray into the room or dining room. Place it on the overbed table or dining table.

Procedure

5 Identify the person. Check the ID bracelet against the dietary card.
6 Drape a napkin across the person's chest and under the chin.
7 Prepare the food for eating.
8 Tell the person what foods are on the tray.
9 Serve foods in the order the person prefers. Alternate between solid and liquid foods. Use a spoon for safety as in Figure 18-11. Allow enough time for chewing. Do not rush the person.
10 Use straws for liquids if the person cannot drink out of a glass or cup. Have one straw for each liquid. Provide a short straw for weak persons. (Persons with dysphagia cannot use straws. Give thickened liquid with a spoon.)
11 Converse with the person in a pleasant manner.
12 Encourage him or her to eat as much as possible.
13 Wipe the person's mouth with a napkin.
14 Note how much and which foods were eaten.
15 Measure and record intake if ordered.
16 Remove the tray.
17 Take the person back to his or her room if the person ate in a dining room.
18 Provide oral hygiene. (Wear gloves for this step.)

Post-Procedure

19 Provide for comfort.
20 Place the signal light within reach.
21 Raise or lower bed rails. Follow the care plan.
22 Wash your hands.
23 Report your observations to the nurse:
   a The amount and kind of food eaten
   b Complaints of nausea or dysphagia (difficulty or discomfort in swallowing)

ENTERAL NUTRITION

Persons who cannot chew or swallow often require enteral nutrition. **Enteral nutrition** is giving nutrients through the gastrointestinal tract *(enteral)*. Formula is given through a feeding tube inserted into the stomach or small intestine. (**Gavage** is another term for tube feeding.)

- A **nasogastric (NG) tube** is inserted through the nose *(naso)* into the stomach *(gastro)* (Fig. 18-12). A doctor or an RN performs the procedure.
- A **nasointestinal tube** is inserted through the nose into the duodenum or jejunum of the small intestine (Fig. 18-13). A doctor or an RN performs the procedure.
- A **gastrostomy** is an opening *(stomy)* into the stomach *(gastro)* (Fig. 18-14). The opening is created surgically.
- A **jejunostomy** is an opening *(stomy)* into the middle part of the small intestine *(jejunum)* (Fig. 18-15). The opening is created surgically.

- A **percutaneous endoscopic gastrostomy (PEG) tube** is inserted with an endoscope. An endoscope is a lighted instrument *(scope)*. It allows the doctor to see inside a body cavity or organ *(endo)*. The endoscope allows the doctor to see inside the stomach. The doctor inserts the endoscope through the person's mouth and esophagus and into the stomach. A stab or puncture wound *(stomy)* is made through *(per)* the skin *(cutaneous)* and into the stomach *(gastro)*. A tube is inserted into the stomach through the stab wound (Fig. 18-16).

Feeding tubes are used when food cannot pass normally from the mouth into the esophagus and then into the stomach. Cancer of the head, neck, or esophagus is a common cause. So is trauma or surgery to the face, mouth, head, or neck. Coma is another reason for tube feedings. So is dysphagia caused by paralysis. Some persons with dementia no longer know how to eat and may require tube feedings. Gastrostomy, jejunostomy, and PEG feedings are used for long-term enteral nutrition. The ostomy may be temporary or permanent.

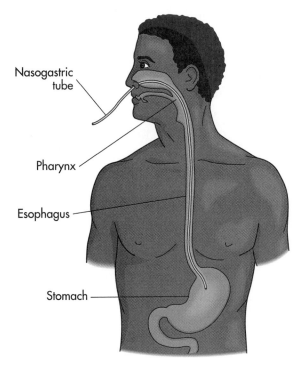

Fig. 18-12 A nasogastric tube is inserted through the nose and esophagus into the stomach.

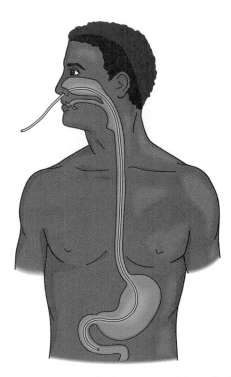

Fig. 18-13 A nasointestinal tube is inserted through the nose into the duodenum or jejunum of the small intestine.

Fig. 18-14 A gastrostomy tube.

Fig. 18-15 A jejunostomy tube.

Fig. 18-16 A percutaneous endoscopic gastrostomy.

Fig. 18-17 A, A tube feeding is given with a syringe. **B,** Formula drips from a feeding bag into the feeding tube.

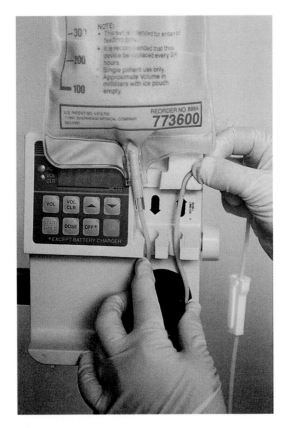

Fig. 18-18 Feeding pump. *(From Potter PA, Perry AG: Fundamentals of nursing: concepts, process, and practice, ed 4, St Louis, 1997, Mosby.)*

FORMULAS

The doctor orders the type of formula and the amount to give. Most formulas contain protein, carbohydrates, fat, vitamins, and minerals. Commercial formulas are common. Sometimes formula is prepared by the dietary department.

SCHEDULED AND CONTINUOUS FEEDINGS

The doctor orders scheduled or continuous feedings. Scheduled feedings usually are given four times a day with a syringe or feeding bag (Fig. 18-17). Usually about 400 ml is given over 20 minutes during a scheduled feeding. The amount and rate are like eating a regular meal.

Continuous feedings require electronic feeding pumps (Fig. 18-18). Nasointestinal and jejunostomy tube feedings are always continuous.

Formula is given at room temperature. Cold fluids can cause cramping. Sometimes continuous feedings are kept cold with ice chips around the container. Otherwise microbes grow in warm formula. The formula warms to room temperature as it drips from the bag and passes through the connecting tubing to the feeding tube. The nurse adds formula to continuous feedings every 3 to 4 hours.

PREVENTING ASPIRATION

Aspiration is a major complication of nasogastric and nasointestinal tubes. Remember, **aspiration** is the breathing of fluid or an object into the lungs. It can cause pneumonia and death. Nasogastric and nasointestinal tubes are passed through the esophagus and then into the stomach or small intestine. During insertion, the tube can slip into the respiratory tract. This causes aspiration. An x-ray is the best way to determine tube placement. One is taken after the doctor or RN inserts the tube.

After insertion, the tube can move out of place from coughing, sneezing, vomiting, suctioning, and poor positioning. The tube can move from the stomach or intestines into the esophagus and then into the respiratory tract. *Therefore the RN checks tube placement before every scheduled tube feeding.* With continuous tube feedings, the RN checks tube placement every 4 to 8 hours. To assess tube placement, the RN attaches a syringe to the tube and aspirates gastrointestinal secretions. Then the RN measures the pH of the secretions.

Aspiration also occurs from regurgitation. **Regurgitation** is the backward flow of food from the stomach into the mouth. This can occur with nasogastric, gastrostomy, and PEG tubes. Delayed stomach emptying and overfeeding are common causes of regurgitation. To prevent regurgitation, the person sits or is in semi-Fowler's position for the feeding. The person remains in this position for at least 1 hour after the feeding. This promotes movement of the formula through the gastrointestinal system and prevents aspiration. The left side-lying position is avoided. This position prevents the stomach from emptying.

The risk of regurgitation is less with nasointestinal and jejunostomy tubes. Formula passes directly into the small intestine. Also, formula is given at a slow rate. Remember, during digestion, food slowly passes from the stomach to the small intestine. The stomach handles larger amounts of food at one time than does the small intestine.

Observations. The nurse must be alert to signs and symptoms of aspiration. Other complications include diarrhea, constipation, and delayed stomach emptying. You must report the following to the nurse immediately:

- Nausea
- Discomfort during the tube feeding
- Vomiting
- Diarrhea
- Distended (enlarged and swollen) abdomen
- Coughing
- Complaints of indigestion or heart burn
- Redness, swelling, drainage, odor, or pain at the ostomy site
- Elevated temperature
- Signs and symptoms of respiratory distress (see Chapter 27)
- Increased pulse rate
- Complaints of flatulence (see Chapter 17)

Fig. 18-19 The feeding tube is taped to the nose.

COMFORT MEASURES

The person with a feeding tube is usually NPO. (*NPO* is the abbreviation for the Latin term *nils per os*, which means nothing by mouth.) Dry mouth, dry lips, and sore throat are sources of discomfort. Some persons are allowed hard candy or gum. The person's nursing care plan will likely include frequent oral hygiene, lubricant for the lips, and mouth rinses. The nose and nostrils also are cleaned every 4 to 8 hours as directed by the nurse and care plan.

Nasogastric and nasointestinal tubes can irritate and cause pressure on the nose. Sometimes they alter the shape of the nostrils or cause pressure ulcers. Securing the tube helps prevent these problems. Use tape or a tube holder to secure the tube to the nose (Fig. 18-19). Tube holders have foam cushions that prevent pressure on the nose. They also eliminate the need for retaping, which irritates the nose. The tube also is secured to the person's gown. Loop a rubber band around the tube. Then pin the rubber band to the person's gown with a safety pin. Or tape the tube to the gown.

OTHER METHODS FOR MEETING NUTRITIONAL NEEDS

Sometimes other methods are used to meet a person's nutritional needs. IV therapy is common. **Hyperalimentation** is the intravenous administration of a solution highly concentrated with proteins, carbohydrates, vitamins, and minerals. Fat also can be added. The solution is far more nutritious than a regular IV solution. Hyperalimentation is used for seriously ill and injured persons. *You are never responsible for administering or regulating hyperalimentation solutions.*

FLUID BALANCE

After oxygen, water is the most important physical need for survival. Death can result from an inadequate water intake or from excessive fluid loss. Water enters the body through fluids and foods. Water is lost through the urine and feces, through the skin as perspiration, and through the lungs with expiration. Fluid balance must be maintained for health. There must be a balance between the amount of fluid taken in and the amount lost.

The amount of fluid taken in (**intake**) and the amount lost (**output**) must be equal. If fluid intake exceeds fluid output, body tissues swell with water. This is called **edema**. Edema is common in people with heart and kidney diseases. **Dehydration** is a decrease in the amount of water in the tissues. It results when fluid output exceeds intake. Inadequate fluid intake, vomiting, diarrhea, bleeding, excessive sweating, and increased urine production are common causes of dehydration.

NORMAL REQUIREMENTS

An adult needs 1500 ml of water daily to survive. Approximately 2000 to 2500 ml of fluid per day is required to maintain a normal fluid balance. The water requirement increases with hot weather, exercise, fever, and illness. Excessive fluid losses also increase the water requirement. *(See Focus on Children box and Focus on Older Persons box.)*

Focus On... CHILDREN

Minimum daily water requirements vary with age. Infants and young children have more body water. They need more fluids than do adults. Excessive fluid losses cannot be tolerated and will quickly cause death in an infant or child.

Focus On... OLDER PERSONS

The amount of body water decreases with age. Older persons also are at risk for diseases that affect fluid balance. Examples include heart disease, kidney disease, cancer, and diabetes mellitus. Many older persons also take drugs that affect fluid balance. Some drugs cause the body to lose fluids. Others cause the body to retain water. The older person is at risk for dehydration and edema.

SPECIAL ORDERS

The doctor may order the amount of fluid a person can have during a 24-hour period. This is done to maintain fluid balance. Special orders include *encourage fluids*, *restrict fluids*, and *nothing by mouth*. Special orders are noted in the person's care plan.

- *Encourage fluids*—the person drinks increased amounts of fluid. The *encourage fluids* order may be general or for a specific amount. Records are kept of the intake. A variety of allowed fluids are provided. They are kept within the person's reach and served at the correct temperature. Frequently offer fluids to persons who cannot feed themselves.
- *Restrict fluids*—fluids are limited to a certain amount. Fluids are offered in small amounts and in small containers. The water pitcher is removed from the room or kept out of sight. Accurate intake records are kept. The person needs frequent oral hygiene. Oral hygiene helps keep mucous membranes of the mouth moist.
- *Nothing by mouth*—the person cannot eat or drink anything. *NPO* is the abbreviation for the Latin term *nils per os*, which means nothing by mouth. Persons are usually NPO before and after surgery, before some laboratory tests and x-ray procedures, and in the treatment of certain illnesses. An NPO sign is posted above the bed. The water pitcher and glass are removed. Frequent oral hygiene is allowed, but the person cannot swallow any fluid. The person is kept NPO 6 to 8 hours before some surgeries, laboratory tests and x-ray procedures.

INTAKE AND OUTPUT RECORDS

The doctor or RN may want a person's fluid intake and output measured. This involves keeping intake and output (I&O) records. I&O records are used to evaluate fluid balance and kidney function. They are used also to plan and evaluate medical treatment. I&O records are kept when the person has special fluid orders. Many diseases and injuries also require measuring output.

All fluids taken by mouth are measured. So are fluids given in IV therapy and tube feedings. The obvious fluids are measured: water, milk, coffee, tea, juices, soups, and soft drinks. So are soft and semisolid foods such as ice cream, sherbet, custard, pudding, creamed cereals, gelatin, and Popsicles. Output to measure includes urine, vomitus, diarrhea, and wound drainage.

Measuring Intake and Output. Intake and output are measured in milliliters (ml) or in cubic centimeters (cc). These metric system measurements are equal in amount. One ounce equals 30 ml. A pint is about 500 ml. There are about 1000 ml in a quart. You need to know the fluid capacity of bowls, dishes, cups, pitchers, glasses, and other containers used to serve fluids. Most I&O records have tables for use in measuring intake (Fig. 18-20).

A **graduate** is used to measure fluids. A graduate is a measuring container. It is like a measuring cup but larger. Some graduates are marked in ounces and in milliliters or cubic centimeters (Fig. 18-21, p. 466). A graduate is used to measure leftover fluids, urine, vomitus, and drainage from suction (see Chapter 25). Plastic urinals, kidney basins, and other receptacles are often marked in amounts.

Fig. 18-20 An intake and output record. (*Courtesy Evangelical Lutheran Society, Sioux Falls, SD.*)

An I&O record is usually kept at the bedside. Whenever fluid is ingested or output is measured, the amount is recorded in the appropriate column (see Fig. 18-20). The amounts are totaled at the end of the shift. The total amount for the shift is recorded in the person's chart. The person's I&O are also communicated to the next shift during the end-of-shift report. Intake through IV therapy or tube feedings is recorded and reported by the nurse.

The purpose of measuring intake and output is explained to the person. How the person can take part is also explained. Some persons measure and record their own intake. Family members may help. The urinal, commode, bedpan, or specimen pan is used for voiding. The toilet is not used. Remind the person not to put toilet tissue into the receptacle.

Medical asepsis, Standard Precautions, and the Bloodborne Pathogen Standard are followed when measuring output.

Fig. 18-21 A graduate calibrated in milliliters.

Measuring Intake and Output

NNAAP™

QUALITY OF LIFE

Remember to:
- Knock before entering the person's room
- Address the person by name
- Introduce yourself by name and title

Pre-Procedure

1 Explain the procedure to the person.
2 Collect the following:
- Intake and output (I&O) record
- Graduates (one for intake and one for output)
- Gloves
3 Place the I&O record at the bedside.

Procedure

4 Measure intake as follows:
  a Wash your hands.
  b Put on gloves.
  c Pour liquid that is remaining in a container into the graduate used to measure intake.
  d Measure the amount at eye level.
  e Check the amount of the serving on the I&O record.
  f Subtract the remaining amount from the full serving amount.
  g Repeat steps 4c through 4f for each liquid.
  h Add the amounts from 4g together. Record the time and amount on the I&O record.

5 Measure output as follows:
  a Wash your hands.
  b Put on gloves.
  c Pour the fluid into the graduate used to measure output.
  d Measure the amount at eye level.
  e Record the amount on the I&O record.
  f Empty the graduate into the toilet, and flush.
  g Rinse and return the graduate to its proper place.
  h Clean and rinse the bedpan, urinal, kidney basin, or other drainage container. Return it to its proper place.

Post-Procedure

6 Remove the gloves, and wash your hands.
7 Report your observations to the nurse.

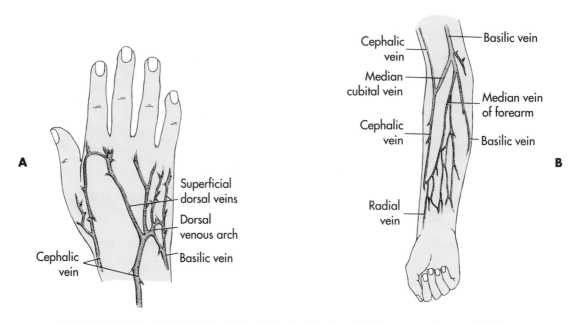

Fig. 18-22 Peripheral IV sites for adults. **A,** Back of the hand. **B,** Forearm and antecubital space. *(From Potter PA, Perry AG: Fundamentals of nursing: concepts, process, and practice, ed 4, St Louis, 1997, Mosby).*

PROVIDING DRINKING WATER

Patients and residents need fresh drinking water. Fresh water is usually provided during the day and evening and whenever the water pitcher is empty. Before passing drinking water you need to know about any special orders. Some persons are NPO, on restricted fluids, or not allowed ice. The rules of medical asepsis are practiced when passing drinking water. Follow the agency's procedure for providing fresh drinking water.

IV THERAPY

Intravenous (IV) therapy is the administration of fluids into a vein. A needle or catheter is inserted into a vein. Fluids enter the needle or catheter and go directly into the person's circulation. *IV* and *IV infusion* also refer to IV therapy. Doctors order IV therapy to:

- Provide needed fluids when the person cannot take fluids by mouth
- Replace minerals and vitamins lost because of illness or injury
- Provide sugar for energy
- Administer drugs and blood

IV therapy is given in hospital, outpatient, subacute care, long-term care, and home settings. RNs are responsible for IV therapy. They start and maintain the infusion according to the doctor's orders. RNs also give IV drugs and administer blood. State laws vary regarding the role of LPNs/LVNs in IV therapy. They also vary regarding the role of assistive personnel.

SITES

Peripheral IV sites and central venous sites are used for IV therapy. Periphery comes from the Greek words that mean around (*peri*) a boundary (*phery*). The boundary is the center of the body near the heart. Therefore *peripheral IV sites* are located away from the center of the body. Arm and hand veins are common IV sites for adults. The back of the hand and forearm are useful sites (Fig. 18-22, *A*). Veins in the antecubital space (crease of the elbow) are sometimes used (Fig. 18-22, *B*). Foot veins also are sites but are avoided if possible. They are small and easily irritated. *(See Focus on Children box.)*

Focus On... CHILDREN

Scalp and dorsal foot veins (Fig. 18-23) are the peripheral sites for infants. *Dorsal* means on the back of something. Dorsal foot veins are on the back of the foot. Hand and arm veins also are used.

Fig. 18-23 The scalp and foot provide peripheral IV sites in infants.

The subclavian vein and the internal jugular vein are *central venous sites.* These sites are close to the heart. A doctor inserts a long catheter into a central vein. The catheter tip is then threaded into the superior vena cava or right atrium (Fig. 18-24, *A* and *B*). The catheter is called a *central venous catheter* or *central line.* The cephalic and basilic veins in the arm also are used. Catheters inserted into these sites are called *peripherally inserted central catheters (PICC).* Inserted into the cephalic or basilic vein, the catheter tip is threaded into the subclavian vein or the superior vena cava (Fig. 18-24, *C*). Doctors and specially trained RNs insert PICCs.

Central venous sites are used to give large amounts of fluid and for long-term IV therapy. They also are used to give IV drugs that irritate the peripheral veins. Sometimes surgery is necessary to insert a central venous catheter. *(See Focus on Home Care box.)*

> **Focus On... HOME CARE**
>
> Patients can receive IV therapy in their homes. These persons often have central venous catheters. The RN teaches the patient and family about giving drugs and managing the catheter.

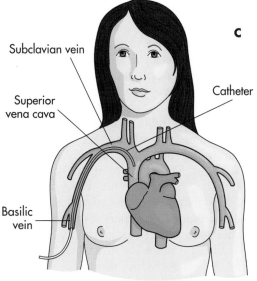

Fig. 18-24 Central venous sites. **A,** Subclavian vein. The catheter tip is in the right atrium. **B,** Internal jugular vein. The catheter tip is in the superior vena cava. C, Basilic vein. This is a peripherally inserted central catheter (PICC).

Fig. 18-25 Equipment for IV therapy.

Fig. 18-26 **A,** Intravenous catheter. **B,** Butterfly needle.

EQUIPMENT

The basic equipment used in IV therapy includes the solution container, IV needle or catheter, infusion set (tubing), and IV pole (Fig. 18-25):

- The solution container is a plastic bag or glass bottle. Plastic bags are common.
- A catheter or needle is inserted into a vein. An intravenous catheter is a plastic tube (Fig. 18-26, *A*). A needle fits over or is inside the catheter for insertion. After insertion, the needle is removed. Butterfly needles also are used (Fig. 18-26, *B*).
- The infusion set (tubing) connects the solution bag to the catheter or needle (see Fig. 18- 25). Fluid drips from the solution bag into the *drip chamber.* The RN uses the *clamp* to regulate the flow rate.
- The fluid bag hangs from the IV pole or ceiling hook. *IV standard* is another name for an IV pole. IV poles are portable or part of the bed. If portable, they are kept in the supply area. An IV pole is brought to the bedside when IV therapy is started. If part of the bed, the pole is stored under the bed frame. The pole is attached to the head, foot, or side of the bed when needed.

FLOW RATE

The flow rate is measured in drops per minute. The abbreviation *gtt* means drops. It comes from the Latin word *guttae* ,which means *drops.*

The doctor orders the amount of fluid to give and amount of time in which to give it in. With this information, the RN calculates the flow rate. The **flow rate** is the number of drops per minute (gtt/min).

The RN sets the clamp for the flow rate. Electronic infusion devices are often used to control the flow rate (Fig. 18-27). An alarm sounds if a problem occurs with the flow rate. Tell the nurse immediately if you hear the alarm. *Never change the position of the clamp or adjust any controls on infusion pumps.*

You assist the RN with IV therapy by checking the flow rate. The RN tells you the number of drops per minute. Check the flow rate by counting the number of drops in 1 full minute (Fig. 18-28). Tell the RN immediately if:

- No fluid is dripping
- The rate is too fast
- The rate is too slow

Also check the time tape on the IV bag (Fig. 18-29). The time tape shows how much fluid is to be given over a period of time. For example, the doctor orders 1000 ml of fluid to be given over 8 hours. The RN marks the tape in eight 1-hour intervals. To check if fluid is being given on time, the fluid line is compared

Fig. 18-27 Electronic infusion pump. *(From Elkin MK, Perry AG, Potter PA: Nursing interventions and clinical skills, ed 2, St Louis, 1996, Mosby.)*

Fig. 18-28 The flow rate is checked by counting the number of drops per minute.

with the time line on the tape. If the fluid line is above or below the time line, the flow rate is too slow or too fast. Tell the RN immediately if too much or too little fluid was given.

The person can suffer serious harm if the rate is too fast or too slow. Changes in flow rate can occur from position changes. Kinked tubes and lying on the tubing also are common problems.

ASSISTING THE RN

You assist the RN with meeting the hygiene and activity needs of persons with IVs. *You are never responsible for starting or maintaining an IV infusion. Nor do you regulate the flow rate or change IV solution containers. You never administer blood or IV medications.* However, you assist the RN in providing safe care. The safety measures in Box 18-6 on p. 472 are important. Complications can occur from IV therapy. Report any of the signs and symptoms listed in Box 18-7 on p. 472 to the RN immediately.

Remember, contact with blood is likely. Always practice Standard Precautions and follow the Blood-borne Pathogen Standard.

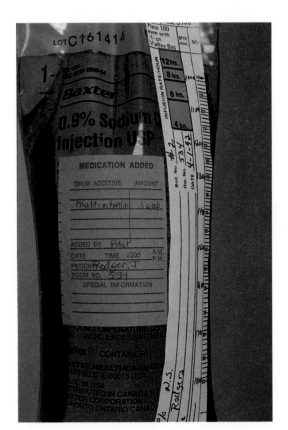

Fig. 18-29 Time tape applied to an IV bag. *(From Elkin MK, Perry AG, Potter PA: Nursing interventions and clinical skills, ed 2, St Louis, 2000, Mosby.)*

Box 18-6	Safety Measures for IV Therapy

- Always practice Standard Precautions and follow the Bloodborne Pathogen Standard.
- Do not move the needle or catheter. The position of the IV needle or catheter must be maintained when assisting a person. If the needle or catheter is moved, it may come out of the vein. Then fluid flows into the tissues (infiltration) or the flow stops.
- Follow the safety measures for restraints if a restraint is used. Sometimes the nurse splints or restrains the extremity to prevent movement of the part (Fig. 18-30). This helps prevent the needle or catheter from moving.
- Be careful not to move the needle or catheter when changing a gown.
- Protect the IV container, tubing, and needle or catheter when ambulating the person. Portable IV standards are rolled along next to the person (Fig. 18-31).
- Assist the person with turning and repositioning. The IV bag is moved to the side of the bed on which the person is lying. Always allow enough slack in the tubing. The needle dislodges if pressure is exerted by the tubing.
- Notify the RN immediately if bleeding occurs from the insertion site. Follow Standard Precautions and the Bloodborne Pathogen Standard.
- Notify the RN immediately of any signs and symptoms listed in Box 18-7.

Box 18-7	Signs and Symptoms of IV Therapy Complications

Local—at the IV site
- Bleeding
- Puffiness or swelling
- Pale or reddened skin
- Complaints of pain at or above the IV site
- Hot or cold skin near the site

Systemic—involving the whole body
- Fever
- Itching
- Drop in blood pressure
- Tachycardia (pulse rate more than 100 beats per minute)
- Irregular pulse
- Cyanosis
- Changes in mental function
- Loss of consciousness
- Difficulty breathing (dyspnea)
- Shortness of breath
- Decreasing or no urine output
- Chest pain
- Nausea
- Confusion

Fig. 18-30 An armboard prevents movement at an IV site. *(From Elkin MK, Perry AG, Potter PA: Nursing interventions and clinical skills, ed 2, St Louis, 2000, Mosby.)*

CROSS-TRAINING OPPORTUNITIES

In some agencies, nursing assistants are cross-trained as dietary aides. Dietary aides work in the dietary department. They serve food, prepare trays, and deliver trays to the nursing units. Dietary aides can also distribute and collect menus on the nursing units.

Fig. 18-31 A person ambulating with an IV.

Circle the BEST answer.

1. Nutrition is
   A. Fats, proteins, carbohydrates, vitamins, and minerals
   B. The many processes involved in the ingestion, digestion, absorption, and use of food and fluids by the body
   C. The Food Guide Pyramid
   D. The balance between calories taken in and used by the body

2. The Food Guide Pyramid encourages
   A. A low-fat diet
   B. A high-fat diet
   C. A low-fiber diet
   D. A low-salt diet

3. How many daily servings of breads, cereals, rice, and pasta are recommended?
   A. 6 to 11
   B. 3 to 5
   C. 2 to 4
   D. 2 to 3

4. How many daily servings of the meat group are recommended?
   A. 6 to 11
   B. 3 to 5
   C. 2 to 4
   D. 2 to 3

5. Which food groups contain the most fat?
   A. Breads, cereal, rice, and pasta
   B. Fruits
   C. Milk, yogurt, and cheese
   D. Meat, poultry, fish, dry beans, eggs, and nuts

6. Fats, oils, and sweets
   A. Should be used in moderate amounts
   B. Are low in calories
   C. Should be used sparingly
   D. Have great nutritional value

7. Protein is needed for
   A. Tissue growth and repair
   B. Energy and the fiber for bowel elimination
   C. Body heat and the protection of organs from injury
   D. Improving the taste of food

8. Which foods provide the *most* protein?
   A. Butter and cream
   B. Tomatoes and potatoes
   C. Meats and fish
   D. Corn and lettuce

9. Sodium-restricted diets are usually ordered for the following persons *except* those with
   A. Diabetes mellitus
   B. Heart disease
   C. Kidney disease
   D. Liver disease

10. Mr. Bonner is on a sodium-restricted diet. He asks for some salt for his chicken. You should
    A. Bring him the salt
    B. Tell the nurse
    C. Remind him that added salt is not allowed on his diet
    D. Ignore the request

11. For persons with diabetes mellitus, diet planning involves controlling the amount of
    A. Water
    B. Sodium
    C. Carbohydrates
    D. Nutrients

12. Which statement about feeding a person is *false*?
    A. Ask if he or she wants to pray before eating.
    B. A fork is used to feed the person.
    C. The person is asked the order in which to serve foods.
    D. Engage the person in a pleasant conversation.

13. To prevent regurgitation after a tubing feeding, the person is positioned
    A. In semi-Fowler's position for 30 minutes after the feeding
    B. In semi-Fowler's position for 1 hour after the feeding
    C. In the left side-lying position for 30 minutes after the feeding
    D. In the left side-lying position for 1 hour after the feeding

14. A person with a feeding tube is usually
    A. Allowed a regular diet
    B. On bedrest
    C. NPO
    D. In a coma

15. Adult fluid requirements for normal fluid balance are about
    A. 1000 to 1500 ml daily
    B. 1500 to 2000 ml daily
    C. 2000 to 2500 ml daily
    D. 2500 to 3000 ml daily

16. A person is NPO. You should
    A. Provide a variety of fluids
    B. Offer fluids in small amounts and small containers
    C. Remove the water pitcher and glass
    D. Prevent the person from having oral hygiene

17. Which are *not* counted as liquid foods?
    A. Coffee, tea, juices, and soft drinks
    B. Butter, spaghetti sauce, and melted cheese
    C. Ice cream, sherbet, custard, and pudding
    D. Jello, Popsicles, soup, and creamed cereals

18. You note that the IV flow rate is too slow. You must
    A. Tell the RN immediately
    B. Adjust the flow rate
    C. Reposition the person
    D. Clamp the tubing

19. A person is bleeding from an IV site. You should
    A. Remove the IV catheter or needle
    B. Apply direct pressure
    C. Call for the RN immediately
    D. Apply a dressing to the site

20. You observe the following in a person receiving IV therapy. Which is not a sign of IV therapy complications?
    A. Swelling at the IV site
    B. Changes in mental function or confusion
    C. Polyuria
    D. Changes in blood pressure, pulse, and respirations

The answers to these questions are on p. 836.

MEASURING VITAL SIGNS

OBJECTIVES

Define the key terms listed in this chapter

Explain why vital signs are measured

List the factors affecting vital signs

Identify the normal ranges of oral, rectal, axillary, and tympanic membrane temperatures

Know when to take oral, rectal, axillary, and tympanic membrane temperatures

Identify the sites for taking a pulse

Describe normal respirations

Describe the factors affecting blood pressure

Describe the practices that are followed when measuring blood pressure

Know the normal pulse, respiration, and blood pressure ranges for different age-groups

Perform the procedures described in this chapter

KEY TERMS

apical-radial pulse Taking the apical and radial pulses at the same time

blood pressure The amount of force exerted against the walls of an artery by the blood

body temperature The amount of heat in the body that is a balance between the amount of heat produced and the amount lost by the body

bradycardia A slow *(brady)* heart rate *(cardia)*; the rate is less than 60 beats per minute

diastole The period of heart muscle relaxation

diastolic pressure The pressure in the arteries when the heart is at rest

hypertension Persistent blood pressure measurements above the normal systolic (140 mm Hg) or diastolic (90 mm Hg) pressures

hypotension A condition in which the systolic blood pressure is below 90 mm Hg and the diastolic pressure is below 60 mm Hg

pulse The beat of the heart felt at an artery as a wave of blood passes through the artery

pulse deficit The difference between the apical and radial pulse rates

pulse rate The number of heartbeats or pulses felt in 1 minute

respiration The act of breathing air into (inhalation) and out of (exhalation) the lungs

sphygmomanometer The instrument used to measure blood pressure

stethoscope An instrument used to listen to the sounds produced by the heart, lungs, and other body organs

systole The period of heart muscle contraction

systolic pressure The amount of force it takes to pump blood out of the heart into the arterial circulation

tachycardia A rapid *(tachy)* heart rate *(cardia)*; the heart rate is over 100 beats per minute

vital signs Temperature, pulse, respirations, and blood pressure

Vital signs reflect the function of three body processes essential for life: regulation of body temperature, breathing, and heart function. The four **vital signs** of body function are temperature, pulse, respirations, and blood pressure.

MEASURING AND REPORTING VITAL SIGNS

A person's vital signs vary within certain limits during any 24-hour period. Many factors affect vital signs. They include sleep, activity, eating, weather, noise, exercise, drugs, anger, fear, anxiety, and illness. Vital signs are measured to detect changes in normal body function. They tell about a person's response to treatment. They often signal life-threatening events. Vital signs are part of the assessment step of the nursing process. Vital signs are measured:

- During physical examinations
- When a person is admitted to a health care agency
- Several times a day for hospital patients and patients in subacute care units
- Before and after surgery
- Before and after complex procedures or diagnostic tests
- After some nursing procedures or measures, such as ambulation
- When drugs are taken that affect the respiratory or circulatory system
- Whenever the person complains of pain, fainting, shortness of breath, rapid heart rate, or not feeling well
- As required by a nursing center resident's care plan

Vital signs show even minor changes in a person's condition. Accuracy is essential in measuring, recording, and reporting vital signs. If unsure of your measurements, promptly ask the nurse to take them again. Unless otherwise ordered, take vital signs with the person lying or sitting. The person is at rest when vital signs are measured. Immediately report to the nurse:

- Any vital sign that is changed from a previous measurement

- Vital signs above the normal range
- Vital signs below the normal range

Many agencies have *temp boards* or *TPR books*. These are divided into columns. Names are listed down the left side of the page. The other columns are for times (such as 0800, 1200, 1600, 2000). Vital signs are recorded on the line in the column appropriate for the person and time. In some agencies, changed or abnormal vital signs are circled in red. The nurse or doctor compares current and previous measurements.

BODY TEMPERATURE

Body temperature is the amount of heat in the body. It is a balance between the amount of heat produced and the amount lost by the body. Heat is produced as cells use food for energy. It is lost through the skin, breathing, urine, and feces. Body temperature remains fairly stable. It is lower in the morning and higher in the afternoon and evening. Factors affecting body temperature include age, weather, exercise, pregnancy, the menstrual cycle, emotions, stress, and illness.

NORMAL BODY TEMPERATURE

Temperature is measured using the Fahrenheit (F) and Centigrade or Celsius (C) scales. Common sites for measuring body temperature are the mouth, rectum, axilla (underarm), and ear (tympanic membrane). Normal body temperature depends on the site and usually stays within a normal range (Table 19-1).

Thermometers are used to measure temperature. Glass and disposable thermometers are common in homes. So are tympanic thermometers. Electronic and tympanic thermometers are common in hospitals and nursing centers. Glass and disposable thermometers also are used for persons requiring isolation. (*See Focus on Older Persons box below* and *Focus on Children box on p. 478.*)

Focus On... OLDER PERSONS

Older persons generally have lower body temperatures than younger adults. An oral temperature of 98.6° F may signal fever in an older person.

Table 19-1	Normal Body Temperatures	
Site	**Baseline**	**Normal Range**
Oral	98.6° F (37° C)	97.6° to 99.6° F (36.5° to 37.5° C)
Rectal	99.6° F (37.5° C)	98.6° to 100.6° F (37.0° to 38.1° C)
Axillary	97.6° F (36.5° C)	96.6° to 98.6° F (35.9° to 37.0° C)
Tympanic membrane	98.6° F (37° C)	98.6° F (37° C)

Focus On... CHILDREN

Pacifier thermometers are available. They are used for children under 5 years of age. The pacifier thermometer has four parts: a storage cover, a nipple with a sensor, a digital display, and an on and off switch. Temperature is measured in about 5 minutes.

To use the thermometer:

- Remove it from the storage case.
- Check the pacifier for cracks or holes. These can occur if the child bites or chews on the thermometer. Discard the thermometer if it is not intact.
- Turn it on by pressing the on/off switch.
- Place the pacifier in the child's mouth. Hold and cuddle the child.
- Read the digital display on the front of the pacifier when the thermometer beeps.
- Clean the thermometer with a disinfectant such as alcohol. Or wash it with soap and water. Do not use boiling water, the dishwasher, or a sterilizer to clean the thermometer.
- Wipe the thermometer dry.
- Return it to the storage case.
- Discard the thermometer when the battery has run out.

Pacifier thermometers are available in stores for home use.

GLASS THERMOMETERS

The glass thermometer (clinical thermometer) is a hollow glass tube with a mercury-filled bulb (Fig. 19-1). When heated, the mercury expands and rises in the tube. The mercury contracts and moves down the tube when cooled.

Long- or slender-tip thermometers are used for oral and axillary temperatures. So are thermometers with stubby and pear-shaped tips. Rectal thermometers have stubby tips that are color coded in red.

Glass thermometers are reusable. However, they have the following disadvantages:

- They take a long time to register—3 to 10 minutes depending on the site. Oral temperatures take 2 to 3 minutes, rectal temperatures take at least 2 minutes, and axillary temperatures take 5 to 10 minutes.
- They break easily. Broken rectal thermometers can injure the rectum and colon.
- The person may bite down on an oral thermometer and cause it to break. Cuts to the oral mucous membranes are risks. Any swallowed mercury can cause mercury poisoning.
- *NOTE: If a glass thermometer breaks, you must report it to the nurse immediately. Mercury is a hazardous substance and requires special disposal procedures. Do*

not touch the mercury, and do not let the person do so. The agency must follow special procedures for handling all hazardous materials. See Chapter 9.

How to Read a Glass Thermometer. Fahrenheit thermometers have long and short lines. Every other long line is marked in an even degree from 94° to 108° F. The short lines indicate 0.2 (two tenths) of a degree (Fig. 19-2, *A*).

Centigrade thermometers also have long and short lines. Each long line represents 1 degree, from 34° to 42° C. Each short line represents 0.1 (one tenth) of a degree (Fig. 19-2, *B*).

Do the following to read a glass thermometer:

- Hold the thermometer at the stem (Fig. 19-3). Bring it to eye level.
- Rotate the thermometer until you can see both the numbers and the long and short lines.
- Turn the thermometer back and forth slowly until you see the silver (or red) mercury line.
- Read the thermometer to the nearest degree (long line). Read the nearest tenth of a degree (short line)—an even number if you are using a Fahrenheit thermometer.

Using a Glass Thermometer. The thermometer is inserted into the mouth, rectum, or axilla. Each area has many microbes. Therefore each person has a thermometer. This prevents the spread of microbes and infection. The following measures are practiced when using a glass thermometer:

- Use only the person's thermometer.
- Rinse the thermometer under cold running water if it was soaking in a disinfectant. Use tissues to dry it from the stem to the bulb end.
- Check the thermometer for breaks and chips.
- Shake down the thermometer so the mercury is below the lines and numbers. Hold the thermometer at the stem. Stand away from walls, tables, or other hard surfaces. Flex and snap your wrist until the mercury is shaken down (Fig. 19-4).
- Clean and store the thermometer following agency policy. Wipe it with tissues first to remove mucus or feces. Do not use hot water for cleaning. It causes the mercury to expand so much that the thermometer could break. After cleaning, rinse the thermometer under cold running water. Then store it in a case or a container filled with disinfectant solution.
- Use plastic covers following agency policy (Fig. 19-5). A cover is used once and then discarded. The thermometer is inserted into a cover, and the temperature taken. The cover is removed to read the thermometer. The thermometer never touches the person.
- Practice medical asepsis and Standard Precautions.

Fig. 19-1 Types of glass thermometers. **A,** The long or slender tip. **B,** The stubby tip (rectal thermometer). **C,** The pear-shaped tip.

98.6

37.0

Fig. 19-2 **A,** Fahrenheit thermometer. The mercury level is at 98.6° F. **B,** Centigrade thermometer. The mercury level is at 37.0° C.

Fig. 19-3 The thermometer is held at the stem. It is read at eye level.

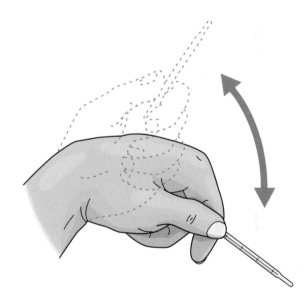

Fig. 19-4 The wrist is snapped to shake down the thermometer.

Fig. 19-5 **A,** The thermometer is inserted into a plastic cover. **B,** The person's temperature is taken with the thermometer in the plastic cover.

▶ **Taking Oral Temperatures.** Oral temperatures are usually taken on older children and adults. The glass thermometer remains in place 2 to 3 minutes or as required by agency policy. Temperatures are not taken orally if the person:

- Is an infant or a child younger than 4 or 5 years
- Is unconscious
- Has had surgery or an injury to the face, neck, nose, or mouth

- Is receiving oxygen
- Breathes through the mouth
- Has a nasogastric tube in place
- Is delirious, restless, confused, or disoriented
- Is paralyzed on one side of the body
- Has a sore mouth
- Has a history of convulsive disorders

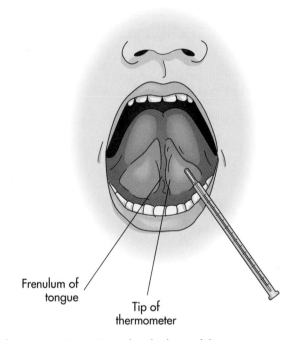

Frenulum of tongue

Tip of thermometer

Fig. 19-6 The thermometer is positioned at the base of the tongue next to the frenulum.

Taking an Oral Temperature With a Glass Thermometer

NNAAP™

QUALITY OF LIFE

Remember to:
- Knock before entering the person's room
- Address the person by name
- Introduce yourself by name and title

Pre-Procedure

1 Explain the procedure to the person. Ask him or her not to eat, drink, smoke, or chew gum for at least 20 minutes.
2 Collect the following:
   - Oral thermometer and holder
   - Tissues
   - Plastic covers if used
   - Gloves
3 Wash your hands.
4 Identify the person. Check the ID bracelet against the assignment sheet.
5 Provide for privacy.

Procedure

6 Put on the gloves.
7 Rinse the thermometer in cold water if it was soaking in a disinfectant solution. Dry it with tissues.
8 Check the thermometer for breaks or chips.
9 Shake down the thermometer.
10 Place a plastic cover on the thermometer if used.
11 Ask the person to moisten his or her lips.
12 Place the bulb end of the thermometer under the person's tongue (Fig. 19-6).
13 Ask the person to close his or her lips around the thermometer to hold it in place. Ask the person not to talk while the thermometer is in place. Also remind the person not to bite down on the thermometer.
14 Leave the thermometer in place for 2 to 3 minutes or as required by agency policy.
15 Remove the thermometer by grasping the stem.
16 Use tissues to remove the plastic cover. Wipe the thermometer with a tissue from the stem to the bulb end if no cover was used.
17 Read the thermometer.
18 Record the person's name and temperature on your note pad or assignment sheet.
19 Shake down the thermometer.
20 Clean the thermometer according to agency policy.

Post-Procedure

21 Provide for comfort.
22 Place the signal light within reach.
23 Unscreen the person.
24 Remove the gloves, and wash your hands.
25 Report any abnormal temperature to the nurse. Record the measurement in the proper place.

▶ **Taking Rectal Temperatures.** Rectal temperatures are taken when the oral route cannot be used. Rectal temperatures are not taken if the person has diarrhea or a rectal disorder or injury or has had rectal surgery. Rectal temperatures are also dangerous for persons with heart disease. The thermometer can stimulate the vagus nerve in the rectum. This nerve also affects the heart. Stimulation of the vagus nerve slows the heart rate. The heart rate can slow to dangerous levels in some persons.

The rectal thermometer is lubricated for easy insertion and to prevent tissue injury. The thermometer is held in place so it is not lost into the rectum or broken. A glass thermometer remains in the rectum for 2 minutes or as required by agency policy.

Privacy is important when taking rectal temperatures. The buttocks and anus are exposed. Many people are embarrassed by the procedure.

Fig. 19-7 The rectal temperature is taken with the patient in Sims' position. The buttock is raised to expose the anus.

Taking a Rectal Temperature With a Glass Thermometer

QUALITY OF LIFE

Remember to:
- Knock before entering the person's room
- Address the person by name
- Introduce yourself by name and title

Pre-Procedure

1 Explain the procedure to the person.
2 Collect the following:
  - Rectal thermometer and holder
  - Toilet tissue
  - Plastic covers if used
  - Gloves
  - Water-soluble lubricant
3 Wash your hands.
4 Identify the person. Check the ID bracelet against the assignment sheet.
5 Provide for privacy.

Procedure

6 Rinse the thermometer in cold water if it was soaking in a disinfectant solution. Dry it with tissues.
7 Check the thermometer for breaks or chips.
8 Shake down the thermometer.
9 Place a plastic cover on the thermometer if used.
10 Position the person in Sims' position.
11 Put on the gloves.
12 Put a small amount of lubricant on a tissue. Lubricate the bulb end of the thermometer.
13 Fold back top linens to expose the anal area.
14 Raise the upper buttock to expose the anus (Fig. 19-7).
15 Insert the thermometer 1 inch into the rectum. Do not force the thermometer. Remember, glass thermometers can break.
16 Hold it in place for 2 minutes or as required by the agency.
17 Remove the thermometer.
18 Remove the plastic cover. Wipe the thermometer with tissues from the stem to the bulb end if no cover was used.
19 Place the used toilet tissue on a paper towel or several thicknesses of toilet tissue. Place the thermometer on clean toilet tissue.
20 Wipe the anal area to remove excess lubricant and any feces. Cover the person.
21 Provide for comfort.
22 Place the signal light within reach.
23 Dispose of tissue.
24 Read the thermometer. Record the person's name and temperature on your note pad or assignment sheet. Write *R* to indicate a rectal temperature.
25 Shake down the thermometer.
26 Clean the thermometer according to agency policy.
27 Remove the gloves, and wash your hands.

Post-Procedure

28 Unscreen the person.
29 Report any abnormal temperature. Record the measurement with an *R* in the proper place.

▶ **Taking Axillary Temperatures.** Axillary temperatures are less reliable than oral, rectal, or tympanic membrane temperatures. They are used when the other routes cannot be used. The axilla must be dry for the measurement. This site is not used right after bathing. The thermometer is held in place to maintain proper position. A glass thermometer is held in place for 5 to 10 minutes or as required by agency policy.

Thermometer

Fig. 19-8 The thermometer is held in place in the axilla by bringing the person's arm over the chest.

Taking an Axillary Temperature With a Glass Thermometer

QUALITY OF LIFE

Remember to:
- Knock before entering the person's room
- Address the person by name
- Introduce yourself by name and title

Pre-Procedure

1 Explain the procedure to the person.
2 Collect the following:
   - Oral glass thermometer and holder
   - Plastic covers if used
   - Tissues
   - Towel
3 Wash your hands.
4 Identify the person. Check the ID bracelet against the assignment sheet.
5 Provide for privacy.

Procedure

6 Rinse the thermometer in cold water if it was soaking in a disinfectant solution. Dry it with tissues.
7 Check the thermometer for breaks or chips.
8 Shake down the thermometer.
9 Place a plastic cover on the thermometer if used.
10 Help the person remove an arm from the gown. Do not expose the person.
11 Dry the axilla with the towel.
12 Place the bulb end of the thermometer in the center of the axilla.
13 Ask the person to place the arm over the chest to hold the thermometer in place (Fig. 19-8). Hold it and the arm in place if he or she cannot help or if the person is an infant or child.
14 Leave the thermometer in place for 5 to 10 minutes or as required by agency policy.
15 Remove the thermometer from the plastic cover. Wipe it with tissues from the stem to the bulb end if no cover was used.
16 Read the thermometer.
17 Record the person's name and temperature with an *A* (for axillary temperature) on your note pad or assignment sheet.
18 Help the person put the gown back on.
19 Provide for comfort.
20 Place the signal light within reach.
21 Shake down the thermometer.
22 Rinse and wash the thermometer. Place it in the holder with disinfectant or in a plastic cover.

Post-Procedure

23 Unscreen the person.
24 Follow agency policy for soiled linen.
25 Wash your hands.
26 Report any abnormal temperature. Record the measurement with an *A* in the proper place.

► ELECTRONIC THERMOMETERS

Electronic thermometers are battery operated. They measure temperature in a few seconds. The temperature is displayed on the front of the instrument. Some models have a battery charger. The hand-held unit is kept in a battery charger when not in use.

Electronic thermometers have oral and rectal probes. A disposable cover (sheath) covers the probe. Disposable probe covers are used once and then discarded. This helps prevent the spread of infection. Medical asepsis and Standard Precautions also help prevent the spread of infection.

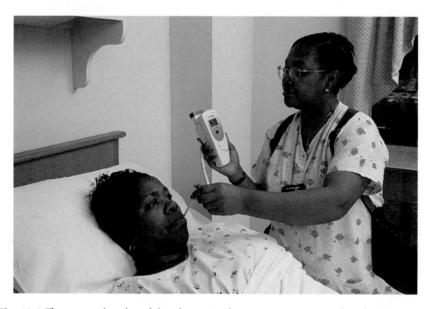

Fig. 19-9 The covered probe of the electronic thermometer is inserted under the tongue.

Taking a Temperature With an Electronic Thermometer

Pre-Procedure

1. Explain the procedure to the person. Ask him or her not to eat, drink, smoke, or chew gum for at least 20 minutes if you will take an oral temperature.
2. Collect the following:
   - Electronic thermometer
   - Probe (blue for an oral or axillary temperature; red for a rectal temperature)
   - Disposable probe covers
   - Toilet tissue (for a rectal temperature)
   - Water-soluble lubricant (for a rectal temperature)
   - Gloves
3. Plug the probe into the thermometer.
4. Wash your hands.
5. Identify the person. Check the ID bracelet against the assignment sheet.

Procedure

6. Provide for privacy. Position the person for an oral, rectal, or axillary temperature.
7. Put on gloves if contact with blood, body fluids, secretions, or excretions is likely.
8. Insert the probe into a probe cover.
9. For an *oral temperature*:
   a. Ask the person to open the mouth and raise the tongue.
   b. Place the covered probe at the base of the tongue on either side (Fig. 19-9).
   c. Ask the person to lower the tongue and close the mouth.

   For a *rectal temperature*:
   a. Lubricate the end of the covered probe using the lubricant on the toilet tissue.
   b. Fold back top linens to expose the anal area.
   c. Raise the upper buttock to expose the anus.
   d. Insert the probe $1/_2$ inch into the rectum.

   For an *axillary temperature*:
   a. Help the person remove an arm from the gown. Do not expose the person.
   b. Dry the axilla with the towel.
   c. Place the covered probe in the axilla. Place the person's arm over the chest.
10. Hold the probe in place until you hear a tone or see a flashing or steady light.
11. Read the temperature on the display.
12. Remove the probe. Press the eject button to discard the cover.
13. Record the person's name and temperature on your note pad or assignment sheet.
14. Return the probe to the holder.
15. Provide for comfort. Help the person put the gown back on if an axillary temperature was taken. For a *rectal temperature*:
    a. Wipe the anal area with tissue to remove lubricant.
    b. Cover the person.
    c. Discard used toilet tissue.
    d. Remove the gloves.

Post-Procedure

16. Place the signal light within reach.
17. Unscreen the person.
18. Remove the gloves, and wash your hands.
19. Return the thermometer to the charging unit.
20. Wash your hands.
21. Report any abnormal temperature. Record the measurement in the proper place. Note if an oral, rectal, or axillary temperature was taken.

► TYMPANIC MEMBRANE THERMOMETERS

Tympanic membrane thermometers measure temperature at the tympanic membrane in the ear (Fig. 19-10). The covered probe is gently inserted into the ear. The temperature is measured in 1 to 3 seconds. These thermometers are battery operated and use disposable probe covers. They must be kept charged.

Tympanic membrane thermometers are comfortable for the person. They are not invasive like rectal thermometers. They are useful for children because of their speed and comfort. The ear has fewer microbes than the mouth or rectum. Therefore the risk of spreading infection is reduced. These thermometers are not used if there is drainage from the ear.

Fig. 19-10 Tympanic membrane thermometer.

Fig. 19-11 A, The ear is pulled back and, B, the tympanic membrane thermometer probe is inserted into the ear canal.

Taking a Tympanic Membrane Temperature

QUALITY OF LIFE

Remember to:
- Knock before entering the person's room
- Address the person by name
- Introduce yourself by name and title

Pre-Procedure

1 Explain the procedure to the person.
2 Get the tympanic membrane thermometer and a probe cover.
3 Wash your hands.
4 Identify the person. Check the ID bracelet against the assignment sheet.
5 Provide for privacy.

Procedure

6 Ask the person to turn his or her head so the ear is in front of you.
7 Insert the probe gently. Pull back on the ear to straighten the ear canal (Fig. 19-11).
8 Start the thermometer.
9 Read the measurement when you hear a tone or see a flashing light.
10 Remove the probe from the ear.
11 Record the person's name and temperature on your note pad or assignment sheet. Note that a tympanic temperature was taken.
12 Press the eject button, and discard the probe.

Post-Procedure

13 Provide for comfort.
14 Place the signal light within reach.
15 Unscreen the person.
16 Return the thermometer to the charging unit.
17 Wash your hands.
18 Report any abnormal temperature. Record the measurement in the proper place. Note that a tympanic membrane temperature was taken.

DISPOSABLE ORAL THERMOMETERS

Disposable oral thermometers have small chemical dots (Fig. 19-12). The dots change color when heated by the body. Each dot must be heated to a certain temperature before it changes color. These thermometers are used only once. They measure temperature in 45 to 60 seconds.

TEMPERATURE-SENSITIVE TAPE

Temperature-sensitive tape changes color in response to body heat. The tape is applied to the forehead or abdomen. It shows if the temperature is normal or above normal. Exact body temperature is not measured. The color change takes about 15 seconds.

PULSE

Arteries carry blood from the heart to all parts of the body (Box 19-1). The **pulse** is defined as the beat of the heart felt at an artery as a wave of blood passes through the artery. A pulse can be felt every time the heart beats.

Box 19-1	Review: Structure and Function of the Heart and Blood Vessels

The heart is a muscle. It pumps blood through the blood vessels to the tissues and cells. The heart lies in the middle to lower part of the chest cavity toward the left side (Fig.19-13).

The heart has four chambers (see Fig. 6-15). Upper chambers receive blood and are called the *atria*. The right atrium receives blood from body tissues. The left atrium receives blood from the lungs. Lower chambers are called *ventricles*. Ventricles pump blood. The right ventricle pumps blood to the lungs for oxygen. The left ventricle pumps blood to all parts of the body.

There are two phases of heart action. During *diastole*, the resting phase, heart chambers fill with blood. During *systole*, the working phase, the heart contracts. Blood is pumped through the blood vessels when the heart contracts.

Blood flows to body tissues and cells through the blood vessels. *Arteries* carry blood away from the heart. Arterial blood is rich in oxygen. The *aorta* is the largest artery. The aorta receives blood directly from the left ventricle. The aorta branches into other arteries that carry blood to all parts of the body (Fig. 19-14). *Veins* return blood to the heart.

See Chapter 6 for more detailed information.

Fig. 19-12 A, Disposable oral thermometer with chemical dots. **B,** The dots change color when the temperature is taken.

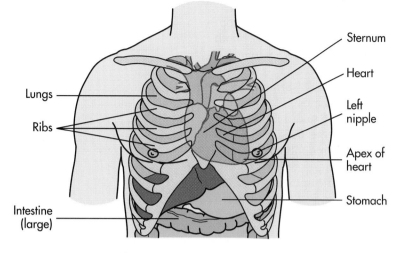

Fig. 19-13 Location of the heart.

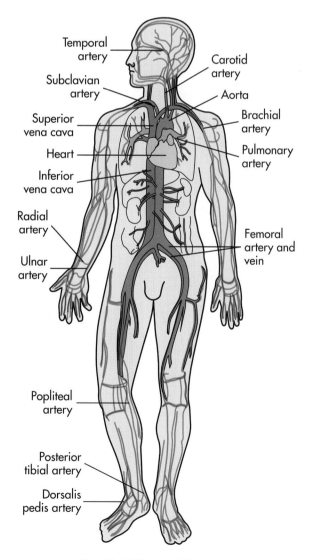

Fig. 19-14 The arterial system.

SITES FOR TAKING A PULSE

The temporal, carotid, brachial, radial, femoral, popliteal, and dorsalis pedis (pedal) pulses are on both sides of the body (Fig. 19-15). Pulses are easy to feel at these sites.

The arteries are close to the body's surface and lie over a bone. The radial site is used most often because it is easy to reach and find. You can take a radial pulse without disturbing or exposing the person. The carotid pulse is taken during cardiopulmonary resuscitation (CPR) and other emergencies (see Chapter 36).

The apical pulse is felt over the apex of the heart. The apex is at the tip of the heart, just below the left nipple. The apical pulse is taken with a stethoscope.

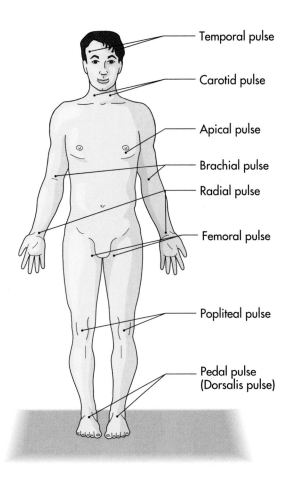

Temporal pulse

Carotid pulse

Apical pulse

Brachial pulse

Radial pulse

Femoral pulse

Popliteal pulse

Pedal pulse
(Dorsalis pulse)

Fig. 19-15 The pulse sites.

USING A STETHOSCOPE

A **stethoscope** is an instrument used to listen to the sounds produced by the heart, lungs, and other body organs (Fig. 19-16). It is used to take the apical pulse and to measure blood pressure. The stethoscope amplifies the sounds for easy hearing.

Stethoscopes are in contact with many persons and health team members. Therefore infection control is important. The earpieces and diaphragm are cleaned before and after use. Cleaning prevents the spread of microbes.

The following measures are practiced when using a stethoscope:

- Wipe the earpieces and diaphragm with alcohol wipes between each use.
- Warm the diaphragm in your hand (Fig. 19-17).
- Place the earpiece tips in your ears so the bend of the tips points forward. Earpieces should fit snugly to block out external noises. They should not cause pain or ear discomfort.
- Place the diaphragm over the artery. Hold it in place as in Figure 19-18.
- Prevent noise. Do not let anything touch the tubing. Ask the person to be silent during the procedure.
- Wipe the earpiece tips and diaphragm with alcohol wipes after the procedure.

Fig. 19-17 The diaphragm of the stethoscope is warmed in the palm of the hand.

Fig. 19-18 The stethoscope is held in place with the fingertips of the index and middle fingers.

Earpieces
Binaurals
Rubber or plastic tubing
Bell
Chestpiece
Diaphragm

Fig. 19-16 Parts of a stethoscope.

PULSE RATE

The **pulse rate** is the number of heartbeats or pulses felt in 1 minute. The rate varies for different age-groups (Table 19-2). The pulse rate is affected by many factors. They include elevated body temperature (fever), exercise, fear, anger, anxiety, excitement, heat, position, and pain. These and other factors cause the heart to beat faster. Some drugs also increase the pulse rate. Other drugs slow down the pulse.

The adult pulse rate is between 60 and 100 beats per minute. A rate of less than 60 or more than 100 is considered abnormal. **Tachycardia** is a rapid *(tachy)* heart rate *(cardia)*. The heart rate is more than 100 beats per minute. **Bradycardia** is a slow *(brady)* heart rate *(cardia)*. The rate is less than 60 beats per minute. Report abnormal rates to the nurse immediately.

RHYTHM AND FORCE OF THE PULSE

The rhythm of the pulse should be regular. That is, a pulse should be felt in a pattern. The same time interval should occur between beats. An irregular pulse occurs when the beats are unevenly spaced or beats are skipped (Fig. 19-19).

The force of the pulse relates to its strength. A forceful pulse is easy to feel and is described as strong, full, or bounding. Pulses that are hard to feel are described as weak, thready, or feeble.

Electronic blood pressure equipment can also count pulses. The pulse rate is displayed along with the blood pressure. However, no information is given about the rhythm and force of the pulse. If electronic blood pressure equipment is used, you still need to feel the pulse to determine rhythm and force.

Table 19-2	Pulse Ranges for Different Ages
Age	**Pulse Rates per Minute**
Birth to 4 weeks	80-180
4 weeks to 1 year	80-160
1 to 2 years	80-130
2 to 6 years	80-120
6 to 12 years	70-110
12 years and older	60-100

Fig. 19-19 A, The electrocardiogram shows a regular pulse. The beats occur at regular intervals. **B,** The beats in this electrocardiogram occur at irregular intervals. *(From Atwood S, Stanton C, Storey J: Introduction to basic cardiac dysrhythmias, ed 2, St Louis, 1996, Mosby.)*

TAKING A RADIAL PULSE

The radial pulse is used for routine vital signs. The pulse is felt by placing the first three fingers of one hand against the radial artery. The radial artery is on the thumb side of the wrist (Fig. 19-20). Do not use your thumb to take a pulse; it has a pulse of its own. You could mistake the pulse in your thumb for the person's pulse. Count the pulse for 30 seconds. Then multiply the number by 2 to get the number of beats per minute. If the pulse is irregular, count the pulse for 1 full minute.

Some agencies require that all radial pulses be taken for 1 full minute. Follow your agency's policy.

Fig. 19-20 The middle three fingers are used to locate the radial pulse on the thumb side of the wrist.

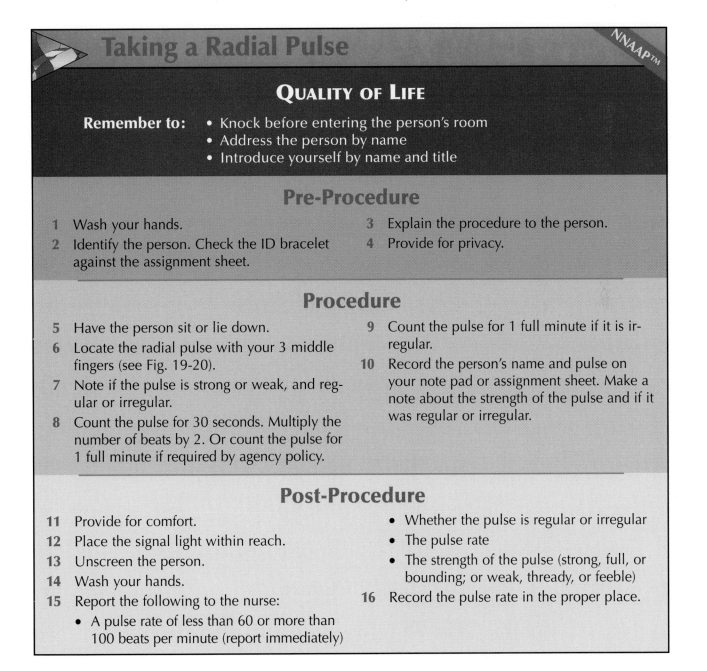

Taking a Radial Pulse

NNAAP™

QUALITY OF LIFE

Remember to:
- Knock before entering the person's room
- Address the person by name
- Introduce yourself by name and title

Pre-Procedure

1 Wash your hands.
2 Identify the person. Check the ID bracelet against the assignment sheet.
3 Explain the procedure to the person.
4 Provide for privacy.

Procedure

5 Have the person sit or lie down.
6 Locate the radial pulse with your 3 middle fingers (see Fig. 19-20).
7 Note if the pulse is strong or weak, and regular or irregular.
8 Count the pulse for 30 seconds. Multiply the number of beats by 2. Or count the pulse for 1 full minute if required by agency policy.
9 Count the pulse for 1 full minute if it is irregular.
10 Record the person's name and pulse on your note pad or assignment sheet. Make a note about the strength of the pulse and if it was regular or irregular.

Post-Procedure

11 Provide for comfort.
12 Place the signal light within reach.
13 Unscreen the person.
14 Wash your hands.
15 Report the following to the nurse:
- A pulse rate of less than 60 or more than 100 beats per minute (report immediately)
- Whether the pulse is regular or irregular
- The pulse rate
- The strength of the pulse (strong, full, or bounding; or weak, thready, or feeble)

16 Record the pulse rate in the proper place.

▶ TAKING AN APICAL PULSE

The apical pulse is taken with a stethoscope. This method is used on infants and children up to about 3 years of age. Apical pulses are also taken on adults who have heart disease or who take drugs that affect the heart. The apical pulse is on the left side of the chest slightly below the nipple (Fig. 19-21). The apical pulse is counted for 1 full minute.

The heartbeat normally sounds like a *lub-dub*. Each *lub-dub* is counted as 1 beat. Do not count the *lub* as 1 beat and the *dub* as another.

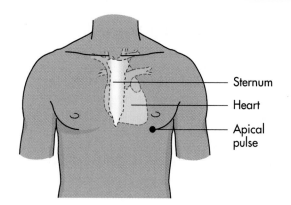

Fig. 19-21 The apical pulse is located 2 to 3 inches to the left of the sternum (breastbone) and below the left nipple.

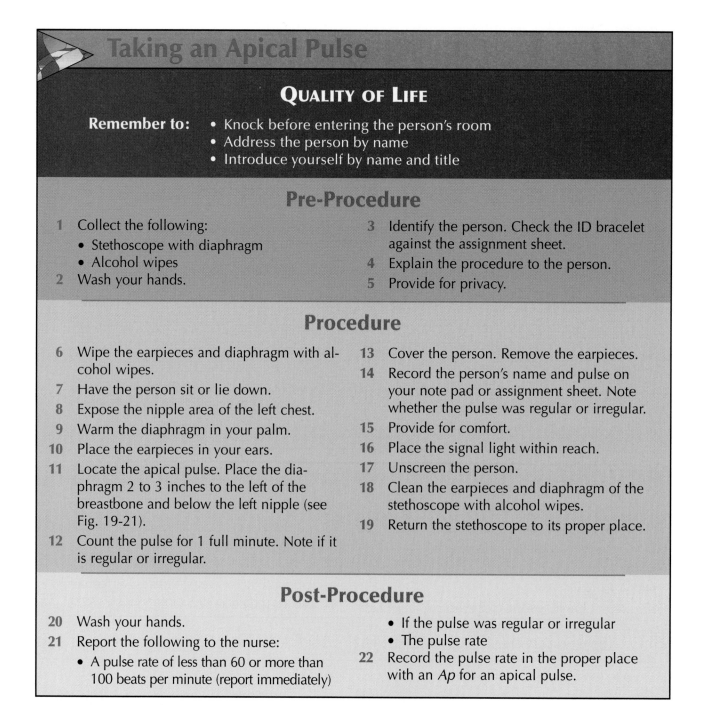

Taking an Apical Pulse

QUALITY OF LIFE

Remember to:
- Knock before entering the person's room
- Address the person by name
- Introduce yourself by name and title

Pre-Procedure

1 Collect the following:
- Stethoscope with diaphragm
- Alcohol wipes
2 Wash your hands.

3 Identify the person. Check the ID bracelet against the assignment sheet.
4 Explain the procedure to the person.
5 Provide for privacy.

Procedure

6 Wipe the earpieces and diaphragm with alcohol wipes.
7 Have the person sit or lie down.
8 Expose the nipple area of the left chest.
9 Warm the diaphragm in your palm.
10 Place the earpieces in your ears.
11 Locate the apical pulse. Place the diaphragm 2 to 3 inches to the left of the breastbone and below the left nipple (see Fig. 19-21).
12 Count the pulse for 1 full minute. Note if it is regular or irregular.

13 Cover the person. Remove the earpieces.
14 Record the person's name and pulse on your note pad or assignment sheet. Note whether the pulse was regular or irregular.
15 Provide for comfort.
16 Place the signal light within reach.
17 Unscreen the person.
18 Clean the earpieces and diaphragm of the stethoscope with alcohol wipes.
19 Return the stethoscope to its proper place.

Post-Procedure

20 Wash your hands.
21 Report the following to the nurse:
- A pulse rate of less than 60 or more than 100 beats per minute (report immediately)

- If the pulse was regular or irregular
- The pulse rate
22 Record the pulse rate in the proper place with an *Ap* for an apical pulse.

▶ TAKING AN APICAL-RADIAL PULSE

The apical and radial pulse rates should be equal. Sometimes heart contractions are not strong enough to create pulses in the radial artery. The radial pulse may be less than the apical pulse. This may occur in people with heart disease. To see if there is a difference between the apical and radial rates, two staff members take the pulses as the same time. This is called an **apical-radial pulse.** The **pulse deficit** is the difference between the apical and radial pulse rates. To obtain the pulse deficit, subtract the radial rate from the apical rate. The apical pulse rate is never less than the radial pulse rate.

Fig. 19-22 Taking an apical-radial pulse. One worker takes the apical pulse, and the other takes the radial pulse.

Taking an Apical-Radial Pulse

QUALITY OF LIFE

Remember to:
- Knock before entering the person's room
- Address the person by name
- Introduce yourself by name and title

Pre-Procedure

1 Ask a nurse or a nursing assistant to help you.
2 Collect a stethoscope and alcohol wipes.
3 Wash your hands.
4 Identify the person. Check the ID bracelet against the assignment sheet.
5 Explain the procedure to the person.
6 Provide for privacy.

Procedure

7 Wipe the earpieces and diaphragm with the alcohol wipes.
8 Have the person sit or lie down.
9 Warm the diaphragm in your palm.
10 Expose the left nipple area of the chest.
11 Place the earpieces in your ears.
12 Find the apical pulse. Have your co-worker find the radial pulse (Fig. 19-22).
13 Give the signal to begin counting.
14 Count the pulse for 1 full minute.
15 Give the signal to stop counting.
16 Cover the person. Remove the earpieces.
17 Record the apical and radial pulses on your note pad or assignment sheet. Subtract the radial pulse from the apical pulse for the pulse deficit. Note whether the pulse was regular or irregular.
18 Provide for comfort.
19 Place the signal light within reach.
20 Unscreen the person.
21 Clean the earpieces and diaphragm with alcohol wipes.
22 Return the stethoscope to its proper place.

Post-Procedure

23 Wash your hands.
24 Report the following to the nurse:
- An apical pulse rate of less than 60 or more than 100 beats per minute (report immediately)
- The apical and radial pulse rates
- The pulse deficit
- If the pulse was regular or irregular

25 Record the pulses in the proper place. Indicate that an apical-radial pulse was taken.

▶ RESPIRATIONS

Respiration is the act of breathing air into the lungs (inhalation) and out of the lungs (exhalation). Oxygen is taken into the lungs during inhalation. Carbon dioxide is moved out of the lungs during exhalation. Each respiration involves one inhalation and one exhalation. The chest rises during inhalation and falls during exhalation. See Box 19-2 for a review of the respiratory system.

The healthy adult has 10 to 20 respirations per minute. The respiratory rate is affected by many of the factors that affect body temperature and pulse. Heart and respiratory diseases usually cause an increased number of respirations per minute.

Respirations are normally quiet, effortless, and regular. Both sides of the chest rise and fall equally. See Chapter 27 for abnormal respiratory patterns.

Respirations are counted when the person is at rest. The person is positioned so you can see the chest rise and fall. To a certain extent, the depth and rate of breathing can be voluntarily controlled. People tend to change breathing patterns when they know their respirations are being counted. Therefore the person should be unaware that you are counting respirations.

Respirations are counted right after taking a pulse. Keep your fingers or stethoscope over the pulse site. (The person assumes you are still taking the pulse.) Count respirations by watching the rise and fall of the chest. Count them for 30 seconds. Then multiply the number by 2 for the total number of respirations in 1 minute. If an abnormal pattern is noted, count the respirations for 1 full minute. (*See Focus on Children box.*)

⬤ Focus On... CHILDREN

Infants and children have higher respiratory rates than adults (Table 19-3). Count an infant's respirations for 1 minute.

Box 19-2 | The Respiratory System: Review of Structure and Function

Oxygen is needed for survival. Every cell needs oxygen. The respiratory system brings oxygen into the lungs and eliminates carbon dioxide. The process of supplying the cells with oxygen and removing carbon dioxide from them is called *respiration*. Respiration involves *inhalation* (breathing in) and *exhalation* (breathing out). The terms *inspiration* (breathing in) and *expiration* (breathing out) are also used. The respiratory system is shown in Figure 19-23.

Air enters the body through the *nose*. The air then passes into the *pharynx* (throat), a tube-shaped passageway for both air and food. Air passes from the pharynx into the *larynx* (the voice box). Air passes from the larynx into the *trachea* (the windpipe). The trachea divides at its lower end into the *right bronchus* and *left bronchus*. Each bronchus enters a lung. On entering the lungs, the bronchi further divide several times into smaller branches called *bronchioles*. Eventually the bronchioles subdivide and end in tiny one-cell air sacs called *alveoli*. They are supplied by capillaries. Oxygen and carbon dioxide are exchanged between the alveoli and capillaries. Blood in the capillaries picks up oxygen from the alveoli. Then the blood is returned to the left side of the heart and pumped to the rest of the body. Alveoli pick up carbon dioxide from the capillaries for exhalation.

Each lung is divided into lobes. The right lung has three lobes; the left lung has two. The lungs are separated from the abdominal cavity by a muscle called the *diaphragm*. A bony framework consisting of the ribs, sternum, and vertebrae protects the lungs.

Table 19-3 | Normal Respiratory Rates for Children

Age	Respirations per Minute
Newborn	35
1 to 11 months	30
2 years	25
4 years	23
6 years	21
8 years	20
10 years	19
12 years	19
14 years	18
16 years	17
18 years	16-18

From Wong DL: *Whaley & Wong's nursing care of infants and children*, ed 6, St Louis, 1999, Mosby.

Counting Respirations

NNAAP™

Procedure

1   Continue to hold the wrist after taking the radial pulse. Keep the stethoscope in place if you took an apical pulse.

2   Do not tell the person you are counting respirations.

3   Begin counting when the chest rises. Count each rise and fall of the chest as 1 respiration.

4   Observe if respirations are regular and if both sides of the chest rise equally. Also note the depth of respirations and if the person has any pain or difficulty in breathing.

5   Count respirations for 30 seconds. Multiply the number by 2.

6   Count respirations for 1 full minute if they are abnormal or irregular.

7   Record respiratory rate, and other observations on your note pad or assignment sheet.

Post-Procedure

8   Provide for comfort.

9   Place the signal light within reach.

10   Wash your hands.

11   Report the following to the nurse:
   • The respiratory rate
   • Equality and depth of respirations
   • If the respirations were regular or irregular
   • If the person experienced pain or difficulty in breathing
   • Any respiratory noises
   • Any abnormal respiratory patterns (see Chapter 27)

12   Record the respiratory rate in the proper place.

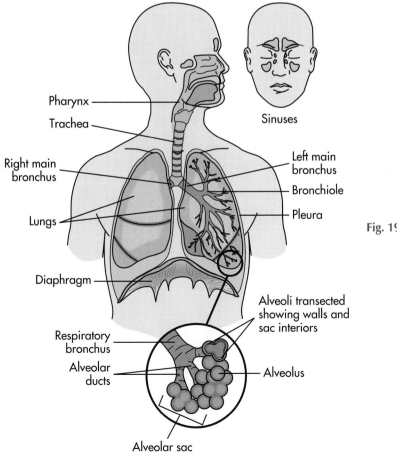

Fig. 19-23 The respiratory system.

Pharynx

Trachea

Sinuses

Right main bronchus

Left main bronchus

Bronchiole

Lungs

Pleura

Diaphragm

Alveoli transected showing walls and sac interiors

Respiratory bronchus

Alveolar ducts

Alveolus

Alveolar sac

BLOOD PRESSURE

Blood pressure is the amount of force exerted against the walls of an artery by the blood. Blood pressure is controlled by:

- The force of heart contractions
- The amount of blood pumped with each heartbeat
- How easily the blood flows through the blood vessels

The period of heart muscle contraction is called **systole.** The period of heart muscle relaxation is called **diastole.**

Both the systolic and diastolic pressures are measured. The **systolic pressure** is the higher pressure. It represents the amount of force needed to pump blood out of the heart into the arterial circulation. The **diastolic pressure** is the lower pressure. It reflects the pressure in the arteries when the heart is at rest. Blood pressure is measured in millimeters (mm) of mercury (Hg). The systolic pressure is recorded over the diastolic pressure. The average adult has a systolic pressure of 120 mm Hg and a diastolic pressure of 80 mm Hg. This is written as 120/80 mm Hg.

FACTORS AFFECTING BLOOD PRESSURE

Blood pressure can change from minute to minute. Such changes are related to the factors described in Box 19-3.

Because it can vary so easily, blood pressure has normal ranges. Systolic pressures between 100 and 140 mm Hg are considered normal. Normal diastolic pressures are between 60 and 90 mm Hg.

Persistent measurements above the normal systolic and diastolic pressures are abnormal. This condition is known as **hypertension.** Report any systolic pressure above 140 mm Hg to the nurse immediately. A diastolic pressure above 90 mm Hg also is reported immediately. Likewise, systolic pressures below 90 mm Hg and diastolic pressures below 60 mm Hg are reported. This is called **hypotension.** Some people normally have low blood pressures. However, hypotension may be a sign of a serious condition that can lead to death if it is not corrected. *(See Focus on Children and Focus on Older Persons boxes in left column on p. 501.)*

Box 19-3 Factors Affecting Blood Pressure

- **Age**—blood pressure increases as a person grows older. It is lowest in infancy and childhood and highest in adulthood. Blood pressure continues to increase with aging.
- **Gender** (male or female)—women usually have lower blood pressures than men. Blood pressures rise in women after menopause.
- **Blood volume**—is the amount of blood in the system. Severe bleeding lowers the blood volume. Therefore the blood pressure lowers. The rapid administration of IV fluids increases the blood volume. The blood pressure rises.
- **Stress**—includes anxiety, fear, and emotions. Heart rate and blood pressure increase as part of the body's response to stress.
- **Pain**—generally increases blood pressure. However, severe pain can cause shock. Blood pressure is seriously low in the state of shock (see Chapter 36).
- **Exercise**—increases heart rate and blood pressure. Blood pressure should not be measured right after exercise.
- **Weight**—blood pressure is higher in overweight persons. The blood pressure lowers with weight loss.
- **Race**—black persons generally have higher blood pressures than white persons do.
- **Diet**—a high-sodium diet increases the amount of water in the body. The extra fluid volume increases blood pressure.
- **Medications**—drugs can be given to raise or lower blood pressure. Other drugs have the side effects of high or low blood pressure.
- **Position**—blood pressure is generally lower when lying down and higher in the standing position. Sudden changes in position can cause sudden changes in blood pressure (orthostatic hypotension). A person who stands suddenly may have a sudden drop in blood pressure. Dizziness and fainting can occur. (See Chapter 20).
- **Smoking**—increases blood pressure. Nicotine in cigarettes causes blood vessels to narrow. The heart must work harder to pump blood through narrowed vessels.
- **Alcohol**—excessive alcohol intake can raise blood pressure.

Fig. 19-24 **A**, Aneroid manometer and cuff. **B**, Mercury manometer and cuff. **C**, Electronic sphygmomanometer.

Focus On... CHILDREN

As with the other vital signs, infants and children have lower blood pressures than adults do. A newborn's blood pressure is usually about 70/55 mm Hg. At 1 year of age the blood pressure increases to 90/55 mm Hg. Blood pressure continues to increase as the child grows older. Adult levels are reached between 14 and 18 years of age.

Blood pressures are not measured routinely in infants and young children. The nurse tells you when to measure their blood pressures.

Focus On... OLDER PERSONS

Arteries narrow and loose their elasticity. The heart has to work harder to pump blood through the vessels. Therefore both the systolic and diastolic pressures are higher in older persons. A blood pressure of 160/90 mm Hg is normal for many older persons. Older persons also are at risk for orthostatic hypotension (see Chapter 20).

EQUIPMENT

A stethoscope and a sphygmomanometer are used to measure blood pressure. The **sphygmomanometer** consists of a cuff and a measuring device. There are three types of sphygmomanometers: aneroid, mercury, and electronic. The aneroid type has a round dial and a needle that points to the calibrations (Fig. 19-24, *A*). The aneroid manometer is small and easy to carry. The mercury manometer is more accurate than the aneroid type. The mercury type has a column of mercury within a calibrated tube (Fig. 19-24, *B*). Many hospitals have wall-mounted mercury sphygmomanometers in patient rooms.

Electronic sphygmomanometers display the systolic and diastolic blood pressures on the front of the instrument (Fig. 19-24, C). The pulse is usually displayed also. The cuff automatically inflates and deflates on some models. Others have automatic deflation only. If electronic blood pressure equipment is used where you work, you need to learn how to use the equipment. Follow the manufacturer's instructions. Electronic devices also are available for home use.

The blood pressure cuff is wrapped around the upper arm. Tubing connects the cuff to the manometer. Another tube connects the cuff to a small hand-held bulb. A valve on the bulb is turned so the cuff inflates as the bulb is squeezed. The inflated cuff causes pressure over the brachial artery. The valve is turned the other way for cuff deflation. Blood pressure is measured as the cuff is deflated.

Focus On... CHILDREN

Pediatric blood pressure cuffs are used for children. Infant and child sizes are available.

Sounds are produced as blood flows through the arteries. The stethoscope is used to listen to the sounds in the brachial artery as the cuff is deflated. Stethoscopes are not needed with electronic sphygmomanometers. (*See Focus on Children box above.*)

▶ MEASURING BLOOD PRESSURE

Blood pressure is normally measured in the brachial artery. Box 19-4 lists the guidelines for measuring blood pressure.

Box 19-4	Guidelines for Measuring Blood Pressure

- Do not take blood pressure on an arm with an IV infusion, a cast, or a dialysis access site. If a person has had breast surgery, blood pressure is not taken on that side. Also avoid taking blood pressure on an injured arm.
- Let the person rest for 10 to 20 minutes before measuring the blood pressure.
- Measure blood pressure with the person sitting or lying. Sometimes the doctor orders measurement of blood pressure in the standing position.
- Apply the cuff to the bare upper arm. Clothing can affect the measurement. Do not apply the cuff over clothing.
- Make sure the cuff is snug. Loose cuffs can cause inaccurate readings.
- Place the diaphragm of the stethoscope firmly over the artery. The entire diaphragm must be in contact with the skin.
- Make sure the room is quiet. Talking, television, radio, and sounds from the hallway can affect an accurate measurement.
- Have the sphygmomanometer clearly visible.
- Locate the radial artery, and then inflate the cuff. When you no longer feel the radial pulse, inflate the cuff another 30 mm Hg. This prevents cuff inflation to an unnecessarily high pressure, which is painful to the person. (You can deflate the cuff at this time and note the point where you feel a pulse. Wait 30 seconds and inflate the cuff 30 mm Hg beyond that point.)
- Measure the systolic and diastolic pressures. Expect to hear the first blood pressure sound at the point where you felt the radial pulse. The first sound is the systolic pressure. The point where the sound disappears is the diastolic pressure.
- Take the blood pressure again if you are not sure of an accurate measurement. Wait 30 to 60 seconds before repeating the measurement.
- Notify the nurse immediately if you cannot hear the blood pressure.

Measuring Blood Pressure

NNAAP™

QUALITY OF LIFE

Remember to:
- Knock before entering the person's room
- Address the person by name
- Introduce yourself by name and title

Pre-Procedure

1 Collect the following:
   - Sphygmomanometer (blood pressure cuff)
   - Stethoscope
   - Alcohol wipes

2 Wash your hands.

3 Identify the person. Check the ID bracelet against the assignment sheet.

4 Explain the procedure to the person.

5 Provide for privacy.

Procedure

6 Wipe the stethoscope earpieces and diaphragm with alcohol wipes.

7 Have the person sit or lie down.

8 Position the person's arm so it is level with the heart. The palm should be up.

9 Stand no more than 3 feet away from the sphygmomanometer. A mercury model should be vertical, on a flat surface, and at eye level. The aneroid type should be directly in front of you.

10 Expose the upper arm.

11 Squeeze the cuff to expel any remaining air. Close the valve on the bulb.

12 Find the brachial artery at the inner aspect of the elbow.

13 Place the arrow on the cuff over the brachial artery (Fig. 19-25, *A*, p. 504). Wrap the cuff around the upper arm at least 1 inch above the elbow. It should be even and snug.

14 Do one of the following:

   a Method 1:
   (1) Place the stethoscope earpieces in your ears.
   (2) Locate the radial artery. Inflate the cuff until you can no longer feel the pulse. Inflate the cuff 30 mm Hg beyond the point where you last felt the pulse.

   b Method 2:
   (1) Locate the radial artery. Inflate the cuff until you can no longer feel the pulse. Inflate the cuff 30 mm Hg beyond the point where you last felt the pulse.
   (2) Deflate the cuff slowly. Note the point when you feel the pulse.
   (3) Wait 30 seconds.
   (4) Place the stethoscope earpieces in your ears.
   (5) Inflate the cuff 30 mm Hg beyond the point where you felt the pulse return.

15 Position the diaphragm over the brachial artery (Fig. 19-25, *B*, p. 504).

16 Deflate the cuff at an even rate of 2 to 4 millimeters per second. Turn the valve counterclockwise to deflate the cuff.

17 Note the point on the scale where you hear the first sound. This is the systolic reading. It should be near the point where the radial pulse disappeared.

18 Continue to deflate the cuff. Note the point where the sound disappears for the diastolic reading.

19 Deflate the cuff completely. Remove it from the person's arm. Remove the stethoscope.

20 Record the person's name and blood pressure on your note pad or assignment sheet.

21 Return the cuff to the case or wall holder.

Continued

Measuring Blood Pressure—cont'd

NNAAP™

Post-Procedure

22 Provide for comfort.

23 Place the signal light within reach.

24 Unscreen the person.

25 Clean the earpieces and diaphragm with alcohol wipes.

26 Return the equipment to its proper place.

27 Wash your hands.

28 Report the blood pressure. Record it in the proper place.

Fig. 19-25 A, The cuff is over the brachial artery. **B,** The diaphragm of the stethoscope is over the brachial artery.

Circle the BEST answer.

1. Which statement is *false?*
   A. The vital signs are temperature, pulse, respirations, and blood pressure.
   B. Vital signs detect changes in body function.
   C. Vital signs change only during illness.
   D. Sleep, exercise, drugs, emotions, and noise affect vital signs.

2. Which temperature should you report immediately?
   A. An oral temperature of 98.4° F
   B. A rectal temperature of 101.6° F
   C. An axillary temperature of 97.6° F
   D. An oral temperature of 99.0° F

3. A rectal temperature is *not* taken when the person
   A. Is unconscious
   B. Is an infant
   C. Has a nasogastric tube
   D. Has had rectal surgery

4. Which gives the *least* accurate measurement of body temperature?
   A. Oral temperature
   B. Rectal temperature
   C. Axillary temperature
   D. Tympanic temperature

5. Which is usually used to take a pulse?
   A. The radial pulse
   B. The apical-radial pulse
   C. The apical pulse
   D. The brachial pulse

6. Which is reported to the nurse immediately?
   A. An adult has a pulse of 120 beats per minute.
   B. An infant has a pulse of 130 beats per minute.
   C. An adult has a pulse of 80 beats per minute.
   D. An adult has a pulse of 64 beats per minute.

7. Which statement about apical-radial pulses is *true?*
   A. The pulse can be taken by one person.
   B. The radial pulse can be greater than the apical pulse.
   C. The apical pulse can be greater than the radial pulse.
   D. The apical and radial pulses are always equal.

8. Normal respirations in an adult are
   A. Between 10 and 20 per minute
   B. Quiet and effortless
   C. Regular with both sides of the chest rising and falling equally
   D. All of the above

9. Respirations are usually counted
   A. After taking the temperature
   B. After taking the pulse
   C. Before taking the pulse
   D. After taking the blood pressure

10. Which blood pressure is normal for an adult?
    A. 88/54 mm Hg
    B. 210/100 mm Hg
    C. 130/82 mm Hg
    D. 152/90 mm Hg

11. When taking a blood pressure, you should do the following *except*
    A. Take the blood pressure in the arm with an IV infusion
    B. Apply the cuff to a bare upper arm
    C. Turn off the television and radio
    D. Locate the brachial artery

12. Which is the systolic blood pressure?
    A. The point at which the pulse is no longer felt
    B. The point where the first sound is heard
    C. The point where the last sound is heard
    D. The point 30 mm Hg above where the pulse was felt

Answers to these questions are on p. 836.

CHAPTER

20

EXERCISE AND ACTIVITY

Define the key terms listed in this chapter

Describe bedrest

Describe the complications of bedrest and how to prevent them

Describe the devices used to support and maintain body alignment

Explain the purpose of a trapeze

Describe range-of-motion exercises

Explain how to help a falling person

Describe four walking aids

Perform the procedures described in this chapter

KEY TERMS

abduction Moving a body part away from the midline of the body

adduction Moving a body part toward the midline of the body

ambulation The act of walking

atrophy A decrease in size or a wasting away of tissue

contracture The lack of joint mobility caused by abnormal shortening of a muscle

dorsiflexion Bending backward

extension Straightening a body part

external rotation Turning the joint outward

flexion Bending a body part

footdrop The foot falls down at the ankle (permanent plantar flexion)

hyperextension Excessive straightening of a body part

internal rotation Turning the joint inward

orthostatic hypotension A drop in *(hypo)* blood pressure when the person stands *(ortho* and *static)*; postural hypotension

plantar flexion The foot *(plantar)* is bent *(flexion)*

postural hypotension Orthostatic hypotension

pronation Turning downward

range of motion (ROM) The movement of a joint to the extent possible without causing pain

rotation Turning the joint

supination Turning upward

syncope A brief loss of consciousness; fainting

Being active is important for physical and mental well-being. Most people move about and function without help. However, illnesses, surgery, injuries, pain, and aging cause weakness and some activity limits. Some people are weak from chronic illnesses. Others are in bed for a long time. Some have permanent paralysis. Some disorders are progressive, causing decreases in activity. Examples include multiple sclerosis, Parkinson's disease, arthritis, and nervous system and muscular disorders (see Chapter 30). Inactivity, whether mild or severe, affects the normal function of every body system. Mental well-being also is affected.

RNs use the nursing process to promote exercise and activity in all persons to the extent possible. An RN assesses and plans for the person's needs. The nursing care plan includes the person's activity level and needed exercises. To assist in promoting exercise and activity, you need to understand:

- Bedrest
- How to prevent complications from bedrest
- How to help persons exercise

BEDREST

Bedrest is ordered by the doctor to treat a person's health problem. Generally bedrest is ordered to:

- Reduce physical activity
- Reduce pain
- Encourage rest
- Regain strength
- Promote healing

The following types of bedrest are common. The person's nursing care plan and your assignment sheet will tell you the activities allowed for each person. Always ask the nurse what bedrest means for each person. Also check with the nurse if you have questions about the person's activity limits.

- *Bedrest*—the person remains in bed but some activities of daily living (ADL) are allowed. Self-feeding, oral hygiene, bathing, shaving, and hair care are often allowed.
- *Strict bedrest*—everything is done for the person. No ADL are allowed.
- *Bedrest with commode privileges*—the person can use the bedside commode for elimination needs.
- *Bedrest with bathroom privileges (bedrest with BRP)*—the person can use the bathroom for elimination needs.

COMPLICATIONS OF BEDREST

Bedrest and lack of exercise and activity can cause serious complications. Every body system is affected. Pressure ulcers, constipation, and fecal impaction can result. Urinary tract infections, renal calculi (kidney stones), blood clots (thrombi), and pneumonia (infection of the lung) [see Chapter 30] can occur.

Contractures and muscle atrophy occur in the musculoskeletal system. A **contracture** is the lack of joint mobility caused by the abnormal shortening of a muscle. The contracted muscle is fixed into position, is deformed, and cannot stretch (Fig. 20-1). Common sites are the fingers, wrists, elbows, toes, ankles, knees, and hips. Contractures can occur also in the neck and spine. The person with a contracture is permanently deformed and disabled. **Atrophy** is the decrease in size or the wasting away of tissue. Muscle atrophy is a decrease in size or a wasting away of muscle (Fig. 20-2). These complications must be prevented to maintain normal body movement.

Orthostatic hypotension and blood clots (see Chapter 24) occur in the cardiovascular system. **Orthostatic hypotension** is a drop in *(hypo)* blood pressure when the person stands *(ortho* and *static)*. When a person moves from lying or sitting to a standing position, the blood pressure drops. The person experiences dizziness, weakness, and spots before the eyes. Syncope can occur. **Syncope** (fainting) is a brief loss of consciousness. (Syncope comes from the Greek word *synkoptein,* which means to cut short.) Orthostatic hypotension also is called **postural hypotension.** *(Postural* relates to posture or standing.) Box 20-1 lists the measures that prevent orthostatic hypotension. Slowly changing positions is an important measure.

Complications from bedrest are prevented by good nursing care. Positioning in good body alignment and range-of-motion exercises are important preventive measures. These are part of the person's care plan.

Fig. 20-2 Muscle atrophy.

Fig. 20-1 A contracture.

Box 20-1	Preventing Orthostatic Hypotension

- Measure blood pressure when the person is supine. Also count the person's pulse and respirations.
- Raise the head of the bed so the person is in Fowler's position. Raise the head of the bed slowly.
  - Ask the person about weakness, dizziness, or spots before the eyes. Lower the head of the bed if these symptoms occur.
  - Measure blood pressure, pulse, and respirations when the person is in Fowler's position.
  - Keep the person in Fowler's position for a short while. Ask the person about weakness, dizziness, or spots before the eyes.
- Assist the person to sit on the side of the bed (see Chapter 11).
  - Ask the person about weakness, dizziness, or spots before the eyes. Assist the person to Fowler's position if any of these symptoms occur.
- Measure blood pressure, pulse, and respirations when the person is sitting on the side of the bed.
- Have the person continue to sit on the side of the bed for a short while.
- Assist the person to stand.
  - Ask the person about weakness, dizziness, or spots before the eyes. Help the person sit on the side of the bed if any of these symptoms occur.
  - Measure blood pressure, pulse, and respirations.
- Help the person sit in a chair or walk as directed by the nurse.
  - Ask the person about weakness, dizziness, or spots before the eyes. If the person is walking, help the person to sit if symptoms occur.
  - Measure blood pressure, pulse, and respirations.
- Report blood pressure, pulse, and respirations to the nurse. Also report other signs or complaints.

POSITIONING

Body alignment and positioning are discussed in Chapter 11. Supportive devices are often used to support and maintain the person in a certain position:

- *Bed boards*—are placed under the mattress. They keep the person in alignment by preventing the mattress from sagging (Fig. 20-3). They are usually made of plywood and are covered with canvas or other material. There are 2 sections so the head of the bed can be raised. One section is for the head of the bed and the other for the foot of the bed.
- *Foot boards*—are placed at the foot of mattresses (Fig. 20-4). They prevent plantar flexion that can lead to footdrop. In **plantar flexion** the foot *(plantar)* is bent *(flexion)*. **Footdrop** is when the foot falls down at the ankle (permanent plantar flexion). The foot board is placed so the soles of the feet are flush against it. The feet are in good alignment as when standing. Foot boards also serve as bed cradles. They keep top linens off the feet.

Fig. 20-3 **A,** Mattress sagging without bed boards. **B,** Bed boards are placed under the mattress. No sagging occurs.

Fig. 20-4 Foot board. Feet are flush with the board to keep them in normal alignment.

- *Trochanter rolls*—prevent the hips and legs from turning outward (external rotation) (Fig. 20-5). They are made from bath blankets. A blanket is folded to the desired length and rolled up. The loose end is placed under the person from the hip to the knee. Then the roll is tucked alongside the body. Pillows or sandbags also are used to keep the hips and knees in alignment.

Fig. 20-5 Trochanter roll made from a bath blanket. It extends from the hip to the knee.

- *Hip abduction wedges*—keep the hips abducted (Fig. 20-6). The wedge is positioned between the person's legs. These are common after hip replacement surgery.

Fig. 20-6 Hip abduction wedge.

- *Hand rolls or hand grips*—prevent contractures of the thumb, fingers, and wrist. Commercial hand rolls are common (Fig. 20-7). Foam rubber sponges, rubber balls, and finger cushions (Fig. 20-8) also are used.

Fig. 20-7 Hand grip. *(Courtesy J. T. Posey Co., Arcadia, Calif.)*

Fig. 20-8 Finger cushion. *(Courtesy J. T. Posey Co., Arcadia, Calif.)*

- *Splints*—keep the elbows, wrists, thumbs, fingers, ankles, and knees in normal position. They are usually secured in place with Velcro. Some have foam padding (Fig. 20-9).
- *Bed cradles*—keep the weight of top linens off the feet (see Fig. 25-5). The weight of top linens can cause footdrop and pressure ulcers.

Fig. 20-9 Splint.

EXERCISE

Exercise helps prevent contractures, muscle atrophy, and other complications of bedrest. Some exercise occurs with activities of daily living and when turning and moving in bed without assistance. Additional exercises are needed for muscles and joints.

A trapeze is used for exercises to strengthen arm muscles. The trapeze is suspended from an overbed frame (Fig. 20-10). The person grasps the bar with both hands to lift the trunk off the bed. The trapeze is also used to move up and turn in bed (see Chapter 11).

Fig. 20-10 Trapeze is used to strengthen the arm muscles.

▶ **Range-of-Motion Exercises.** The movement of a joint to the extent possible without causing pain is the **range of motion (ROM)** of that joint. Range-of-motion exercises involve exercising the joints through their complete range of motion. The exercises are usually done at least twice a day. Range-of-motion exercises are active, passive, or active-assistive:

- *Active* range-of-motion exercises are done by the person.
- *Passive* range-of-motion exercises involve having another person move the joints through their range of motion.
- *Active-assistive* range-of-motion is when the person does the exercises with some help from another person.

Range-of-motion exercises naturally occur during activities of daily living. Bathing, hair care, eating, reaching, and walking all involve joint movements. Persons on bedrest have little activity. Therefore range-of-motion exercises are done. The nurse tells you which joints to exercise and if the exercises are to be active, passive, or active-assistive. Box 20-2 describes the movements involved in range-of-motion exercises. (*See Focus on Children and Focus on Long-Term Care boxes on p. 519.*)

Range-of-motion exercises can cause injury if not done properly. Muscle strain, joint injury, and pain are possible. The rules in Box 20-3 are practiced when performing or assisting with range-of-motion exercises.

Text continued on p. 520

Box 20-2	Joint Movements

Abduction—moving a body part away from the midline of the body
Adduction—moving a body part toward the midline of the body
Extension—straightening a body part
Flexion—bending a body part
Hyperextension—excessive straightening of a body part
Dorsiflexion—bending backward
Rotation—turning the joint
Internal rotation—turning the joint inward
External rotation—turning the joint outward
Plantar flexion—bending the foot down at the ankle
Pronation—turning downward
Supination—turning upward

	Rules for Performing Range-of-Motion
Box 20-3	Exercises

- Exercise only the joints the nurse tells you to exercise.
- Expose only the body part being exercised.
- Use good body mechanics.
- Support the extremity being exercised.
- Move the joint slowly, smoothly, and gently.
- Do not force a joint beyond its present range of motion or to the point of pain.
- *Perform range-of-motion exercises to the neck only if allowed by agency policy.* In some agencies, only physical or occupational therapists do neck exercises. This is because of the danger of neck injuries.

Performing Range-Of-Motion Exercises

NNAAP™

QUALITY OF LIFE

Remember to:
- Knock before entering the person's room
- Address the person by name
- Introduce yourself by name and title

Pre-Procedure

1 Identify the person. Check the ID bracelet against the assignment sheet.

2 Explain the procedure to the person.

3 Wash your hands.

4 Obtain a bath blanket.

5 Provide for privacy.

6 Raise the bed to the best level for good body mechanics. Make sure bed rails are up.

Procedure

7 Lower the bed rail near you.

8 Position the person supine and in good alignment.

9 Cover the person with a bath blanket. Fanfold top linens to the foot of the bed.

10 Exercise the neck *if allowed by your agency and if the RN instructs you to do so* (Fig. 20-11, p. 516):

   a Place your hands over the person's ears to support the head.

   b Flexion—bring the head forward so the chin touches the chest.

   c Extension—straighten the head.

   d Hyperextension—bring the head backward until the chin is pointing up.

   e Rotation—turn the head from side to side.

   f Lateral flexion—move the head to the right and to the left.

   g Repeat flexion, extension, hyperextension, rotation, and lateral flexion 5 times—or the number of times stated on the care plan.

11 Exercise the shoulder (Fig. 20-12, p. 516):

   a Grasp the wrist with one hand and the elbow with the other.

   b Flexion—raise the arm straight in front and over the head.

   c Extension—bring the arm down to the side.

   d Hyperextension—move the arm behind the body. (This can be done if the person is sitting in a straight-back chair or is standing.)

   e Abduction—move the straight arm away from the side of the body.

   f Adduction—move the straight arm to the side of the body.

   g Internal rotation—bend the elbow, and place it at the same level as the shoulder. Move the forearm down toward the body.

   h External rotation—move the forearm toward the head.

   i Repeat flexion, extension, hyperextension, abduction, adduction, and internal and external rotation 5 times—or the number of times stated on the care plan.

12 Exercise the elbow (Fig. 20-13, p. 516):

   a Grasp the person's wrist with one hand and the elbow with the other.

   b Flexion—bend the arm so the same-side shoulder is touched.

   c Extension—straighten the arm.

   d Repeat flexion and extension 5 times. Or the number of times stated on the care plan.

Continued

Performing Range-Of-Motion Exercises—cont'd

NNAAP™

Procedure—cont'd

13 Exercise the forearm (Fig. 20-14, p. 516):

  a Pronation—turn the hand so the palm is down.

  b Supination—turn the hand so the palm is up.

  c Repeat pronation and supination 5 times—or the number of times stated on the care plan.

14 Exercise the wrist (Fig. 20-15, p. 517):

  a Hold the wrist with both of your hands.

  b Flexion—bend the hand down.

  c Extension—straighten the hand.

  d Hyperextension—bend the hand back.

  e Radial flexion—turn the hand toward the thumb.

  f Ulnar flexion—turn the hand toward the little finger.

  g Repeat flexion, extension, hyperextension, and radial and ulnar flexion 5 times—or the number of times stated on the care plan.

15 Exercise the thumb (Fig. 20-16, p. 517):

  a Hold the person's hand with one hand and the thumb with your other hand.

  b Abduction—move the thumb out from the inner part of the index finger.

  c Adduction—move the thumb back next to the index finger.

  d Opposition—touch each fingertip with the thumb.

  e Flexion—bend the thumb into the hand.

  f Extension—move the thumb out to the side of the fingers.

  g Repeat flexion, extension, abduction, adduction, and opposition 5 times—or the number of times stated on the care plan.

16 Exercise the fingers (Fig. 20-17, p. 517):

  a Abduction—spread the fingers and the thumb apart.

  b Adduction—bring the fingers and thumb together.

  c Extension—straighten the fingers so the fingers, hand, and arm are straight.

  d Flexion—make a fist.

  e Repeat abduction, adduction, extension, and flexion 5 times—or the number of times stated on the care plan.

17 Exercise the hip (Fig. 20-18, p. 518):

  a Place one hand under the knee and the other under the ankle to support the leg.

  b Flexion—raise the leg.

  c Extension—straighten the leg.

  d Abduction—move the leg away from the body.

  e Adduction—move the leg toward the other leg.

  f Internal rotation—turn the leg inward.

  g External rotation—turn the leg outward.

  h Repeat flexion, extension, abduction, adduction, and inward and outward rotation 5 times—or the number of times stated on the care plan.

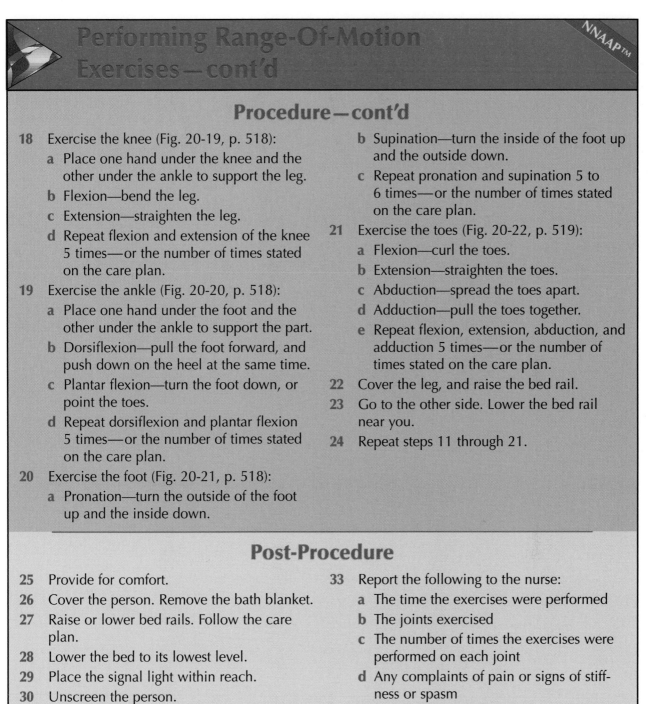

Performing Range-Of-Motion Exercises—cont'd

NNAAP™

Procedure—cont'd

18 Exercise the knee (Fig. 20-19, p. 518):
  a Place one hand under the knee and the other under the ankle to support the leg.
  b Flexion—bend the leg.
  c Extension—straighten the leg.
  d Repeat flexion and extension of the knee 5 times—or the number of times stated on the care plan.

19 Exercise the ankle (Fig. 20-20, p. 518):
  a Place one hand under the foot and the other under the ankle to support the part.
  b Dorsiflexion—pull the foot forward, and push down on the heel at the same time.
  c Plantar flexion—turn the foot down, or point the toes.
  d Repeat dorsiflexion and plantar flexion 5 times—or the number of times stated on the care plan.

20 Exercise the foot (Fig. 20-21, p. 518):
  a Pronation—turn the outside of the foot up and the inside down.

  b Supination—turn the inside of the foot up and the outside down.
  c Repeat pronation and supination 5 to 6 times—or the number of times stated on the care plan.

21 Exercise the toes (Fig. 20-22, p. 519):
  a Flexion—curl the toes.
  b Extension—straighten the toes.
  c Abduction—spread the toes apart.
  d Adduction—pull the toes together.
  e Repeat flexion, extension, abduction, and adduction 5 times—or the number of times stated on the care plan.

22 Cover the leg, and raise the bed rail.
23 Go to the other side. Lower the bed rail near you.
24 Repeat steps 11 through 21.

Post-Procedure

25 Provide for comfort.
26 Cover the person. Remove the bath blanket.
27 Raise or lower bed rails. Follow the care plan.
28 Lower the bed to its lowest level.
29 Place the signal light within reach.
30 Unscreen the person.
31 Return the bath blanket to its proper place.
32 Wash your hands.

33 Report the following to the nurse:
  a The time the exercises were performed
  b The joints exercised
  c The number of times the exercises were performed on each joint
  d Any complaints of pain or signs of stiffness or spasm
  e The degree to which the person participated in the exercises

Flexion Extension Hyperextension

Rotation Lateral flexion

Fig. 20-11 Range-of-motion exercises for the neck.

Flexion

Abduction

Adduction

Extension

Hyperextension

Outward rotation

Inward rotation

Fig. 20-12 Range-of-motion exercises for the shoulder.

Supination Pronation

Fig. 20-13 Range-of-motion exercises for the elbow.

Flexion

Extension

Fig. 20-14 Range-of-motion exercises for the forearm.

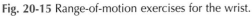

Hyperextension

Ulnar flexion

Extension

Flexion

Radial flexion

Fig. 20-15 Range-of-motion exercises for the wrist.

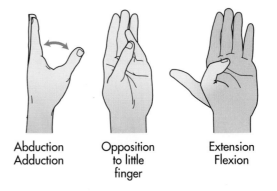

Abduction
Adduction

Opposition
to little
finger

Extension
Flexion

Fig. 20-16 Range-of-motion exercises for the thumb.

Abduction

Adduction

Extension

Flexion

Fig. 20-17 Range-of-motion exercises for the fingers.

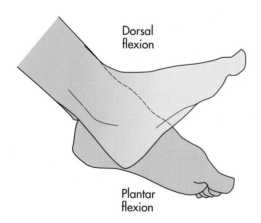

Fig. 20-18 Range-of-motion exercises for the hip.

Fig. 20-19 Range-of-motion exercises for the knee.

Fig. 20-20 Range-of-motion exercises for the ankle.

Fig. 20-21 Range-of-motion exercises for the foot.

Fig. 20-22 Range-of-motion exercises for the toes.

Focus On... CHILDREN

Depending on the child's activity limits, most any play activity promotes active range-of-motion exercises in children. Some examples are:
- Kicking a Mylar balloon or foam rubber ball
- Playing "pat-a-cake" and having the child clap, kick, jump, or do other motions
- Playing basketball using a wastebasket and a foam rubber ball or wadded paper
- Playing video games for finger and hand movements
- Playing with finger paints, clay, or play dough
- Having tricycle or wheelchair races
- Playing "hide and seek" by hiding a toy in the bed or room
- Always check with the nurse for the child's activity limits.

Modified from Wong DL: *Whaley and Wong's nursing care of infants and children*, ed 6, St Louis, 1999, Mosby.

Focus On... LONG-TERM CARE

OBRA requires that nursing centers have an assessment and care planning process to prevent unnecessary reduction in a resident's range of motion. Prevention involves active, active-assistive, or passive range-of-motion exercises. Splints and braces are used if needed.

OBRA also requires activity programs for residents. Recreational activities are important for the physical and mental well-being of older persons. Joints and muscles are exercised, and circulation is stimulated. Recreational activities also provide social opportunities and are mentally stimulating.

The activities must meet the interests and physical, mental, and psychosocial needs of each resident. Bingo, movies, dances, exercise groups, shopping trips, museum trips, concerts, and guest speakers are often arranged. Some centers have gardening activities.

The right to personal choice is protected. The resident chooses which activities to take part in. OBRA requires that activities promote physical, intellectual, social, and emotional well-being. Well-being is promoted when the resident attends activities of personal choice. The resident must not be forced to take part in an activity that has no interest to him or her.

Residents may need help getting to an activity. Some also need help in participating. You must provide assistance as necessary.

▶ AMBULATION

For most persons on bedrest, activity is increased slowly and in steps. First the person dangles (sits on the side of the bed). The next step is to sit in a bedside chair. Walking about in the room and then in the hallway are the next steps. **Ambulation,** the act of walking, is not a problem if complications were prevented. Contractures and muscle atrophy are prevented by proper positioning and exercise.

Some patients and residents are weak and unsteady from bedrest, illness, surgery, or injury. You need to help these persons walk. Use a gait (transfer or safety) belt if the person is weak or unsteady (see Chapter 11). For additional support, the person uses hand rails along the wall. Always check the person for orthostatic hypotension.

Fig. 20-23 Assist with ambulation by walking slightly behind the person's side. Use a gait belt for the person's safety.

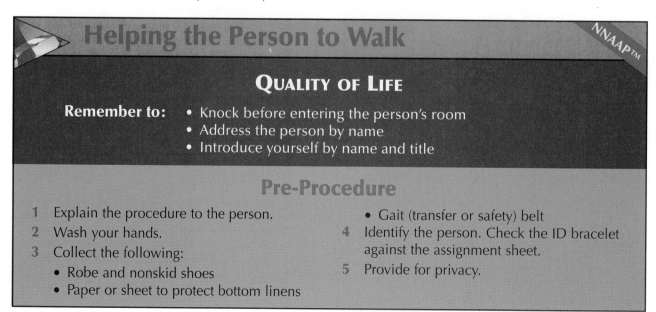

Helping the Person to Walk

NNAAP™

QUALITY OF LIFE

Remember to:
- Knock before entering the person's room
- Address the person by name
- Introduce yourself by name and title

Pre-Procedure

1 Explain the procedure to the person.
2 Wash your hands.
3 Collect the following:
- Robe and nonskid shoes
- Paper or sheet to protect bottom linens

- Gait (transfer or safety) belt
4 Identify the person. Check the ID bracelet against the assignment sheet.
5 Provide for privacy.

Helping the Person to Walk—cont'd

NNAAP™

Procedure

6 Move furniture as needed for moving space for you and the person.

7 Lower the bed to its lowest position. Lock the bed wheels.

8 Fanfold top linens to the foot of the bed.

9 Place the paper or sheet under the person's feet. This protects the bottom sheet from the shoes. Put the shoes on the person.

10 Help the person dangle. (See *Helping the Person Sit on the Side of the Bed,* p. 263.)

11 Help the person put on the robe.

12 Apply the gait belt. (See *Applying a Transfer [Gait] Belt,* p. 264.)

13 Help the person stand:
   a Stand facing the person.
   b Grasp the gait belt at each side.
   c Brace your knees against the person's knees. Block his or her feet with your feet (see Fig. 11-21, *B* on p. 268).
   d Pull the person up into a standing position as you straighten your knees (see Fig. 11-21, *C* on p. 268).

14 Stand slightly behind the person's side while he or she gains balance. Do not let go of the gait belt. Grasp the belt at the side and back.

15 Encourage the person to stand erect with the head up and back straight.

16 Assist the person to walk. Walk to the side and slightly behind the person. Provide support with the gait belt (Fig. 20-23).

17 Encourage the person to walk normally. The heel of the foot strikes the floor first. Discourage shuffling, sliding, or walking on tiptoes.

18 Walk the required distance if the person can tolerate the activity. Do not rush the person.

19 Help the person return to bed:
   a Have the person stand at the side of the bed.
   b Pivot him or her a quarter turn. The backs of the knees should touch the bed.
   c Grasp the sides of the gait belt.
   d Lower the person onto the bed as you bend your knees. Remove the gait belt and robe.
   e Help the person lie down. (See *Helping the Person Sit on the Side of the Bed,* p. 263.)

20 Lower the head of the bed. Help the person to the center of the bed.

21 Remove the shoes, and remove the paper or sheet over the bottom sheet.

Post-Procedure

22 Provide for comfort. Cover the person.

23 Place the signal light within reach.

24 Raise or lower bed rails. Follow the care plan.

25 Return the robe and shoes to their proper place.

26 Return furniture to its proper location.

27 Unscreen the person.

28 Wash your hands.

29 Report the following to the nurse:
   • How well the person tolerated the activity
   • The distance walked

▶ THE FALLING PERSON

A person may start to fall when standing or walking. The person may be weak, lightheaded, or dizzy. Fainting may occur. Falling may be caused by slipping or sliding on spills, waxed floors, throw rugs, or improper shoes (see Chapter 9).

When a person is falling, the tendency is to try to prevent the fall. However, trying to prevent a fall could cause greater harm. You could injure yourself and the person as you twist and strain to stop the fall. Balance is lost as a person is falling. If you try to prevent the fall, you could lose your balance. Thus both you and the person could fall or cause the other person to fall. Head, hip, and knee injuries are common from falls.

If a person starts to fall, ease him or her to the floor. This lets you control the direction of the fall. You can also protect the person's head.

Do not move or allow the person to get up after the fall. Call for a nurse to check the person for injuries. You will need to complete an incident report as required by agency policy.

▶ Helping the Falling Person

Procedure

1. Stand with your feet apart. Keep your back straight.

2. Bring the person close to your body as quickly as possible. Use the gait belt if one is worn. If not, wrap your arms around the person's waist. You can also hold the person under the arms (Fig. 20-24, *A*).

3. Move your leg so the person's buttocks rest on it (Fig. 20-24, *B*). Move the leg near the person.

4. Lower the person to the floor. Let him or her slide down your leg to the floor (Fig. 20-24, *C*). Bend at your hips and knees as you lower the person.

5. Call a nurse to check the person.

6. Help the nurse return the person to bed. Get other staff to help if necessary.

7. Report the following to the nurse:
   - How the fall occurred
   - How far the person walked
   - How activity was tolerated before the fall
   - Any complaints before the fall
   - The amount of assistance needed by the person while walking

8. Complete an incident report.

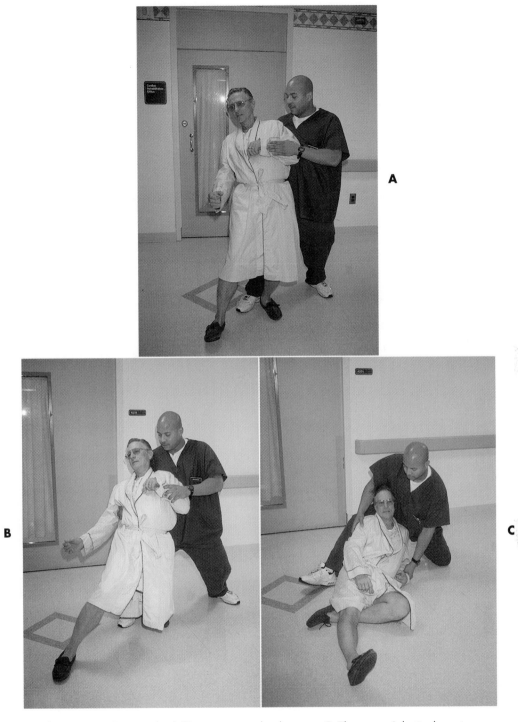

Fig. 20-24 A, Support the falling person under the arms. **B,** The person's buttocks rest on your leg. **C,** Slide the person down your leg to the floor.

WALKING AIDS

Walking aids support the body. They are ordered by the doctor, RN, or physical therapist. The type ordered depends on the person's physical condition, the amount of support needed, and the type of disability. The physical therapist or RN teaches the person to use the walking aid. Its use may be temporary or permanent.

Crutches. Crutches are used when the person cannot use one leg or when one or both legs need to gain strength. Some persons with permanent leg weakness can use crutches. They usually use Lofstrand crutches (Fig. 20-25). These crutches are made of metal. A metal band fits around the forearm. Axillary crutches extend from the underarm (axilla) to the ground (Fig. 20-26). They are made of wood or metal.

Fig. 20-25 Lofstrand crutches. *(From Elkin MK, Perry AG, Potter PA: Nursing interventions and clinical skills, St Louis, 2000, Mosby.)*

Fig. 20-26 Axillary crutches. *(From Elkin MK, Perry AG, Potter PA: Nursing interventions and clinical skills, St Louis, 2000, Mosby.)*

The person learns to crutch walk, climb up and down stairs, and sit and stand. Safety is important. The person on crutches is at risk of falling. The following safety measures are followed:

- The crutches must fit. An RN or physical therapist measures and fits the person with crutches. An improper fit increases the risk of falling and further injury. Back pain, nerve damage, and injuries to the underarms and palms are other risks.
- Crutch tips must be attached to the crutches. They must not be worn down, torn, or wet. Replace worn or torn crutch tips. Dry wet tips with a towel or paper towels.
- Crutches are checked for flaws. Check wooden crutches for cracks and metal crutches for bends. All bolts on both types must be tight.

- Street shoes are worn. They must be flat and have nonskid soles.
- Clothes must fit well. Loose clothing may get caught between the crutches and underarms. Loose clothing can also hang forward and block the person's view of the feet and crutch tips.
- Safety rules to prevent falls are followed (see Chapter 9).
- Crutches are kept where the person can reach them. Place them next to the person's chair or against a wall.
- Know which crutch gait the person uses:
  - Four-point alternating gait (Fig. 20-27)
  - Three-point alternating gait (Fig. 20-28)
  - Two-point alternating gait (Fig. 20-29, p. 526)
  - Swing-to gait (Fig. 20-30, p. 526)
  - Swing-through gait (Fig. 20-31, p. 526)

Fig. 20-27 The four-point alternating gait. The person uses both legs. The right crutch is moved forward and then the left foot. Then the left crutch is moved forward followed by the right foot.

Fig. 20-28 The three-point alternating gait. One leg is used. Both crutches are moved forward. Then the good foot is moved forward.

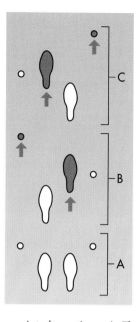

Fig. 20-29 The two-point alternating gait. The person bears some weight on each foot. The left crutch and right foot are moved forward at the same time. Then the right crutch and left foot are moved forward.

Fig. 20-30 Swing-to gait. The person bears some weight on each leg. Both crutches are moved forward. Then the person lifts both legs and swings *to* the crutches.

Fig. 20-31 Swing-through gait. The person bears some weight on each leg. Both crutches are moved forward. Then the person lifts both legs and swings *through* the crutches.

Canes. Canes are used for weakness on one side of the body. They help provide balance and support. There are single-tip and four-point (quad) canes (Fig. 20-32). A cane is held on the *strong side* of the body. (If the left leg is weak, the cane is held in the right hand.) Four-point canes give more support than single-tip canes. However, they are harder to move.

The cane tip is about 6 to 10 inches to the side of the foot and about 6 to 10 inches in front of the foot on the strong side. The grip is level with the hip.

Fig. 20-32 A, Single-tip cane. **B,** Four-point (quad) cane.

The person walks as follows:

Step A: The cane is moved forward 6 to 10 inches (Fig. 20-33, *A*).

Step B: The weak leg (opposite the cane) is moved forward even with the cane (Fig. 20-33, *B*).

Step C: The strong leg is brought forward and ahead of the cane and the weak leg (Fig. 20-33, *C*).

Fig. 20-33 Walking with a cane. **A,** The cane is moved forward about 1 foot. **B,** The leg opposite the cane (weak leg) is brought forward even with the cane. **C,** The leg on the cane side (strong leg) is moved ahead of the cane and the weak leg.

Walkers. A walker is a four-point walking aid (Fig. 20-34). It gives more support than a cane. Many people feel safer and more secure with a walker than with a cane. There are many kinds of walkers. The standard walker is picked up and moved about 6 to 8 inches in front of the person. The person then moves the right foot and then the left foot up to the walker (Fig. 20-35).

A wheeled walker has wheels on the front legs and rubber tips on the back legs. The person pushes the walker ahead about 6 to 8 inches and then walks up to it. The rubber tips prevent the walker from moving while the person is walking or standing.

Baskets, pouches, and trays can be attached to walkers (see Fig. 20-34). The attachment is used to carry needed items. The person is more independent and does not have to rely on others. The attachment also keeps the hands free to grip the walker.

Fig. 20-34 A walker.

Fig. 20-35 Walking with a walker. **A,** The walker is moved about 6 inches in front of the person. **B,** Both feet are moved up to the walker.

Braces. Braces support weak body parts. They also prevent or correct deformities or prevent joint movement. Metal, plastic, or leather is used for braces. A brace is applied over the ankle, knee, or back (Fig. 20-36). An ankle-foot orthosis (AFO) is positioned in the shoe (Fig. 20-37). Then the foot is inserted. The device is secured in place with a Velcro strap.

Bony points under braces are protected. Otherwise skin breakdown can occur. The skin also is kept clean and dry. When you remove a brace, report any sign of redness or skin breakdown (see Chapter 25). Also report complaints of pain or discomfort. The nurse assesses the skin under braces every shift. The care plan tells you when to apply and remove a brace.

Fig. 20-36 Leg brace.

Fig. 20-37 Ankle-foot orthosis (AFO).

Circle the BEST answer.

1. Ms. Porter is on bedrest. Which statement is *false?*
   A. She has orthostatic hypotension.
   B. Bedrest helps reduce pain and promote healing.
   C. Complications of bedrest include pressure ulcers, constipation, and blood clots.
   D. Contractures and muscle atrophy can occur.

2. Which helps to prevent permanent plantar flexion?
   A. Bed boards
   B. A foot board
   C. Trochanter rolls
   D. Hand rolls

3. Which prevents the hip from turning outward?
   A. Bed boards
   B. A foot board
   C. Trochanter roll
   D. All of the above

4. A trapeze is used to
   A. Prevent footdrop
   B. Prevent contractures
   C. Strengthen arm muscles
   D. Strengthen leg muscles

5. Passive range-of-motion exercises are performed by
   A. The person
   B. A health team member
   C. The person with the assistance of another
   D. The person with the use of a trapeze

6. ROM exercises are ordered for Ms. Porter. You should do the following *except*
   A. Support the extremity being exercised
   B. Move the joint slowly, smoothly, and gently
   C. Force the joint through full range of motion
   D. Exercise only the joints indicated by the nurse

7. Flexion involves
   A. Bending the body part
   B. Straightening the body part
   C. Moving the body part toward the body
   D. Moving the body part away from the body

8. Which statement about ambulation is *false?*
   A. A transfer belt is used if the person is weak or unsteady.
   B. The person is allowed to shuffle or slide when walking after bedrest.
   C. Walking aids may be needed permanently or temporarily.
   D. Crutches, canes, walkers, and braces are common walking aids.

9. You are getting a person ready to crutch walk. You should do the following *except*
   A. Check the crutch tips
   B. Have the person wear street shoes
   C. Get any pair of crutches from physical therapy
   D. Tighten the bolts on the crutches

10. A single-tip cane is used
    A. At waist level
    B. On the strong side
    C. On the weak side
    D. On either side

Circle T if the answer is true and F if it is false.

11. T F A single-tip cane and a four-point cane give equal support.

12. T F When a cane is used, the feet are moved first.

13. T F Mr. Parker uses a walker. First he moves the walker in front of him. Then he moves his right foot and left foot forward.

14. T F Mr. Parker starts to fall. You should try to prevent the fall.

15. T F A person has a brace. Bony areas need protection from skin breakdown.

Answers to these questions are on p. 836.

COMFORT, REST, AND SLEEP

Define the key terms listed in this chapter

Explain why comfort, rest, and sleep are important

Describe four types of pain

Explain why pain is a personal experience

Describe the factors that affect pain

List the signs and symptoms of pain

List the nursing measures that relieve pain

Explain why meeting basic needs is important for rest

Describe the nursing measures that promote rest

Identify when rest is needed

Describe the factors that affect sleep

Describe the common sleep disorders

Explain circadian rhythm and how it affects sleep

Describe the stages of sleep

Know the sleep requirements for each age-group

List the nursing measures that promote sleep

List the OBRA requirements for comfort, rest, and sleep

KEY TERMS

acute pain Pain that is felt suddenly from injury, disease, trauma, or surgery; it generally lasts less than 6 months

chronic pain Pain lasting longer than 6 months; it may be constant or occur off and on

circadian rhythm A daily rhythm based on a 24-hour cycle; the day-night cycle or body rhythm

comfort A state of well-being; the person has no physical or emotional pain and is calm and at peace

discomfort To ache, hurt, or be sore; pain

distraction To change the person's center of attention

enuresis Urinary incontinence in bed at night

guided imagery Creating and focusing on an image

insomnia A chronic condition in which the person cannot sleep or stay asleep all night

nonREM sleep NREM sleep

NREM sleep The stage of sleep when there is *no rapid eye movement*; nonREM sleep

pain Discomfort

phantom pain Pain felt in a body part that is no longer there

radiating pain Pain felt at the site of tissue damage and in nearby areas

relaxation To be free from mental or physical stress

REM sleep The stage of sleep when there is *rapid eye movement*

rest To be calm, at ease, and relaxed; to be free of anxiety and stress

sleep A state of unconsciousness, reduced voluntary muscle activity, and lowered metabolism

Comfort, rest, and sleep are needed for well-being. The total person—the physical, emotional, social, and spiritual—is affected by comfort, rest, and sleep problems. People need to be comfortable and free of pain. Discomfort and pain can be physical or emotional. Whatever the cause, discomfort and pain affect rest and sleep. They also decrease function and quality of life.

Rest and sleep restore energy and well-being. Illness and injury increase the need for rest and sleep. The body needs more energy for healing and repair. When a person is ill or injured, more energy than normal is needed to perform daily activities.

COMFORT

Comfort is a state of well-being. There is no physical or emotional pain. The person is calm and at peace. Age, illness, and activity affect comfort. So do factors like temperature, ventilation, noise, odors, and lighting. Those factors are controlled to meet the person's needs (see Chapter 12).

To have **discomfort** or **pain** means to ache, hurt, or be sore. Discomfort is unpleasant. Comfort and discomfort are subjective. That is, you cannot see, hear, touch, or smell the person's comfort or discomfort. You must rely on what the person tells you. You must report complaints to the nurse. The information is used for the nursing process.

Pain is personal. It differs for each person. What *hurts* to one person may *ache* to another. What one person calls *sore*, another may call *aching*. Pain is subjective. If a person complains of pain or discomfort, the person *has* pain or discomfort. You must believe the person. Remember, you cannot see, hear, feel, or smell the pain.

Pain is a warning from the body. It means there is damage to body tissues. Pain often causes the person to seek health care.

TYPES OF PAIN

There are different types of pain. The doctor uses the type of pain when diagnosing. The type of pain also is used in the nursing process:

- **Acute pain** is felt suddenly from injury, disease, trauma, or surgery. There is tissue damage. Acute pain lasts a short time, usually less than 6 months. It decreases with healing.
- **Chronic pain** lasts longer than 6 months. Pain is constant or occurs off and on. There is no longer tissue damage. Chronic pain remains long after healing. Arthritis and cancer are common causes of chronic pain.
- **Radiating pain** is felt at the site of tissue damage and in nearby areas. Pain from a heart attack is often felt in the left side of the chest, left jaw, left shoulder, and left arm. A diseased gallbladder can cause pain in the right upper abdomen, the back, and the right shoulder (Fig. 21-1).
- **Phantom pain** is felt in a body part that is no longer there. A person with an amputated leg may still sense leg pain (see Chapter 30).

FACTORS AFFECTING PAIN

A person may handle pain well one time and poorly the next time. Many factors affect reactions to pain.

Past Experience. We learn from past experiences. They help us know what to do or what to expect. Whether it is going to school, driving a car, taking a test, shopping, having a baby, or caring for children, the past prepares us for similar events at another time. We also learn from the past experiences shared by family and friends.

A person may have had pain before. The severity of pain, its cause, how long it lasted, and if relief occurred all affect the person's current response to pain. Knowing what to expect can help or hinder how the person handles pain.

Some people have not had pain. When pain is felt, the person may be very afraid and anxious. Fear and anxiety affect pain.

Anxiety. Anxiety relates to feelings of fear, dread, worry, and concern. The person feels uneasy and tense. The person may feel troubled or threatened or sense danger. Something is wrong but the person does not know what or why.

Pain and anxiety are related. Pain can cause anxiety. Anxiety increases how much pain the person feels. Lessening anxiety helps reduce pain. For example, the nurse explains to Mr. Smith that he will have pain after surgery. The nurse also explains that he will receive drugs for pain relief. Mr. Smith knows the cause of the pain and what to expect. This helps reduce his anxiety and therefore the amount of pain felt.

Rest and Sleep. Rest and sleep restore energy. They reduce body demands, and the body repairs itself. Lack of needed rest and sleep affects how a person thinks and copes with daily life. Ill and injured persons need more sleep than usual. Many also have pain. Lack of rest and sleep affects how the person deals with pain. Pain seems worse when the person is tired or restless. Also, the person usually pays more attention to pain when tired and unable to rest or sleep.

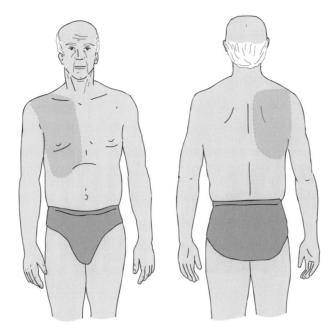

Fig. 21-1 Gallbladder pain radiates to the right upper abdomen, the back, and the right shoulder.

Attention. The more a person thinks about the pain, the worse it can seem. Sometimes pain is so severe that it is all the person thinks about. However, even mild pain can seem worse if the person thinks about it all the time. Pain often seems worse at night. Activity is less, it is quiet, there are no visitors, the radio or television is off, and others are asleep. When unable to sleep, the person has time to think about the pain.

Personal and Family Duties. How a person deals with pain often relates to personal and family obligations. Often pain is ignored if children must be cared for. Some people go to work when having pain. Others deny pain because they fear a serious illness. The illness can interfere with earning money, going to school, or caring for children, a partner, or ill parents.

The Value or Meaning of Pain. Some people view pain as a sign of weakness. It also may mean a serious illness and the need for painful tests and treatments. Therefore pain is ignored or denied. Sometimes pain results in pleasure. The pain of childbirth is one example.

For some persons, pain means not having to work or assume daily routines. Pain is used to avoid certain people or things. Pain is useful for the person. Some people like doting and pampering by others. The person values and wants such attention.

Support From Others. Pain is often easier to deal with when family and friends offer comfort and support. The pain of childbirth is easier when a loving father gives support and encouragement. A child bears pain much better when comforted by a caring mother, father, or other family member. The use of touch by a valued person is very comforting. Just being nearby also helps.

Some people do not have caring family or friends. They must deal with pain alone. Being alone can increase anxiety. It also gives the person more time to think about the pain. Facing pain alone is hard for everyone, especially children and older persons.

Culture. Culture affects how a person responds to pain. (See Caring About Culture [Pain Reactions] box on p. 536.) In some cultures the person in pain is stoic. To be stoic means to show no reaction to joy, sorrow, pleasure, or pain. Strong verbal and nonverbal reactions to pain are seen in other cultures.

Age. (See Focus on Children and Focus on Older Persons boxes on p. 536.)

Caring About Culture

PAIN REACTIONS

People of Mexico and the Philippines may appear stoic in reaction to pain. In the Philippines, pain is viewed as the will of God and that God will give strength to bear the pain.

In Vietnam, pain may be severe before pain relief measures are requested. The people of India accept pain quietly and will accept some relief measures. In China, showing emotion is a weakness of character. Therefore pain is often suppressed. Pain relief measures must be offered more than once before they are accepted. The people of China find it impolite to accept something the first time it is offered.

Remember, individuals may not follow every belief and practice of their culture and religion. Each person is unique. Do not judge the person by your own standards.

Modified from Geissler EM: *Pocket guide to cultural assessment,* ed 2, St Louis, 1998, Mosby.

Focus On... CHILDREN

Children may not understand pain. They know it feels bad. Their pain experiences are fewer. They do not know what to expect. They also have fewer ways of dealing with the pain. Adults can take some pain drugs bought in stores. They also know that heat or cold applications help to relieve pain. They can distract attention away from the pain. Music, working, reading, and hobbies are distracting for some adults. Children do not know how to relieve their own pain. They rely on adults for help.

Infants, toddlers, and preschool children have difficulty alerting adults to pain. Infants cry, fuss, and are restless. Such behaviors also mean hunger and the need for a diaper change. Toddlers and preschool children may not have the words to express pain. Adults must be alert for behaviors and situations that signal pain.

Focus On... OLDER PERSONS

Older persons may have decreased pain sensations. They do not feel pain, or it may not feel severe. This places them at greater risk for undetected disease or injury. Remember, pain occurs with tissue damage. Therefore pain alerts the person to illness or injury. If pain is not felt, the person does not know to seek health care.

Some older persons have many health problems that cause pain. Chronic pain may mask new pain. Older persons may also ignore or deny new pain. They may think it is related to an existing health problem. Like other adults, older persons often deny or ignore pain because of what it may mean.

Thinking and reasoning are affected in some older persons. Some cannot verbally communicate pain. Changes in usual behavior may indicate the person has pain. Nursing staff must be alert for the signs of pain. Always report to the nurse any changes in the person's usual behavior.

SIGNS AND SYMPTOMS

You cannot see, hear, feel, or smell the person's pain. You must rely on what the person tells you. Promptly report to the RN any information you collect about pain. Use the person's exact words when you report and record. The RN needs the following information when assessing the person's pain:

- *Location.* Where is the pain? Ask the person to point to the area of pain (Fig. 21-2). Remember, pain can radiate. Ask the person if the pain is anywhere else and to point to those areas.
- *Onset and duration.* When did the pain start? How long has the pain lasted?
- *Intensity.* Does the person complain of mild, moderate, or severe pain? Ask the person to rate the pain on a scale of 1 to 10, with 10 being the most severe.
- *Description.* Ask the person to describe the pain. Box 21-1 lists some words used to describe pain. Write down what the person says. Use the person's words when reporting to the nurse.
- *Factors causing pain.* These are called *precipitating* factors. To precipitate means to cause. Such factors include moving or turning in bed, coughing or deep breathing, and exercise. Ask what the person was doing before the pain started and when it started.
- *Vital signs.* What are the person's pulse, respirations, and blood pressure? Increases in these vital signs often occur with pain.
- *Other signs and symptoms.* Does the person have other symptoms: dizziness, nausea, vomiting, weakness, numbness or tingling, or others? Box 21-2 lists the signs and symptoms that often occur with pain.

Fig. 21-2 The person points to the area of pain.

Box 21-1	Words Used to Describe Pain

- Aching
- Burning
- Cramping
- Crushing
- Dull
- Gnawing
- Knifelike
- Piercing
- Pressure
- Sharp
- Sore
- Squeezing
- Stabbing
- Throbbing
- Viselike

Box 21-2	Signs and Symptoms of Pain

BODY RESPONSES
- Increased pulse, respirations, and blood pressure
- Sweating (diaphoresis)
- Nausea
- Vomiting
- Pale skin (pallor)

BEHAVIORS
- Changes in speech: slow or rapid; loud or quiet
- Crying
- Gasping
- Grimacing
- Groaning
- Grunting
- Holding the affected body part (splinting)
- Irritability
- Maintaining one position; refusing to move
- Moaning
- Quietness
- Restlessness
- Rubbing
- Screaming

Box 21-3	Nursing Measures to Promote Comfort and Relieve Pain

- Position the person in good body alignment; use pillows for support.
- Keep bed linens tight and wrinkle-free.
- Make sure the person is not lying on drainage tubes.
- Assist the person to the bathroom or commode, or offer the bedpan or urinal.
- Provide blankets for warmth and to prevent chilling.
- Use correct lifting, moving, and turning procedures.
- Wait one-half hour after pain medication was given before performing procedures.
- Give a back massage.
- Provide soft music to distract the person.
- Use touch to provide comfort.
- Allow family members and friends at the bedside as requested by the person.
- Avoid sudden or jarring movements of the bed.
- Handle the person gently.
- Practice safety measures if the person is receiving strong pain medication or sedatives:
  - Keep the bed in the low position.
  - Raise bed rails as directed. Follow the care plan.
  - Check on the person every 10 to 15 minutes.
  - Provide assistance when the person is up.
- Apply heat or cold applications as directed by the nurse (see Chapter 26).
- Provide a calm, quiet, darkened environment.

NURSING MEASURES

The RN uses the nursing process to promote comfort and relieve pain. Box 21-3 lists the nursing measures that are often part of care plans. You learned how to perform most of the measures in earlier chapters (Fig. 21-3, p. 538). You also learned why they are important for comfort.

Other measures are often needed to control pain. These include distraction, relaxation, and guided imagery. Nurses, physical therapists, occupational therapists, and recreational therapists may assist patients and residents with these measures. The nurse may ask you to assist. The nurse instructs you on how to properly perform them.

Distraction means to change the person's center of attention. The person's attention is moved away from the pain. Listening to music, playing games, singing, praying, watching television, and needlework are some ways to distract attention (Fig. 21-4, p. 538).

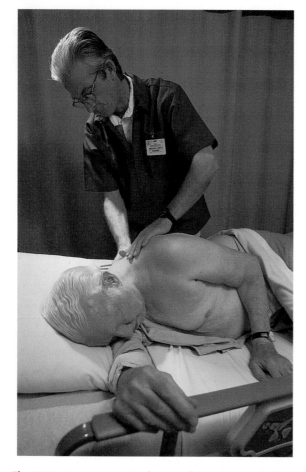

Fig. 21-3 Measures are implemented to relieve pain. The person is positioned in good body alignment with pillows used for support. The room is darkened. Blankets provide warmth. A back massage provides touch and promotes relaxation.

Fig. 21-4 A comforting pet can provide needed distraction from pain.

Relaxation means to be free from mental or physical stress. This state reduces pain and anxiety. The nurse or therapist teaches the person relaxation techniques. The person is taught to breathe deeply and slowly and to contract and relax muscle groups. A comfortable position and a quiet room are important. Box 21-4 is an example of how the nurse teaches the person relaxation.

Guided imagery is creating and focusing on an image. The person is asked to create a pleasant scene. The RN notes this on the care plan so the staff uses the same image with the person. The nurse uses a calm, soft voice when helping the person focus on the image. Soft music, a blanket for warmth, and a darkened room may help. The nurse coaches the person to focus on the image and then to practice relaxation exercises. See Box 21-5 for an example of guided imagery.

Doctors often order drugs to control or relieve pain. Nurses give these drugs. Such drugs can cause orthostatic hypotension, drowsiness, dizziness, and coordination problems. Therefore the person is protected from injury. The nurse and care plan alert you to any needed safety measures. (*See Focus on Children box.*)

Box 21-4	**Relaxation Taught by the Nurse**

Let's begin by finding as comfortable a position as possible. Arms at your side . . . legs uncrossed. . . . Move until you feel at ease. . . . Take a deep breath. Feel your stomach and chest slowly rise. . . . Relax. . . . Now breathe out slowly . . . slowly . . . and relax.

Count to 4, inhaling on 1 and 2, exhaling on 3 and 4. . . . Continue to breathe slowly. . . . Your body is beginning to relax. . . . Think "relax". . . . Feel the parts of your body. . . . Notice any tension in your muscles. . . . Continue to breathe slowly . . . and relax.

Concentrate on your face . . . your jaws . . . your neck. . . . Notice any tightness. . . . Breathe in warmth and relaxation. . . . Concentrate on any tension in your hands. . . . Notice how it feels. . . . Now make a fist—a tight fist! As you begin to exhale, relax your fist. . . . Good! Notice how your hand feels . . . Think "relax". . . . Your hand feels warm . . . heavy or light. . . . Just relax more . . . and more. Now focus on your forearms. . . . Notice any tension. . . . Relax your arms. . . . Feel your body relaxing. . . . Let the feelings of relaxation spread from your fingers and hands through the muscles of your arms.

Modified from Potter PA, Perry AG: *Fundamentals of nursing: concepts, process, and practice,* ed 4, St Louis, 1997, Mosby.

Box 21-5	Guided Imagery

Imagine yourself lying on a cool bed of grass with sounds of rushing water from a nearby stream. It's a balmy day. You turn to see a patch of blue wildflowers in bloom and can smell their fragrance.

Modified from Potter PA, Perry AG: *Fundamentals of nursing: concepts, process, and practice,* ed 4, St Louis, 1997, Mosby.

Focus On... CHILDREN

Pacifiers are often comforting for infants and young children. Favorite toys and blankets also are comforting. So is holding, rocking, touching, and talking or singing to them. Always check with the nurse before picking up and holding a child. Sometimes children are not held for treatment reasons.

Fig. 21-5 Needlework is relaxing for this lady.

REST

Rest means being calm, at ease, and relaxed. The person is free of anxiety and stress. Rest may involve physical inactivity. Or the person may do things that he or she finds calming and relaxing. Examples include reading, music, television, needlework, prayer, gardening, baking, golf, walking, and carpentry (Fig. 21-5).

Basic needs must be met for a person to rest. Thirst, hunger, elimination needs, and pain or discomfort can affect rest. You can promote rest by meeting physical needs. A comfortable position and good body alignment also are important. A quiet setting promotes rest. So does a clean, dry, and wrinkle-free bed. Some people rest easier in a clean, neat, and uncluttered room.

Safety and security needs must be met. The person must feel safe from falling or other injuries. The person is secure with the signal light within reach. Understanding the reasons for treatments also helps the person feel safe. So does knowing how procedures are done. That is why you always explain the procedure before it is performed.

Many persons have rituals or routines before resting. These may include going to the bathroom, brushing teeth, washing the face and hands, praying, having a snack or beverage, locking doors, or making sure children or loved ones are safe at home. The person may want a favorite blanket or afghan. Follow routines and rituals whenever possible.

Love and belonging are important for rest. Visits or telephone calls from family and friends may help the

Fig. 21-6 This nursing center resident reads cards and letters from family and friends.

person relax. The person knows that others care and are concerned. Reading cards and letters may also help the person relax and rest (Fig. 21-6).

Esteem needs relate to feeling good about oneself. A person may find hospital gowns embarrassing. Others fear exposure. Many persons rest better wearing their own gowns or pajamas. Personal appearance also affects esteem. Hair care, being clean and free of body odors, and other hygiene and grooming measures all help people feel good about themselves. If esteem needs are met, the person may rest easier.

Some people are refreshed after resting for 15 or 20 minutes. Others need more time. Health care routines usually allow time for afternoon rest.

Ill or injured persons need to rest more often. Some need to rest during or after a procedure. For example, a bath tires Mr. Smith. So does getting dressed. You need to let him rest before making the bed. Some people need a few hours to complete oral hygiene, bathing, grooming, and dressing. Others need to rest after meals. Do not push the person beyond his or her limits. Allow rest periods as they are needed. Do not rush the person.

Distraction, relaxation, and guided imagery also promote rest. So does a back massage. You must plan and organize care so that the person can rest without interruptions.

The doctor may order bedrest for a person. Bedrest, its complications, and how to prevent complications are presented in Chapter 20.

SLEEP

Sleep is a state of unconsciousness, reduced voluntary muscle activity, and lowered metabolism. An unconscious person is unaware of the environment and cannot respond to people and things in the environment. The unconsciousness is temporary. People awake from sleep. Alarm clocks, voices, and crying babies easily awaken sleeping persons. Voluntary muscles are skeletal muscles. During sleep, there are no voluntary arm or leg movements. Metabolism is the burning of food and energy for use by the body. Less energy is needed during sleep. Thus metabolism is reduced during sleep.

Sleep is a basic need. It lets the mind and body rest. The body saves energy. Body functions slow. Vital signs fall. That is, blood pressure, temperature, and pulse and respiration rates are lower than when awake. Tissue healing and repair occur during sleep. Sleep lowers stress, tension, and anxiety. It refreshes and renews the person. That is, the person regains energy and mental alertness. The person thinks and functions better after needed sleep.

CIRCADIAN RHYTHM

Sleep occurs regularly. It is part of circadian rhythm. Circadian comes from the Latin words *circa* meaning *about* and *dies* meaning *day*. **Circadian rhythm** is a pattern based on a 24-hour cycle. It is a daily rhythm called the *day-night cycle* or *body rhythm*. Functioning is affected by circadian rhythm. Some people function better in the morning. They are more alert and active; they think and react better. Others do better in the evening.

Circadian rhythm includes a sleep-wake cycle. The person's *biological clock* signals the time for sleep and the time to wake up. You have usual times for going to sleep and waking up. You may awaken before the alarm clock goes off. That is all part of your biological clock. Health care agencies often interfere with a person's circadian rhythm and the sleep-wake cycle. Sleep problems easily occur.

Many people work evening and night shifts. They include health care workers, police officers, fire fighters, fast-food workers, and factory workers. Their bodies must adjust to changes in the sleep-wake cycle.

SLEEP CYCLE

There are two phases of sleep. Nonrapid eye movement is **NREM sleep** or **nonREM sleep**. NREM sleep has four stages. Sleep goes from light to deep as the person moves through the four stages.

The rapid eye movement phase is called **REM sleep**. The person is hard to arouse. Mental restoration occurs during REM sleep. Events and problems of the previous day are thought to be reviewed during REM sleep. The person prepares for the next day.

Box 21-6 shows the stages of NREM and REM sleep. There are usually 4 to 6 cycles of NREM and REM sleep during the 7 to 8 hours of sleep each night. Stage 1 of NREM is usually not repeated (Fig. 21-7).

SLEEP REQUIREMENTS

The amount of sleep needed varies for each age-group. The amount needed decreases with age (Table 21-1). Infants need more sleep than toddlers. Toddlers need more than preschool children. School-age children need more than teenagers. Older persons need less sleep than middle-age adults.

Box 21-6	Sleep Cycle

Stage 1: NREM sleep
- Lightest sleep level
- Lasts a few minutes
- Gradual fall in vital signs
- Gradual lowering of metabolism
- Person feels drowsy and relaxed
- Person easily aroused
- Daydreaming feeling after being aroused

Stage 2: NREM sleep
- Sound sleep
- Relaxation increases
- Still easy to arouse
- Lasts 10 to 20 minutes
- Body functions continue to slow

Stage 3: NREM sleep
- First stages of deep sleep
- Hard to arouse the person
- Person rarely moves
- Muscles relax completely
- Vital signs fall
- Lasts 15 to 30 minutes

Stage 4: NREM sleep
- Deepest stage of sleep
- Hard to arouse the person
- Body rests and is restored
- Vital signs much lower than when awake
- Lasts about 15 to 30 minutes
- Sleepwalking and **enuresis** (urinary incontinence in bed at night) may occur

REM sleep
- Vivid, full-color dreaming
- Usually starts 50 to 90 minutes after sleep has begun
- Rapid eye movements
- Blood pressure, pulse, and respirations may fluctuate
- Voluntary muscles are relaxed
- Mental restoration occurs
- Hard to arouse the person
- Lasts about 20 minutes

Modified from Potter PA, Perry AG: *Fundamentals of nursing: Concepts, process, and practice,* ed 4, St Louis, 1997, Mosby.

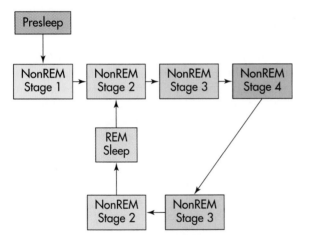

Fig. 21-7 Adult sleep cycle.

Table 21-1	Average Sleep Requirements	
Age-Group		**Hours Per Day**
Newborns (birth to 4 weeks)		14 to 18
Infants (4 weeks to 1 year)		12 to 14
Toddlers (1 to 3 years)		11 to 12
Preschoolers (3 to 6 years)		11 to 12
Middle and late childhood (6 to 12 years)		10 to 11
Adolescents (12 to 18 years)		8 to 9
Young adults (18 to 40 years)		7 to 8
Middle-age adults (40 to 65 years)		7
Older adults (65 years and older)		5 to 7

FACTORS AFFECTING SLEEP

Several factors affect the amount and quality of sleep. Quality relates to how well the person slept and if needed amounts of NREM and REM sleep were obtained.

- *Illness.* Illness increases the need for sleep. However, the signs and symptoms of illness can interfere with sleep. They include pain, nausea, vomiting, coughing, difficulty breathing, diarrhea, frequent voiding, and itching. Treatments and therapies can also interfere with sleep. Often patients and residents are awakened for treatments or medications. Traction or a cast can cause uncomfortable positions. The emotional effects of illness can affect sleep. These include fear, anxiety, and worry.
- *Nutrition.* Weight loss or gain affects sleep. The need for sleep increases with weight gain. It decreases with weight loss. Some foods affect sleep. Those with caffeine (chocolate, coffee, tea, colas) prevent sleep. The protein L-tryptophan tends to help sleep. It is found in milk, cheese, and beef (Fig. 21-8).
- *Exercise.* Exercise is good for the body. It improves health and fitness. Exercise requires energy. The person usually feels good after exercising. Eventually the person tires. Being tired helps the person sleep well at night. Exercising right before bedtime interferes with sleep. Exercise causes the release of substances into the bloodstream that stimulate the body. Therefore there should be at least 2 hours between exercise and bedtime.
- *Environment.* People adjust to their usual sleeping environments. They get used to such things as the bed, pillows, noises in the home or neighborhood, lighting, and a sleeping partner. Any change in the usual environment can affect the amount and quality of sleep.
- *Drugs and other substances.* Some drugs promote sleep. These are commonly called *sleeping pills.* Drugs given for anxiety, depression, and pain may cause the person to sleep. However, these drugs and sleeping pills reduce the length of REM sleep. Remember, mental restoration occurs during REM sleep. Behavior problems and sleep deprivation can occur. Alcohol is a drug. Alcohol tends to cause drowsiness and sleep. However, it interferes with REM sleep. Those under the influence of alcohol may awaken during sleep. Difficulty returning to sleep is common. Some drugs contain caffeine. As stated earlier, caffeine is a stimulant and prevents sleep. Besides in drugs, it is found in coffee, tea, chocolate, and colas. The side effects of some drugs can disrupt sleep. These include frequent voiding and nightmares.

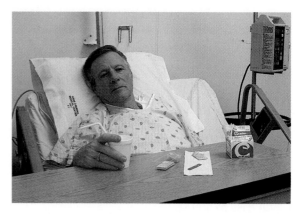

Fig. 21-8 A bedtime snack of milk, cheese, and crackers helps to promote sleep.

- *Life-style changes.* Life-style relates to a person's daily routines and way of living. Work, school, play, and social events are all part of life-style. Life-style changes can affect sleep. Travel, vacation, and social events often affect usual bedtimes and when the person awakens. Children usually stay up later during school holidays. They may sleep later, too. If work hours change, the person needs to change sleep hours. Such changes affect normal sleep-wake cycles and the circadian rhythm.
- *Emotional problems.* Fear, worry, depression, and anxiety affect sleep. These may be caused by work, personal, or family problems. Loss of a close family member or friend is another cause. Money problems are stressful. People may have difficulty falling asleep, or they awaken often. Difficulty getting back to sleep may occur.

SLEEP DISORDERS

Sleep disorders involve repeated sleep problems. The amount and quality of sleep are affected. Sleep disorders affect life-style. Box 21-7 lists the signs and symptoms that occur.

Insomnia. Insomnia is a chronic condition in which the person cannot sleep or stay asleep throughout the night. There are three forms of insomnia:

- Unable to fall asleep
- Unable to stay asleep
- Early awakening and unable to fall back asleep

	Signs and Symptoms
Box 21-7	**of Sleep Disorders**

- Hand tremors
- Slowed responses to questions, conversations, or situations
- Reduced word memory; difficulty finding the right word
- Decreased reasoning and judgment
- Irregular pulse
- Red, puffy eyes
- Dark circles under the eyes
- Moodiness; mood swings
- Disorientation
- Irritability
- Fatigue
- Sleepiness
- Agitation
- Restlessness
- Decreased attention
- Hallucinations (see Chapter 31)
- Coordination problems
- Slurred speech

	Nursing Measures
Box 21-8	**to Promote Sleep**

- Organize care to allow for uninterrupted rest.
- Avoid physical activity before bedtime.
- Encourage the person to avoid tending to business or family matters before bedtime.
- Allow a flexible bedtime. Bedtime is when the person is tired and fatigued—not a certain time.
- Provide a comfortable room temperature.
- Allow the person to take a warm bath or shower.
- Provide a bedtime snack.
- Avoid caffeine (coffee, tea, colas, chocolate).
- Avoid alcoholic beverages.
- Have the person void before going to bed. Make sure incontinent residents are clean and dry. Change a baby's diaper.
- Follow bedtime rituals.
- Make sure the person wears loose-fitting nightwear.
- Provide adequate warmth (blankets, socks) for those who tend to be cold.
- Reduce noise.
- Darken the room by closing shades, blinds, and the privacy curtain. Shut off or dim lights.
- Dim lights in hallways and the nursing unit.
- Make sure linens are clean, dry, and wrinkle-free.
- Position the person in good alignment.
- Support body parts as ordered.
- Make sure the person is in a comfortable position.
- Give a back massage.
- Implement measures to relieve pain.
- Allow the person to read. Read to children.
- Allow the person to listen to music.
- Allow the person to watch television.
- Assist with relaxation exercises as ordered.
- Sit and talk with the person.

Emotional problems are common causes of insomnia. The fear of dying during sleep is another cause. Some people are afraid of not waking up. This may occur after recent heart disease or after being told of a terminal illness. The fear of not being able to sleep is another cause. The physical and emotional discomforts of illness can also cause insomnia.

The RN plans measures to promote sleep. However, the emotional or physical problems causing the insomnia also are treated.

Sleep Deprivation. With sleep deprivation, the amount and quality of sleep are decreased. Sleep is interrupted. NREM and REM sleep stages are not completed. Illness and hospital care are common causes of sleep deprivation. Patients in intensive care units (ICUs) are at great risk. ICU lights are on much of the time. The many care measures and sounds from equipment interfere with sleep. Factors that affect sleep can also lead to sleep deprivation. Sleep deprivation results in many of the signs and symptoms listed in Box 21-7.

Sleepwalking. The person who sleepwalks leaves the bed and walks about. The person is not aware of sleepwalking and has no memory of the event on awakening. Children sleepwalk more than adults. The event may last 3 to 4 minutes or longer.

Stress, fatigue, and some drugs can cause sleepwalking. The person needs protection from injury. The risk of falling is great. Intravenous infusions, catheters, nasogastric tubes, and other tubes are also sources of injury. The tubes or catheters can be pulled out of the body when the person gets out of bed. Guide sleepwalkers back to bed. They startle easily. Awaken them gently.

PROMOTING SLEEP

The RN assesses the person's sleep patterns. Your observations are important. Report any of the signs and symptoms listed in Box 21-7. The RN plans measures to promote sleep (Box 21-8). Check the care plan so that you give the correct care. Also report your observations so the nurse can evaluate if the goal of a regular sleep pattern was met. *(See Focus on Older Persons and Focus on Long-Term Care boxes on p. 544.)*

Focus On ... OLDER PERSONS

Older persons have less energy than younger people. Many older persons take naps during the day. You need to let the person sleep. Organize the person's care to allow uninterrupted naps.

Focus On ... LONG-TERM CARE

OBRA requires that residents receive care that promotes well-being. Comfort, rest, and sleep are necessary for physical, emotional, and mental well-being. OBRA requires that resident rooms be designed and equipped to provide for comfort. The following room requirements under OBRA promote quality of life and comfort, rest, and sleep:

- No more than 4 residents in a room
- Suspended privacy curtain that extends around the bed
- A bed of proper height and size for the resident
- Clean, comfortable mattress
- Linens appropriate to the weather and climate
- Clean and orderly room
- Odor-free room
- Room temperature between 71° and 81° F
- Acceptable noise level
- Adequate ventilation and room humidity
- Appropriate lighting

Many residents have specific rituals and routines before bedtime. They are allowed if safe. The person may perform personal hygiene measures in a certain order. Some residents like to check on friends in the center before going to bed. Some are given the responsibility of turning off lights at bedtime. A bedtime snack may be important. Watching certain television shows in bed may be a bedtime routine. Others may read religious writings, pray, or say a rosary before going to sleep. Whatever the routine or ritual, it is important to the resident.

The resident is involved in planning care. The person is allowed to choose when to nap or sleep. The person also has the right to choose what measures are helpful in promoting comfort, rest, and sleep. You must follow the care plan and the person's wishes.

Some older persons have dementia. Sleep disturbances are common in some types of dementia. Night wandering is common. Restlessness and confusion increase at night. This increases the risk of falls. Quietly and calmly direct the person back to his or her room. Nighttime wandering in a safe and supervised setting is helpful for some people. The measures listed in Box 21-8 also are tried. Specific measures for the person are found in the care plan.

Circle the BEST answer.

1. These statements are about pain. Which is *false?*
   A. Pain is objective. It can be seen, heard, smelled, or felt.
   B. Pain is a warning from the body. It means there is damage to tissues.
   C. Pain is personal. It is different for each person.
   D. Pain is used to make diagnoses.

2. A person complains of pain in the left side of the chest, up into the left jaw, and down to the left shoulder and left arm. This is
   A. Acute pain
   B. Chronic pain
   C. Radiating pain
   D. Phantom pain

3. Mr. Smith complains of pain. You should do the following *except*
   A. Ask him to point to where the pain is felt
   B. Ask him when the pain started
   C. Ask him to describe the pain
   D. Ask to look at the pain

4. The nurse gives Mr. Smith a drug for pain. A procedure is scheduled for this time. You should
   A. Perform the procedure before the medication is given
   B. Perform the procedure right after the medication is given
   C. Wait one-half hour to let the medication take effect
   D. Omit the procedure for the day

5. Mr. Smith is protected from injury after receiving pain medication. You should do the following *except*
   A. Keep the bed in the high position
   B. Raise bed rails as directed
   C. Check on him every 10 to 15 minutes
   D. Provide assistance if he needs to get up

6. Which measure will not help relieve pain?
   A. Providing blankets as needed
   B. Keeping the room well lighted
   C. Providing soft music
   D. Giving a back massage

7. Mr. Smith's care plan has the following nursing measures. Which will *not* help him rest or sleep?
   A. Have him urinate before rest or sleep.
   B. Assist him to assume a comfortable position.
   C. Assist him to ambulate before rest or sleep.
   D. Allow him to choose sleep attire.

8. Mr. Smith tires very easily. His morning care includes a bath, hair care, and getting dressed. His bed is made after he is dressed. When should he rest?
   A. After morning care is completed
   B. After his bath and before hair care
   C. After you make the bed
   D. Whenever he needs to

9. These statements are about sleep. Which is *false?*
   A. Tissue healing and repair occur during sleep.
   B. Voluntary muscle activity increases during sleep.
   C. Sleep refreshes and renews the person.
   D. Ill and injured persons need more sleep than healthy persons do.

10. Mr. Smith was awake several nights when he first entered the hospital. Which is *true?*
    A. His circadian rhythm may be affected.
    B. NREM and REM sleep are affected.
    C. His biological clock will still tell him when to sleep and wake up.
    D. His functioning will not be affected.

11. Mr. Smith is 35 years old. When healthy, he probably needs about
    A. 12 to 14 hours of sleep per day
    B. 8 to 9 hours of sleep per day
    C. 7 to 8 hours of sleep per day
    D. About 6 hours of sleep per day

12. Mr. Smith asks for a snack. He said a friend brought him a chocolate chip cheesecake and some beef summer sausage. He asks for milk with his snack. Which foods will prevent sleep?
    A. Chocolate
    B. Cheese
    C. Milk
    D. Beef

13. Mr. Smith has difficulty sleeping, and he awakens several times during the night. He has difficulty answering your questions and seems moody. His pulse is irregular, and his eyes are red and puffy. He is showing signs of
    A. Insomnia
    B. Sleep deprivation
    C. Enuresis
    D. Distraction

14. These measures are part of Mr. Smith's care plan. Which should you question?
    A. Let Mr. Smith choose his bedtime.
    B. Provide a bedtime snack of hot tea and a cheese sandwich.
    C. Make sure his casted extremity is properly supported.
    D. Follow his bedtime rituals.

Answers to these questions are on p. 837.

CHAPTER

22

ADMISSIONS, TRANSFERS, AND DISCHARGES

Define the key terms listed in this chapter

Describe what occurs in the admitting office

Prepare the person's room

Explain how to admit a person to the nursing unit

Measure height and weight

Explain why a person may be transferred to another agency or nursing unit

Explain how a person is prepared for discharge

Perform the procedures described in this chapter

KEY TERMS

admission Official entry of a person into an agency or nursing unit

discharge Official departure of a person from an agency or nursing unit

transfer Moving a person from one room, nursing unit, or agency to another

Admission to a health care agency causes anxiety and fear. The person and family may worry about the need for treatment or surgery and its outcome. They may fear serious health problems. The fear of pain is very common. People admitted to nursing centers have fears of never returning home. Many people are unfamiliar with health care agencies. They worry about where to go, what to expect, and the strange sights and sounds. They worry about getting meals, finding the bathroom, and how to get help. Similar concerns occur with transfers to other agencies or nursing units. Discharge usually brings relief and happiness. However, the person may need home care.

Admission, transfer, and discharge are critical events. Patients, residents, and families need to feel comfortable and secure. You must be courteous, kind, and respectful.

You will use learning from previous chapters when admitting, transferring, and discharging patients and residents. This includes privacy, confidentiality, reporting and recording, communicating with the health team, and understanding and communicating with the person. Respect for the person and the person's property also applies.

Focus On... LONG-TERM CARE

Many nursing centers have admission coordinators. They make the resident's admission as easy and as simple as possible. Often admission procedures are completed 2 or 3 days before the person enters the center. Identifying information is obtained from the person or family member.

The nursing staff is told of the admission and room assignment before the person arrives. Some residents arrive by ambulance or wheelchair van. The attendants take them directly to their rooms. Some residents arrive by private car. A nurse or nursing assistant takes them to their rooms. Some residents want a family member with them. Then the family also goes to the room. This is a critical and emotional time for the resident and family. They are not separated until they are comfortable doing so. Remember, the center is now the person's home.

At some time after admission, a photograph is taken and the person is given an ID bracelet.

Persons with dementia and their families may need special help during the admission process. The person's confusion may increase in the new setting. He or she may become fearful and agitated and want to leave. The family is also fearful and often feels guilty about admitting the person to a nursing center. The health care team works together to help the resident and family feel safe and welcome.

ADMISSIONS

Except in emergencies, the admission process starts in the admitting office. **Admission** is the official entry of a person into an agency or nursing unit. Admitting staff or a nurse obtains identifying information. This includes the person's full name, age, date of birth, doctor's name, social security number, and religion. The information is recorded on the admission record. The person is given an identification number and an ID bracelet (see Chapter 9). A general consent for treatment is signed at this time.

Admitting office staff notify the nursing unit that a new patient or resident is being admitted. The nursing staff is told the person's room and bed number. Someone from the admitting office brings the person to the nursing unit. Some agencies let the person walk to the nursing unit if able. Most require transport by wheelchair or stretcher. *(See Focus on Long-Term Care box.)*

Fig. 22-1 The room is ready for a person to be admitted.

▶ PREPARING THE ROOM

The room must be ready for the new patient or resident. This is usually your responsibility. Figure 22-1 shows a room prepared for a person's arrival.

▶ Preparing the Person's Room

Pre-Procedure

1 Know which room and bed to prepare. Find out if the person is arriving by wheelchair or stretcher.
2 Wash your hands.
3 Collect the following:
   - Patient or resident pack (contains bath basin, pitcher, cup, and personal care items)
   - Admission checklist (Fig. 22-2, pp. 550-551)
   - Urine specimen container (if a urine specimen is ordered)
   - Sphygmomanometer
   - Stethoscope
   - Gown or pajamas
   - IV pole if needed

Procedure

4 For the person who is ambulatory or arriving by wheelchair:
   a Open the bed.
   b Lower the bed to its lowest position.
5 For the person arriving by stretcher:
   a Make a surgical bed (see Chapter 13)
   b Raise the bed to its highest level.
6 Attach the signal light to the bed linens.
7 Place the sphygmomanometer, stethoscope, and admission checklist on the overbed table.
8 Place the gown or pajamas on the bed.
9 Place the patient pack and specimen container on the bedside stand or overbed table.
10 Make sure towels and washcloths, a bedpan, kidney basin, and urinal (for a male) are in the bedside stand. Get missing items.
11 Wash your hands.

BONELL NURSING UNIT ADMISSION CHECKLIST

For Nursing Assistants

_____ 1. Check the room before resident arrives to see that: _____ room is clean.
_____ bed made _____ straw & H$_2$O pitcher _____ washcloth & hand towel.
_____ 2. Introduce resident to yourself, other residents, and staff. Likes to be called _____.
_____ 3. Orient resident to room and call lights _____.
_____ 4. _____ T. _____ P. _____ R. _____ BP. _____ Wt. _____ Ht.
_____ 5. Fill out Inventory of Personal Effects form _____.
_____ 6. Laundry service: _____ family to do   _____ sign posted at receptacle
                          _____ facility to do   _____ clothes marked
_____ 7. Mark comb, brush, toothbrush, denture cup, dentures, eyeglasses, etc. _____.
_____ 8. Assist in putting personal possessions away _____.

Signature _____ Date _____

For Medical Records Unit Assistant or Charge Nurse

_____ 1. Alert CNA of new admission _____.
_____ 2. Copy Face Sheet and sent to medical records _____ Kitchen (also sent written request).
_____ 3. Order lab work: _____ X-ray   _____ Other
_____ 4. Complete chart: _____.
_____ 5. Place name in the following places: _____ bath schedule   _____ room door
          _____ medicine cabinet   _____ closet door   _____ bed   _____ dresser
          _____ daily census   _____ daily report   _____ wheelchair   _____ towel rack
_____ 6. Place name tag on resident.

Signature _____ Date _____

For Social Services

_____ 1. Take 2 pictures.
_____ 2. _____ Desire beauty shop   _____ Barber shop
_____ 3. Placement of door badge.

Signature _____ Date _____

For Admitting Nurse

_____ 1. Talked with resident of Philosophy of Independence and of going to dining room for meals.
_____ 2. Complete Nursing Assessment, Pain Assessment, Braden, Bladder Assessment, and Safety Assessment. Send communique to P.T. for a Rehab Assessment one week prior to Care Conference.
_____ 3. Determine allergies.
_____ 4. Remove all medication from room.
_____ 5. Make out nursing care plan and aide assignment sheet.
_____ 6. Chart admission remarks—(date, time, admitted from, with whom, mode of transportation, mobility, (V.S., etc.).
_____ 7. Check Physicians Orders: clarify orders, obtain missing Dx (i.e.: catheter, psych Dx), write treatment on treatment profile sheet.
_____ 8. Call Pharmacy, inform them of Pay Status, order medication if needed. Write medication on medication profile sheet.
_____ 9. Obtain V.S. × each shift × 3 days.
_____ 10. Chart each shift × 3 days.
_____ 11. Schedule Glucose monitoring next AM.
_____ 12. Obtain order for 2-step TB test.
_____ 13. Place name on daily census and 24 hour report. Place name on resident roster along with pertinent data.
_____ 14. Supply Care Enrollment form.
_____ 15. Write name in lab book.

Signature _____ Date _____

Fig. 22-2 An admission checklist. _(Courtesy Bonell Good Samaritan Center, Greeley, Colo.)_

Discharge Checklist

_____ 1. Physician order received _____.

_____ 2. Responsible party notified _____, who _____.

_____ 3. Update MDS for discharge; make 2 copies _____.

     a. _____ one for resident

     b. _____ one for Medical Records

_____ 4. Complete Discharge Summary and Post Discharge Plan GSS #227.

_____ 5. If discharge to hospital or other health care facility, transfer form filled out _____.

_____ 6. If discharged to home, a discharge form filled out_____. Was a home health care agency ordered and contracted? _____.

_____ 7. Discharge instructions: Medications (for home) special instructions _____; other written instructions _____ (retain a copy)·

     a. _____ equipment _____ .

     b. _____ dietary instructions _____ .

_____ 8. Document on Nurses Notes the time of discharge, on the above information, document dispensation of all medications, and on the physical, mental, and psychosocial assessment of resident.

_____ 9. Place name on daily census for discharge _____ and on daily report _____, and remove from Resident Roster.

_____ 10. Remove name from bath list _____.

_____ 11. Notify kitchen _____.

_____ 12. Notify housekeeping _____.

_____ 13. Confirm forwarding address _____ and notify finance of discharge and address.

_____ 14. Send chart to Medical Records _____.

_____ 15. Place Schedule II, III, IV, and V count sheets and unused medications in locked Narcotic cupboard in medication room. Inform Nurse Manager.

_____ 16. Notify Pharmacy _____ Date _____ Time _____·

_____ 17. Inventory of personal effects reviewed, and disposition noted on Inventory of Personal Effects form.

_____ 18. Place discharge information in OPUS Book and Lab Book.

Signature _____ Date _____

Fig. 22-2, cont'd For legend see opposite page.

ADMITTING THE PERSON

A nurse usually greets and admits the person. It may be your responsibility if the person has no serious discomfort or distress. The admission record is used to find out the person's name. When you greet the person, call him or her by name. Introduce yourself by name and title to the person and to family members who may be present (Fig. 22-3).

Admission procedures involve:

- Completing an admission checklist
- Weighing and measuring the person
- Obtaining a urine specimen if one is ordered
- Orienting the person to the room, nursing unit, and the agency
  (*See Focus on Long-Term Care box.*)

Fig. 22-3 The nursing assistant introduces herself to the person and family member.

Focus On... LONG-TERM CARE

The resident needs to feel comfortable, safe, and secure. Avoid rushing into admission procedures. Rather, treat the resident and family as if they are guests in your home. Offer them a cup of coffee, tea, or other beverage. Visit with them, and tell them some of the many good things about the center. This is a good time to introduce the person's roommate. You can also introduce the person to other residents in nearby rooms. Write down their names for the new resident. Remembering names is hard for many people. When the family leaves, it is important that the resident know others. By being introduced to others, the new resident is not left in the awkward position of not knowing anyone. Other residents are a source of great comfort and support to the new resident. They understand, better than any staff member, what it is like to enter a nursing center.

Remember, the center is the person's home. You need to help the resident make the room as homelike as possible. You can help the person unpack. The person might need help hanging clothes and putting things in drawers. The person might want to hang pictures or display photographs. You need to show caring and compassion. Do all that you can to help the person feel safe, comfortable, and secure.

When the resident is comfortable, the admission procedures are completed. A nurse or social worker explains the resident's rights to the resident and family. They are also given a booklet explaining these rights.

Admitting the Person

QUALITY OF LIFE

Remember to:
- Knock before entering the person's room
- Address the person by name
- Introduce yourself by name and title

Pre-Procedure

1 Wash your hands.

2 Prepare the room.

Admitting the Person—cont'd

Procedure—cont'd

3 Greet the person by name. Ask if he or she prefers a certain name.

4 Introduce yourself to the person and relatives or friends who may be present. Give your title, and explain that you assist the nurses in giving care.

5 Introduce the roommate.

6 Call for a nurse immediately if the person complains of any severe pain or appears to be in distress.

7 Proceed if the person's condition does not present an immediate or serious problem.

8 Provide for privacy. Ask family members or friends to leave the room. Tell them how much time you need and where they can wait comfortably. (Allow a family member or friend to stay if the person prefers.)

9 Have a hospital patient put on a gown or pajamas. Assist as needed. (A nursing center resident can stay dressed if his or her condition permits.)

10 Provide for comfort. He or she should be in bed or in a chair as directed by the nurse.

11 Complete the admission checklist (see Fig. 22-2). This includes measuring vital signs (see Chapter 19) and measuring height and weight.

12 Complete a clothing and valuables list (see Chapter 9).

13 Hang clothes in the closet. Put personal items in the drawers and bedside stand.

14 Explain any ordered activity limits.

15 Obtain a urine specimen if ordered (see Chapter 16).

16 Take the specimen to the storage area or laboratory. Clean equipment, and wash your hands.

17 Orient the person to the area:

a Give names of the nurses.

b Identify items in the bedside stand. Explain the purpose of each item.

c Show how the signal light is used.

d Show how to operate the bed and television controls.

e Explain how to make telephone calls. Place the phone within reach.

f Explain visiting hours and policies.

g Describe the location of the nurses' station, lounge, chapel, dining room, gift shop, and other important areas.

h Explain other services: newspaper, library, activities, educational programs, religious services, and others.

i Identify other staff: workers from x-ray, laboratory, housekeeping, dietary, and physical therapy, as well as students and others.

j Explain when meals and nourishments are served.

18 Fill the water pitcher if oral fluids are allowed.

19 Place the signal light within reach. Place other controls and needed items within reach.

20 Keep the bed in its lowest position.

21 Raise or lower bed rails. Follow the care plan.

22 Unscreen the person.

23 Clean used equipment. Discard used disposable items. Wash your hands.

24 Provide a denture container if needed. Label it with the person's name and room number.

25 Label personal property and personal care equipment for the nursing center resident. Items are labeled with the person's name.

Post-Procedure

26 Wash your hands.

27 Report your observations to the nurse.

▶ **Measuring Height and Weight.** Height and weight are measured on admission. The person wears only a gown or pajamas. Clothes add weight. Shoes or slippers also add weight and add to the height measurement. The person urinates before being weighed. A full bladder affects the weight measurement. If a urine specimen is needed, collect it at this time.

Standing, chair, and lift scales are used (Fig. 22-4). Chair and lift scales are used for persons who cannot stand. The manufacturer's instructions and agency procedures are followed when using a chair or lift scale.

(See Focus on Children box.)

Focus On... CHILDREN

Birth weight serves as the baseline for measuring an infant's growth. The RN also uses the weight measurements for the nursing process. Weighing infants is described in Chapter 35.

Length, not height, is measured in children younger than 2 years. The child lies on a measuring board or on a paper. Two people hold the child still. One holds the head still, and the other extends and holds the legs still. The measurement is taken from the top of the head to the heels. If using paper, mark the paper at the head and heels. Measure the distance between the two points.

A **B** **C**

Fig. 22-4 Types of scales. **A,** Standing scale. **B,** Chair scale. **C,** Lift scale.

Measuring Height and Weight

NNAAP™

QUALITY OF LIFE

Remember to:
- Knock before entering the person's room
- Address the person by name
- Introduce yourself by name and title

Pre-Procedure

1 Explain the procedure to the person.
2 Ask the person to urinate.
3 Wash your hands.
4 Collect the following:
- Scale (standing, chair, wheelchair, or lift scale)
- Paper towels

5 Identify the person. Check the ID bracelet against the assignment sheet.
6 Provide for privacy.

Procedure

7 Standing scale:
   a Place the paper towels on the scale platform.
   b Raise the height rod.
   c Have the person remove the robe and slippers. Assist as needed.
   d Help the person stand on the scale platform. Arms are at the sides.
   e Move the weights until the balance pointer is in the middle (Fig. 22-5, p. 556).
   f Record the weight on your note pad or assignment sheet.
   g Ask the person to stand very straight.
   h Lower the height rod until it rests on the person's head (Fig. 22-6, p. 556).
   i Record the height on your note pad or assignment sheet.
8 Chair scale:
   a Help the person transfer from the wheelchair to the chair scale (see *Transferring a Person to a Chair or Wheelchair,* p. 266).
   b Place the person's feet on the foot platform (see Fig. 22-4, *B*).

   c Move the weights until the balance pointer is in the middle.
   d Record the weight on your notepad or assignment sheet.
9 Lift scale:
   a Attach the sling and chains to the lift.
   b Place both weights on zero.
   c Level and balance the scale according to the manufacturer's instructions.
   d Remove the sling from the scale.
   e Place the person on the sling, and attach it to the lift. Raise the resident about 4 inches off the bed (see *Using a Mechanical Lift,* p. 272).
   f Move the weights until the balance pointer is in the middle.
   g Record the weight on your notepad or assignment sheet.
   h Lower the person to the bed.
   i Remove the sling.
10 Help the person put on the robe and slippers if he or she will be up. Help the person back to bed if necessary.

Post-Procedure

11 Provide for comfort.
12 Place the signal light within reach.
13 Raise or lower bed rails. Follow the care plan.
14 Unscreen the person.

15 Discard the paper towels.
16 Return the scale to its storage area.
17 Wash your hands.
18 Report and record the measurements.

Fig. 22-5 Weighing a person. **A,** The person is weighed. **B,** The weight is read when the balance pointer is in the middle.

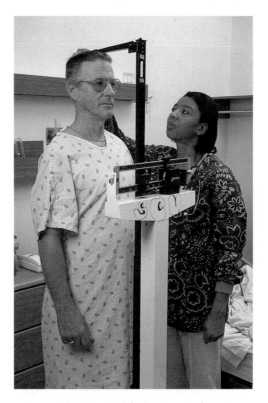

Fig. 22-6 Height is measured.

Measuring Height: The Person in Bed or a Wheelchair

QUALITY OF LIFE

Remember to:
- Knock before entering the person's room
- Address the person by name
- Introduce yourself by name and title

Pre-Procedure

1 Explain the procedure to the person.
2 Wash your hands.
3 Collect a measuring tape and ruler.
4 Ask a co-worker to help you.
5 Provide for privacy.

Procedure

6 Position the person supine if this position is allowed.
7 Have your co-worker hold the end of the measuring tape at the person's heel.
8 Pull the measuring tape alongside the person's body until it extends past the head.
9 Place the ruler flat across the top of the person's head. It should extend from the resident's head to the measuring tape. Make sure the ruler is level (Fig. 22-7).
10 Record the height on your notepad or assignment sheet.
11 Assist the person back to the wheelchair if appropriate.

Post-Procedure

12 Provide for comfort.
13 Raise or lower bed rails if the person stays in bed. Follow the care plan.
14 Place the signal light within reach.
15 Unscreen the person.
16 Return equipment to its proper location.
17 Wash your hands.
18 Report and record the height.

Fig. 22-7 The person is measured in bed. The ruler extends from the top of his head to his heel.

► TRANSFERS

A **transfer** is moving a person from one room, nursing unit, or agency (hospital, nursing center, or hospice) to another. Transfers are usually related to changes in condition. The person may or may not welcome the transfer. Sometimes the person requests a room change. Room changes may be necessary if roommates do not get along.

Reasons for the transfer are explained by the doctor, nurse, or social worker. The family and business office are notified. You may assist in the transfer or carry out the entire procedure. The person is usually transported by wheelchair or stretcher. Sometimes the bed is used.

► Transferring the Person to Another Nursing Unit

QUALITY OF LIFE

Remember to:
- Knock before entering the person's room
- Address the person by name
- Introduce yourself by name and title

Pre-Procedure

1. Find out where the person is going. Ask if the bed, a wheelchair, or a stretcher will be used.
2. Explain the procedure to the person.
3. Get a stretcher or wheelchair, bath blanket, and a utility cart if needed.
4. Wash your hands.

Procedure

5. Identify the person. Check the ID bracelet against the transfer slip.
6. Collect the person's belongings and bedside equipment. Place them on the utility cart for transport.
7. Assist the person to the wheelchair or stretcher. Cover the person with a bath blanket.
8. Transport the person to the assigned place.
9. Introduce the person to the receiving nurse.
10. Help transfer the person from the wheelchair or stretcher into bed or a chair. Help position the person.
11. Bring the person's belongings and equipment to the new room. Help put them away.
12. Report the following to the receiving nurse:
    a How the person tolerated the transfer
    b That a nurse will bring the person's chart, care plan, Kardex, and medications

Post-Procedure

13. Return the wheelchair or stretcher and the utility cart to the storage area.
14. Wash your hands.
15. Report the following to the nurse:
    - The time of transfer
    - Where the person was taken
    - How the person was transferred (bed, wheelchair, or stretcher)
    - How the person tolerated the transfer
    - Who received the person
    - Any other observations
16. Strip the bed, clean the unit, and make a closed bed. (This may be done by housekeeping staff.)
17. Wash your hands.

▶ DISCHARGES

Discharge is usually planned a few days in advance. **Discharge** is the official departure of a person from an agency or nursing unit. This is a happy time if the person is going home. Some people are discharged to another hospital or to a nursing center. Some need home care. They may have other fears and concerns. The doctor, nurse, dietitian, social worker, and other health team members plan the person's discharge. They teach the person and family about diet, exercise, and needed drugs. They also teach about dressing changes and treatments. Home care and special therapy and equipment are arranged. So is a doctor's appointment.

You will often help persons pack belongings and change into street clothes. You also transport persons out of the agency. The nurse tells you when to start the discharge procedure. The doctor must write a discharge order before the person is allowed to leave. The nurse tells you when the person can leave and how to transport him or her. Usually a wheelchair is used. Some agencies let the person walk. Occasionally a person or resident leaves by ambulance. The ambulance attendants bring the stretcher to the room.

Financial arrangements are made on admission or before discharge. Before leaving the agency, the person or family makes arrangements at the business office for payment.

Always use good communication skills when assisting with a person's discharge. Wish the person and family well as they leave the agency.

A person may want to leave the agency without the doctor's permission. You must notify the nurse immediately if the person expresses the wish or intent to leave. The nurse handles this situation.

▶ Discharging the Person

QUALITY OF LIFE

Remember to:
- Knock before entering the person's room
- Address the person by name
- Introduce yourself by name and title

Pre-Procedure

1 Make sure the person is to be discharged. Find out if transportation arrangements were made.

2 Explain the procedure to the person.

Procedure

3 Wash your hands.

4 Identify the person. Check the ID bracelet against the discharge slip.

5 Provide for privacy.

6 Help the person dress as needed.

7 Help the person pack. Check all drawers and closets to make sure all items are collected.

8 Check off the clothing list. Ask the person to sign the form indicating that all clothing has been returned.

9 Tell the nurse that the person is ready for the final visit. The nurse:
   a Gives prescriptions written by the doctor
   b Provides discharge instructions
   c Gets valuables from the safe

10 Get a wheelchair and a utility cart for the person's belongings. Ask a co-worker to help you.

Discharging the Person—cont'd

Procedure

11 Bring the wheelchair to the bedside, and lock the wheels. Lock the bed wheels. Lower the bed to its lowest position.

12 Assist the person into the wheelchair.

13 Unlock the wheels.

14 Take the person to the exit area. Lock the wheels of the wheelchair.

15 Help the person out of the wheelchair and into the car (Fig. 22-8).

16 Help put the belongings into the car.

Post-Procedure

17 Return the wheelchair and cart to the storage area.

18 Wash your hands.

19 Report the following to the nurse:
- The time of discharge
- How the person was transported
- Who accompanied the person
- The person's destination
- Any other observations

20 Strip the bed, clean the unit, and make a closed bed. (This may be done by housekeeping staff.)

21 Wash your hands.

Fig. 22-8 The person is being discharged.

Circle T if the answer is true and F if it is false.

1. T F The person's identifying information is obtained on arrival to the nursing unit.

2. T F The person is usually transported to the nursing unit by wheelchair or stretcher.

3. T F The bed is opened when preparing the room for the person.

4. T F The person is greeted by name when being admitted to the nursing unit.

5. T F A person complains of pain. The complaint is reported after the admission checklist is completed.

6. T F A urine specimen may be needed on admission.

7. T F You help orient the person to the new environment.

8. T F A robe and slippers are worn when the person is weighed and measured.

9. T F A list is made of clothing and valuables during the admission process.

10. T F A person's condition may require a transfer to another nursing unit.

11. T F A doctor's order is required for discharge from the agency.

12. T F You provide the person with instructions about diet and drugs.

Answers to these questions are on p. 837.

ASSISTING WITH THE PHYSICAL EXAMINATION

Define the key terms listed in this chapter

Explain what to do before, after, and during a physical examination

Identify the equipment used during a physical examination

Describe how to prepare a person for an examination

Describe four examination positions and how to drape the person for each position

Explain the rules for assisting with a physical examination

Perform the procedure described in this chapter

KEY TERMS

dorsal recumbent position The back-lying examination position; the legs are together

horizontal recumbent position The dorsal recumbent position

knee-chest position The person kneels and rests the body on the knees and chest; the head is turned to one side, the arms are above the head or flexed at the elbows, the back is straight, and the body is flexed about 90 degrees at the hips

laryngeal mirror An instrument used to examine the mouth, teeth, and throat

lithotomy position The person is in a back-lying position, the hips are brought down to the edge of the examination table, the knees are flexed, the hips are externally rotated, and the feet are supported in stirrups

nasal speculum An instrument used to examine the inside of the nose

ophthalmoscope A lighted instrument used to examine the internal structures of the eye

otoscope A lighted instrument used to examine the external ear and the eardrum (tympanic membrane)

percussion hammer An instrument used to tap body parts to test reflexes; reflex hammer

Sims' position A position sometimes used to examine the rectum or vagina

tuning fork An instrument used to test hearing

vaginal speculum An instrument used to open the vagina so that it and the cervix can be examined

Physical examinations are usually done by doctors. Many RNs also perform them. They are done for many reasons. Routine health examinations are done to promote health. Preemployment physicals are done to determine fitness for work. Physical examinations are also used to diagnose and treat disease. You may be asked to assist a doctor or RN with a physical examination.

YOUR RESPONSIBILITIES

Your responsibilities depend on the agency's policies and procedures. The examiner's preferences also af-

fect what you are expected to do. You may do some or all of the following:

- Collect linens for draping the person and for the procedure.
- Collect equipment and supplies used for the examination.
- Prepare the room for the examination.
- Transport the person to and from the examination room.
- Provide enough lighting.
- Measure vital signs, height, and weight.
- Position and drape the person for the examination.
- Hand equipment and instruments to the examiner.

- Label specimen containers.
- Dispose of soiled linen, and discard used disposable supplies.
- Clean reusable equipment after the examination.
- Help the person dress or assume a comfortable position after the examination.

EQUIPMENT

Some equipment and supplies used in a physical examination are used for nursing care. You may recognize some of the instruments. You need to know the instruments in Figure 23-1:

- **Ophthalmoscope**—a lighted instrument used to examine the internal structures of the eye.
- **Otoscope**—used to examine the external ear and the eardrum (tympanic membrane). The otoscope is a lighted instrument. Some scopes have interchangeable parts. They are changed into an ophthalmoscope or otoscope.
- **Percussion hammer**—used to tap body parts to test reflexes. It is also called a *reflex hammer*.
- **Vaginal speculum**—used to open the vagina so it and the cervix can be examined.
- **Nasal speculum**—used to examine the inside of the nose.
- **Tuning fork**—vibrated to test hearing.
- **Laryngeal mirror**—used to examine the mouth, teeth, and throat.

Many agencies have examination trays in the central supply department. If not, collect needed items. Items listed in *Preparing the Person for an Examination*, p. 566 usually are used for an examination. They are arranged on a tray or table for the examiner.

Fig. 23-1 Instruments used for a physical examination.

▶ PREPARING THE PERSON

The physical examination causes anxiety for many people. They are concerned about possible findings. Other factors can add to their anxiety. These include discomfort, embarrassment, the fear of exposure, and not knowing the procedure. You need to be sensitive to the person's feelings and concerns. The person is prepared physically and psychologically for the examination. The RN explains the purpose of the examination and what to expect. This could be your responsibility, depending on the situation and the agency. *(See Focus on Long-Term Care box.)*

Usually all clothes are removed for a complete physical examination. The person is covered with a drape. It may be a disposable paper drape, a bath blanket, a sheet, or a drawsheet. Usually a hospital gown is worn. It reduces the feeling of nakedness and the fear of exposure. Explain to the person that there is little exposure during the examination. The person needs to understand that some exposure is necessary to examine the body. However, only the body part being examined is exposed. You must screen the person and close the door to the room. This further protects the person's right to privacy. *(See Focus on Children box.)*

The person urinates before the examination. An empty bladder is necessary for the examiner to feel the abdominal organs. A full bladder can change the normal position and shape of organs. It can also cause discomfort, especially when the abdominal organs are felt. If a urine specimen is needed, obtain it at this time. Explain how to collect the specimen, and label the container properly (see Chapter 16).

Warmth is a major concern during the examination. The person is protected from chilling, especially if ill, an older person, or a child. An extra bath blanket should be nearby. Also take measures to prevent drafts.

The examiner may want height, weight, and vital signs measured. These are obtained before the examination starts. They are recorded on the examination form. The person is then positioned and draped for the examination.

Focus On... LONG-TERM CARE

The resident's quality of life must be promoted. The resident has the right to personal choice. The doctor or RN is responsible for informing the resident about the examination. Reasons for the examination are given. The resident is told who will do the examination and when it will be done. The procedure is explained. The resident must give consent. The resident may want a different examiner. Or the resident may want a family member present. Some residents may want the examination results explained with a family member present. All of these are part of the resident's right to personal choice.

Focus On... CHILDREN

Toddlers, preschool children, and school-age children are allowed to wear underpants during the examination. The underpants are lowered or removed as necessary during the procedure.

Preparing the Person for an Examination

QUALITY OF LIFE

Remember to:
- Knock before entering the person's room
- Address the person by name
- Introduce yourself by name and title

Pre-Procedure

1 Explain the procedure to the person.
2 Wash your hands.
3 Assemble the following items on a tray at the bedside or in the examination room:
- Flashlight
- Sphygmomanometer
- Stethoscope
- Thermometer
- Tongue depressors (blades)
- Laryngeal mirror
- Ophthalmoscope
- Otoscope
- Nasal speculum
- Percussion (reflex) hammer
- Tuning fork
- Tape measure
- Gloves
- Water-soluble lubricant
- Vaginal speculum
- Cotton-tipped applicators
- Specimen containers and labels
- Disposable bag
- Emesis basin
- Towel
- Bath blanket
- Tissues
- Drape (sheet, bath blanket, drawsheet, or disposable drape)
- Paper towels
- Cotton balls
- Waterproof bed protector
- Eye chart (Snellen chart)
- Slides
- Gown
- Alcohol wipes
- Wastebasket
- Container for soiled instruments
- Marking pencils or pens

4 Identify the person. Check the ID bracelet against the assignment sheet.
5 Provide for privacy.

Procedure

6 Ask the person to put on the gown. Instruct him or her to remove all clothes. Assist as necessary.
7 Ask the person to urinate. If the person is not ambulatory, offer the bedpan or urinal. Provide for privacy.
8 Transport the person to the examination room.
9 Weigh and measure the person (see Chapter 22).
10 Help the person get on the examination table. Have him or her use a stool if neces-

sary. Omit this step if the examination will be done in the person's room.
11 Position the person as directed. Raise the bed to its highest level. Raise the bed rails if the person is in bed.
12 Drape the person.
13 Place a bed protector under the buttocks.
14 Arrange for adequate lighting.
15 Turn on the signal light for the RN or examiner. Do not leave the person unattended.

Fig. 23-2 Positioning and draping for the physical examination. **A,** Dorsal recumbent position. **B,** Lithotomy position. **C,** Knee-chest position. **D,** Sims' position.

POSITIONING AND DRAPING

The person may have to assume a special position for the examination. Some examination positions (Fig. 23-2) are uncomfortable and embarrassing. The examiner tells you how to position the person. Help the person assume and maintain the position. But first explain the following to the person:

- The need for the position
- How the position is assumed
- How the body is draped
- How long the person can expect to stay in the position

The **dorsal recumbent (horizontal recumbent)** or supine position is used to examine the abdomen, anterior chest, and breasts. The person is supine with the legs together. If the perineal area is to be examined, the knees are flexed and hips externally rotated (see Fig. 23-2, *A*). The person is draped as for perineal care (see *Giving Female Perineal Care,* p. 345).

The **lithotomy position** (Fig. 23-2, *B*) is used to examine the vagina. The person lies on her back, and her hips are brought to the edge of the examination table. The knees are flexed, and the hips externally rotated. The feet are supported in stirrups. The person is draped as for the dorsal recumbent position. Some agencies provide socks to cover the feet and calves.

The **knee-chest position** (Fig. 23-2, *C*) is used to examine the rectum. Sometimes it is used to examine the vagina. The person kneels on the bed or examination table. Then the person rests his or her body on the knees and chest. The head is turned to one side, and the arms are above the head or flexed at the elbows. The back is straight, and the body is flexed about 90 degrees at the hips. The person wears a gown and sometimes socks. The drape is applied in a diamond shape to cover the back, buttocks, and thighs. *(See Focus on Older Persons box, in left column on p. 568.)*

The **Sims' position** (Fig. 23-2, *D*) is sometimes used to examine the rectum or vagina. The drape is applied in a diamond shape. The corner near the examiner is folded back to expose the rectum or vagina.

Focus On... OLDER PERSONS

The knee-chest position is rarely used for older persons. They usually assume the side-lying position for examination of the rectum.

ASSISTING WITH THE EXAMINATION

You may be asked to prepare, position, and drape the person. You may also be asked to assist the doctor or RN during the examination. When assisting with the examination, follow the rules in Box 23-1. *(See Focus on Children box and Focus on Older Persons box at right.)*

AFTER THE EXAMINATION

After the examination the person is taken back to the room. In a clinic, the person dresses in the examination room. Assist as needed. Lubricant is used for the vaginal or rectal examination. The area is wiped or cleaned before the person dresses or returns to the room.

Used disposable items are put in a waste container. Examples are bed protectors, paper drapes, tongue blades, applicators, and cotton balls. These supplies are replaced so the tray is ready for the next examination. Reusable items are cleaned according to agency policy and returned to the tray. This includes the otoscope and ophthalmoscope tips, speculum, and stethoscope. The examination table is covered with a clean drawsheet or paper. All specimens are labeled and sent to the laboratory with a requisition slip. The person's unit or examination room should be neat and orderly after the examination. Follow agency policy for soiled linens.

CROSS-TRAINING OPPORTUNITIES

Physical examinations often involve laboratory tests and electrocardiograms (ECG or EKG). These tests are used by the doctor to diagnose a person's health problems and to evaluate care. You may be cross-trained to assist with or to perform these special procedures. They are done by phlebotomists and EKG or ECG technicians:

- *Phlebotomist*—draws blood from people for laboratory study. Blood is taken from a vein. Phlebotomy is the process of withdrawing blood from a vein. Phlebotomists work in the laboratory. They are given on-the-job training or take a course at a community college, technical school, or vocational school.
- *EKG or ECG technician*—takes electrocardiograms (see Fig. 24-2). Training is given on the job. Some community colleges, technical schools, and vocational schools offer EKG or ECG courses.

Box 23-1 Rules for Assisting With the Physical Examination

- Wash your hands before and after the examination.
- Provide for privacy. This is done by screening, closing doors, and draping. Expose only the body part being examined.
- Assist the person in assuming positions as directed by the examiner.
- Place instruments and equipment in a handy location for the examiner.
- Stay in the room when a female is examined (unless you are a male). When a woman is examined by a man, another female is in the room. This is for the legal protection of the woman and the male examiner. A female attendant also adds to the psychological comfort of the woman. A female examiner may want a male attendant present when she examines a male. This also is for her legal protection.
- Protect the person from falling.
- Anticipate the examiner's need for equipment.
- Place paper or paper towels on the floor if the person is asked to stand.
- Practice medical asepsis and Standard Precautions. Also follow the Bloodborne Pathogen Standard.

Focus On... CHILDREN

The examination of an infant or child is like an adult examination. However, a parent is present. The parent may need to hold the infant or child still during some parts of the procedure if the infant or child is uncooperative. Being kept still may frighten an infant. The child may also fear separation from the parent. Some children fear being physically harmed during the examination. A calm, comforting manner helps both the child and the parent. Remember, the parent may be anxious too.

The equipment needed is like that used for the adult examination. Toys are used to assess development. Vaginal speculums are not used.

Focus On... OLDER PERSONS

Some older persons have dementia. Persons with dementia may resist the examiner's efforts. The person may be agitated and physically aggressive because of confusion and fear. The person who refuses or actively resists an examination is not restrained or forced to have the procedure. The person may react better at another time. Having a family member present may calm the person. The person's rights are always respected.

Circle the BEST answer.

1. The otoscope is used to
   A. Examine the internal structures of the eye
   B. Examine the external ear and the eardrum
   C. Test reflexes
   D. Open the vagina

2. You are preparing Mrs. Janz for an examination. You should do the following *except*
   A. Have her urinate
   B. Ask her to undress
   C. Drape her
   D. Go tell the nurse when Mrs. Janz is ready

3. Which part of Mrs. Janz's examination can you do?
   A. Examine her eyes and ears
   B. Inspect her mouth, teeth, and throat
   C. Measure her height, weight, and vital signs
   D. Observe her perineum and rectum

4. Mrs. Janz is supine. Her hips are flexed and externally rotated. Her feet are supported in stirrups. She is in the
   A. Dorsal recumbent position
   B. Lithotomy position
   C. Knee-chest position
   D. Sims' position

5. You will assist with Mrs. Janz's examination. Which is *false*?
   A. Handwashing is done before and after the examination.
   B. Instruments are placed near the examiner.
   C. You leave the room when Mrs. Janz is examined.
   D. Provide for privacy by screening, closing the door, and proper draping.

Answers to these questions are on p. 837.

THE PERSON HAVING SURGERY

Define the key terms listed in this chapter

Describe the common fears and concerns of surgical patients

Explain how people are physically and psychologically prepared for surgery

Describe how to prepare a room for the postoperative patient

List the signs and symptoms to report to the nurse postoperatively

Explain how circulation is stimulated after surgery

Describe how to meet hygiene, nutrition, fluid, and elimination needs after surgery

Perform the procedures described in this chapter

KEY TERMS

anesthesia The loss of feeling or sensation produced by a drug

douche Vaginal irrigation

elective surgery Scheduled surgery a person chooses to have at a certain time

embolus A blood clot (thrombus) that travels through the vascular system until it lodges in a distant blood vessel

emergency surgery Unscheduled surgery done immediately to save the person's life or limb

general anesthesia Unconsciousness and the loss of feeling or sensation produced by a drug

local anesthesia The loss of sensation in a small area, produced by a drug injected at the specific site

postoperative After surgery

preoperative Before surgery

regional anesthesia The loss of sensation or feeling in a large area of the body, produced by the injection of a drug; the person does not lose consciousness

thrombus A blood clot

urgent surgery Surgery necessary for the person's health; it must be done soon to prevent further damage or disease

vaginal irrigation The introduction of a fluid into the vagina and the immediate return of the fluid; douche

Surgery is done for many reasons. Common reasons include removing a diseased organ or body part, removing a tumor, or repairing injured tissue. Surgery is done also to diagnose a disease, improve appearance, and relieve symptoms.

Many surgeries require hospital stays. The person is admitted before the surgery and stays for a few or several days after the surgery. However, ambulatory surgery (outpatient surgery, one-day surgery, same-day surgery) is quite common. It does not require an overnight hospital stay. The person is in the hospital less than 23 hours. Many outpatient surgeries are done in clinics or surgical centers that are part of hospitals or doctors' offices.

Surgeries are elective, urgent, or emergency:

- **Elective surgery** is done for the person's well-being. It is not lifesaving and may not be necessary for the person's health. The surgery is scheduled anywhere from 1 day to months in advance. Cosmetic surgery—surgery to improve appearance—is often elective surgery.
- **Urgent surgery** is needed for the person's health. It must be done soon to prevent further damage or disease. Cancer surgery and coronary artery bypass surgery are examples.
- **Emergency surgery** is done immediately to save a person's life or limb. The need is sudden and unexpected. Accidents, stabbings, and bullet wounds often require emergency surgery.

The fear of . . .
- Cancer
- Disfigurement and scarring
- Disability
- Pain during surgery
- Dying during surgery
- Anesthesia and its effects
- Going to sleep or not waking up after surgery
- Exposure
- Severe pain or discomfort after surgery
- Tubes, needles, and other equipment used for care
- Complications
- Prolonged recovery
- More surgery or treatments
- Separation from family and friends

Concern about . . .
- Caring for children and other family members
- Pets or plants
- The house, lawn, and garden
- Monthly bills, loan payments, mortgages, or rent
- Insurance coverage for hospital and doctor bills

The person is prepared for what happens before, during, and after surgery. This involves physical and psychological preparation. Nurses and doctors prepare the person for the surgical experience.

In hospitals you will have contact with patients before and after surgery. In nursing centers many residents are recovering from surgery. Many postoperative patients need home care.

PSYCHOLOGICAL CARE

Illness or injury causes many fears and concerns (Box 24-1). Surgery increases these fears. The person's deepest and worst fears are often felt. How would you feel if you needed surgery tomorrow? Would you fear cancer or the loss of an organ or body part? Would you have fears about pain or death? Who will care for your children and your home? Who will earn money while you are in the hospital? Imagine you are in an accident. You wake up hours later. You are told that your right leg was amputated during surgery.

Feelings are affected by past experiences. Some persons have had surgery before. Others have not. Family and friends usually share their surgical experiences with the patient. Their experiences also can affect the patient. Most people know about tragic surgical events—surgery on the wrong person, surgery on the wrong body part, instruments left in the body, death during surgery. Some people do not talk about their fears and concerns. They may cry, be quiet and

withdrawn, or constantly talk about other things. Some pace or are very cheerful.

Psychological preparation is important. You must respect the person's fears and concerns. The health team must show the person warmth, sensitivity, and caring.

PATIENT INFORMATION

The doctor explains the need for surgery to the patient and family. They are told about the surgical procedure, risks, and possible complications. Risks from not having surgery are also explained. Information is given about who will do the surgery, when it is scheduled, and how long it will take. The person and family may have questions about the surgery and what to expect. Questions and misunderstandings are cleared up. Instructions about care also are given. All information before surgery is given by the doctor or nurse.

After surgery the doctor tells the patient and the family about the results. The doctor decides what and when to tell them. Often the health team knows before the person does. Patients and families are usually anxious to know the results. They often ask you, nurses, and other health workers. Often they ask if reports are back from the laboratory or what the reports say. Knowing what the person was told is very important. You do not tell of any diagnosis. Nor do you give incomplete or inaccurate information. The nurse tells you what and when the person and family were told.

YOUR ROLE

You can assist in the psychological care of the surgical patient. Do the following if you are involved in preoperative and postoperative care:

- Listen to the person who voices fears or concerns about surgery.
- Refer any questions about the surgery or its results to the nurse.
- Explain to the person procedures you will perform and why they are being done.
- Follow the rules of communication (see Chapter 4).
- Use verbal and nonverbal communication (see Chapter 5).
- Perform procedures and tasks with skill and ease.
- Report to the nurse verbal and nonverbal signs of patient fear or anxiety.
- Report to the nurse a person's request to see a member of the clergy.

THE PREOPERATIVE PERIOD

The **preoperative** (before surgery) period may be many days or just a few minutes. If time permits, the person is prepared psychologically and physically for the effects of anesthesia and surgery. Good preoperative preparation prevents complications after surgery.

Fig. 24-1 Recovery room.

Fig. 24-2 An electrocardiogram is taken.

 Focus On... CHILDREN

The child and parents are prepared for the surgery. Often play is used to help the child understand what will happen. For example, anatomical dolls are used to show the site of surgery. A tour of the operating and recovery rooms also is common. The child and parents are introduced to the nursing staff who will care for the child.

PREOPERATIVE TEACHING

A nurse does the preoperative teaching. The nurse explains what to expect before and after surgery. Teaching includes the following:

- *Preoperative activities*—This includes tests and their purpose, skin preparation, personal care, and the purpose and effects of preoperative drugs.
- *Deep breathing, coughing, and leg exercises*—These are taught and practiced. After surgery, they are done every 1 or 2 hours when the person is awake.
- *The recovery room*—This is where the person wakes up (Fig. 24-1). Care in the recovery room is explained.
- *Vital signs*—These are taken frequently until stable.
- *Food and fluids*—The person is NPO and has an IV infusion after surgery. The doctor orders food and oral fluids when the person's condition is stable.
- *Turning and repositioning*—The person usually is turned and repositioned every 2 hours after surgery.
- *Early ambulation*—Usually the person walks as soon as possible after surgery.
- *Pain*—The person is told about the type and amount of pain to expect and about drugs for pain relief.
- *Needed treatments and equipment*—The person also may need a urinary catheter, NG tube, oxygen, wound suction, a cast, or traction.
- *Position restrictions*—Some surgeries require certain positions. For example, the hip is abducted after hip replacement surgery (see Chapter 30).

(See Focus on Children box.)

SPECIAL TESTS

Before surgery the doctor orders tests to evaluate the person's circulatory, respiratory, and urinary systems. These tests include a chest x-ray, a complete blood count (CBC), and urinalysis. An electrocardiogram (ECG or EKG) detects any cardiac (heart) problems (Fig. 24-2). If blood loss is expected, the person's blood is tested to determine blood type. This is called *type and crossmatch*. Other tests depend on the person's condition and the surgery. The person is prepared for the tests as needed. The results must be on the chart by the time of surgery.

NUTRITION AND FLUIDS

A light meal is usually allowed. Then the person is NPO 6 to 8 hours before the surgery. These measures reduce the risk of vomiting and aspiration during anesthesia and after surgery. An NPO sign is placed in the person's room. Remember, the water pitcher and glass are removed when the person is NPO.

ELIMINATION

Abdominal surgeries usually require a preoperative enema. Cleansing enemas are common before intestinal surgeries. Remember, feces contain microbes. When the intestine is opened, feces can spill into the sterile abdominal cavity. To prevent this contamination, cleansing enemas are given to clear the colon of feces.

Enemas are also given when straining or a bowel movement could cause postoperative problems. Such problems include pain, severe bleeding (hemorrhage), or stress on the operative area. The doctor orders what enema to give and when.

Some surgeries require catheters. For pelvic and abdominal surgeries, the bladder must be empty. A full bladder is easily injured during surgery. Catheters also allow accurate output measurements during and after surgery.

PERSONAL CARE

Personal care before surgery usually involves the following:

- A complete bed bath, shower, or tub bath is taken. A special soap or cleanser may be ordered. A shampoo is included. The bath and shampoo reduce the number of microbes on the body at the time of surgery.
- Makeup and nail polish are removed. The skin, lips, and nail beds are observed for color and circulation during and after surgery.
- Long hair is braided. All hairpins, clips, combs, and similar items are removed. So are wigs and hairpieces. Some agencies have both men and women wear surgical caps. A cap keeps hair out of the face and the operative area.
- Oral hygiene is performed to promote comfort. Being NPO causes thirst and a dry mouth. The person must not swallow any water during oral hygiene. (See Focus on Children box.)
- Dentures are removed. They are removed before preoperative medications are given. They are cleaned and kept moist in a denture cup. They are kept in a safe place. Some people do not like being seen without their dentures. Let them wear their dentures as long as possible. This promotes the person's sense of dignity and esteem.

VALUABLES

Valuables are removed for safekeeping. These include dentures, glasses, contact lenses, hearing aids, and jewelry. Artificial eyes and limbs also are removed. These items are easily lost or broken during surgery. Transfers to the operating room (OR), recovery room, and back to the person's room also present safety risks. A note is made on the person's chart about the valuables removed and where they are kept. The person may want to wear a wedding band or religious medal. The item is secured in place with gauze or tape according to agency policy.

Focus On... CHILDREN

Check for loose teeth when giving oral hygiene. Report any loose teeth to the nurse. The nurse notes the observation on the preoperative checklist and informs the OR staff. A loose tooth can fall out during anesthesia. The child can aspirate the tooth.

▶ SKIN PREPARATION

The skin and hair shafts contain microbes that could enter the body through the surgical incision. A serious infection could result. The skin cannot be sterilized. However, a *skin prep* can reduce the number of microbes.

Agency policy and the surgeon's preferences determine the area to be prepared for a specific surgery (Fig. 24-3). The incision site and a large area around the area are *prepped*.

The skin prep is done right before the surgery. It is done in the person's room or in the OR. Hair is removed by applying a depilatory (cream hair remover) or shaving.

Disposable prep kits are used for shaving. A kit has a razor, a sponge filled with soap, a basin, and a drape and towel (Fig. 24-4, p. 577). The skin is lathered with soap. Then the skin is shaved in the direction of hair growth (Fig. 24-5, p. 577). Any skin break is a possible infection site. If you do a skin prep, be very careful not to cut, scratch, or nick the skin. Standard Precautions and the Bloodborne Pathogen Standard are followed.

Text continued on p. 579

Fig. 24-3 Skin preparation sites. The *shaded area* indicates the area to shave. **A,** Abdominal surgery. **B,** Chest or thoracic surgery. **C,** Open-heart surgery. **D,** Breast surgery. **E,** Perineal surgery. **F,** Cervical spine surgery. **G,** Kidney surgery. **H,** Knee surgery.

Continued

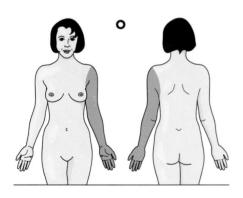

Fig. 24-3, cont'd I, Hip and thigh surgery. **J,** Lower leg and foot surgery. **K,** Complete lower extremity surgery. **L,** Abdominal and leg surgery. **M,** Upper arm surgery. **N,** Lower arm surgery. **O,** Elbow surgery.

Fig. 24-4 Skin prep kit.

Fig. 24-5 The skin is held taut. Shaving is done in the direction of hair growth.

The Surgical Skin Prep

QUALITY OF LIFE

Remember to:
- Knock before entering the person's room
- Address the person by name
- Introduce yourself by name and title

Pre-Procedure

1 Explain the procedure to the person.
2 Wash your hands.
3 Collect the following:
  - Disposable skin prep kit
  - Bath blanket
  - Warm water
  - Gloves
  - Waterproof pad
  - Bath towel
4 Identify the person. Check the ID bracelet against the assignment sheet.
5 Provide for privacy.

Procedure

6 Make sure you have good lighting. There should be no glares or shadows.
7 Raise the bed to the best level for good body mechanics. Lower the bed rail near you.
8 Cover the person with a bath blanket. Fan-fold top linens to the foot of the bed.
9 Place the waterproof pad under the area you will shave.
10 Open the skin prep kit.
11 Position the person for the skin prep. Drape him or her with the disposable drape.
12 Add warm water to the basin. Put on the gloves.
13 Apply soap to the skin with the sponge. Work up a good lather.
14 Hold the skin taut. Shave in the direction of hair growth (see Fig. 24-5).
15 Shave outward from the center, using short strokes.
16 Rinse the razor often.
17 Check to see that the entire area is free of hair. Also check for cuts, scratches, or nicks.
18 Rinse the skin thoroughly. Pat dry.
19 Remove the drape and waterproof pad. Remove the gloves.
20 Return top linens. Remove the bath blanket.

Post-Procedure

21 Provide for comfort.
22 Lower the bed to its lowest position.
23 Raise or lower bed rails. Follow the care plan.
24 Place the signal light within reach.
25 Unscreen the person.
26 Return equipment to its proper place.
27 Discard supplies and soiled linen following agency policy.
28 Wash your hands.
29 Report the following to the nurse:
  - The time the procedure was completed
  - The area prepared
  - Any cuts, nicks, or scratches
  - Any other observations

▶ VAGINAL IRRIGATION

A **vaginal irrigation (douche)** is the introduction of a fluid into the vagina and the immediate return of the fluid. For vaginal surgeries, doctors order douches to clean the vagina preoperatively. They also are ordered to relieve pain and inflammation and to clean the vagina of discharge. Drugs, heat, and cold can be applied by vaginal irrigation. You do not perform the procedure if heat, cold, or a drug is applied. (Giving a vaginal irrigation is not a nursing assistant function in some agencies.)

Vaginal irrigations are not done during menstruation. Nor are they done during late pregnancy or during the first 6 to 8 weeks after childbirth. Douching after intercourse is not a birth control method. Normally, douching is not necessary. The vaginal secretions cleanse the vagina naturally and protect it from infection.

The woman voids before the procedure to empty the bladder of urine. A full bladder can cause discomfort during the procedure. If ambulatory, the woman uses the bathroom. Otherwise she uses the bedpan or commode.

A disposable kit has a container, connecting tubing, and nozzle. The plastic nozzle is checked for chips and cracks, which could cause vaginal injury. The person is positioned on her back for the procedure. The nozzle is gently inserted backward and upward (Fig. 24-6). This follows the angle of the vagina when the person is in the back-lying position.

Vaginal irrigations require touching and exposure of the genital area. The genital area is a sexual area. The person is protected from sexual abuse. You also must protect yourself from being accused of sexual abuse. Remember, some people do not like being touched. The purpose of the touch can be interpreted the wrong way. Culture, religion, and personal values and beliefs affect the meaning of touch. You must perform the procedure in a competent and professional manner. Explain the procedure to the person, and get the person's consent to proceed. Also protect the right to privacy. Exposure of the person is a form of sexual abuse. How you communicate with the person deserves special attention. You must be careful what you say and do. Some words have different meanings to different people. Your nonverbal communication is important. Follow the principles of communication to protect the person and yourself.

Fig. 24-6 Vaginal irrigation. **A,** Position of the woman. **B,** Solution is used to cleanse the vulva. **C,** Solution flows through a nozzle inserted into the vagina. The nozzle is inserted 3 to 4 inches. **D,** The head of the bed is elevated to allow solution to drain from the vagina.

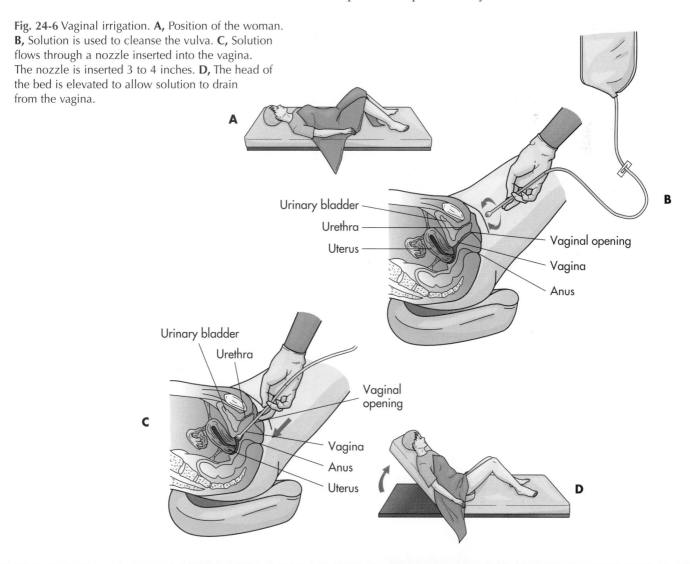

Giving a Vaginal Irrigation

QUALITY OF LIFE

Remember to:
- Knock before entering the person's room
- Address the person by name
- Introduce yourself by name and title

Pre-Procedure

1 Explain the procedure to the person.
2 Wash your hands.
3 Collect the following:
   - Disposable vaginal irrigation kit
   - 1000 ml of the irrigation solution
   - Bath thermometer
   - Bath blanket
   - Bedpan
   - Toilet tissue
   - Waterproof pad
   - Gloves
   - IV pole
   - Water pitcher
   - Equipment for perineal care
4 Identify the person. Check the ID bracelet against the assignment sheet.
5 Provide for privacy.
6 Ask the woman to void. Assist her to the bathroom or commode. Or provide the bedpan.
7 Wash your hands.
8 Raise the bed to the best level for good body mechanics. Make sure bed rails are up.

Procedure

9 Warm the irrigation solution to body temperature or 105° F (40.5° C) as directed by the nurse. If the solution was prepared by central supply, set the container in a basin of hot water. Allow it to warm.
10 Do the following to warm a tap water solution:
   a Fill the pitcher with 1000 ml of warm water.
   b Measure the water temperature.
   c Adjust the water temperature as needed.
11 Cover the person with a bath blanket. Fanfold the top linens to the foot of the bed.
12 Help the person to a back-lying position. Drape her with the bath blanket as for perineal care.
13 Place the waterproof pad under her buttocks.
14 Put on the gloves.
15 Provide perineal care (see *Giving Female Perineal Care,* p. 345).
16 Position her on the bedpan.
17 Clamp the irrigation tubing. Pour the solution into the irrigation container.
18 Hang the container from the IV pole. It should be 12 inches above the vagina.
19 Position the nozzle over the vulva. Unclamp the tubing. Let some solution run over the perineal area.
20 Insert the nozzle 3 to 4 inches into the vagina (see Fig. 24-6). Rotate the nozzle gently during the procedure.
21 Clamp the tubing when the container is empty. Remove the nozzle.
22 Place the tubing in the irrigation container.
23 Raise the head of the bed. This lets solution drain from the vagina into the bedpan.
24 Help her lie down again.
25 Remove the bedpan. Dry the perineal area with toilet tissue.
26 Raise the bed rail.
27 Take the bedpan into the bathroom. Clean and return it to its proper place.
28 Remove the waterproof pad.
29 Discard used disposable items.
30 Change damp linen. Remove the gloves.

Giving a Vaginal Irrigation—cont'd

Post-Procedure

31 Provide for comfort.

32 Return top linens, and remove the bath blanket.

33 Lower the bed to its lowest position.

34 Raise or lower bed rails. Follow the care plan.

35 Place the signal light within reach.

36 Unscreen the person.

37 Wash your hands.

38 Report the following to the nurse:
- The time the irrigation was given
- The amount, type, and temperature of the solution
- The person's response
- The character of the returned solution
- Any other observations

THE CONSENT FOR SURGERY

Before surgery is done, the person must give permission. The person signs an *operative permit* or *surgical consent*. The consent is signed when the person understands the information given by the doctor. Sometimes the person's spouse or nearest relative is also required to sign the consent. A parent or legal guardian signs for a minor child. The legal guardian signs for a person who is mentally incompetent. The doctor is responsible for securing the person's written consent. However, this responsibility is often delegated to the RN. *You are never responsible for obtaining the person's written consent for surgery.*

THE PREOPERATIVE CHECKLIST

A preoperative checklist (Fig. 24-7, p. 582) is placed on the front of the person's chart. The RN makes sure the checklist is completed. The person is ready for surgery when the list is complete. The nurse may ask you to do some things on the list. Promptly report when you complete each task. Also report any observations. Except for the bed rails, the entire checklist is completed before preoperative drugs are given.

PREOPERATIVE MEDICATION

About 45 minutes to 1 hour before surgery, the preoperative medications are given. One drug helps the person relax and feel drowsy. The other dries up respiratory secretions to prevent aspiration. Drowsiness, lightheadedness, thirst, and dry mouth are normal and expected.

Falls and accidents are prevented after the drugs are given. Bed rails are raised, and the person is not allowed out of bed. Therefore the person voids before the drugs are given. After the drugs are given, the bedpan or urinal is used for voiding. Smoking is not allowed. The person can fall asleep while smoking.

The bed is kept in the lowest position or raised to the highest position following agency policy. Move furniture out of the way to make room for the stretcher. Also clean off the overbed table and the bedside stand. This prevents damage to equipment and valuables. Raise the bed to the highest position for transferring the patient from the bed to a stretcher.

TRANSPORT TO THE OPERATING ROOM

A nurse or an OR attendant brings a stretcher to the room. The patient is transferred onto the stretcher and covered with a bath blanket. The blanket provides warmth and prevents exposure. Falling is prevented. Safety straps are secured and the side rails raised. A small pillow is sometimes placed under the person's head for comfort.

Identification checks are made. Then the person's chart is given to the OR staff member.

The nurse responsible for preoperative care may go with the person to the OR entrance. Often the family also is allowed to go this far. *(See Focus on Children box.)*

Focus On... CHILDREN

Some agencies allow a parent to be with the child while anesthesia is given. The parent stays in the OR until the child is asleep.

OSF

ST. JOSEPH MEDICAL CENTER

2200 E. Washington Street, Bloomington, Illinois 61701
Phone (309) 662-3311

PRE-OPERATIVE CHECKLIST

DATE OF SURGERY: _____

CHART PREPARATION	ADEQUATE INITIAL HERE	NOT ADEQUATE INITIAL HERE AND EXPLAIN
1. HISTORY AND PHYSICAL ON CHART HT. _____ WT. _____		
2. SURGICAL CONSENT ON CHART, SIGNED		
3. CONSENT FOR ADM BLOOD/BLOOD PROD.		
4. PREGNANCY TEST OBTAINED WHEN INDICATED		
5. URINALYSIS REPORT ON CHART		
6. BLOOD WORK TYPE _____		
7. TYPE AND CROSSMATCH		
8. CHEST X-RAY REPORT ON CHART		
9. EKG REPORT ON CHART READ _____		
10. KNOWN ALLERGIES AND SENSITIVITIES NOTED ON CHART		
11. KNOWN EXPOSURE AND/OR ALLERGY TO **LATEX** NOTED ON CHART		

PATIENT PREPARATION	ADEQUATE INITIAL HERE	NOT ADEQUATE INITIAL HERE AND EXPLAIN
12. FAMILY NOTIFIED OF SURGERY NAME _____ DATE/TIME _____		
13. PATIENT IDENTIFICATION ON WRIST		
14. ALL PROSTHESIS REMOVED (INCLUDING DENTURES, WIGS, HAIRPINS, CONTACT LENSES, COSMETICS, NAIL POLISH, ARTIFICIAL EYES, LIMBS, ETC.)		
15. ALL JEWELRY REMOVED		
16. CLOTHING REMOVED EXCEPT HOSPITAL GOWN WITH TIES		
17. SURGICAL PREP DONE		
18. TIME OF LAST MEAL OR FLUIDS _____ TIME		
19. PRE-OP TPR AND BP: T_____ P_____ R _____ BP_____		
20. VOIDED TIME _____ OR FOLEY		
21. PRE-OP IV AND/OR ANTIBIOTIC: TIME:		

	DRUG	DOSAGE	ROUTE

PREOPERATIVE MEDICATION GIVEN,_____   TIME _____ GIVEN BY _____

☐ SIDE RAILS UP

READY FOR O.R.   DATE _____   TIME _____   SIGNATURE _____

PATIENT IDENTIFIED BY TRANSPORTER AND STAFF NURSE   TIME _____

FLOOR NURSE
SIGNATURE _____   OR TRANSPORTER
SIGNATURE _____   OR NURSE
SIGNATURE _____

IDENTIFICATION OF INITIALS			
INITIALS	SIGNATURE	INITIALS	SIGNATURE

Fig. 24-7 Preoperative checklist. (Courtesy OSF St. Joseph Medical Center, Bloomington, Ill.)

ANESTHESIA

Anesthesia is the loss of feeling or sensation produced by a drug. There are three types of anesthesia:

- **General anesthesia** produces unconsciousness and the loss of feeling or sensation. A drug is given intravenously, or a gas is inhaled.
- **Regional anesthesia** produces loss of sensation or feeling in a large area of the body. The person does not lose consciousness. A drug is injected into a body part.
- **Local anesthesia** produces loss of sensation in a small area. A drug is injected at the specific site.

Anesthetics are given by specially educated doctors and nurses. An *anesthesiologist* is a doctor who specializes in the administration of anesthetics. An *anesthetist* is an RN who has had advanced study in the administration of anesthetics.

THE POSTOPERATIVE PERIOD

After surgery **(postoperative)** the person is taken to the recovery room (RR). This is often called the postanesthesia room (PAR) or postanesthesia care unit (PACU). The recovery room is near the OR. There the person recovers from the anesthetic. This can take 1 to 2 hours. The person is watched very closely. Vital signs are taken and observations are made often. The person leaves the recovery room when:

- Vital signs are stable.
- The person has good respiratory function.
- The person can respond and call for help when it is needed.

The doctor gives the transfer order when appropriate.

PREPARING THE PERSON'S ROOM

The room must be ready for the person's return from the recovery room. A surgical bed is made (see Chapter 13). Equipment and supplies needed for the person's care are brought to the room. The nurse tells you if special measures and equipment are needed. The room is prepared after the person is taken to the OR. Preparations include:

- Making a surgical bed
- Placing equipment and supplies in the room:
  - Thermometer
  - Stethoscope
  - Sphygmomanometer
  - Kidney basin
  - Tissues
  - Waterproof bed protector
  - Vital signs flow sheet

  - I&O record
  - IV pole
  - Other items as directed by the nurse
- Raising the bed to its highest position
- Lowering bed rails
- Moving furniture out of the way for the stretcher

RETURN FROM THE RECOVERY ROOM

The recovery room nurse calls the nursing unit when the person is ready for transfer. The person is transported by the recovery room nurses. A nurse meets the person on the nursing unit, and the person is transferred from the stretcher to bed. Assist as needed in the transfer. Also help position the person.

Vital signs are taken and observations made. They are compared with those reported by the recovery room nurse. The nurse checks dressings for bleeding. Catheters, IV infusions, and other tube placement and function are checked. Bed rails are raised, and the signal light is placed within the person's reach. Necessary care and treatments are given. Then the family can see the person.

MEASUREMENTS AND OBSERVATIONS

Often you will measure vital signs and observe the person's condition. Vital signs are usually measured:

- Every 15 minutes the first hour
- Every 30 minutes for 1 to 2 hours
- Every hour for 4 hours
- Then every 4 hours

The nurse tells you how often to check the person. This is an important function. Always be alert for the signs and symptoms listed in Box 24-2 on p. 584. Report them to the nurse immediately.

POSITIONING

Proper positioning promotes comfort and prevents complications. The type of surgery affects positioning. Position restrictions may be ordered. The person is usually positioned for easy and comfortable breathing. Also, stress on the incision is prevented. When the person is supine, the head of the bed is usually raised slightly. The person's head may be turned to the side. These positions prevent aspiration if vomiting occurs.

Repositioning every 1 to 2 hours helps prevent respiratory and circulatory complications. It may be painful to turn. Provide support, and turn the person with smooth, gentle motions. Pillows and other positioning devices are often used (see Chapters 11 and 20).

The nurse tells you when to reposition the person and the positions allowed. Usually you assist the nurse. Sometimes you turn and reposition the person yourself. This occurs when the person's condition is stable and care is simple. *(See Focus on Older Persons box at bottom left on p. 584.)*

Box 24-2	Postoperative Observations

- Choking
- A drop or rise in blood pressure
- Bright red blood from the incision, drainage tubes, or suction tubes
- A pulse rate of more than 100 or less than 60 beats per minute
- A weak or irregular pulse
- A rise or drop in body temperature
- Hypoxia (see Chapter 27)
- The need for upper airway suctioning (tachypnea, dyspnea, moist-sounding respirations or gurgling, restlessness, cyanosis)
- Shallow, slow breathing
- Rapid, gasping, or difficult respirations
- Weak cough
- Complaints of thirst
- Restlessness
- Cold, moist, clammy, or pale skin
- Cyanosis of the lips or nails
- Increased drainage on or under dressings or on bed linens (including draw sheets, bottom sheets, and pillowcases)
- Complaints of pain or nausea
- Vomiting
- Confusion or disorientation
- Other measurements and observations:
  - The amount, character, and time of the first voiding after surgery
  - Intake and output
  - IV flow rate
  - The appearance of drainage from a urinary catheter, NG tube, or wound suction
  - Any other observation that can mean a change in the person's condition

Focus On... OLDER PERSONS

Many older persons have stiff and painful joints. Sore muscles, bones, and joints occur from positioning on the operating room table. Remember to turn and reposition older persons slowly and gently.

COUGHING AND DEEP BREATHING

Respiratory complications are prevented. There are two major complications. One is *pneumonia*—an inflammation and infection in the lung. The other is *atelectasis*—the collapse of a portion of the lung. Coughing and deep breathing exercises and incentive spirometry help prevent these complications (see Chapter 27). *(See the first Focus on Older Persons box below.)*

STIMULATING CIRCULATION

After surgery, circulation must be stimulated. This is especially true for blood flow in the legs. If blood flow is sluggish, blood clots may form. Blood clots **(thrombi)** can form in the deep leg veins (Fig. 24-8, *A*). A blood clot **(thrombus)** can break loose and travel through the bloodstream. It then becomes an embolus. An **embolus** is a blood clot that travels through the vascular system until it lodges in a distant vessel (Fig. 24-8, *B*). An embolus from a vein eventually lodges in the lungs (pulmonary embolus). A pulmonary embolus can cause severe respiratory problems and death. *(See the second Focus on Older Persons box below.)*

Leg Exercises. Leg exercises increase venous blood flow. Therefore they help prevent thrombi. Leg exercises are easy to do. You assist if the person is weak. If the person had leg surgery, a doctor's order is needed for the exercises. The nurse tells you when to do the exercises. They are done with the person supine. They are done at least every 1 or 2 hours while the person is awake. The following exercises are done 5 times:

- Ask the person to make circles with the toes. This rotates the ankles.
- Have the person dorsiflex and plantar flex the feet (see Chapter 20).
- Have the person flex and extend one knee and then the other (Fig. 24-9).
- Ask the person to raise and lower one leg off the bed (Fig. 24-10). Repeat this exercise with the other leg.

Focus On... OLDER PERSONS

The changes of aging increase the older person's risk for respiratory complications. Respiratory muscles are weaker. Lung tissue is less elastic. The person has less strength for coughing. Coughing, deep breathing, and incentive spirometry are very important.

Focus On... OLDER PERSONS

Older persons are at risk for thrombi and emboli. Blood is pumped through the body with less force. Circulation is already sluggish.

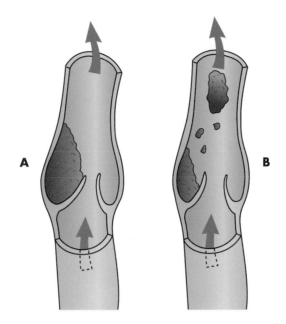

Fig. 24-8 A, A blood clot is attached to the wall of a vein. The *arrows* show the direction of blood flow. **B,** Part of the thrombus has broken off and has become an embolus. The embolus will travel in the bloodstream until it lodges in a distant vessel.

Fig. 24-9 The knee is flexed and then extended during postoperative leg exercises.

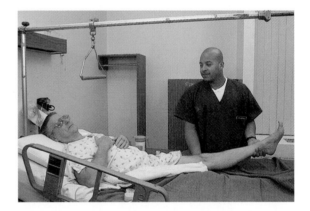

Fig. 24-10 The patient is assisted with raising and lowering the leg.

▶ **Elastic Stockings.** Elastic stockings help prevent thrombi. The elastic exerts pressure on the veins, promoting venous blood flow to the heart. Elastic stockings are often ordered for postoperative patients and for those with heart disease and circulatory disorders. Bedrest and pregnancy are also reasons for elastic stockings. Affected persons can develop blood clots (thrombi).

The stockings come in many sizes. Thigh-high or knee-high lengths are available. The nurse measures the person to determine the correct size. The stockings are removed at least twice each day. They are applied before the person gets out of bed. Otherwise the person's legs can swell from sitting or standing. Stockings are difficult to apply when the legs are swollen.

Fig. 24-11 Applying elastic stockings. **A,** The stocking is turned inside out down to the heel. **B,** The stocking is slipped over the toes, foot, and heel. **C,** The stocking turns right side out as it is pulled up over the leg.

Applying Elastic Stockings

NNAAP™

QUALITY OF LIFE

Remember to:
- Knock before entering the person's room
- Address the person by name
- Introduce yourself by name and title

Pre-Procedure

1 Explain the procedure to the person.
2 Wash your hands.
3 Obtain elastic stockings in the correct size.
4 Identify the person. Check the ID bracelet against the assignment sheet.
5 Provide for privacy.
6 Raise the bed to the best level for good body mechanics. Make sure bed rails are up.

Procedure

7 Lower the bed rail near you.
8 Position the person supine.
9 Expose the legs. Fanfold top linens back toward the person.
10 Turn the stocking inside out down to the heel (Fig. 24-11, A).
11 Slip the foot of the stocking over the toes, foot, and heel (Fig. 24-11, B).
12 Grasp the stocking top. Slip it over the foot and heel, and pull it up the leg. It turns right side out as it is pulled up the leg. The stocking should be even and snug (Fig. 24-11, C).
13 Make sure the stocking is not twisted and has no creases or wrinkles.
14 Repeat steps 10 through 13 for the other leg.
15 Return top linens to their proper position.

Post-Procedure

16 Provide for comfort.
17 Lower the bed to its lowest position.
18 Raise or lower bed rails. Follow the care plan.
19 Place the signal light within reach.
20 Unscreen the person.
21 Wash your hands.
22 Report that you applied the stockings. Report the time of application.

▶ **Elastic Bandages.** Bandages are applied to an extremity. They have the same purposes as elastic stockings. They also provide support and reduce swelling from musculoskeletal injuries. The bandage is applied from the lower (*distal*) part of the extremity to the top (*proximal*) part. The nurse gives you directions about the area to bandage. When applying bandages:

- Use the correct size. Use the proper length and width to bandage the extremity.
- Position the extremity in good alignment.
- Face the person during the procedure.
- Expose fingers or toes if possible. This allows circulation checks.
- Apply the bandage with firm, even pressure.
- Check the color and temperature of the extremity every hour.
- Reapply a loose, wrinkled, moist, or soiled bandage.

Fig. 24-12 Applying an elastic bandage. **A,** The roll of the elastic bandage is up. The loose end is at the bottom. **B,** The bandage is applied to the smallest part with two circular turns. **C,** The bandage is applied with spiral turns in an upward direction.

Applying Elastic Bandages

QUALITY OF LIFE

Remember to:
- Knock before entering the person's room
- Address the person by name
- Introduce yourself by name and title

Pre-Procedure

1. Explain the procedure to the person.
2. Wash your hands.
3. Collect the following:
   - Elastic bandage (the nurse tells you what size)
   - Tape or metal clips
4. Identify the person. Check the ID bracelet against the assignment sheet.
5. Provide for privacy.
6. Raise the bed to the best level for good body mechanics. Make sure bed rails are up.

Procedure

7. Lower the bed rail near you.
8. Help the person to a comfortable position. Expose the part to be bandaged.
9. Make sure the area is clean and dry.
10. Hold the bandage so the roll is up and the loose end is on the bottom (Fig. 24-12, *A*).
11. Apply the bandage to the smallest part of the wrist, ankle, or knee.
12. Make two circular turns around the part (Fig. 24-12, *B*).
13. Make overlapping spiral turns in an upward direction. Each turn should overlap about $^2/_3$ of the previous turn (Fig. 24-12, *C*).
14. Apply the bandage smoothly with firm, even pressure. It should not be tight.
15. Tape or clip the end of the bandage to hold it in place. The clip must not be under the body part.
16. Check the fingers or toes for cold or cyanosis. Also check for complaints of pain, numbness, or tingling. Remove the bandage if any are noted. Report your observations to the nurse.

Post-Procedure

17. Provide for comfort.
18. Place the signal light within reach.
19. Lower the bed.
20. Raise or lower bed rails. Follow the care plan.
21. Unscreen the person.
22. Wash your hands.
23. Report the following to the nurse:
    - The time the bandage was applied
    - The site of the application
    - Any other observations

Sequential Compression Devices (SCD). A sequential compression device is a sleeve that is wrapped around the leg. Made of cloth or plastic, it is secured in place with Velcro. The device is attached to a pump. The pump inflates the device with air. This promotes venous blood flow to the heart by causing pressure on the veins. Then the pump deflates the device. After deflation, the device is inflated again. Inflation and deflation sequence is repeated as ordered by the doctor.

EARLY AMBULATION

Early ambulation prevents postoperative circulatory complications such as thrombi. It also prevents pneumonia, atelectasis, constipation, and urinary tract infections. The person usually ambulates the day of surgery. The person dangles first. Blood pressure and pulse are measured. If they are stable, the person is assisted out of bed. Usually the person does not walk very far—just a few feet in the room. Distance increases as the person gains strength.

The nurse tells you when to ambulate the person. Usually you assist the nurse the first time.

WOUND HEALING

The incision needs protection. Healing is promoted and infection prevented. Sterile dressing changes are done by the doctor or nurse. Some states let assistive personnel do simple dressing changes. Wound healing is discussed in Chapter 25.

NUTRITION AND FLUIDS

The person has an IV infusion on return from the OR. Continued IV therapy depends on the type of surgery and the person's condition. Anesthesia can cause nausea and vomiting. The person's diet progresses from NPO to clear liquids, to full liquids, to a light diet, to a regular diet. The diet is ordered by the doctor. Frequent oral hygiene is important when the person is NPO.

Some patients have nasogastric (NG) tubes (see Chapter 18). Often the NG tube is attached to suction to keep the stomach empty. The person is NPO and receives IV therapy.

ELIMINATION

Anesthesia, the surgery, and being NPO affect normal bowel and urinary elimination. Drugs for pain relief can cause constipation. The measures to promote elimination are practiced as directed by the nurse (see Chapters 16 and 17).

Intake and output are measured postoperatively. The person must urinate within 8 hours after surgery. Report the time and amount of the person's first voiding. If the person does not void within 8 hours, a catheterization is usually ordered. Some patients have catheters after surgery. See Chapter 16 for care of the person with a catheter.

Fluid intake and return to a regular diet are needed for bowel elimination. Suppositories or enemas may be ordered for constipation. Rectal tubes may be ordered for flatulence.

COMFORT AND REST

Pain is common after surgery. The degree of pain depends on the extent of surgery, incision site, and the presence of drainage tubes, casts, or other devices. Positioning during surgery can cause muscle strains and discomfort. The doctor orders drugs for pain relief. The RN uses the nursing process to promote comfort and rest. Many of the measures listed in Chapter 21 are part of the person's care plan.

PERSONAL HYGIENE

Personal hygiene is important for the person's physical and mental well-being. Wound drainage and skin prep solutions can irritate the skin and cause discomfort. NPO causes a dry mouth and breath odors. Moist, clammy skin from blood pressure changes or elevated body temperatures also cause discomfort. Frequent oral hygiene, hair care, and a complete bed bath the day after surgery help refresh and renew the person physically and psychologically. The gown is changed whenever it becomes wet or soiled.

Circle the BEST answer.

1. Which is *true* of elective surgery?
   A. The surgery is done immediately.
   B. The need for surgery is sudden and unexpected.
   C. Surgery is scheduled for a later date.
   D. General anesthesia is always used.

2. Mr. Long said he was afraid of surgery. He might show his fear by
   A. Being quiet and withdrawn
   B. Crying
   C. Pacing or being unusually cheerful
   D. All of the above

3. You can assist in Mr. Long's psychological preparation by explaining
   A. The reason for the surgery
   B. The procedures you are doing
   C. The risks and possible complications of surgery
   D. What to expect during the preoperative and postoperative periods

4. Preoperatively, Mr. Long is
   A. NPO
   B. Allowed only water
   C. Given a regular breakfast
   D. Given a tube feeding

5. Cleansing enemas are ordered for Mr. Long preoperatively. The enemas are given
   A. To clean the colon of feces
   B. To prevent bleeding
   C. To relieve flatus
   D. To prevent pain

6. Mr. Long's skin prep is done preoperatively to
   A. Completely bathe the body
   B. Sterilize the skin
   C. Reduce the number of microbes on the skin
   D. Destroy nonpathogens and pathogens

7. When shaving the skin before surgery
   A. Shave in the direction opposite of hair growth
   B. Shave toward the center of the specific area
   C. Be careful not to cut, scratch, or nick the skin
   D. Use an electric razor

8. Mr. Long's preoperative medication was given. He
   A. Must remain in bed
   B. Is allowed to smoke with supervision
   C. Can use the commode to void
   D. Is allowed only sips of water

9. General anesthesia
   A. Is a specially educated nurse
   B. Produces unconsciousness and the loss of feeling or sensation
   C. Is a specially educated doctor
   D. Produces loss of sensation or feeling in a body part

10. Mr. Long must cough and deep breathe after surgery to prevent
    A. Bleeding
    B. A pulmonary embolus
    C. Respiratory complications
    D. Pain and discomfort

11. Leg exercises are ordered for Mr. Long. Which is *false?*
    A. Leg exercises stimulate circulation.
    B. Leg exercises prevent thrombi.
    C. Leg exercises are done 5 times every 1 or 2 hours.
    D. Leg exercises are done only for leg surgery.

12. Postoperatively, Mr. Long's position is changed
    A. Every 2 hours
    B. Every 3 hours
    C. Every 4 hours
    D. Every shift

13. Mr. Long wears elastic stockings to
    A. Prevent blood clots
    B. Hold dressings in place
    C. Reduce swelling after musculoskeletal injury
    D. All of the above

14. When applying an elastic bandage
    A. The extremity is in good alignment
    B. The fingers or toes are covered if possible
    C. It is applied from the largest to the smallest part of the extremity
    D. It is applied from the upper to the lower part of the extremity

Circle **T** if the answer is true and **F** if it is false.

15. T F Hair is kept out of the face for surgery by using pins, clips, or combs.

16. T F Nail polish is removed before surgery.

17. T F Women can wear makeup to surgery.

18. T F Pajamas are worn to the operating room.

19. T F Contact lenses are removed before surgery.

20. T F A surgical bed is made for the person's return from the recovery room.

21. T F A drop in a person's blood pressure is reported to the nurse immediately.

22. T F The person ambulates the first time the day after surgery.

23. T F Intake and output are measured after surgery.

24. T F A surgical patient should urinate within 8 hours after surgery.

Answers to these questions are on p. 837.

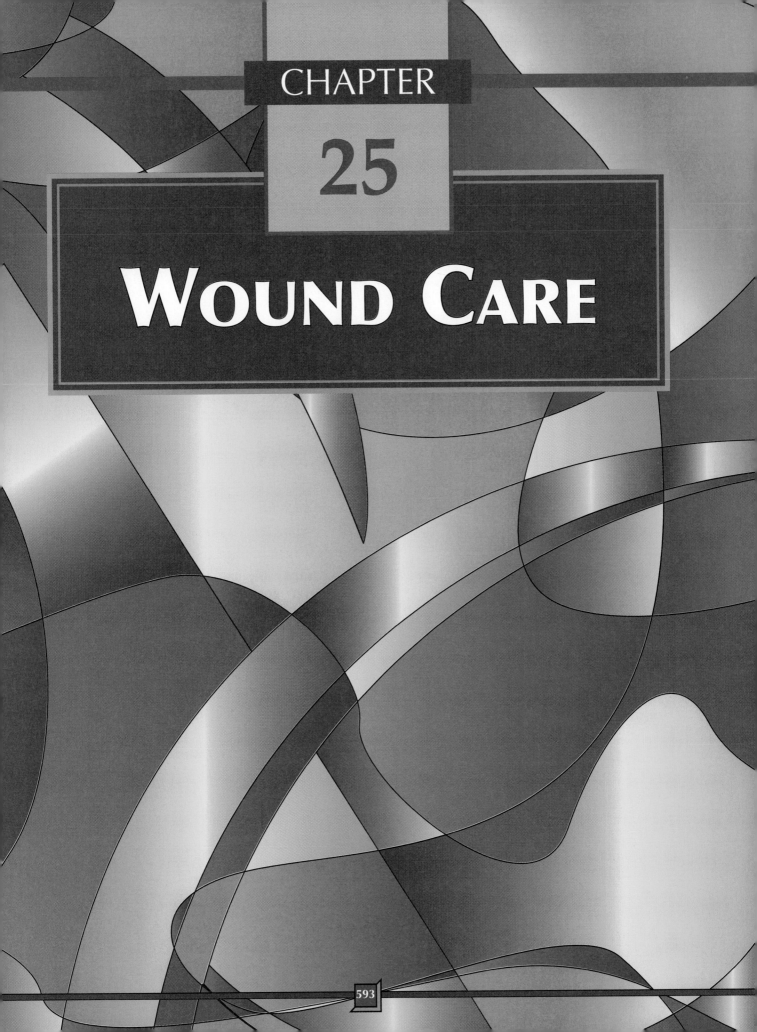

CHAPTER

25

WOUND CARE

OBJECTIVES

Define the key terms listed in this chapter

Describe the different types of wounds

Describe the signs, symptoms, and causes of pressure ulcers and circulatory ulcers

Identify the pressure points in each body position

Describe how to prevent pressure ulcers and circulatory ulcers

Describe the process, types, and complications of wound healing

Describe the observations to make about a wound

Describe the different types of wound drainage

Explain how to measure wound drainage

Explain how to secure dressings

Explain the rules for applying dressings

Explain the rules for cleaning wounds and drain sites

Explain the purpose of binders and how to apply them

Describe how to meet the basic needs of persons with wounds

Perform the procedure described in this chapter

KEY TERMS

abrasion A partial-thickness wound caused by the scraping away or rubbing of the skin

arterial ulcer An open wound on the lower legs and feet caused by decreased blood flow through the arteries

bedsore A pressure ulcer, pressure sore, or decubitus ulcer

chronic wound A wound that does not heal easily

circulatory ulcer An open wound on the lower legs and feet caused by a decrease in blood flow through the arteries and veins; vascular ulcer

clean wound A wound that is not infected; microbes have not entered the wound

clean-contaminated wound A wound occurring from the surgical entry of the urinary, reproductive, respiratory, or gastrointestinal system

closed wound A wound in which tissues are injured but the skin is not broken

contaminated wound A wound with a high risk of infection

contusion A closed wound caused by a blow to the body

decubitus ulcer A pressure ulcer, pressure sore, or bedsore

dehiscence The separation of wound layers

dirty wound An infected wound

epidermal stripping Removing the epidermis (outer skin layer) with tape

evisceration The separation of the wound along with the protrusion of abdominal organs

full-thickness wound The dermis, epidermis, and subcutaneous tissue are penetrated; muscle and bone may be involved

gangrene A condition in which there is death of tissue

hematoma The collection of blood under the skin and tissues

hemorrhage The excessive loss of blood in a short period of time

incision An open wound with clean, straight edges; usually intentionally produced with a sharp instrument

infected wound A wound containing large amounts of bacteria and that shows signs of infection; a dirty wound

intentional wound A wound created for therapy

KEY TERMS *continued*

laceration An open wound with torn tissues and jagged edges

open wound The skin or mucous membrane is broken

partial-thickness wound A wound in which the dermis and epidermis of the skin are broken

penetrating wound An open wound in which the skin and underlying tissues are pierced

pressure sore A bedsore, decubitus ulcer, or pressure ulcer

pressure ulcer Any injury caused by unrelieved pressure; a decubitus ulcer, bedsore, or pressure sore

puncture wound An open wound made by a sharp object; entry of the skin and underlying tissues may be intentional or unintentional

purulent drainage Thick green, yellow, or brown drainage

sanguineous drainage Bloody drainage *(sanguis)*

serosanguineous drainage Thin, watery drainage *(sero)* that is blood-tinged *(sanguineous)*

serous drainage Clear, watery fluid *(serum)*

shock The condition that results when there is not enough blood supply to organs and tissues

skin tear A break or rip in the skin that separates the epidermis from the underlying tissues

stasis ulcer An open wound caused by poor blood return to the heart from the legs and feet; venous ulcer

trauma An accident or violent act that injures the skin, mucous membranes, bones, and internal organs

unintentional wound A wound resulting from trauma

vascular ulcer A circulatory ulcer

venous ulcer A stasis ulcer

wound A break in the skin or mucous membrane

A **wound** is a break in the skin or mucous membrane. Wounds result from many causes. A surgical incision leaves a wound. Often wounds result from **trauma**—an accident or violent act that injures the skin, mucous membranes, bones, and internal organs. Falls, vehicle accidents, gun shots, stabbings, and other violent acts are sources of trauma. Human and animal bites, burns, and frostbite are other types of trauma. Pressure ulcers (pressure sores) are wounds that occur from poor skin care and immobility. Circulatory ulcers are caused by a decrease in blood flow through the arteries and veins.

The wound is a portal of entry for microbes. Thus infection is a major threat. Wound care involves preventing infection and preventing further injury to the wound and surrounding tissues. Preventing blood loss and pain also are important.

Your role in wound care depends on state law, your job description, and the person's condition. Whatever your role, you need to know the types of wounds, how wounds heal, and the measures that promote wound healing. A review of surgical asepsis is useful before studying this chapter (see Chapter 10).

TYPES OF WOUNDS

Wounds are described in many ways. They are intentional or unintentional, open or closed, clean or dirty, and partial-thickness or full-thickness. **Intentional wounds** are created for therapy. Surgical incisions and venipunctures for starting IV therapy or for collecting blood specimens are examples. **Unintentional wounds** result from trauma. Falls, vehicle accidents, gun shots, stabbings, and other violent acts are sources of unintentional wounds.

A wound is open or closed. An **open wound** is when the skin or mucous membrane is broken. Intentional and most unintentional wounds are open. In a **closed wound**, tissues are injured but the skin is not broken. Bruises, twists, and sprains are examples of closed wounds.

Contamination is another factor in describing wounds. A **clean wound** is not infected, and microbes have not entered the wound. Closed wounds are usually clean. So are intentional wounds created under surgically aseptic conditions. In addition, the urinary, respiratory, and gastrointestinal systems are not entered. A **clean-contaminated wound** occurs from the surgical entry of the reproductive, respiratory, or gastrointestinal system. These systems are not sterile and contain normal flora. A **contaminated wound** has a high risk of infection. Unintentional wounds generally are contaminated. Wound contamination also occurs from breaks in surgical asepsis and spillage of intestinal contents. Tissues may show signs of inflammation. An **infected wound (dirty wound)** contains large amounts of bacteria and shows signs of infection. Examples include old wounds, surgical incisions into infected areas, and traumatic injuries that rupture the bowel. A **chronic wound** is one that does not heal easily. Pressure ulcers and circulatory ulcers are examples.

Partial or full thickness describes a wound's depth. In a **partial-thickness wound** the dermis and epidermis of the skin are broken. The dermis, epidermis, and subcutaneous tissue are penetrated in a **full-thickness wound**. Muscle and bone may be involved.

Wounds also are described by their cause:

- **Abrasion**—a partial-thickness wound caused by the scraping away or rubbing of the skin
- **Contusion**—a closed wound caused by a blow to the body
- **Incision**—an open wound with clean, straight edges; usually intentionally produced with a sharp instrument
- **Laceration**—an open wound with torn tissues and jagged edges
- **Penetrating wound**—an open wound in which the skin and underlying tissues are pierced
- **Puncture wound**—an open wound made by a sharp object; entry of the skin and underlying tissues may be intentional or unintentional

(See Focus on Older Persons box below.)

Focus On... OLDER PERSONS

Older persons have thin and fragile skin. Therefore they are at risk for skin tears. A **skin tear** is a break or rip in the skin that separates the epidermis (top layer) from the underlying tissues. Skin tears commonly occur on the hands, arms, and lower legs.

Skin tears are caused by shearing (see Chapter 11), pulling, or pressure on the skin. Bumping a hand, arm, or leg on a bed rail, wheelchair, or other hard surface can cause a skin tear. They also result from holding the person's arm or leg too tight. Even buttons and zippers can cause skin tears. Skin tears are painful. They provide a portal of entry for microbes. Wound complications can develop. Notify the nurse immediately if you cause or find a skin tear.

To prevent skin tears:
- Keep your fingernails short and filed smoothly.
- Keep the residents' fingernails short and filed smoothly. Report long and tough toenails to the nurse.
- Do not wear rings with large stones.
- Encourage the person to wear long-sleeved shirts, blouses, or sweaters and long pants.
- Handle the person gently during lifting, moving, transfer, bathing, and dressing procedures.

PRESSURE ULCERS

A **pressure ulcer (decubitus ulcer, bedsore, pressure sore)** is any injury caused by unrelieved pressure. It usually occurs over a bony prominence. Prominence means to stick out. Therefore a bony prominence is an area where the bone sticks out or projects out from the flat surface of the body. The shoulder blades, elbows, hip bones, sacrum, knees, ankle bones, heels, and toes are bony prominences (Fig. 25-1). *(See Focus on Older Persons box below.)*

CAUSES

Pressure, friction, and shearing are common causes of skin breakdown and pressure ulcers. Other factors include breaks in the skin, poor circulation to an area, moisture, dry skin, and irritation by urine and feces.

Pressure occurs when the skin over a bony prominence is squeezed between hard surfaces. The bone itself is one hard surface. The other is usually the mattress or chair seat. The squeezing or pressure prevents blood flow to the skin and underlying tissues. Lack of blood flow means oxygen and nutrients cannot get to the cells. Therefore the involved skin and tissues die (Fig. 24-2, p. 598).

Friction scrapes the skin. An open area, the scrape is a portal of entry for microbes. The open area needs to heal. A good blood supply to the area is necessary. Infection is prevented so healing occurs. A poor blood supply or an infection can lead to a pressure ulcer.

Shearing is when the skin sticks to a surface (usually the bed or chair) and deeper tissues move downward (see Fig. 11-7). This occurs when a person is sitting in a chair or in Fowler's position. Shearing occurs when the person slides down in the bed or chair. Blood vessels and tissues are damaged. Therefore blood flow to the area is reduced.

Focus On... OLDER PERSONS

Older and disabled persons are at great risk for pressure ulcers. Their skin is easily injured. Causes included age-related skin changes, chronic disease, and general debility.

Fig. 25-1 Pressure points. **A,** The supine position. **B,** The lateral position. **C,** The prone position. **D,** Fowler's position. **E,** The sitting position.

Fig. 25-2 A pressure ulcer.

Box 25-1   Stages of Pressure Ulcers

Stage 1 The skin is red. The color does not return to normal when the skin is relieved of pressure (Fig. 25-3, *A*).

Stage 2 The skin cracks, blisters, or peels (Fig. 25-3, *B*). There may be a shallow crater.

Stage 3 The skin is gone, and the underlying tissues are exposed (Fig. 25-3, *C*). The exposed tissue is damaged. There may be drainage from the area.

Stage 4 Muscle and bone are exposed and damaged (Fig. 25-3, *D*). Drainage is likely.

Focus On... CHILDREN

Infants and children also are at risk for pressure ulcers. Pressure, friction, and shearing are causes. Epidermal stripping is another cause, especially in newborns. **Epidermal stripping** is removing the epidermis (outer skin layer) with tape. Remember, newborns have fragile skin. Risk factors for pressure ulcers in infants and children include poor mobility, lack of bowel and bladder control (incontinence), and poor nutrition. Infection is another risk factor.

PERSONS AT RISK

Persons at risk for pressure ulcers are those who:

- Are confined to bed or chair
- Are unable to move
- Have loss of bowel or bladder control
- Have poor nutrition
- Have altered mental awareness
- Have problems sensing pain or pressure
- Have circulatory problems
- Are older, obese, very thin, or malnourished
- *(See Focus on Children box.)*

SIGNS OF PRESSURE ULCERS

The first sign of a pressure ulcer is pale skin or a reddened area. The person may complain of pain, burning, or tingling in the area. Some do not feel anything unusual. Box 25-1 describes the four stages of pressure ulcer development.

SITES

Pressure ulcers usually occur over bony areas. The bony areas are called *pressure points* because they bear the weight of the body in a certain position. Pressure from body weight can reduce the blood supply to the area. Figure 25-1 shows the pressure points for the bed positions and the sitting position. In obese people, pressure ulcers can develop in areas where skin is in contact with skin. Friction results when this occurs. Pressure ulcers can develop between abdominal folds, the legs, and the buttocks and underneath the breasts.

PREVENTION

Preventing pressure ulcers is much easier than trying to heal them. Good nursing care, cleanliness, and skin care are essential. The measures listed in Box 25-2 on p. 600 help prevent skin breakdown and pressure ulcers. You must follow the person's care plan.

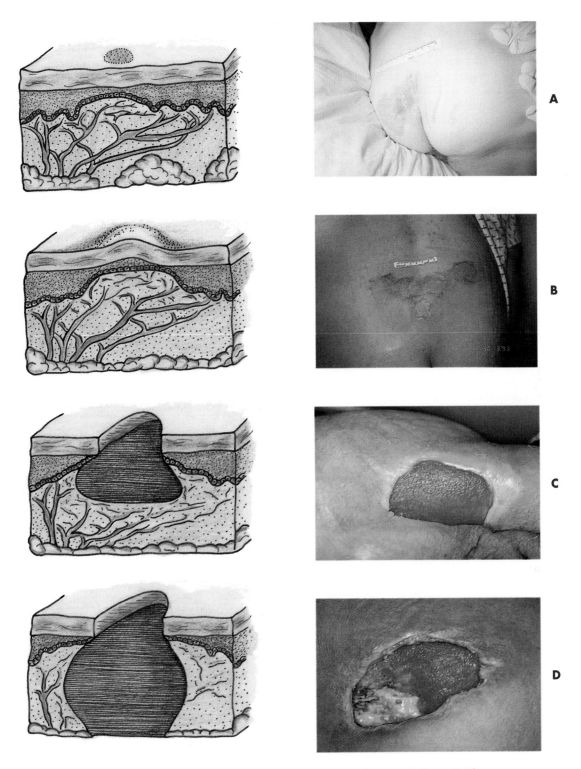

Fig. 25-3 Stages of pressure ulcers. **A,** Stage 1. **B,** Stage 2. **C,** Stage 3. **D,** Stage 4. *(Courtesy Laurel Wiersema-Bryant, RN, MSN, Clinical Nurse Specialist, Barnes-Jewish Hospital, St Louis, Mo.)*

Box 25-2   Measures to Prevent Pressure Ulcers

- Reposition the person at least every 2 hours or as scheduled in the person's care plan. Some persons are repositioned every 15 minutes. Use pillows for support as instructed by the nurse. The 30-degree lateral position is recommended (Fig. 25-4).
- Prevent shearing and friction during lifting and moving procedures.
- Prevent shearing by not raising the head of the bed more than 30 degrees. Follow the care plan.
- Prevent friction by applying a thin layer of cornstarch to the bottom sheets.
- Provide good skin care. The skin must be clean and dry after bathing. The skin is free of moisture from urine, feces, perspiration, and wound drainage.
- Minimize skin exposure to moisture. Check incontinent persons (those without bowel or bladder control) often. Also check persons who perspire heavily and those with wound drainage. Change linens and clothing as needed, and provide good skin care.
- Check with the nurse before using soap. Remember, soap can dry and irritate the skin.
- Apply a moisturizer to dry areas such as the hands, elbows, legs, ankles, and heels. The nurse tells you what to use and the areas that need attention.
- Give a back massage when repositioning the person. Do not massage bony areas.
- Keep linens clean, dry, and free of wrinkles.
- Apply powder where skin touches skin.
- Do not irritate the skin. Avoid scrubbing or vigorous rubbing when bathing or drying the person.
- Avoid massaging over pressure points. *Never rub or massage reddened areas.*
- Use pillows and blankets to prevent skin from being in contact with skin and to reduce moisture and friction.
- Keep the heels off the bed. Use pillows or other devices as instructed by the nurse. Place the pillows or devices under the lower legs from midcalf to the ankles.
- Use protective devices as instructed by the nurse and the care plan.
- Remind persons sitting in chairs to shift their positions every 15 minutes. This decreases pressure on bony points.
- Report any signs of skin breakdown or pressure ulcers immediately to the nurse.

Fig. 25-4 The 30-degree lateral position. Pillows are placed under the head, shoulder, and leg. This position inclines (lifts up) the hip to avoid pressure on the hip. The person does not lie on the hip as in the side-lying position. *(From Bryant et al: Pressure ulcer. In Bryant RA, ed: Acute chronic wounds: nursing management, St Louis, 1992, Mosby.)*

TREATMENT

The doctor directs pressure ulcer treatment. Wound care products, drugs, treatments, and special equipment are ordered to promote healing. The nurse and nursing care plan tell you about a person's treatment. The following protective devices often are ordered to prevent and treat pressure ulcers.

- *Bed cradle*—A bed cradle (Anderson frame) is a metal frame placed on the bed and over the person. Top linens are brought over the cradle to prevent pressure on the legs and feet (Fig. 25-5). Top linens are tucked in at the bottom of the mattress and mitered. They are also tucked under both sides of the mattress to protect the person from air drafts and chilling. *(See Focus on Home Care box.)*

- *Elbow protectors*—Elbow protectors are made of foam rubber or sheepskin. They fit the shape of the elbow (Fig. 25-7) and are secured in place with straps. Friction is prevented between the bed and the elbow.
- *Heel elevators*—Pillows or special cushions are used to raise the heels off the bed (Fig. 25-8). Special braces and splints also are used to keep pressure off the heels.

Focus On ... HOME CARE

A cardboard box is useful as a bed cradle (Fig. 25-6). The nurse tells you how to line the box to prevent pressure on the heels.

Fig. 25-5 A bed cradle is placed on top of the bed. Linens are brought over the top of the cradle.

Fig. 25-7 Elbow protector.

Fig. 25-8 Heel elevator.

Fig. 25-6 A box serves as a bed cradle. It keeps top linens off the person's feet.

- *Flotation pads*—Flotation pads or cushions (Fig. 25-9) are like water beds. They are made of a gel-like substance. The outer case is heavy plastic. They are used for chairs and wheelchairs. The pad is placed in a pillowcase so the plastic does not touch the skin.
- *Eggcrate-like mattress*—The eggcrate-like mattress is a foam pad that looks like an egg carton (Fig. 25-10). Peaks in the mattress distribute the person's weight more evenly. The eggcrate-like mattress is placed on top of the regular mattress. Only a bottom sheet covers the eggcrate-like mattress. Before the bottom sheet is put on, the eggcrate-like mattress is put in a special cover. The cover protects against moisture and soiling.

- *Special beds*—Some beds have air flowing through the mattresses (Fig. 25-11). The *person floats* on the mattress. Body weight is distributed evenly. There is little pressure on bony parts. Another type of bed allows repositioning without moving the person. Depending on the bed, the person is turned to the prone or supine position or tilted various degrees. Body alignment does not change. Pressure points change as the position changes. There is little friction. Some beds constantly rotate from side to side. These beds are useful for persons with spinal cord injuries.
- *Other equipment*—Trochanter rolls and footboards also are used to prevent and treat pressure ulcers. These are described in Chapter 20.

Fig. 25-9 Flotation pad.

Fig. 25-10 Eggcrate-like mattress on the bed.

Fig. 25-11 Air flotation bed.

CIRCULATORY ULCERS

Some people have diseases that affect blood flow to and from the legs and feet. Such poor circulation can lead to pain, open wounds, and swelling of tissues (edema). Infection and gangrene can result from the open wound and poor circulation. **Gangrene** is a condition in which there is death of tissue (see Chapter 30).

The doctor directs the person's care. The RN uses the nursing process to meet the person's needs. Preventing skin breakdown on the legs and feet is very important.

CIRCULATORY ULCERS

Circulatory ulcers (vascular ulcers) are caused by a decrease in blood flow through arteries or veins. Persons with diseases affecting the blood vessels are at risk for these ulcers on the legs and feet. These wounds are painful and hard to heal.

STASIS ULCERS

Stasis ulcers (venous ulcers) are open wounds caused by poor blood return to the heart from the legs and feet (Fig. 25-12). Valves in the leg veins do not close efficiently. Therefore the veins do not pump blood back to the heart normally. This causes blood and fluid to collect in the legs and feet. Small veins in the skin can rupture. Remember, hemoglobin gives blood its red color. When the veins rupture, hemoglobin is released into the tissues. This causes the skin to turn brown. The skin is also dry, leathery, and hard. Itching is common.

The heels and inner aspect of the ankles are common sites for stasis ulcers. These ulcers can occur from skin injury. Scratching is a common cause. Or the ulcers occur spontaneously. The ulcers are painful and make walking difficult. Healing is slow, and infection is a great risk.

Preventing skin breakdown is important. Good skin care and good positioning are important. The person should avoid wearing tight clothing that can interfere with circulation. Injury to the feet and legs is avoided. The doctor may order elastic stockings or elastic bandages (see Chapter 24). Professional foot care is important.

ARTERIAL ULCERS

Arterial ulcers are open wounds on the legs and feet caused by poor blood flow through the arteries. The leg and foot may feel cold and look blue and shiny. The ulcer is often painful at rest. Pain is usually worse at night.

These ulcers are caused by diseases or injuries that decrease arterial blood flow to the legs and feet. High blood pressure and diabetes are common causes. So are narrowed arteries from aging. Smoking is another risk factor.

Arterial ulcers are found between the toes, on top of the toes, and on the outer side of the ankle. The heels are common sites for persons on bedrest. Arterial ulcers can occur in pressure sites from shoes that fit poorly.

The doctor directs the person's treatment. The disease causing the ulcer is treated. Drugs, wound care, and a walking program are ordered. Professional foot care is important. You need to follow the care plan and prevent further injury.

WOUND HEALING

The healing process has three phases:

- *Inflammatory phase* (3 days). Bleeding stops, and a scab forms over the wound. The scab protects microbes from entering the wound. Blood supply to the wound increases. The blood brings nutrients and healing substances. Because blood supply increases, signs and symptoms of inflammation appear: redness, swelling, heat or warmth, and pain. Loss of function may occur.
- *Proliferative phase* (day 3 to day 21). Proliferate means to multiply rapidly. During this phase, tissue cells multiply to repair the wound.
- *Maturation phase* (day 21 to 1 or 2 years). The scar gains strength. The red, raised scar eventually becomes thin and pale.

TYPES OF WOUND HEALING

The healing process occurs through primary intention, secondary intention, or tertiary intention. With *primary intention (first intention, primary closure)*, the wound edges are brought together. Sutures (stitches), staples, clips, or adhesive strips close the wound. Doctors now have special glues to close wounds.

Secondary intention (second intention) is used for contaminated and infected wounds. Wounds are cleaned

Fig. 25-12 Stasis ulcer.

and dead tissue removed. Wound edges are not brought together, and the wound gaps. Healing occurs naturally. However, healing takes longer and leaves a larger scar. The threat of infection is great.

Tertiary intention *(third intention, delayed intention)* involves leaving a wound open and then closing it later. Thus tertiary intention combines secondary and primary intention. Infection and poor circulation are common reasons for tertiary intention.

COMPLICATIONS OF WOUND HEALING

Many factors affect the healing process and increase the risk of complications. The type of wound is one factor. Other factors include the person's age, general health, nutrition, and life-style. Good circulation is important. Age, smoking, circulatory disease, and diabetes all affect circulation. Certain drugs (Coumadin and heparin) can prolong bleeding. Tissue growth and repair require adequate protein in the diet. Infection is a risk for persons with immune system changes and for those taking antibiotics. Antibiotics kill pathogens. Specific antibiotics kill specific pathogens. In doing so, an environment may be created that allows other pathogens to grow and multiply.

Hemorrhage. Hemorrhage is the excessive loss of blood in a short period of time (see Chapter 36). If the bleeding is not stopped, death results. Hemorrhage may be internal or external. Internal hemorrhage cannot be seen. Bleeding occurs inside the body into tissues and body cavities. A hematoma may form. A **hematoma** is a collection of blood under the skin and tissues. The area appears swollen and has a reddish-blue color. Shock, vomiting blood, coughing up blood, and loss of consciousness are signs of internal hemorrhage.

You can see external bleeding. Bloody drainage and dressings soaked with blood are common signs. Remember, gravity causes fluid to flow down. Therefore blood can flow down and collect under the part. Always check under the body part for the pooling of blood. As with internal hemorrhage, shock can occur.

Shock results when there is not enough blood supply to organs and tissues (see Chapter 36). Signs and symptoms include low or falling blood pressure, a rapid and weak pulse, and rapid respirations. The skin is cold, moist, and pale. The person is restless and may complain of thirst. Confusion and loss of consciousness occur as shock worsens.

Hemorrhage and shock are emergencies. Immediately notify the nurse, and assist as requested. Remember to practice Standard Precautions and follow the Bloodborne Pathogen Standard when in contact with blood. Gloves are always worn. Gowns, masks, and eye protection are necessary when blood splashes and splatters are likely.

Infection. Wound contamination can occur during or after the injury. Trauma is a common source of contaminated wounds. Surgical wounds can be contaminated during or after surgery. An infected wound appears inflamed (reddened) and has drainage. The wound is painful and tender. The person has a fever.

Dehiscence. Dehiscence is the separation of the wound layers (Fig. 25-13). Separation may involve the skin layer or underlying tissues. Abdominal wounds are most commonly affected. Coughing, vomiting, and abdominal distention place stress on the wound. The person often describes the sensation of the wound popping open.

Evisceration. Evisceration is the separation of the wound along with the protrusion of abdominal organs (Fig. 25-14). Causes are the same as for dehiscence.

Dehiscence and evisceration are surgical emergencies. The wound is covered with large sterile dressings saturated with sterile saline. You must notify the nurse immediately, and assist in preparing the person for surgery.

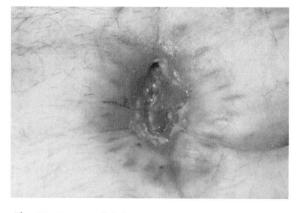

Fig. 25-13 Wound dehiscence. *(Courtesy Morison M: A colour guide to the nursing management of wounds, London, 1992, Wolfe Medical Publishers.)*

Fig. 25-14 Wound evisceration. *(From Mosby's medical, nursing, & allied health dictionary, ed 4, St Louis, 1994, Mosby.)*

WOUND APPEARANCE

During the healing process, doctors and nurses routinely observe the wound and its drainage. They observe for healing and complications. You need to make certain observations when assisting with wound care. You report your observations to the nurse, and record them according to agency policy. Box 25-3 lists the wound observations that you need to make. (*See Focus on Home Care box.*)

Box 25-3   Wound Observations

Wound location
- Multiple wounds may exist from surgery or trauma.

Wound size and depth (measure in centimeters)
- *Size:* measure from top to bottom and side to side.
- *Depth:* (1) insert a sterile swab inside the deepest part of the wound; (2) remove the swab, and measure the distance on the swab. *Measure depth only when the wound is open and with the nurse's supervision.*
- Use the same ruler when measuring the wound.

Wound appearance
- Is the wound red and swollen?
- Is the area around the wound warm to touch?
- Are sutures, staples, or clips intact or broken?
- Are wound edges closed or separated? Did the wound break open?

Drainage
- Is the drainage serous, sanguineous, serosanguineous, or purulent?
- What is the amount of drainage?

Odor
- Does the wound or drainage have an odor?

Surrounding skin
- Is surrounding skin intact?
- What is the color of surrounding skin?
- Are surrounding tissues swollen?

 Focus On... HOME CARE

The RN may ask you to take photographs of wounds. The photograph helps the RN with wound assessment and evaluation. Before taking a photograph, make sure the person has signed a consent for photography. (The RN is responsible for obtaining the consent.) If you use a Polaroid camera, write the person's name and the date and time on the back of the photo. If using regular film, note the frame number, the person's name, and the date and time in the person's record.

The photograph does not replace making accurate observations as listed in Box 25-3.

WOUND DRAINAGE

During injury and the inflammatory phase of wound healing, fluid and cells escape from the tissues. The amount of drainage may be small or large, depending on wound size and location. Bleeding and infection also affect the amount and kind of drainage. Wound drainage is observed and measured.

Major types of wound drainage are as follows:

- **Serous drainage**—clear, watery fluid (Fig. 25-15, *A*). The fluid in a blister is serous. *Serous* comes from the word *serum,* which is the clear, thin, fluid portion of the blood. Serum does not contain blood cells or platelets.
- **Sanguineous drainage**— bloody drainage (Fig. 25-15, *B*). Sanguineous comes from the Latin word *sanguis,* which means blood. The amount and color of sanguineous drainage is important. Hemorrhage is suspected when large amounts are present. Bright drainage indicates fresh bleeding. Older bleeding is darker.
- **Serosanguineous drainage**— thin, watery drainage (*sero*) that is blood-tinged (*sanguineous*) (Fig. 25-15, *C*).
- **Purulent drainage**—thick drainage that is green, yellow, or brown (Fig. 25-15, *D*).

Drainage must leave the wound for healing to occur. If drainage is trapped inside the wound, underlying tissues swell. The wound may heal at the skin level, but underlying tissues do not close. This can lead to infection and other complications.

When large amounts of drainage are expected, the doctor inserts a drain. A *Penrose drain* is a rubber tube that drains onto a dressing (Fig. 25-16, p. 606). Because the Penrose drain opens onto the dressing, it is an open drain and a portal of entry for microbes.

Fig. 25-15 Wound drainage. **A,** Serous drainage. **B,** Sanguineous drainage. **C,** Serosanguineous drainage. **D,** Purulent drainage. (From Potter PA, Perry AG: *Fundamentals of nursing: concepts, process, and practice,* ed 4, St Louis, 1997, Mosby.)

Fig. 25-16 A Penrose drain. The safety pin prevents the drain from slipping into the wound. *(From Potter PA, Perry, AG: Fundamentals of nursing: concepts, process, and practice, ed 4, St Louis, 1997, Mosby.)*

Fig. 25-17 A Hemovac. Drains are sutured to the wound and connected to the reservoir. *(From Elkin MK, Perry AG, Potter PA: Nursing interventions and clinical skills, ed 2, St Louis, 2000, Mosby.)*

Fig. 25-18 The Jackson-Pratt drainage system. *(From Elkin MK, Perry AG, Potter PA: Nursing interventions and clinical skills, ed 2, St Louis, 2000, Mosby.)*

Closed drainage systems prevent microbes from entering the wound. A drainage tube is placed in the wound and attached to suction. The Hemovac (Fig. 25-17) and Jackson-Pratt (Fig. 25-18) systems are examples. Other systems are used depending on the type of wound, its size, and its location.

Drainage is measured in three ways:

- Noting the number and size of dressings with drainage. The amount and kind of drainage is described. Are dressings saturated? Is drainage on just part of the dressing? If so, which part? Is drainage through some or all layers of the dressing?
- Weighing dressings before applying them to the wound. The weight of each dressing is noted. Dressings are weighed after removal. The weight of the dry dressing is subtracted from the wet dressing (wet dressings weigh more).
- Measuring the amount of drainage in the collecting receptacle if closed drainage is used.

DRESSINGS

Wound dressings have many functions. They protect wounds from injury and microbes. Drainage is absorbed and removed along with dead tissue. Dressings can promote comfort and cover unsightly wounds. They also provide a moist environment for wound healing. When bleeding is a problem, pressure dressings help control bleeding.

The type and size of dressing used depend on many factors. These include the type of wound, its size and location; amount of drainage; and the presence or absence of infection. The dressing's function and the frequency of dressing changes are other factors. The doctor and nurse choose the best type of dressing for each wound.

TYPES OF DRESSINGS

Dressings are described by the material used and application method. Many products are available for dressing wounds. The follow materials are common:

- Gauze—comes in squares, rectangles, pads, and rolls (Fig. 25-19). Gauze dressings absorb moisture.
- Nonadherent gauze—is a gauze dressing with a nonstick surface. The dressing does not stick to the wound and removes easily without injuring tissue.
- Transparent adhesive film—prevents fluids and bacteria from reaching the wound but air can. The wound is kept moist. Drainage is not absorbed. The transparent film allows wound observation.

Some dressings contain special agents to promote wound healing. If you assist with the dressing change, the nurse explains its use to you.

Fig. 25-19 Gauze dressings. **A,** 4 × 4. **B,** Gauze roll. **C,** Abdominal pad (ABD). **D,** 2 × 2.

Fig. 25-20 Tape is applied at the top, middle, and bottom of the dressing. Note that the tape extends several inches beyond both sides of the dressing.

Dressing application methods involve dry and wet dressings:

- *Dry-to-dry dressing* (usually called a *dry dressing*)—dry gauze dressing is placed over the wound. Additional dressings are placed on top of the first dressing as needed. Drainage is absorbed by the dressing and is removed with the dressing. A dry dressing can stick to the wound. The dressing is removed carefully to prevent tissue injury and discomfort.
- *Wet-to-dry dressing*—a gauze dressing saturated with a solution is applied over the wound. Additional dressings are applied as needed. These dressings are also moistened with solution. The solution softens dead tissue in the wound. The dead tissue is absorbed by the dressing and is removed with the dressing. The dressings are removed when dry.
- *Wet-to-wet dressing*—gauze dressings saturated with solution are placed in the wound. The dressing is kept moist.

SECURING DRESSINGS

Dressings must be secure over wounds. Bacteria can enter the wound and drainage can escape if the dressing is dislodged. Tape and Montgomery ties are commonly used to secure dressings. Binders and bandages also hold dressings in place.

Tape. Adhesive, paper, plastic, and elastic tapes are available. Adhesive tape sticks well to the skin. However, the adhesive part can remain on the skin and is hard to remove. The adhesive can irritate the skin. Sometimes skin is removed with the tape, causing an abrasion. Many people are allergic to adhesive tape. Paper and plastic tapes are nonallergenic. This means that they do not cause allergic reactions. Elastic tape allows movement of the body part.

Fig. 25-21 Montgomery ties.

Tape is applied to secure the top, middle, and bottom of the dressing (Fig. 25-20). The tape extends several inches beyond each side of the dressing. *The tape must not encircle the entire body part. If swelling occurs, circulation to the part is impaired.*

Montgomery Ties. Montgomery ties (Fig. 25-21) are used for large dressings and when frequent dressing changes are needed. A Montgomery tie consists of an adhesive strip and a cloth tie. When the dressing is in place, the adhesive strips are placed on both sides of the dressing. Then the cloth ties are secured over the dressing. Two or three Montgomery ties may be needed on each side. The cloth ties are undone for the dressing change. The adhesive strips are not removed unless soiled.

(See Focus on Children and Focus on Older Persons boxes on p. 608.)

Focus On... CHILDREN

Children are often afraid of dressing changes. Tape removal is often painful for them. The wound's appearance can be frightening. A calm, cooperative child is important to prevent contamination of the sterile field. A parent or caregiver holds the child so the wound can be reached with ease. Letting the child hold or play with a favorite toy is often comforting.

Focus On... OLDER PERSONS

Older persons have thin, fragile skin. Skin tears must be prevented. Extreme care is necessary when removing tape.

▶ APPLYING DRESSINGS

The doctor usually does the first dressing change after surgery. The nurse follows the doctor's order for dressing changes. Your job description may allow you to apply simple, dry, nonsterile dressings to uncomplicated wounds and to assist the nurse with complex wounds. The nurse tells you when to change a dressing and what supplies to use. Box 25-4 lists the rules for applying dressings. *(See Focus On Home Care box.)*

Box 25-4	**Rules for Applying Dry Nonsterile Dressings**

- Make sure your state allows assistive personnel to perform the procedure.
- Make sure the procedure is in your job description.
- Apply dressings only under the nurse's direction and supervision.
- Review the procedure with the nurse.
- Allow pain medications time to take effect. The person may experience discomfort during the dressing change. The nurse gives the medication and tells you how long to wait.
- Provide for the person's fluid and elimination needs before starting the procedure.
- Collect all needed equipment and supplies before you begin.
- Control your nonverbal communication. Wound odors, appearance, and drainage may be unpleasant. Do not communicate your thoughts and reactions to the person.
- Remove soiled dressings so that the underside of the dressing is away from the person's sight. The drainage and its odor may upset the person.
- Do not force the person to look at the wound. A wound can affect the person's body image and esteem. The nurse helps the person deal with the wound.
- Practice Standard Precautions and follow the Bloodborne Pathogen Standard. Wear personal protective equipment as necessary.
- Wear clean, disposable gloves.
- Remove tape by pulling the tape toward the wound.
- Remove dressings gently to prevent pain and discomfort. The dressing may stick to the wound and surrounding skin.

Focus On... HOME CARE

Make sure you have the necessary supplies before leaving the agency. The RN may ask you to telephone him or her after removing the old dressings. During this telephone call, you report your observations to the RN. Then the RN gives you instructions about how to proceed.

Applying a Dry Nonsterile Dressing

Pre-Procedure

1. Review the procedure with the nurse.
2. Explain to the person what you are going to do.
3. Allow time for pain medication to take effect.
4. Provide for the person's fluid and elimination needs.
5. Wash your hands.
6. Collect needed equipment:
   - Gloves
   - Personal protective equipment as needed
   - Tape or Montgomery ties as directed by the nurse
   - Dressings as directed by the nurse
   - Adhesive remover
   - Scissors
   - Leakproof plastic bag
   - Bath blanket
7. Identify the person. Check the ID bracelet against the assignment sheet.
8. Provide for privacy. Close the door and privacy curtain.
9. Arrange furniture for your work surface. You should not have to reach over or turn your back on the work surface.
10. Raise the bed to a level for good body mechanics. Make sure bed rails are up.

Procedure

11. Lower the bed rail near you.
12. Help the person to a comfortable position.
13. Cover the person with a bath blanket. Fanfold top linens to the foot of the bed.
14. Expose the affected body part.
15. Remind the person not to touch supplies or the wound.
16. Make a cuff on the plastic bag. Place the bag within easy reach.
17. Put on the clean gown and mask if needed.
18. Put on the gloves.
19. Undo Montgomery ties or remove tape:
    a. *Montgomery ties:* fold ties away from the wound.
    b. *Tape:* hold the skin down, and gently pull the tape toward the wound.
20. Remove adhesive from the skin if necessary. Wet a 4 x 4 gauze dressing with the adhesive remover. Clean away from the wound.
21. Remove gauze dressings starting with the top dressing. Keep the soiled side of the dressing away from the person's sight. Place dressings in the plastic bag. Do not let the dressings touch the outside of the bag.
22. Remove the dressing directly over the wound very gently. The dressing may stick to the wound or drain.
23. Observe the wound, drain site, and wound drainage (see Box 25-3).
24. Remove the gloves. Discard them into the plastic bag.
25. Wash your hands. Raise the bed rail when you leave the bedside, and lower it upon your return.
26. Put on clean gloves.
27. Open the dressings.
28. Cut the length of tape needed.
29. Apply dressings over the wound as directed by the nurse.
30. Secure the dressings in place. Use tape (see Fig. 25-20) or Montgomery ties (see Fig. 25-21).
31. Remove your gloves. Discard them in the plastic bag.

Applying a Dry Nonsterile Dressing—cont'd

Post-Procedure

32 Provide for comfort. Cover the person with the top linens, and remove the bath blanket.

33 Place the signal light within the person's reach.

34 Lower the bed to its lowest position.

35 Raise or lower bed rails. Follow the care plan.

36 Unscreen the person.

37 Discard supplies into the plastic bag. Discard the plastic bag according to agency policy.

38 Clean your work surface following the Bloodborne Pathogen Standard. Return furniture to its proper place.

39 Wash your hands.

40 Report your observations to the nurse.

BINDERS

Binders are applied to the abdomen, chest, or perineal areas. Binders promote healing because they:

- Support wounds and hold dressings in place
- Reduce or prevent swelling by promoting circulation
- Promote comfort
- Prevent injury

They must be applied properly. Incorrect application can cause severe discomfort, skin irritation, and circulatory and respiratory complications. The binder's effectiveness and the person's safety depend on correct application. Box 25-5 lists the rules for applying these binders:

- *Straight abdominal binders*—provide abdominal support and hold dressings in place (Fig. 25-22). The binder is a rectangle. The binder is applied with the person supine. The top part is positioned at the person's waist. The lower part is over the hips. The binder is secured in place with pins, hooks, or Velcro.
- *Breast binders*—support the breasts after breast surgery (Fig. 25-23). They also apply pressure to the breasts after childbirth. If the mother does not breast-feed, pressure from the binder helps dry up the milk in the breasts. The binder also promotes comfort and provides support to swollen breasts after childbirth. The woman is supine when the breast binder is applied. The binder is pulled snugly across the chest and secured in place.

Box 25-5	Rules for Applying Binders

- Apply the binder so that firm, even pressure is exerted over the area.
- Apply the binder so it is snug but does not interfere with breathing or circulation.
- Position the person in good alignment when the binder is applied.
- Reapply the binder if it becomes loose, wrinkled, or out of position or causes discomfort.
- Secure pins so they point away from incisional areas.
- Change binders that are moist or soiled to prevent the growth of microbes.

Fig. 25-22 Straight abdominal binder.

Fig. 25-23 Breast binder.

Fig. 25-24 A, Single T binder. **B,** Double T binder.

- *T binders*—are used to secure dressings in place after rectal and perineal surgeries. The single T binder is used for women (Fig. 25-24, *A*). The double T binder is used for men (Fig. 25-24, *B*). If perineal dressings are large, women may need double T binders. To apply a T binder, the waistbands are brought around the waist and pinned at the front. The tails are brought between the person's legs and up to the waistband. They are pinned in place at the waistband.

HEAT AND COLD APPLICATIONS

Heat and cold applications are often ordered for wound care. Heat and cold applications are ordered by doctors to promote healing, promote comfort, and reduce tissue swelling. Heat and cold applications are discussed in Chapter 26.

THE PERSON'S BASIC NEEDS

This chapter focuses on wounds. However, you must remember that it is the *person* who has the wound. The wound, which can affect the person's basic needs, is only one aspect of the person's care.

You must remember that the person is recovering from surgery or trauma. The wound is a source of pain and discomfort. The wound and the pain may interfere with breathing and moving. Turning, repositioning, and ambulating may be painful. You must handle the person gently and allow pain medications to take effect before giving care.

Good nutrition is needed for healing. However, pain and discomfort can affect the person's appetite. So can odors from wound drainage. Remove soiled dressings promptly from the room, use room deodorizers, and keep drainage containers out of the person's sight. If the person has a taste for certain foods or beverages, report this information to the nurse.

Infection is always a threat. You must practice Standard Precautions and follow the Bloodborne Pathogen Standard. Also, observe the wound and the person carefully for signs and symptoms of infection.

Delayed healing is a risk for persons who are older or obese or have poor nutrition. Poor circulation and diabetes also affect healing. These conditions are risk factors for infection.

Many fears affect the person's sense of safety and security. The person fears scarring, disfigurement, delayed healing, and infection. Fears about the wound "popping open" are common. Costly medical bills are another concern. Continued hospital care, home care, or long-term care may be needed.

Victims of violence have many other concerns. Future attacks, finding and convicting the attacker, and fear for family members is common. Victims of domestic violence, child abuse, and elderly abuse often hide the true source of their injuries.

The person's wound may be large or small. It may be visible to others—on the face, arms, or legs—or hidden by clothing. Wound drainage may have unpleasant odors. The wound may be extensive and disfiguring. It may affect the person's ability to perform sexually or the person's sense of being sexually attractive. The amputation of a finger, hand, arm, toe, foot, or leg can affect the person's function, everyday activities, and job. Eye injuries can affect vision. Abdominal trauma and surgery can affect eating and elimination.

Whatever the location or size of the wound, physical function and body image are affected. The person's sense of love and belonging and self-esteem are affected. You must be sensitive to the person's feelings. The person may be sad and tearful or angry and hostile. Adjustment may be difficult and rehabilitation necessary. You must be gentle and kind, give thoughtful care, and practice good communication techniques. Other health team members— social workers, psychiatrists, and the clergy—may be involved in the person's care.

Circle the BEST answer.

1. Sally Jones fell off her bike. She has a laceration on her right leg. Which is *false?*
   A. She has an open wound.
   B. She has an infected wound.
   C. She has a contaminated wound.
   D. She has an unintentional wound.

2. A person had rectal surgery. What type of wound does the person have?
   A. A clean wound
   B. A dirty wound
   C. A clean-contaminated wound
   D. A contaminated wound

3. The skin and underlying tissues are pierced. This is
   A. A penetrating wound
   B. An incision
   C. A contusion
   D. An abrasion

4. Which can cause skin tears?
   A. Keeping your nails trimmed and smooth
   B. Dressing the person in clothing with long sleeves and pants
   C. Wearing rings
   D. Handling the person gently

5. Which can cause pressure ulcers?
   A. Repositioning the person every 2 hours
   B. Scrubbing and rubbing the skin
   C. Applying lotion to dry areas
   D. Keeping linens clean, dry, and wrinkle-free

6. Which are *not* used to treat pressure ulcers?
   A. Special beds
   B. Waterbeds and flotation pads
   C. Plastic drawsheets and waterproof pads
   D. Heel elevators and elbow protectors

7. A person has a stasis ulcer. These measures are in the person's care plan. Which should you question?
   A. Use elastic garters to hold socks in place.
   B. Do not cut or trim toenails.
   C. Avoid injury to the person's legs.
   D. Apply elastic stockings.

8. A person is at risk for arterial ulcers. Which is *not* a common site for arterial ulcers?
   A. Between the toes
   B. On top of the toes
   C. On the outer side of the ankle
   D. Behind the knee

9. A wound appears red and swollen. The area around it is warm to touch. These are signs of
   A. The inflammatory phase of wound healing
   B. The proliferative phase of wound healing
   C. Healing by primary intention
   D. Healing by secondary intention

10. A wound is healing by primary intention. The nurse notes that the wound is separating. This is called
    A. Dehiscence
    B. Tertiary intention
    C. Evisceration
    D. Hematoma

11. You note a clear, watery drainage from a wound. This drainage is called
    A. Purulent drainage
    B. Serous drainage
    C. Sero-purulent drainage
    D. Serosanguineous drainage

12. You note large amounts of sanguineous drainage in a Hemovac. Which is *true?*
    A. The person is bleeding.
    B. You need to notify the doctor.
    C. The person has an infection.
    D. The person has a Penrose drain.

13. A dressing does the following *except*
    A. Protect the wound from injury
    B. Absorb drainage
    C. Provide a moist environment for wound healing
    D. Support the wound and reduce swelling

14. You are securing a dressing with tape. Tape is applied
    A. Around the entire part
    B. To the top and bottom of the dressing
    C. To the top, middle, and bottom of the dressing
    D. As the person prefers

15. Mr. Moore has an abdominal binder. The binder is used to
    A. Prevent blood clots
    B. Prevent wound infection
    C. Provide support and hold dressings in place
    D. Decrease circulation and swelling

Answers to these questions are on p. 837.

HEAT AND COLD APPLICATIONS

Define the key terms listed in this chapter

Identify the purposes, effects, and complications of heat and cold applications

Identify the persons at risk for complications from heat and cold applications

Explain the differences between moist and dry heat and cold applications

Describe the rules for the application of heat and cold

Explain how cooling and warming blankets are used

Perform the procedures described in this chapter

KEY TERMS

constrict To narrow

cyanosis Bluish skin color

dilate To expand or open wider

hyperthermia A body temperature *(thermia)* that is much higher *(hyper)* than the person's normal range

hypothermia A very low *(hypo)* body temperature *(thermia)*

Doctors order heat and cold applications to promote healing and comfort. These applications also reduce tissue swelling. Heat and cold have opposite effects on body function. Severe injuries and changes in body function can occur. The risks are great. You must thoroughly understand the purposes, effects, and complications of heat and cold applications.

In some agencies, only nurses apply heat and cold. Other agencies let assistive personnel apply heat and cold. Before you perform these procedures, make sure that:

- Your state allows you to perform the procedure
- The procedure is in your job description
- You have the necessary training
- You are familiar with the equipment
- You review the procedure with a nurse
- A nurse is available to answer questions and to supervise you

HEAT APPLICATIONS

Heat applications can be applied to almost any body part. They are often used for musculoskeletal injuries or problems (sprains, arthritis). Heat applications are used to:

- Relieve pain
- Relax muscles

- Promote healing
- Reduce tissue swelling
- Decrease joint stiffness

EFFECTS

When heat is applied to the skin, blood vessels in the area dilate. **Dilate** means to expand or open wider (Fig. 26-1, p. 616). More blood flows through the vessels. The tissues have more oxygen and nutrients for healing. Excess fluid is removed from the area faster. The skin is reddened and feels warm.

COMPLICATIONS

High temperatures can cause burns. Pain, excessive redness, and blisters are danger signs. Report these signs immediately. Also observe for pale skin. When heat is applied too long, blood vessels **constrict** (narrow) (see Fig. 26-1, *C*). Blood flow decreases when vessels constrict. This reduces the amount of blood for the tissues. Tissue damage occurs, and the skin is pale.

Fair-skinned people are at great risk for complications. Their delicate and fragile skin is easily burned. Persons with difficulty sensing heat or pain are also at risk. Nervous system damage, loss of consciousness, and circulatory disorders interfere with sensation. So do confusion and strong pain medications.

Persons with metal implants are at risk. Metal conducts heat. Deep tissues can be burned. Pacemakers and joint replacements are made of metal. Heat is not applied in the area of the implant.

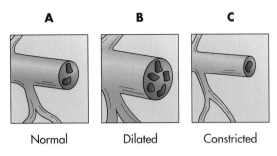

A   **B**   **C**

Normal   Dilated   Constricted

Fig. 26-1 A, Blood vessel under normal conditions. **B,** Dilated blood vessel. **C,** Constricted blood vessel.

Heat is not applied to a pregnant woman's abdomen. The heat can affect fetal growth.

(See Focus on Children box and Focus on Older Persons box.)

Moist and Dry Applications

A *moist heat application* means that water is in contact with the skin. Water conducts heat. The effects from moist heat are greater and occur faster than from dry heat applications. Heat penetrates deeper with a moist application. To prevent injury, moist heat applications have lower (cooler) temperatures than dry heat applications.

Water is not in contact with the skin with *dry heat applications.* Dry heat has advantages:
- The application stays at the desired temperature longer.
- Dry heat does not penetrate as deeply as moist heat.

Because water is not used, dry heat needs higher (hotter) temperatures to achieve the desired effect. Therefore burns are still a risk.

The person is protected from injury during local heat applications. Practice the rules in Box 26-1 to prevent burns and other complications.

Focus On... CHILDREN

Infants and young children also have fragile skin. They are at risk for burns. They need careful observation. Always respond to infants and young children who are crying. Crying is a way of communicating pain.

Focus On... OLDER PERSONS

Older persons have thin and fragile skin. They also are at risk for burns. Other changes from aging and health problems increase the risk for burns. They include circulatory and nervous system changes. Some drugs also affect the older person's ability to sense pain. Confused persons and those with dementia may not recognize pain. Look for changes in the person's behavior. Behavior changes can signal pain.

Box 26-1	Rules for Applying Heat and Cold

- Know how to operate equipment used in the procedure.
- Measure the temperature of moist applications. Use a bath thermometer.
- Follow agency policies for safe temperature ranges. See Table 26-1 for guidelines.
- Do not apply *very hot* (above 106° to 115° F, or 41.1° to 46.1° C) applications. Tissue damage can occur. A nurse applies *very hot* applications.
- Ask the nurse what the temperature of the application should be:
  - Heat—cooler temperatures are used for persons at risk.
  - Cold—warmer temperatures are used for persons at risk.
- Know the precise site of the application. Ask the nurse to show you the site.
- Cover dry heat or cold applications before applying them. Use a flannel cover, towel, or pillowcase according to agency policy.

- Observe the skin for signs of complications. Immediately report the following to the nurse:
  - Complaints of pain, numbness, or burning
  - Excessive redness
  - Blisters
  - Pale, white, or gray skin
  - Cyanosis (bluish skin color)
  - Shivering
- Do not let the person change the temperature of the application.
- Ask the nurse how long to leave the application in place. Carefully watch the time. Heat and cold are applied for no longer than 20 minutes.
- Follow the rules of electrical safety when using electrical appliances to apply heat.
- Expose only the body part where you will apply heat or cold. Provide for privacy through proper draping and screening.
- Place the signal light within the person's reach.

Table 26-1	Heat and Cold Temperature Ranges	
Temperature	**Farenheit Range**	**Centigrade Range**
Very hot	106° to 115° F	41.1° to 46.1° C
Hot	98° to 106° F	36.6° to 41.1° C
Warm	93° to 98° F	33.8° to 36.6° C
Tepid	80° to 93° F	26.6° to 33.8° C
Cool	65° to 80° F	18.3° to 26.6° C
Cold	50° to 65° F	10.0° to 18.3° C

Modified from Perry AG, Potter PA: *Clinical nursing skills and techniques*, ed 4, St Louis, 1998, Mosby.

▶ HOT COMPRESSES AND PACKS

Hot compresses and packs are moist heat applications. They consist of a washcloth, small towel, or gauze dressing. A compress is applied to a small area. Packs are applied to large areas.

The application is left in place for 20 minutes. Sometimes an aquathermia pad is applied over the compress or pack. This maintains the temperature of the compress or pack.

Fig. 26-2 A hot compress is covered with plastic and a bath towel. These keep the compress warm.

Applying Hot Compresses

QUALITY OF LIFE

Remember to:
- Knock before entering the person's room
- Address the person by name
- Introduce yourself by name and title

Pre-Procedure

1 Explain the procedure to the person.
2 Wash your hands.
3 Collect the following:
- Basin
- Bath thermometer
- Small towl, washcloth, or gauze squares
- Plastic wrap or aquathermia pad
- Ties, tape, or rolled gauze
- Bath towel
- Waterproof bed protector
4 Identify the person. Check the ID bracelet against the assignment sheet.
5 Provide for privacy.

Procedure

6 Place the protector under the body part.
7 Fill the basin ½ to ⅔ full with hot water as directed by the nurse.
8 Place the compress in the water.
9 Wring out the compress.
10 Apply the compress. Note the time.
11 Cover the compress quickly. Do one of the following as directed by the nurse:
- a Cover it with plastic wrap and then with a bath towel (Fig. 26-2). Secure the towel in place with ties, tape, or rolled gauze.
- b Cover it with an aquathermia pad, see p. 624.
12 Place the signal light within reach. Raise or lower bed rails. Follow the care plan.
13 Check the area every 5 minutes. Check for redness and complaints of pain, discomfort, or numbness. Remove the compress if any occur. Tell the nurse immediately.
14 Change the compress if cooling occurs.
15 Remove the compress after 20 minutes or as directed by the nurse. Pat the area dry with a towel.

Post-Procedure

16 Provide for comfort.
17 Unscreen the person.
18 Raise or lower bed rails. Follow the care plan.
19 Place the signal light within reach.
20 Clean equipment. Discard disposable items.
21 Follow agency policy for soiled linen.
22 Wash your hands.
23 Report the following to the nurse:
- Time, site, and length of the application
- Observations of the skin
- The person's response

▷ **Commercial Compresses.** Sterile commercial compresses are premoistened and packaged in foil. An infrared lamp is used to heat the wrapped compress as instructed by the manufacturer. The lamp is kept in the clean utility room, treatment room, medication room, or the person's room.

Commercial compresses are sterile. Sometimes doctors order them for nonsterile compresses. RNs may decide they are needed in certain situations. Commercial compresses are costly and are used only when necessary.

Applying a Commercial Compress

QUALITY OF LIFE

Remember to:
- Knock before entering the person's room
- Address the person by name
- Introduce yourself by name and title

Pre-Procedure

1 Explain the procedure to the person.
2 Wash your hands.
3 Collect the following:
- Commercial compress
- Infrared lamp
- Towel
- Ties, tape, or rolled gauze
- Waterproof bed protector
- Aquathermia pad (if ordered)

4 Heat the compress following the manufacturer's instructions.
5 Identify the person. Check the ID bracelet against the assignment sheet.
6 Provide for privacy.

Procedure

7 Place the bed protector under the body part.
8 Open the foil-wrapped compress.
9 Apply the compress quickly. Use the outside of the foil to pick up and apply the compress.
10 Cover the compress with a towel.
11 Secure the towel in place with ties, tape, or rolled gauze.
12 Apply the aquathermia pad (if ordered). See *Applying an Aquathermia Pad,* p. 625.

13 Place the signal light within reach. Raise or lower bed rails. Follow the care plan.
14 Check the area every 5 minutes. Check for redness and complaints of pain, discomfort, or numbness. Remove the compress if any occur. Tell the nurse immediately.
15 Change the compress if cooling occurs.
16 Remove the compress after 20 minutes or as directed by the nurse. Pat the area dry with the towel. (If the bed rail is up, lower it for this step.)

Post-Procedure

17 Follow steps 16 through 23 in *Applying Hot Compresses.*

▶ HOT SOAKS

A hot soak involves putting the body part into water. This usually is used for smaller parts, such as a hand, lower arm, foot, or lower leg (Fig. 26-3). Sometimes larger areas are soaked (arm, leg, or torso). Then a tub is used. The soak lasts 15 to 20 minutes. The person's comfort and body alignment are maintained during the hot soak.

Fig. 26-3 The hot soak.

The Hot Soak

QUALITY OF LIFE

Remember to:
- Knock before entering the person's room
- Address the person by name
- Introduce yourself by name and title

Pre-Procedure

1 Explain the procedure to the person.
2 Wash your hands.
3 Collect the following:
- Water basin or an arm or foot bath
- Bath thermometer
- Bath blanket
- Waterproof pads
4 Identify the person. Check the ID bracelet against the assignment sheet.
5 Provide for privacy.

Procedure

6 Position the person for the treatment. Place the signal light within reach.
7 Place a waterproof pad under the area.
8 Fill the container $1/2$ full with hot water as directed by the nurse. Measure water temperature.
9 Expose the area. Avoid unnecessary exposure.
10 Place the part into the water. Pad the edge of the container with a towel. Note the time.
11 Cover the person with a bath blanket for extra warmth.
12 Check the area every 5 minutes. Check for redness and complaints of pain, numbness, or discomfort. Remove the part from the soak if any of these complications occur. Wrap the part in a towel, and tell the nurse immediately.
13 Check water temperature every 5 minutes. Change water as necessary. Wrap the part in a towel while changing the water.
14 Remove the part from the water in 15 to 20 minutes. Pat dry with a towel.

Post-Procedure

15 Follow steps 16 through 23 in *Applying Hot Compresses.*

▶ THE SITZ BATH

The sitz bath involves immersing the perineal and rectal areas areas in warm or hot water for 20 minutes. (*Sitz* means *seat* in German.) Sitz baths are used to clean perineal or anal wounds. They also are used to promote healing, relieve pain and soreness, increase circulation, and stimulate voiding. They are common after rectal or female pelvic surgery, for hemorrhoids, and after childbirth.

The disposable plastic sitz bath fits onto the toilet seat (Fig. 26-4). A sitz tub is a built-in fixture with a deep seat. The person sits in a seat filled with water (Fig. 26-5).

Blood flow to the perineal and rectal areas increases. Therefore less blood flows to other body parts. The person may become weak or feel faint. Drowsiness can occur from the treatment's relaxing effect. Observe the person for signs of weakness, faintness, or fatigue. Also protect the person from injury. Check the person often, keep the signal light within reach, and prevent chills and burns.

Fig. 26-4 The disposable sitz bath.

Fig. 26-5 The built-in sitz bath.

Assisting the Person to Take a Sitz Bath

QUALITY OF LIFE

Remember to:
- Knock before entering the person's room
- Address the person by name
- Introduce yourself by name and title

Pre-Procedure

1 Explain the procedure to the person.
2 Wash your hands.
3 Collect the following:
   - Disposable sitz bath or wheelchair if the built-in sitz bath is used
   - Bath thermometer
   - Large water container
   - Two bath blankets, bath towels, and a clean gown
   - Footstool if the person is short
   - Disinfectant solution
   - Utility gloves
4 Identify the person. Check the ID bracelet against the assignment sheet.
5 Provide for privacy.

Procedure

6 Do one of the following:
   a Place the disposable sitz bath on the toilet seat.
   b Transport the person by wheelchair to the sitz bath room.
7 Fill the sitz bath $\frac{2}{3}$ full with water as directed by the nurse. Measure water temperature.
8 Use bath towels to pad the metal parts that will be in contact with the person.
9 Raise the gown, and secure it above the waist.
10 Help the person sit in the sitz bath.
11 Place a bath blanket around the shoulders. Place another over the legs for warmth.
12 Provide a footstool if the edge of the sitz bath causes pressure under the knees.
13 Make sure the signal light is within reach, and provide for comfort.
14 Stay with a person who is weak or unsteady.
15 Check the person every 5 minutes for complaints of weakness, faintness, and drowsiness. Check for a rapid pulse. If any occur, get assistance to help the person back to bed.
16 Help the person out of the sitz bath after 20 minutes or as directed by the nurse.
17 Assist the person with drying and dressing.
18 Assist the person back to bed.

Post-Procedure

19 Provide for comfort.
20 Unscreen the person.
21 Place the signal light within reach.
22 Raise or lower bed rails. Follow the care plan.
23 Clean the sitz bath with disinfectant solution. Wear utility gloves for this step.
24 Return reusable items to their proper place. Follow agency policy for soiled linen.
25 Wash your hands.
26 Report your observations to the nurse.

THE AQUATHERMIA PAD

The aquathermia pad (Aqua-K, K-Pad) is an electric device used for dry heat. Tubes inside the pad are filled with distilled water. A bedside heating unit also is filled with distilled water. The heated water flows to the pad through a connecting hose (Fig. 26-6). Another hose returns water to the heating unit. The water is re-heated and returned back into the pad.

The heating unit is kept level with the pad and connecting hoses. Water must flow freely. Hoses must be free of kinks and air bubbles. The temperature is set at 105°F (40.5°C) with a key. Then the key is removed. This prevents anyone from changing the temperature. The temperature is often set in the central supply department. The key is kept in that department.

The following safety measures are practiced:

- Follow electrical safety precautions (see Chapter 9).
- Check the device for damage or other flaws.
- Place the heating unit on an even, uncluttered surface. This prevents it from being knocked over or knocked off of the surface.
- Use a flannel cover to insulate the pad. It also absorbs perspiration at the application site. (Some agencies use a towel or pillowcase.)
- Secure the pad in place with ties, tape, or rolled gauze. Do not use pins. They can puncture the pad and cause leaking.
- Do not place the pad under the person or under a body part. This prevents the escape of heat. Burns can result if heat cannot escape.
- *(See Focus on Home Care box.)*

Fig. 26-6 The aquathermia pad and heating unit.

Focus On... HOME CARE

Many people have heating pads with electric coils made of wire. These coils present fire hazards if they break. Burns are a great risk because the temperature is easily adjusted. Always make sure the heating pad is in good repair. Check the temperature often to make sure the patient has not changed it.

Another type of pad serves as a heating pad or a cold application. This pad is filled with a special fluid. The pad is kept in the freezer until needed. If used as a heating pad, the pad is heated in a microwave oven following the manufacturer's instructions. The pad, whether used for heat or cold, is secured in place with attached Velcro straps.

Applying an Aquathermia Pad

QUALITY OF LIFE

Remember to:
- Knock before entering the person's room
- Address the person by name
- Introduce yourself by name and title

Pre-Procedure

1 Explain the procedure to the person.
2 Wash your hands.
3 Collect the following:
   - Aquathermia pad and heating unit
   - Distilled water
   - Flannel cover, pillowcase, or towel
   - Ties, tape, or rolled gauze
4 Identify the person. Check the ID bracelet against the assignment sheet.
5 Provide for privacy.

Procedure

6 Fill the heating unit $^2/_3$ full with distilled water.
7 Remove air bubbles. Place the pad and tubing below the heating unit. Tilt the unit from side to side.
8 Set the temperature as instructed by the nurse (usually 105° F or 40.5° C). Remove the key (give it to the nurse when you complete the procedure).
9 Place the pad in the cover.
10 Plug in the unit. Let water warm to the desired temperature.
11 Set the heating unit on the bedside stand. Keep the pad and connecting hoses level with the unit. Hoses must not have kinks.
12 Apply the pad to the part. Note the time.
13 Secure the pad in place with ties, tape, or rolled gauze. Do not use pins.
14 Unscreen the person. Place the signal light within reach.
15 Raise or lower bed rails. Follow the care plan.
16 Check the skin for redness, swelling, and blisters. Ask about pain, discomfort, or decreased sensation. Remove the pad if any occur. Tell the nurse immediately.
17 Remove the pad at the specified time. (If the bed rail is up, lower it for this step.)

Post-Procedure

18 Follow steps 16 through 23 in *Applying Hot Compresses*.

COLD APPLICATIONS

Cold applications are often used to treat sprains and fractures. They reduce pain, prevent swelling, and decrease circulation and bleeding. Cold cools the body when fever is present.

EFFECTS

Cold has the opposite effect of heat. When cold is applied to the skin, blood vessels constrict (see Fig. 26-1, C). Decreased blood flow results. Less oxygen and nutrients are carried to the tissues. Cold applications are useful right after injury. The decreased circulation reduces the amount of bleeding. The amount of fluid collecting in tissues is also reduced. Cold has a numbing effect on the skin. This helps reduce or relieve pain in the part.

COMPLICATIONS

Complications include pain, burns and blisters, and **cyanosis** (bluish skin color). Burns and blisters tend to occur from intense cold. They also occur when dry cold applications are in direct contact with the skin. When cold is applied for a long time, blood vessels dilate. Blood flow increases. The prolonged application of cold has the same effects as local heat applications.

Fair-skinned persons have fragile skin. They are at great risk for complications. So are persons with mental or sensory impairments. *(See Focus on Children box and Focus on Older Persons box.)*

> **Focus On... CHILDREN**
>
> As with hot applications, infants and children are at risk for complications from cold applications. Check the child often.

> **Focus On... OLDER PERSONS**
>
> As with hot applications, older persons are at risk for complications from cold applications. Check the person often.

MOIST AND DRY APPLICATIONS

Cold applications are moist or dry. The ice bag and ice collar are dry cold applications. The cold compress is a moist application. Moist cold applications penetrate deeper than dry ones. Therefore temperatures of moist applications are not as cold as dry applications.

Injuries from cold applications are prevented. See the rules listed in Box 26-1.

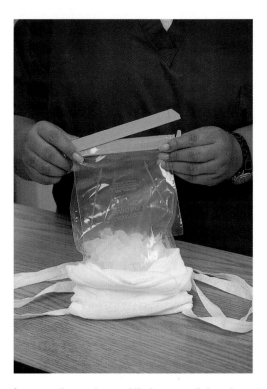

Fig. 26-7 The ice bag is filled $\frac{1}{2}$ to $\frac{2}{3}$ full with ice.

ICE BAGS, ICE COLLARS, AND DISPOSABLE COLD PACKS

An ice bag and ice collar are dry cold applications. Ice collars are applied to the neck. The bag or collar is filled with crushed ice. Then it is placed in a cover. If the cover becomes moist, it is removed and a dry one applied.

Commercial ice bags are kept frozen until needed. They are refrozen for reuse. Covers are also needed with ice collars or commercial ice bags.

Disposable cold packs are used once and discarded. They come in many sizes. Some have an outer covering allowing direct application to the skin. Otherwise a cover is used. *(See Focus on Home Care box.)*

Focus On... HOME CARE

Disposable ice packs are common in home settings. They are kept in the freezer until needed. A bag of frozen peas or corn is useful as an ice bag. So are plastic bags. After filling the bag with ice, close the bag securely to prevent leaks. Then wrap the pack, bag of peas or corn, or plastic bag in a towel, dish cloth, or pillowcase.

Applying an Ice Bag, Ice Collar, or Disposable Cold Pack

QUALITY OF LIFE

Remember to:
- Knock before entering the person's room
- Address the person by name
- Introduce yourself by name and title

Pre-Procedure

1 Explain the procedure to the person.
2 Wash your hands.
3 Collect a disposable cold pack or the following:
- Ice bag or collar
- Crushed ice
- Flannel cover, towel, or pillowcase
- Paper towels
4 Apply an ice bag or collar:
  a Fill the ice bag with water. Put in the stopper. Turn the bag upside down to check for leaks.
  b Empty the bag.
  c Fill the bag $\frac{1}{2}$ to $\frac{2}{3}$ full with crushed ice or ice chips (Fig. 26-7).

  d Remove excess air. Bend, twist, or squeeze the bag; or press it against a firm surface.
  e Place the cap or stopper on securely.
  f Dry the bag with the paper towels.
  g Place the bag in the cover.
5 Apply a disposable cold pack:
  a Squeeze, knead, or strike the cold pack as directed by the manufacturer. This releases cold.
  b Place the bag in the cover.
6 Identify the person. Check the ID bracelet against the assignment sheet.

Procedure

7 Provide for privacy.
8 Apply the ice bag. Secure it in place with ties, tape, or rolled gauze. Note the time.
9 Place the signal light within reach. Raise or lower bed rails. Follow the care plan.
10 Check the skin every 10 minutes. Check for

blisters; pale, white, or gray skin; cyanosis; and shivering. Ask about numbness, pain, or burning. Remove the bag if any occur. Tell the nurse immediately.
11 Remove the bag after 20 minutes or as directed by the nurse.

Post-Procedure

12 Follow steps 16 through 23 in *Applying Hot Compresses.*

► COLD COMPRESSES

Applying a cold compress is like applying a hot compress. The cold compress is a moist application. Moist cold compresses are left in place no longer than 20 minutes.

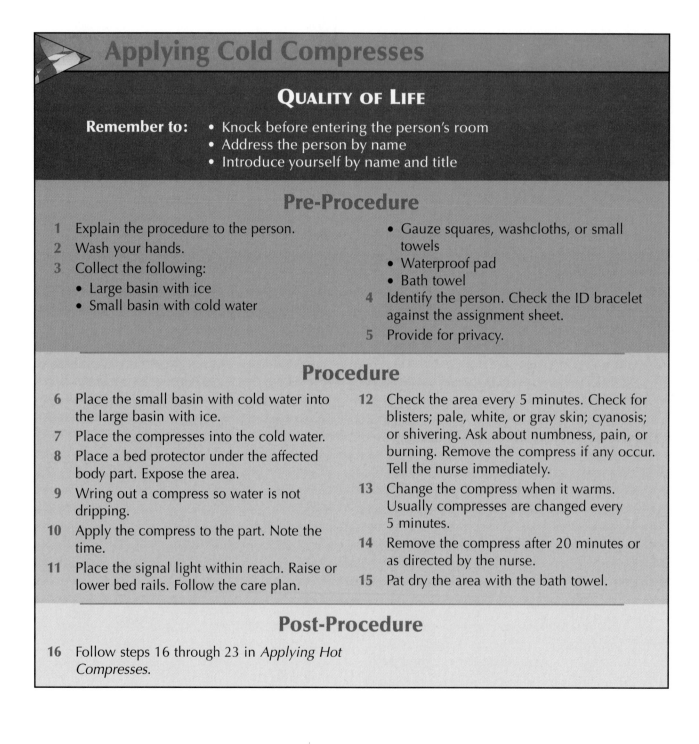

► Applying Cold Compresses

QUALITY OF LIFE

Remember to:
- Knock before entering the person's room
- Address the person by name
- Introduce yourself by name and title

Pre-Procedure

1 Explain the procedure to the person.
2 Wash your hands.
3 Collect the following:
   - Large basin with ice
   - Small basin with cold water
   - Gauze squares, washcloths, or small towels
   - Waterproof pad
   - Bath towel
4 Identify the person. Check the ID bracelet against the assignment sheet.
5 Provide for privacy.

Procedure

6 Place the small basin with cold water into the large basin with ice.
7 Place the compresses into the cold water.
8 Place a bed protector under the affected body part. Expose the area.
9 Wring out a compress so water is not dripping.
10 Apply the compress to the part. Note the time.
11 Place the signal light within reach. Raise or lower bed rails. Follow the care plan.
12 Check the area every 5 minutes. Check for blisters; pale, white, or gray skin; cyanosis; or shivering. Ask about numbness, pain, or burning. Remove the compress if any occur. Tell the nurse immediately.
13 Change the compress when it warms. Usually compresses are changed every 5 minutes.
14 Remove the compress after 20 minutes or as directed by the nurse.
15 Pat dry the area with the bath towel.

Post-Procedure

16 Follow steps 16 through 23 in *Applying Hot Compresses.*

COOLING AND WARMING BLANKETS

Hyperthermia is a body temperature *(thermia)* that is much higher *(hyper)* than the person's normal range. Usually body temperature is greater than 103° F (39.4° C). It is often called *heat stroke* when caused by hot weather temperatures. Other causes include illness, dehydration, and not being able to perspire. Lowering the person's body temperature is necessary. Otherwise death can occur. The doctor orders ice packs applied to the person's head, neck, underarms, and groin. Sometimes cooling blankets are used alone or with ice packs.

A cooling blanket is an electric device. Made of rubber or plastic, the device has tubes filled with distilled water or other fluid. The fluid circulates through the tubes. The blanket is placed on the person's bed and covered with a sheet. The blanket is turned on to the cool setting and allowed to cool. The person lies on the blanket. The person's vital signs are measured often. Rapid and excess cooling are prevented.

Hypothermia is a very low *(hypo)* body temperature *(thermia)*. Body temperature is less than 95° F (35° C). Cold weather temperatures are a common cause. The person must be warmed to prevent death. The person's treatment may include a warming blanket. A warming blanket is the same as a cooling blanket except that the temperature is turned to warm. Vital signs are checked often to prevent rapid or excess warming.

When used to cool the body, the device is called a *hypothermia blanket.* When used to warm the body, it is called a *hyperthermia blanket.* The device has warm and cool settings.

(See Focus on Children box.)

Focus On... CHILDREN

Infants and children are at great risk for rapid changes in body temperature. They are observed closely. Body temperature is measured according to the nurse's instructions. Always report the measurement immediately. Also report any changes in vital signs or in the child's condition.

Circle the BEST answer.

1. Local heat has the following effects *except*
   A. Pain relief
   B. Muscle relaxation
   C. Healing
   D. Decreased blood flow

2. Which is the greatest threat from heat applications?
   A. Infection
   B. Burns
   C. Chilling
   D. Pressure ulcers

3. Who has the greatest risk of complications from local heat applications?
   A. A 10-year-old boy
   B. A teenager
   C. A 40-year-old woman
   D. An older person

4. These statements are about moist heat applications. Which is *false?*
   A. Water is in contact with the skin.
   B. The effects of moist heat are less than with a dry heat application.
   C. Moist heat penetrates deeper than dry heat.
   D. The temperature of a moist heat application is lower than a dry heat application.

5. The temperature of a hot application is usually between
   A. 80° and 93° F
   B. 93° and 98° F
   C. 98° and 106° F
   D. 106° and 115° F

6. These statements are about sitz baths. Which is *false?*
   A. The perineal and rectal areas are immersed in warm or hot water for 20 minutes.
   B. The sitz bath lasts 25 to 30 minutes.
   C. They clean the perineum, relieve pain, increase circulation, or stimulate voiding.
   D. Weakness and fainting can occur.

7. Mrs. Parks is using an aquathermia pad. Which is *false?*
   A. The aquathermia pad is a dry heat application.
   B. The temperature of an aquathermia pad is usually set at 105° F.
   C. Electrical safety precautions are practiced.
   D. Pins secure the pad in place.

8. Local cold applications
   A. Reduce pain, prevent swelling, and decrease circulation
   B. Dilate blood vessels
   C. Prevent the spread of microbes
   D. All of the above

9. Which is *not* a complication of local cold applications?
   A. Pain
   B. Burns and blisters
   C. Cyanosis
   D. Infection

10. Before applying an ice bag
    A. Place the bag in a freezer
    B. Measure the temperature of the bag
    C. Place the bag in a cover
    D. Ask the person to void

11. Moist cold compresses are left in place no longer than
    A. 20 minutes
    B. 30 minutes
    C. 45 minutes
    D. 60 minutes

12. A cooling blanket is used for
    A. Hypothermia
    B. Hyperthermia
    C. Cyanosis
    D. Shivering

Answers to these questions are on p. 837.

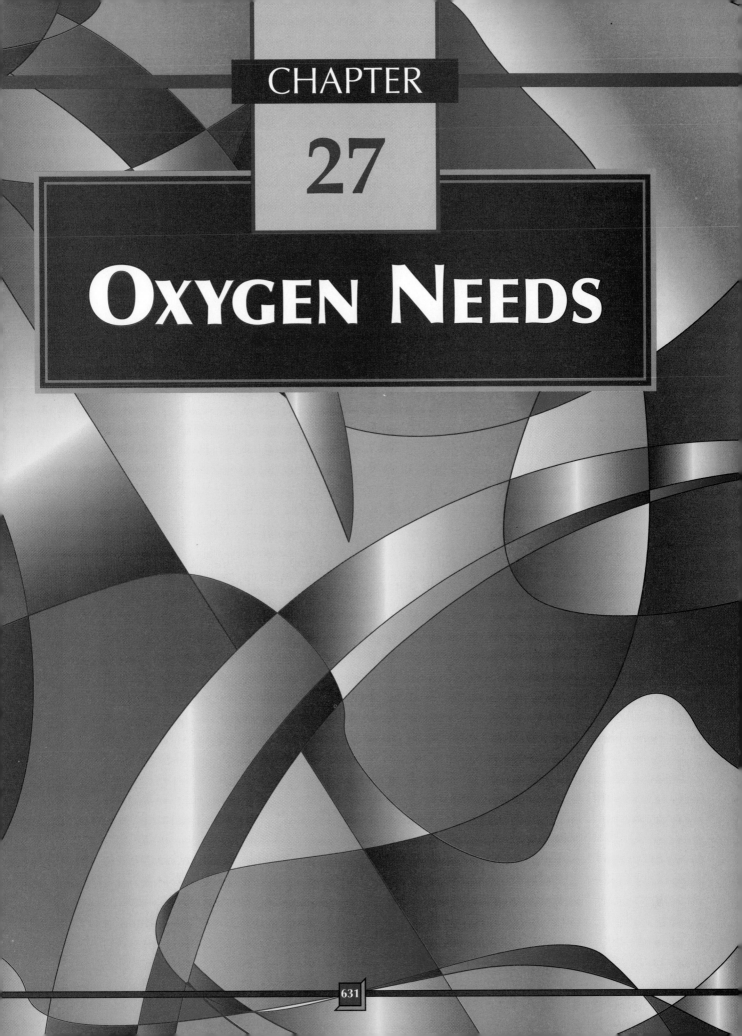

CHAPTER
27

OXYGEN NEEDS

Define the key terms listed in this chapter

Describe the factors affecting oxygen needs

Identify the signs and symptoms of hypoxia and altered respiratory function

Described the tests used to diagnose respiratory problems

Explain how positioning, coughing and deep breathing, and incentive spirometry promote oxygenation

Describe the devices used to administer oxygen

Explain how to safely assist with oxygen therapy

Explain how to assist in the care of persons with artificial airways

Describe the safety measures for oral suctioning

Explain how to assist in the care of persons on mechanical ventilation

Explain how to assist in the care of persons with chest tubes

Perform the procedures described in this chapter

KEY TERMS

allergy A sensitivity to a substance that causes the body to react with signs and symptoms

apnea The lack or absence *(a)* of breathing *(pnea)*

Biot's respirations Irregular breathing with periods of apnea; respirations may be slow and deep or rapid and shallow

bradypnea Slow *(brady)* breathing *(pnea)*; respirations are fewer than 10 per minute

Cheyne-Stokes Respirations gradually increase in rate and depth and then become shallow and slow; breathing may stop *(apnea)* for 10 to 20 seconds

dyspnea Difficult, labored, or painful *(dys)* breathing *(pnea)*

hemoptysis Bloody *(hemo)* sputum *(ptysis* meaning "to spit")

hemothorax The collection of blood *(hemo)* in the pleural space *(thorax)*

hyperventilation Respirations that are rapid *(hyper)* and deeper than normal

hypoventilation Respirations that are slow *(hypo)*, shallow, and sometimes irregular

hypoxemia A reduced amount *(hypo)* of oxygen *(ox)* in the blood *(emia)*

hypoxia A deficiency *(hypo)* of oxygen in the cells *(oxia)*

intubation The process of inserting an artificial airway

Kussmaul's respirations Very deep and rapid respirations; a sign of diabetic coma

mechanical ventilation Using a machine to move air into and out of the lungs

orthopnea Being able to breathe *(pnea)* deeply and comfortably only while sitting or standing *(ortho)*

orthopneic position Sitting up in bed *(ortho)* and leaning forward over the bedside table

oxygen concentration The amount of hemoglobin that contains oxygen (O_2)

pleural effusion The escape and collection of fluid *(effusion)* in the pleural space

pneumothorax The collection of air *(pneumo)* in the pleural space *(thorax)*

pollutant A harmful chemical or substance in the air or water

respiratory arrest Breathing stops

respiratory depression Slow, weak respirations that occur at a rate of fewer than 12 per minute; respirations are not deep enough to bring enough air into the lungs

sputum Expectorated mucus

suction The process of withdrawing or sucking up fluid (secretions)

tachypnea Rapid *(tachy)* breathing *(pnea)*; respirations are usually more than 24 per minute

Oxygen (O_2) is a tasteless, odorless, and colorless gas. It is a basic need and is necessary for survival. Death occurs within minutes if a person stops breathing. Serious illnesses occur without enough oxygen. Illness, surgery, and injuries affect the amount of oxygen in the blood and cells. Often you will assist nurses in giving care to persons with oxygen needs. You need to know how to give safe and effective care. See Box 27-1 for a review of the respiratory system.

FACTORS AFFECTING OXYGEN NEEDS

The respiratory and cardiovascular systems must function properly for cells to get enough oxygen. Any disease, injury, or surgery involving these systems affects the body's ability to take in oxygen and deliver it to the cells. Each body system depends on the other. Altered function of any system (for example, the nervous, musculoskeletal, or urinary system) affects the body's ability to meet its oxygen needs. Major factors affecting oxygen needs are:

- *Respiratory system status*—Structures must be intact and functioning. The airway must be open (patent). Alveoli must exchange O_2 and carbon dioxide (CO_2).
- *Cardiovascular system function*—Blood must flow freely to and from the heart. Narrowed vessels affect the delivery of oxygen-rich blood to the cells and blood return to the heart. Capillaries and cells must exchange O_2 and CO_2.
- *Red blood cell count*—The blood must have enough red blood cells (RBCs). RBCs contain hemoglobin, which picks up oxygen in the lungs and carries it to the cells. The bone marrow must produce enough RBCs. Poor diet, chemotherapy, and leukemia affect bone marrow function. Blood loss also reduces the number of RBCs.
- *Intact nervous system*—Nervous system diseases and injuries can affect respiratory muscle function. Breathing may be difficult or impossible. Brain damage affects respiratory rate, rhythm, and depth. Narcotics and depressant drugs are chemicals that affect the brain. They slow respirations. The amount of O_2 and CO_2 in the blood also affects brain function. Respirations increase when O_2 is lacking. The body tries to bring in more oxygen. Respirations also increase when CO_2 increases. The body tries to get rid of CO_2.
- *Aging*—Respiratory muscles weaken, and lung tissue becomes less elastic. Strength for coughing decreases. Coughing and removing secretions from the upper airway are important. Otherwise, upper respiratory tract infections can lead to *pneumonia* (inflammation of the lung). Older persons are at risk for respiratory complications after surgery.

Box 27-1	The Respiratory System: Review of Structure and Function

Oxygen is needed for survival. Every cell needs oxygen. The respiratory system brings oxygen into the lungs and eliminates carbon dioxide. The process of supplying the cells with oxygen and removing carbon dioxide from them is called *respiration*. Respiration involves *inhalation* (breathing in) and *exhalation* (breathing out). The terms *inspiration* (breathing in) and *expiration* (breathing out) also are used. The respiratory system is shown in Figure 27-1 on p. 634.

Air enters the body through the *nose*. The air then passes into the *pharynx* (throat), a tube-shaped passageway for both air and food. Air passes from the pharynx into the *larynx* (the voice box). Air passes from the larynx into the *trachea* (the windpipe). The trachea divides at its lower end into the *right bronchus* and *left bronchus*. Each bronchus enters a lung. On entering the lungs, the bronchi further divide several times into smaller branches called *bronchioles*. Eventually the bronchioles subdivide and end in tiny one-cell air sacs called *alveoli*. They are supplied by capillaries. Oxygen and carbon dioxide are exchanged between the alveoli and capillaries. Blood in the capillaries picks up oxygen from the alveoli. Then the blood is returned to the left side of the heart and pumped to the rest of the body. Alveoli pick up carbon dioxide from the capillaries for exhalation.

Each lung is divided into lobes. The right lung has three lobes; the left lung has two. The lungs are separated from the abdominal cavity by a muscle called the *diaphragm*. A bony framework consisting of the ribs, sternum, and vertebrae protects the lungs.

- *Exercise*—Oxygen needs increase with exercise. Normally, respiratory rate and depth increase to bring enough O_2 into the lungs. Persons with heart and respiratory diseases may have enough oxygen at rest. However, even slight activity can increase their oxygen needs. Their bodies may not be able to bring in oxygen and to deliver it to cells.
- *Fever*—Oxygen needs increase. As with exercise, respiratory rate and depth must increase to meet the body's needs.
- *Pain*—Pain increases the need for oxygen. Respirations increase to meet this need. However, chest and abdominal injuries and surgeries often involve the respiratory muscles. This interferes with breathing in and out.

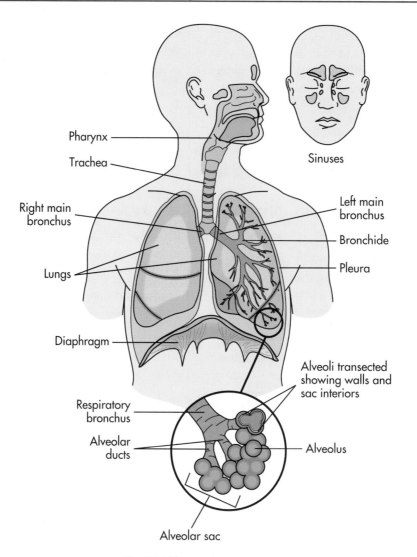

Pharynx
Trachea
Right main bronchus
Lungs
Diaphragm
Sinuses
Left main bronchus
Bronchide
Pleura
Alveoli transected showing walls and sac interiors
Respiratory bronchus
Alveolar ducts
Alveolus
Alveolar sac

Fig. 27-1 The respiratory system.

- *Medications*—Some drugs depress the respiratory center in the brain. **Respiratory depression** is slow, weak respirations at a rate of fewer than 12 per minute. Respirations are too shallow to bring enough air into the lungs. **Respiratory arrest** is when breathing stops. Narcotics such as morphine and Demerol can have these effects. (The word narcotic comes from the Greek word *narkoun.* It means stupor or to be numb.) These drugs are given in safe amounts for severe pain. Substance abusers are at risk for respiratory depression and respiratory arrest from overdoses of narcotics and depressants. Narcotics include opium, heroin, and methadone. Depressant drugs include barbiturates (Nembutal, phenobarbital, secobarbital, Tuinal, and others) and the benzodiazepines (Dalmane, diazepam, Halcion, Librium, Tranxene, Valium, Xanax, and others).

- *Smoking*—Smoking causes lung cancer and chronic obstructive pulmonary disease (COPD). It is a risk factor for coronary artery disease.

- *Allergies*—An **allergy** is a sensitivity to a substance that causes the body to react with signs and symptoms. Respiratory signs and symptoms include runny nose, wheezing, and congestion. Mucous membranes in the upper airway swell. With severe swelling, the airway closes. Shock and death are risks. Pollens, dust, foods, drugs, and cigarette smoke often cause allergies. Persons with allergies are at risk for chronic bronchitis and asthma.

- *Pollutant exposure*—A **pollutant** is a harmful chemical or substance in the air or water. Dust, fumes, toxins, asbestos, coal dust, and sawdust are some air pollutants. They damage the lungs. Pollutant exposure occurs in home, work, and community settings.

- *Nutrition*—Good nutrition is needed for red blood cell production. RBCs live about 3 or 4 months. New ones must replace those that die off. The body needs iron and vitamins (vitamin B_{12}, vitamin C, and folic acid) to produce RBCs.

- *Substance abuse*—Alcohol depresses the brain. Excessive amounts reduce the cough reflex and increase the risk of aspiration. Obstructed airway and pneumonia are risks from aspiration. Respiratory depression and respiratory arrest are risks when narcotics and depressant drugs are abused.

ALTERED RESPIRATORY FUNCTION

Respiratory system function involves three processes. Air moves into and out of the lungs. Oxygen and carbon dioxide are exchanged at the alveoli. The blood transports O_2 to the cells and removes CO_2 from them. Respiratory function is altered if even one process is affected. (See Box 27-1.)

HYPOXIA

Hypoxia is a deficiency *(hypo)* of oxygen in the cells *(oxia)*. Cells do not receive enough oxygen. Therefore they do not function properly. Hypoxia is caused by any illness, disease, injury, or surgery affecting respiratory function. The brain is very sensitive to inadequate oxygen. Restlessness is an early sign of hypoxia. So are dizziness and disorientation. Report signs and symptoms of hypoxia to the nurse immediately (Box 27-2).

Hypoxia is life threatening. The heart, brain, and other organs must receive enough oxygen to function. Oxygen is given, and treatment is directed at the cause of the hypoxia.

ABNORMAL RESPIRATIONS

Normal respirations occur between 12 and 20 times per minute in the adult. Infants and children have faster rates. Respirations are normally quiet, effortless, and regular. Both sides of the chest rise and fall equally. The following breathing patterns are abnormal:

- **Tachypnea**—rapid *(tachy)* breathing *(pnea)*. Respirations are usually more than 24 per minute. Fever, exercise, pain, pregnancy, airway obstruction, and hypoxemia are common causes. **Hypoxemia** is a reduced amount *(hypo)* of oxygen *(ox)* in the blood *(emia)*.
- **Bradypnea**—slow *(brady)* breathing *(pnea)*. Respirations are fewer than 10 per minute. Bradypnea is seen with drug overdoses and central nervous system disorders.
- **Apnea**—the lack or absence *(a)* of breathing *(pnea)*. It occurs in cardiac arrest and respiratory arrest. Sleep apnea and periodic apnea of newborns are other types of apnea.
- **Hypoventilation**—respirations that are slow *(hypo)*, shallow, and sometimes irregular. Lung disorders affecting the alveoli are common causes. Pneumonia is an example. Other causes include obesity, airway obstruction, drug side effects, and nervous system and musculoskeletal disorders affecting the respiratory muscles.

Box 27-2	**Signs and Symptoms of Hypoxia**

- Restlessness
- Dizziness
- Disorientation
- Confusion
- Behavior and personality changes
- Difficulty concentrating and following directions
- Apprehension
- Anxiety
- Fatigue
- Agitation
- Increased pulse rate
- Increased rate and depth of respirations
- Sitting position, often leaning forward
- Cyanosis (bluish color to the skin, lips, mucous membranes, and nail beds)
- Dyspnea

- **Hyperventilation**—respirations that are rapid *(hyper)* and deeper than normal. Its many causes include asthma, emphysema, infection, fever, central nervous system disorders, hypoxia, anxiety, pain, and some drugs.
- **Dyspnea**—difficult, labored, or painful *(dys)* breathing *(pnea)*. Heart disease, exercise, and anxiety are common causes.
- **Cheyne-Stokes**—respirations gradually increase in rate and depth and then become shallow and slow. Breathing may stop (apnea) for 10 to 20 seconds. Drug overdose, heart failure, renal failure, and brain disorders are common causes. These respirations are common when death is near.
- **Orthopnea**—breathing *(pnea)* deeply and comfortably only while sitting or standing *(ortho)*. Common causes include emphysema, asthma, pneumonia, angina pectoris, and other heart and respiratory disorders.
- **Biot's respirations**—irregular breathing with periods of apnea. Respirations are slow and deep or rapid and shallow. They occur with central nervous system disorders.
- **Kussmaul's respirations**—very deep and rapid respirations. They are a sign of diabetic coma.

ASSISTING WITH ASSESSMENT AND DIAGNOSTIC TESTING

Altered respiratory function may be an acute or chronic problem. Doctors and nurses are always alert for altered respiratory function. Report your observations to the nurse promptly and accurately (Box 27-3, p. 636). Quick action is necessary to meet the person's oxygen needs. Measures are taken to correct the situation and prevent the problem from getting worse.

Box 27-3   Signs and Symptoms of Altered Respiratory Function

- Signs and symptoms of hypoxia (see Box 27-2)
- Any abnormal breathing pattern
- Complaints of shortness of breath or being "winded" or "short-winded"
- Cough (note frequency and time of day)
  - Dry and hacking
  - Harsh and barking
  - Productive (produces sputum) or nonproductive
- Sputum
  - Color—clear, white, yellow, green, brown, or red
  - Odor—none or foul odor
  - Consistency—thick, watery, or frothy (with bubbles or foam)
  - **Hemoptysis**—bloody *(hemo)* sputum *(ptysis* meaning "to spit"); note if the sputum is bright red, dark red, blood tinged, or streaked with blood
- Noisy respirations
  - Wheezing
  - Wet-sounding respirations
  - Crowing sounds
- Chest pain
  - Note location
  - Constant or intermittent (comes and goes)
  - Person's description (stabbing, knifelike, aching)
  - What makes it worse (movement, coughing, yawning, sneezing, sighing, deep breathing)
- Cyanosis
  - Skin
  - Mucous membranes
  - Lips
  - Nail beds
- Changes in vital signs
- Body position
  - Sitting upright
  - Leaning forward or hunched over a table

The doctor orders tests to determine the cause of altered respiratory function. The following tests are common. You are likely to assist with pulse oximetry and in collecting sputum specimens.

- *Chest x-ray (CXR)*—An x-ray is taken of the chest. It is used to evaluate changes in the lungs. All clothing and jewelry from the waist to the neck are removed. The person wears a hospital gown.
- *Lung scan*—The lungs are scanned to see what areas are not getting air or blood. The person inhales radioactive gas and is injected with a radioisotope. *Radioactive* means to give off radiation. A *radioisotope* is an element that gives off radiation. Lung tissue getting air and blood flow "take up" the radioactive substances. A scanner senses areas

with radioactive substances. As when having a chest x-ray, the person removes all clothing and jewelry from the waist to the neck. A hospital gown is worn.

- *Bronchoscopy*—A scope *(scopy)* is passed into the trachea and bronchi *(broncho)*. The doctor inspects the larynx, trachea, and bronchi for bleeding and tumors. The doctor can take tissue samples (biopsy) or remove mucus plugs and foreign objects. The person is NPO 6 to 8 hours before the procedure. This reduces the danger of vomiting and aspiration. A local or general anesthetic is given. After the procedure, the person is NPO and watched carefully until the gag and swallow reflexes return. They usually return in about 2 hours. Preoperative and postoperative care are given as directed by the RN.
- *Thoracentesis*—The pleura *(thora)* is punctured, and air or fluid is aspirated *(centesis)* from it. The doctor inserts a needle through the chest wall into the pleural sac. Injury or disease can cause the pleural sac to fill with air, blood, or fluid. This affects respiratory function. The procedure is done also to remove fluid for laboratory study or to inject anticancer drugs into the pleural sac. The procedure takes a few minutes. Vital signs are taken before a local anesthetic is given. The person sits up and leans forward and is asked not to talk, cough, or move suddenly (Fig. 27-2). Postprocedure care involves applying a dressing to the puncture site and taking vital signs. A chest x-ray is taken to check for lung damage. The person is checked often for shortness of breath, dyspnea, cough, sputum, chest pain, cyanosis, vital sign changes, and other respiratory signs and symptoms.
- *Pulmonary function tests*—Tests measure the amount of air moving into and out of the lungs (volume) and how much air the lungs can hold (capacity). The person takes as deep a breath as possible. Using a mouthpiece, the person blows into a machine (Fig. 27-3). The tests are used to evaluate persons at risk for lung diseases or postoperative pulmonary complications. They also are used to measure the progress of lung disease and its treatment. Fatigue is common after the tests. The person should rest after the procedure.
- *Arterial blood gases (ABGs)*—A radial or femoral artery is punctured to obtain arterial blood. Laboratory tests measure the amount of oxygen in the blood. Hemorrhage from the artery must be prevented. Pressure is applied to the artery for at least 5 minutes after the procedure. Pressure is applied longer if the person has blood clotting problems. The procedure is done by a specially trained nurse, respiratory therapist, or laboratory technician.

Fig. 27-2 The person is positioned for a thoracentesis. *(From Wilson SF, Thompson JM: Respiratory Disorders, St Louis, 1990, Mosby.)*

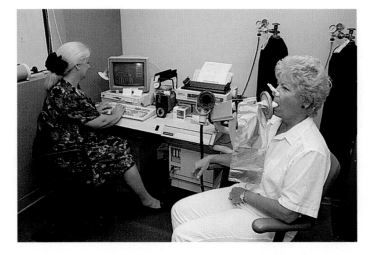

Fig. 27-3 Pulmonary function testing.

► **Pulse Oximetry.** Pulse oximetry measures *(metry)* oxygen *(oxi)* concentration in arterial blood. **Oxygen concentration** is the amount (percent) of hemoglobin that contains oxygen. The normal range is 95% to 100%. For example, if 97% of all the hemoglobin (100%) carries O_2, tissues get enough oxygen. If only 90% of the hemoglobin contains O_2, tissues do not get enough oxygen to function. Measurements are used to prevent hypoxia and to evaluate treatment.

A sensor (or probe) is attached to the person's finger, toe, earlobe, nose, or forehead (Fig. 27-4). Two light beams on one side of the sensor pass through the tissues. A detector on the other side measures the amount of light passing through the tissues. The oximeter receives this information and measures the oxygen concentration. The value and the person's pulse rate are displayed on the monitor. Oximeters have alarms. The alarms sound if oxygen concentration is low, the pulse is too fast or slow, or other problems occur.

A good sensor site is needed. The nurse tells you what site to use based on the person's condition. Swollen sites are avoided. So are sites with breaks in the skin. Finger and toe sites are avoided in persons with poor circulation.

Bright light, dark nail polish, and movements affect measurements. Place a towel over the sensor to block bright light. Remove nail polish, or use another site. Movements from shivering, seizures, or tremors affect finger sensors. The earlobe is a better site for these problems. Blood pressure cuffs affect blood flow. If using a finger site, do not measure blood pressure on that side.

Report and record measurements accurately. Use the abbreviation SpO_2 when recording the oxygen concentration value (S=saturation, p=pulse, O_2=oxygen). Also, report and record:

- The date and time
- What the person was doing at the time of the measurement
- Oxygen flow rate and the device used
- Reason for the measurement (routine or change in the person's condition)
- Other observations

Pulse oximetry does not lessen the need for good observations. The person's condition can change rapidly. You assist the nurse in observing for signs and symptoms of hypoxia.

(See Focus on Children box, Focus on Older Persons box, and Focus on Home Care box.)

Fig. 27-4 A, A pulse oximetry sensor is attached to a person's finger. **B,** The sensor is attached to an infant's great toe. *(B from Wong DL:* Whaley & Wong's nursing care of infants and children, *ed 6, St Louis, 1999, Mosby.)*

Ⓞ **Focus On... CHILDREN**

The sensor is attached to the sole of a foot, palm of the hand, finger, toe, or earlobe (see Fig. 27-4, B). If the child moves a lot, the earlobe is a better site.

Ⓞ **Focus On... OLDER PERSONS**

Older persons often have poor circulation from aging or vascular disease. Blood flow to the toe or finger may be poor. Use the ear, nose, or forehead site.

Ⓞ **Focus On... HOME CARE**

Small, hand-held oximetry units are available for home use. Instead of constant monitoring, oxygen concentration is often measured with vital signs. Because it is portable and used for many patients, you must make sure the pulse oximeter is accurate. After applying the sensor, check the person's pulse (radial or apical) and compare it with the displayed pulse. The pulse rates should be the same.

Using a Pulse Oximeter

QUALITY OF LIFE

Remember to:
- Knock before entering the person's room
- Address the person by name
- Introduce yourself by name and title

Pre-Procedure

1 Review the procedure with the nurse.
2 Ask the nurse what site to use.
3 Explain the procedure to the person.
4 Collect the following:
   a Oximeter and sensor
   b Nail polish remover
   c Cotton balls
   d SpO$_2$ flow sheet
   e Tape
   f Towel
5 Identify the person. Check the ID bracelet against the assignment sheet.
6 Provide for privacy.

Procedure

7 Provide for comfort.
8 Remove nail polish using a cotton ball. (If a toe site is used, remove any nail polish).
9 Dry the site with a towel.
10 Clip or tape the sensor to the site.
11 Turn on the oximeter.
12 Check the person's pulse (apical or radial), and compare it with the pulse on the display. The pulses should be equal. Tell the nurse if the pulses are not equal.
13 Read the SpO$_2$ on the display. Note the value on the flow sheet.
14 Leave the sensor in place for continuous monitoring. Otherwise, turn off the oximeter and remove the sensor.

Post-Procedure

15 Provide for comfort.
16 Place the signal light within the person's reach.
17 Raise or lower bed rails. Follow the care plan.
18 Unscreen the person.
19 Return the pulse oximeter to its proper place if continuous monitoring is not ordered.
20 Wash your hands.
21 Report the SpO$_2$ and your other observations to the nurse.

▶ **Collecting Sputum Specimens.** Respiratory disorders cause the lungs, bronchi, and trachea to secrete mucus. The mucus is called **sputum** when expectorated (expelled) through the mouth. Sputum is different from saliva. Saliva is a thin, clear liquid produced by the salivary glands in the mouth. Saliva is often called "spit."

Sputum specimens are studied for blood, microbes, and abnormal cells. The person coughs up sputum from the bronchi and trachea. This is often painful and difficult. Specimen collection is easier in the early morning when secretions are coughed up upon awakening. The person rinses the mouth with water. Rinsing decreases saliva and removes food particles. Mouthwash is not used before the procedure. It destroys some of the microbes in the mouth.

Collecting a sputum specimen can embarrass the person. Coughing and expectorating sounds can upset or nauseate other persons nearby. Also, sputum is unpleasant to look at. For these reasons, privacy is important. The specimen container is covered and placed in a bag. Some agencies use sputum containers that conceal the contents. Always follow Standard Precautions and the Bloodborne Pathogen Standard when collecting a sputum specimen.

(See Focus on Children box and Focus on Older Persons box.)

Focus On... CHILDREN

Breathing treatments and suctioning are often needed to produce a sputum specimen in infants and small children. The RN or respiratory therapist gives the breathing treatment. The nurse suctions the trachea for the sputum specimen. The infant or child is likely to be uncooperative during suctioning. You can assist by holding the child's head and arms still.

Focus On... OLDER PERSONS

Older persons may not have the strength to cough up sputum. Coughing is easier after postural drainage. Postural drainage involves draining secretions by gravity. Gravity causes fluids to flow down. Different positions are used depending on what part of the lungs to drain (Fig. 27-5). The nurse or respiratory therapist is responsible for postural drainage.

Fig. 27-5 Some positions used for postural drainage. **A,** Draining the right upper lobe. **B,** Draining the right middle lobe. **C,** Draining the right lower lobe. *(From Potter PA, Perry AG: Fundamentals of nursing: concepts, process, and practice, ed 4, St Louis, 1997, Mosby.)*

Fig. 27-6 The person expectorates into the center of the specimen container.

Collecting a Sputum Specimen

QUALITY OF LIFE

Remember to:
- Knock before entering the person's room
- Address the person by name
- Introduce yourself by name and title

Pre-Procedure

1 Explain the procedure to the person.
2 Wash your hands.
3 Collect the following:
   - Sputum specimen container
   - Tissues
   - Label
   - Laboratory requisition
   - Disposable bag
   - Gloves

Procedure

4 Label the container.
5 Identify the person. Check the ID bracelet against the requisition slip.
6 Provide for privacy. If able, the person goes into the bathroom to obtain the specimen.
7 Ask the person to rinse the mouth out with clear water.
7 Put on the gloves.
9 Have the person hold the container. Only the outside of the container is touched.
10 Ask the person to cover the mouth and nose with tissues when coughing.

11 Ask him or her to take 2 or 3 deep breaths and cough up the sputum.
12 Have the person expectorate directly into the container (Fig. 27-6). Sputum should not touch the outside of the container.
13 Collect 1 to 2 tablespoons of sputum unless told to collect more.
14 Put the lid on the container immediately.
15 Place the container in the bag. Attach the requisition to the bag.
16 Remove the gloves.

Post-Procedure

17 Provide for comfort.
18 Place the signal light within reach.
19 Unscreen the person.
20 Wash your hands.
21 Take the bag to the laboratory.
22 Wash your hands.

23 Report the following to the nurse:
   - The time the specimen was collected and taken to the laboratory
   - The amount of sputum collected
   - How easily the person raised the sputum
   - The consistency and appearance of sputum (see Box 27-3)
   - Any other observations

PROMOTING OXYGENATION

For the body to get enough oxygen, air must move deeply into the lungs. Air must reach the alveoli for the exchange of oxygen and carbon dioxide with the blood. Disease and injury can prevent air from reaching the alveoli. Secretions can congest lung tissue and the airway. Pain, immobility, and narcotics interfere with deep breathing and coughing up secretions. Therefore secretions collect in the respiratory system. They interfere with air movement and alveolar function in the affected part of the lung. Secretions also provide an environment for microbes. Infection is a threat.

The RN plans measures to meet the person's oxygen needs. The following measures are often included in nursing care plans.

POSITIONING

Breathing is usually easier in semi-Fowler's and Fowler's position. Persons with difficulty breathing often prefer to sit up in bed and lean forward over the overbed table. This is called the **orthopneic position.** *Ortho* means sitting or standing; *pnea* means breathing. You can increase the person's comfort by placing a pillow on the overbed table (Fig. 27-7).

Frequent position changes are important. Unless the doctor limits positioning, the person must not lie on one side for a long time. This prevents lung expansion on that side and allows secretions to pool. Position changes are usually done at least every 2 hours. You must follow the person's care plan.

► COUGHING AND DEEP BREATHING

Mucus is removed by coughing. Deep breathing promotes air movement into most parts of the lungs. Coughing and deep breathing exercises are helpful for persons with respiratory disorders. They are routinely done after surgery and are important for persons on bedrest. The exercises are painful after injury or surgery. The person may be afraid of breaking open an incision while coughing.

Coughing and deep breathing help prevent pneumonia and atelectasis. *Atelectasis* is the collapse of a portion of the lung. It occurs when mucus collects in the airway. Air cannot get to a part of the lung, and the lung collapses.

The frequency of coughing and deep breathing varies. Some doctors order the exercises every 1 or 2 hours while the person is awake. Others want them done 4 times a day. The nurse tells you when coughing and deep breathing are done. You are told how many deep breaths and coughs the person should do. You must follow the person's care plan.

Fig. 27-7 The person is in the orthopneic position. Note that a pillow is on the overbed table for the person's comfort.

Assisting With Coughing and Deep Breathing Exercises

QUALITY OF LIFE

Remember to:
- Knock before entering the person's room
- Address the person by name
- Introduce yourself by name and title

Pre-Procedure

1 Explain the procedure to the person.

2 Identify the person. Check the ID bracelet against the assignment sheet.

3 Provide for privacy.

Procedure

4 Help the person to a comfortable sitting position: dangling, semi-Fowler's, or Fowler's.

5 Have the person deep breathe:

 a Have the person place the hands over the rib cage (Fig. 27-8, p. 644).

 b Ask the person to exhale. Explain that when exhaling, the ribs should move as far down as possible.

 c Have the person take a deep breath. It should be as deep as possible. Remind the person to inhale through the nose.

 d Ask the person to hold the breath for 3 seconds.

 e Ask the person to exhale slowly through pursed lips (Fig. 27-9, p. 644). The person should exhale until the ribs move as far down as possible.

 f Repeat this step 4 more times.

6 Ask the person to cough:

 a Have the person interlace the fingers over the incision (Fig. 27-10, A, p. 644). The person can also hold a small pillow or folded towel over the incision (Fig. 27-10, B, p. 644).

 b Have the person take in a deep breath as in step 5.

 c Ask the person to cough strongly twice with the mouth open.

Post-Procedure

7 Provide for comfort.

8 Raise or lower bed rails. Follow the care plan.

9 Place the signal light within reach.

10 Unscreen the person.

11 Report your observations to the nurse:
- The number of times the person coughed and deep breathed
- How the person tolerated the procedure

Fig. 27-8 The hands are over the rib cage for deep breathing.

Fig. 27-9 The person inhales through the nose and exhales through pursed lips during the deep-breathing exercise.

Fig. 27-10 The person supports an incision for the coughing exercise. **A,** Fingers are interlaced over the incision. **B,** A small pillow is held over the incision.

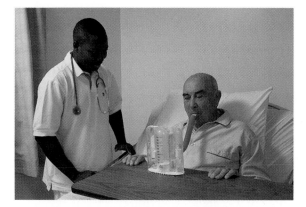

Fig. 27-11 The persons uses a spirometer.

INCENTIVE SPIROMETRY

Incentive means to give encouragement. A *spirometer* is a machine that measures the amount (volume) of air inhaled. Thus incentive spirometry involves encouraging the person to inhale until reaching a preset volume of air. Balls or bars in the spirometer allow the person to see the movement of air when inhaling (Fig. 27-11).

The spirometer is placed upright. The person exhales normally and then seals the lips around a mouthpiece. The person takes in a slow, deep breath until the balls rise to the desired height. The breath is held for 2 to 6 seconds to keep the balls floating. Then the person removes the mouthpiece and exhales slowly. The person may cough at this time. The nurse tells you how often the person needs incentive spirometry and how many breaths the person needs to take. The information also is in the care plan. Follow agency policy for cleaning and replacing disposable mouthpieces.

ASSISTING WITH OXYGEN THERAPY

Disease, injury, and surgery often interfere with breathing. The amount of oxygen in the blood may be less than normal (hypoxemia). If so, the doctor orders supplemental oxygen.

Oxygen is treated as a drug. The doctor orders the amount of oxygen to give and the device to use. The order also states if oxygen is given continuously or intermittently (periodically). *Continuous oxygen therapy* means that the oxygen is never stopped. That is, the administration of oxygen is not interrupted for any reason. *Intermittent oxygen therapy* is for symptom relief. Chest pain and exercise are common reasons for intermittent oxygen. The oxygen helps relieve chest pain. Persons with chronic respiratory diseases may have enough oxygen at rest. With mild exercise or activities of daily living, they become short of breath. Oxygen helps to relieve the shortness of breath.

Fig. 27-12 Wall oxygen outlet.

You are not responsible for administering oxygen. The nurse and respiratory therapist start and maintain oxygen therapy. You assist the nurse in providing safe care to persons receiving oxygen.

OXYGEN SOURCES

Oxygen is supplied through wall outlets, oxygen tanks, and oxygen concentrators. With the wall outlet (Fig. 27-12), O_2 is piped into each patient or resident unit. Each unit is connected to a centrally located oxygen supply.

The oxygen tank is portable. It is brought to the person's unit when the doctor orders oxygen therapy. Small tanks are used during emergencies and transfers. Some ambulatory persons need continuous oxygen. Portable tanks are used when walking (Fig. 27-13, p. 646). The gauge on the tank tell how much oxygen is left in the tank (Fig. 27-14, p. 646). Tell the nurse if the oxygen in the tank is low.

Oxygen concentrators (Fig. 27-15, p. 646) do not need an oxygen source (wall outlet or tank). The concentrator removes oxygen from the air. A power source is needed. If the concentrator is not portable, moving about is limited. The person stays close to the machine. A portable oxygen tank is needed in case of a power failure and for mobility.

Liquid oxygen systems also are used (Fig. 27-16, p. 464). A portable unit is filled from a stationary unit. The portable unit will last as long as 8 hours. A liquid content indicator tells you when the unit needs

Fig. 27-13 The person uses a portable oxygen tank during ambulation.

Fig. 27-14 The gauge shows the amount of oxygen remaining in the tank.

Fig. 27-15 Oxygen concentrator.

Fig. 27-16 Liquid oxygen system.

> ### Focus On... HOME CARE
>
> Oxygen tanks, oxygen concentrators, and liquid oxygen systems are used in home care. The source ordered depends on the person's needs. The source is supplied by a medical supply company. Keep the company's name and phone number near the telephone.
>
> The patient and family must practice safety measures where oxygen is used and stored. The safety measures to prevent fire are practiced (Box 27-4). Also, the oxygen source and oxygen tubing are kept away from open flames and heat sources. These include candles, stoves, heating ducts, radiators, heating pipes, space heaters, and kerosene heaters and lamps. Keep a fire extinguisher in the room. If a fire occurs, turn off the oxygen. Then get the person and other family members out of the home and call the fire department.

refilling. Tell the nurse if the liquid oxygen in the tank is low. The portable unit can be worn over the shoulder. This allows the person to be mobile. Liquid oxygen is very cold. If touched, it can cause the skin to freeze. Never tamper with the equipment. Doing so is unsafe and could damage the equipment. Follow agency policies and procedures and the manufacturer's instructions when working with liquid oxygen.

(See Focus on Home Care box.)

Box 27-4	Safety Rules for Fire and Using Oxygen

- Place "No Smoking" signs in the room and on the room door.
- Remove smoking materials from the room (cigarettes, cigars, pipes, matches, lighters).
- Remove materials from the room that ignite easily (alcohol, nail polish remover, oils, greases).
- Keep oxygen tanks away from heat sources.
- Turn off electrical items before unplugging them.
- Use electrical equipment that is in good repair (e.g., razor, radio, TV).
- Use only electrical equipment with three-prong plugs.
- Do not use materials that cause static electricity (wool and synthetic fabrics).

Fig. 27-18 Simple face mask.

Fig. 27-17 Nasal cannula.

Fig. 27-19 Partial-rebreathing face mask.

DEVICES USED TO ADMINISTER OXYGEN

The doctor orders the device used to administer oxygen. These devices are common:

- **Nasal cannula** (Fig. 27-17)—two prongs project from the tubing. The prongs are inserted a short distance into the nostrils. The prongs point downward. This prevents drying of the sinuses. An elastic headband or tubing brought behind the ears keeps the cannula in place. The person can eat and talk with a cannula in place. Nasal irritation occurs with tight prongs. Pressure on the ears is possible.
- **Simple face mask** (Fig. 27-18)—covers the nose and mouth. The mask has small holes in the sides. Carbon dioxide escapes during exhalation. Room air enters during inhalation.
- **Partial-rebreathing mask** (Fig. 27-19)—a reservoir bag is added to the simple face mask. The bag is for exhaled air. With inhalation, the person inhales oxygen and some of the exhaled air. Some room air also is inhaled. The bag should not totally deflate when the person inhales.

Fig. 27-20 Nonrebreathing face mask.

- **Nonrebreathing face mask** (Fig. 27-20)—prevents exhaled air from entering the reservoir bag. Exhaled air leaves through holes in the mask. When the person inhales, oxygen from the reservoir bag is inhaled. The bag must not totally collapse during exhalation.

Fig. 27-21 Venturi mask.

- **Venturi mask** (Fig. 27-21)—allows precise amounts of oxygen to be given. Color-coded adaptors indicate the amount of oxygen delivered.

Special care is needed when masks are used. Masks make talking difficult. Listen carefully to what the person is saying. Moisture can build up under masks. Keep the person's face clean and dry to help prevent irritation from the mask. Masks are removed for eating. Usually oxygen is administered by nasal cannula during meals.

OXYGEN FLOW RATES

The amount of oxygen given is called the *flow rate*. This is ordered by the doctor. The flow rate is measured in liters per minute (L/min). The flow rate is anywhere from 2 to 15 liters of oxygen per minute. The flowmeter (see Fig. 27-12) is set for the desired rate. This is done by the nurse or respiratory therapist.

The nurse tells you what the flow rate is for the person. This information also is found in the care plan. When giving care and checking patients and residents, always check the flow rate. Tell the nurse immediately if the flow rate is too high or too low. A nurse or respiratory therapists adjust the flow rate. Some states and agencies let assistive personnel adjust oxygen flow rates.

Fig. 27-22 Oxygen administration system with humidifier.

▶ PREPARING FOR OXYGEN ADMINISTRATION

The nurse may ask you to set up the oxygen administration system (Fig. 27-22). The nurse tells you the following:

- The person's name and room and bed number
- The oxygen administration device ordered
- If humidification was ordered

Oxygen is a dry gas. If not humidified (made moist), oxygen dries the airway's mucous membranes. Distilled water is added to the humidifier to create water vapor. Oxygen tubing is attached to the humidifier. Oxygen picks up water vapor as it flows into the system. Bubbling in the humidifier means water vapor is being produced. If humidification is not ordered, distilled water and the humidifier are not used.

Before performing this procedure, make sure that:

- Your state allows assistive personnel to perform the procedure.
- The procedure is in your job description.
- You have the necessary education and training.
- A nurse is available to answer questions and to supervise you.

Setting Up for Oxygen Administration

QUALITY OF LIFE

Remember to:
- Knock before entering the person's room
- Address the person by name
- Introduce yourself by name and title

Pre-Procedure

1 Review the doctor's orders with the nurse.
2 Wash your hands.
3 Collect the following:
- Oxygen administration device with connecting tubing
- Flowmeter
- Humidifier (if ordered)
- Distilled water (if using a humidifier)
4 Identify the person. Check the ID bracelet against the assignment sheet.
5 Explain to the person what you are going to do.

Procedure

6 Make sure the flowmeter is in the *OFF* position.
7 Attach the flowmeter to the wall outlet.
8 Fill the humidifier with distilled water.
9 Attach the humidifier to the bottom of the flowmeter.
10 Attach the oxygen administration device and connecting tubing to the humidifier. *Do not set the flowmeter or apply the oxygen administration device on the person.*

Post-Procedure

11 Discard packaging.
12 Make sure the cap is securely on the distilled water. Store it according to agency policy.
13 Provide for comfort.
14 Place the signal light within reach.
15 Tell the nurse that you completed the procedure. *The nurse will:*
a *Turn on the oxygen and set the flow rate*
b *Apply the oxygen administration device on the person*
16 Wash your hands.

OXYGEN SAFETY

Remember, you assist the nurse with oxygen therapy. You are not responsible for administering oxygen. You do not adjust the flow rate unless allowed by your state and agency. However, you must give safe care to persons receiving oxygen. Box 27-5 on p. 650 lists the rules for assisting with oxygen therapy. Also follow the rules in Box 27-4.

Box 27-5	Safety Rules for Oxygen Therapy

- Never remove the device (cannula, mask) used to administer oxygen.
- Make sure the oxygen administration device is secure but not tight.
- Check for signs of irritation from the device. Check behind the ears, under the nose (cannula), and around the face (mask).
- Never shut off oxygen flow from the wall outlet, tank, or oxygen concentrator.
- Do not adjust the flow rate unless allowed by your state and agency.
- Notify the nurse immediately if the flow rate is too high or too low.
- Make sure the humidifier is bubbling. Notify the nurse immediately if the humidifier is not bubbling.
- Tape connecting tubing to the person's gown. Tubing must be secured in place.
- Make sure there are no kinks in the tubing.
- Make sure the person is not lying on any part of the tubing.
- Report signs and symptoms of hypoxia, respiratory distress, or abnormal breathing patterns to the nurse immediately (see Boxes 27-2 and 27-3).
- Give oral hygiene as directed by the nurse. Follow the care plan.
- Make sure the device is clean and free of mucus.
- Maintain an adequate water level in the humidifier.

ARTIFICIAL AIRWAYS

Artificial airways keep the airway patent (open). They are used when:

- The airway is obstructed from disease, injury, secretions, or aspiration
- The person is semiconscious or unconscious
- The person is recovering from anesthesia
- The person needs mechanical ventilation

Intubation is the process of inserting an artificial airway. Usually plastic, disposable airways are used. They come in adult, pediatric, and infant sizes. The following airways are common:

- *Oropharyngeal airway*—is inserted through the mouth and into the pharynx (Fig. 27-23, *A*). A nurse or respiratory therapist can insert the airway.
- *Nasopharyngeal airway*—is inserted through a nostril and into the pharynx (Fig. 27-23, *B*). A nurse or respiratory therapist can insert the airway.
- *Endotracheal tube*—is inserted through the mouth or nose and into the trachea (Fig. 27- 23, *C*). A doctor or RN with special training intubates using a lighted scope. A balloon (called a *cuff*) at the end of the tube is inflated to keep the airway in place.

Fig. 27-23 Artificial airways. **A,** Oropharyngeal airway. **B,** Nasopharnygeal airway. **C,** Endotracheal tube. **D,** Tracheostomy tube.

- *Tracheostomy tube*—is inserted through a surgical incision *(ostomy)* into the trachea *(tracheal)* (Fig. 27-23, *D*). Some tracheostomy tubes have cuffs. The cuff is inflated to keep the tube in place. The tracheostomy is done by a doctor.

You assist the nurse in caring for persons with artificial airways. The person's vital signs are checked often. The person is observed for hypoxia and other respiratory signs and symptoms. If an airway comes out or is dislodged, tell the nurse immediately. The person needs frequent oral hygiene. The nurse tells you when and how to perform oral hygiene. This information also is in the care plan.

Talking is hard with oropharyngeal and nasopharyngeal airways. Persons with endotracheal tubes cannot speak. Some tracheostomy tubes allow the person to speak. Paper and pencils, Magic Slates, communication boards, and hand signals are ways to communiate.

Gagging and choking sensations are common with artificial airways. Imagine something in your mouth, nose, or throat. The person needs comforting and reassurance. Remind the person that the airway helps breathing. Use touch to show you care.

TRACHEOSTOMIES

Tracheostomies are temporary or permanent. They are temporary when the person requires mechanical ventilation. They are permanent when airway structures are surgically removed. Some cancers require removing airway structures. Sometimes a permanent tracheostomy is required when severe trauma injures the airway. *(See Focus on Children box.)*

Tracheostomy tubes are made of plastic or metal. A tracheostomy tube has three parts (Fig. 27-24): the outer tube, the inner tube, and the obturator. *Cannula* is another word for tube. The inner and outer tubes are often called the *inner* and *outer* cannulas.

The obturator has a rounded end. It is used to insert the outer cannula. After the outer cannula is inserted, the obturator is removed. (The obturator is placed within easy reach in case the tracheostomy tube falls out and needs to be reinserted. It is taped to the wall

Fig. 27-24 Parts of a tracheostomy tube.

or bedside stand.) The inner cannula is inserted and locked in place. The outer cannula is secured in place with ties around the person's neck or a Velcro collar. The inner cannula is removed for cleaning and mucus removal. This keeps the airway patent. The outer cannula is not removed.

Some plastic tracheostomy tubes do not have inner cannulas. These are used for persons who are suctioned often. With frequent suctioning, mucus does not stick to the cannula.

The cuffed tracheostomy tube provides a seal between the cannula and the trachea (see Fig. 27-23, *D*). This type is used with mechanical ventilation. The cuff prevents air from leaking around the tube. It also prevents aspiration. A nurse or respiratory therapist inflates and deflates the cuff.

Securing tracheostomy tubes in place is important. The tube must not come out (extubation). If not secured properly, the tube could come out with coughing or if pulled on. Damage to the airway is possible if the tube is loose and moves up and down in the trachea.

The tracheostomy tube must remain patent (open). Some persons can cough secretions up and out of the tracheostomy. Others require suctioning. *Call for the nurse if the person shows signs and symptoms of hypoxia or respiratory distress. Also call the nurse if the outer cannula comes out.*

Measures are needed to prevent aspiration. Nothing can enter the stoma. Otherwise the person can aspirate. The nurse teaches the person and family the following:

- Make sure dressings do not have loose gauze or lint.
- Keep the stoma or tube covered when outside. Wear a stoma cover, scarf, or shirt or blouse that buttons at the neck. The cover prevents dust, insects, and other small particles from entering the stoma.

- Take tub baths instead of showers. If showers are taken, wear a shower guard and use a hand-held nozzle. Direct water away from the stoma.
- Be careful when shampooing. Ask another person to help you.
- Cover the stoma when shaving.
- Do not swim. Water will enter the tube or stoma.
- Wear a medical alert bracelet. Also carry a medical alert ID card.

Tracheostomy Care. Tracheostomy care involves cleaning the inner cannula, cleaning the stoma, and applying clean ties or Velcro collar. Cleaning the inner cannula removes mucus. This keeps the airway patent. A clean stoma and clean ties or collar help prevent infection at the tracheostomy site. Cleaning the stoma also helps prevent skin breakdown.

Some inner cannulas are disposable. They are used once and then discarded. The inner cannula is not cleaned. A new one is inserted.

The nurse may ask you to assist with tracheostomy care. It may be done daily or every 8 to 12 hours. Tracheostomy care is done when there are excess secretions, the ties or collar is soiled, or the dressing is soiled or moist. When the ties are removed, you must hold the outer cannula in place. The ties or collar must be secure but not tight. A finger should slide under the ties or collar (Fig. 27-25). Standard Precautions and the Bloodborne Pathogen Standard are followed when assisting the nurse. *(See Focus on Children box.)*

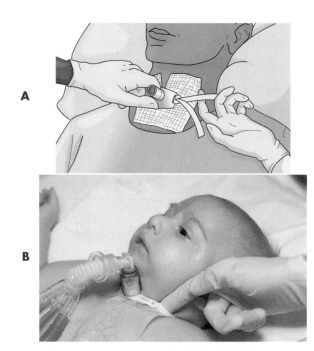

Fig. 27-25 A, A finger is inserted under the ties. **B,** For children, only a fingertip is inserted under the ties. *(B from Wong DL:* Whaley & Wong's nursing care of infants and children, *ed 6, St Louis, 1999, Mosby).*

Focus On... CHILDREN

As with adults, the ties must be secure but not tight. Only a fingertip should slide under the ties (see Fig. 27-25, B). Ties are too loose if you can slide your whole finger under them.

When assisting with tracheostomy care, you must hold the child still. Position the child's head so that the neck is slightly extended.

SUCTIONING THE AIRWAY

Injury and illness often cause secretions to collect in the upper airway. Removing the secretions is necessary so air can flow into and out of the airway. Retained secretions obstruct the airway. They provide an environment for microbes and interfere with oxygen and carbon dioxide exchange. Hypoxia occurs if secretions are not removed. Usually coughing removes the secretions. Sometimes the person cannot cough or the cough is too weak to remove secretions. Then suctioning is necessary.

Suction is the process of withdrawing or sucking up fluid (secretions). A tube is connected to a suction source (wall outlet or suction machine) at one end and to a suction catheter at the other end. The catheter is inserted into the airway. Secretions are withdrawn through the catheter.

SUCTIONING ROUTES

The nose, mouth, and pharynx make up the upper airway. The trachea and bronchi are the lower parts of the airway.

The *oropharyngeal* route involves suctioning the mouth *(oral)* and pharynx *(pharyngeal)*. The suction catheter is passed through the mouth and into the pharynx. The *nasopharyngeal* route involves suctioning the nose *(nasal)* and pharynx *(pharyngeal)*. The suction catheter is passed through the nose and into the pharynx. These routes are used for persons who cannot expectorate or swallow secretions after coughing.

Lower airway suctioning is done through an endotracheal tube or a tracheostomy tube.

SAFETY MEASURES

If not done correctly, suctioning can seriously harm the person. Suctioning removes oxygen from the airway. Therefore the person does not get a fresh supply of oxygen during suctioning. Hypoxia and life-threatening complications can arise from the respiratory, cardiovascular, and nervous systems. Cardiac arrest can occur. Infection and injury to the airway's mucous membranes also are possible. The nurse may ask you to assist with suctioning. Therefore you need to understand the principles and safety measures involved in safe suctioning. These are described in Box 27-6.

<table>
<tr><td>

Box 27-6

Principles and Safety Measures for Suctioning

- Review the procedure with the nurse. Know what the nurse expects you to do.
- Suctioning is done as needed *(prn)*. Coughing and signs and symptoms of respiratory distress signal the need for suctioning. The nurse tells you what signs to look for in each person. Suctioning is not done at scheduled intervals.
- Standard Precautions and the Bloodborne Pathogen Standard are followed. Remember, secretions can contain blood and are potentially infectious.
- The mouth is clean, not sterile. Microbes enter the mouth through breathing, eating, and drinking. Sterile technique is not required for oropharyngeal suctioning.
- Sterile technique is used when suctioning a tracheostomy (see Chapter 10).
- The nurse tells you what catheter size to collect. Airway injury can occur if the catheter is too large.
- Suction is not applied while inserting the catheter. When suction is applied, air is sucked out of the person's airway.
- The catheter is cleared with water or saline after removal.
- The catheter is inserted smoothly. This helps prevent injury to the mucous membranes.
- The suction catheter is passed (inserted) no more than 3 times. The risk of injury and hypoxia increases each time the suction catheter is passed.
- Check the person's pulse, respirations, and pulse oximeter measurement before, during, and after the procedure. Also observe the person's level of consciousness. Call for the nurse immediately if any of the following occur:
  - A drop in pulse rate or a pulse rate less than 60 beats per minute
  - Irregular cardiac rhythms
  - A drop or rise in blood pressure
  - Respiratory distress
  - A drop in the SpO_2

</td></tr>
</table>

OROPHARYNGEAL SUCTIONING

For oropharyngeal suctioning, one complete cycle involves inserting the catheter, suctioning, and removing the catheter. A suction cycle takes no more than 10 to 15 seconds to complete. (Hold your breath during the suction cycle. This helps you experience what the person feels during suctioning.)

Some people have large amounts of thick secretions. The Yankauer suction catheter often is used for these persons (Fig. 27-26). It is larger and stiffer than other suction catheters.

Hypoxia is a risk during suctioning. Remember, the person does not receive oxygen when the suction catheter is inserted. Also, suction removes air out of the airway. Therefore the person's lungs are hyperventilated before suctioning a tracheostomy. To *hyperventilate* means to give extra (hyper) breaths (ventilate). This is done with a manual resuscitation or Ambu bag (Fig. 27-27). The Ambu bag is attached to an oxygen source. Then the oxygen delivery device is removed from the tracheostomy tube. The Ambu bag is attached to the tracheostomy tube. The bag is compressed (squeezed) as the person inhales. Three to five breaths are given as directed by the nurse or respiratory therapist.

Fig. 27-26 The Yankauer suction catheter.

Fig. 27-27 The Ambu bag. Two hands are used to compress the bag.

Focus On... CHILDREN

Suctioning procedures may frighten children. They need clear explanations about the procedure. As with other procedures, you may need to hold the child still. This is done by controlling the child's head and arm movements.

Always make sure needed suction equipment and supplies are at the bedside. When the person needs suctioning, you do not have time to collect supplies from the supply area.

(See Focus on Children box.)

Remember, an oxygen source is attached to the Ambu bag. Oxygen is treated like a drug. Assistive personnel do not administer drugs. Therefore you need to check if your state and agency allow you to use an Ambu bag attached to an oxygen source.

Some agencies limit suctioning to 10 seconds. Others allow 10 to 15 seconds for the suction cycle (inserting the catheter, applying suction, and removing the catheter). *(See Focus on Children box.)*

MECHANICAL VENTILATION

Weak muscle effort, airway obstruction, and damaged lung tissue cause hypoxia. Central nervous system diseases and injuries can affect the respiratory center in the brain. Nerve damage can interfere with messages being sent between the lungs and the brain. Drug overdose can depress the brain. These and other respiratory problems are so severe that some people cannot breathe on their own. Or they cannot maintain enough oxygen in the blood. These persons often need mechanical ventilation. **Mechanical ventilation** is using a machine to move air into and out of the lungs (Fig. 27-28). Oxygen enters the lungs, and carbon dioxide leaves the lungs.

Persons on mechanical ventilation have artificial airways. Depending on the person's problems, an endotracheal tube or tracheostomy tube is used. You assist the nurse with the person's care.

Ventilators have alarms that warn when something is wrong. One alarm is for when the person gets disconnected from the ventilator. *When any alarm sounds, first check to see if the person's endotracheal tube or tracheostomy tube is attached to the ventilator. If it is disconnected, attach the tube to the ventilator.* Then notify the nurse immediately about the alarm. Do not reset alarms. Remember, the person is on a ventilator because of respiratory difficulties. The person can die if not connected to the ventilator.

Persons needing mechanical ventilation are seriously ill. They often have other problems and injuries. Their reactions to mechanical ventilation are many. Some are confused, disoriented, or unable to think clearly. Many are frightened by the machine and fear dying. Some feel relief when their bodies get enough oxygen. Many fear having to remain on the machine for life. Mechanical ventilation can be painful for those with chest injuries or chest surgery. Tubes and hoses restrict movement, adding to the person's discomfort.

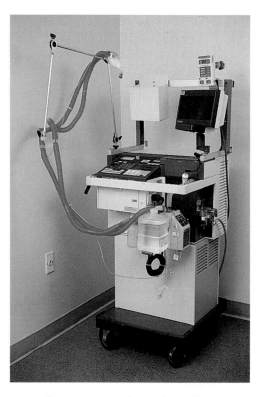

Fig. 27-28 A mechanical ventilator.

The nurse may ask you to assist with the person's care. Box 27-7 lists important aspects of the person's care. *(See Focus on Long-Term Care box and Focus on Home Care box.)*

| Box 27-7 | Care of Persons Receiving Mechanical Ventilation |

- Keep the signal light within the person's reach.
- Make sure there is enough slack on hoses and connecting tubing. They should not pull on the endotracheal or tracheostomy tube.
- Answer signal lights promptly. Remember, the person depends on others for basic needs.
- Explain who you are and what you are going to do whenever you enter the room.
- Orient the person to day, date, and time.
- Tell the nurse immediately if the person shows signs of respiratory distress or discomfort.
- Do not change any settings on the ventilator or reset alarms.
- Provide a means of communication. Remember, the person on mechanical ventilation cannot talk.
- Use established hand or eye signals for "yes" and "no." All health team members (nursing staff, doctors, respiratory therapists, and others) and the family must use the same signals. Otherwise, communication does not occur.
- Ask questions that have simple answers. The person may not have the strength to write out long responses.

- Be careful what you say when within the person's hearing distance. The person may pay close attention to what is being said. Do not say anything that could upset the person.
- Watch your nonverbal communication. Although seriously ill and unable to speak, the person may be very aware of nonverbal messages. Avoid communicating worry and concern to the person.
- Take time to comfort and reassure the person. Tell the person what you are going to do and why. Also tell the person about such things as the weather, pleasant news events, and gifts and cards.
- Meet the person's basic needs for personal and oral hygiene, elimination, and activity (repositioning, range-of-motion exercises, sitting in a chair) as directed by the nurse.
- Apply a moist wash cloth or lubricant to the person's lips as directed by the nurse. This helps prevent the lips from drying and cracking.
- Use touch to reassure and comfort the person.
- Tell the peZrson when you are leaving the room and when you will be back.

CHEST TUBES

When the chest is entered, air, blood, or fluid can collect in the pleural space (sac or cavity). Chest entry occurs with chest surgery or injury. **Pneumothorax** is the collection of air *(pneumo)* in the pleural space *(thorax)*. **Hemothorax** is the collection of blood *(hemo)* in the pleural space *(thorax)*. **Pleural effusion** is the escape and collection of fluid (effusion) in the pleural space.

Pressure caused by the collection of air, blood, or fluid collapses the lung. Air cannot reach the affected aveoli. O_2 and CO_2 are not exchanged at the alveoli. Respiratory distress and hypoxia result. Sometimes there is pressure on the heart. This affects the heart's ability to pump blood and is a life-threatening problem.

The doctor inserts chest tubes to remove the air, fluid, or blood (Fig. 27-29). The sterile procedure is done in surgery, in the emergency room, or at the bedside. A nurse assists with the procedure.

The chest tubes are attached to a drainage system (Fig. 27-30, p. 656). The system must be airtight so that air does not enter the pleural space. Water-seal drainage is used to keep the system airtight (Fig. 27-31, p. 656). This is done as follows:

- A chest tube is attached to connecting tubing.
- Connecting tubing is then attached to a tube in the drainage container.
- The tube in the drainage container extends under water. The water prevents air from entering the chest tube and then the pleural space.

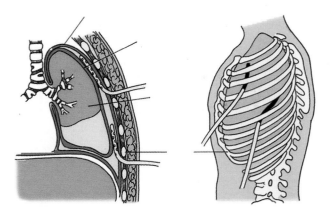

Fig. 27-29 Chest tubes inserted into the pleural space. *(From Elkin MK, Perry AG, Potter PA: Nursing interventions and clinical skills, ed 2, St Louis, 2000, Mosby.)*

A one-, two-, or three-bottle system or a disposable system is used (see Fig. 27-31). Disposable systems are common. Bottles are shown in Figure 27-31 to give you a clearer understanding of how the system works. Sometimes suction is applied to the drainage system. See Box 27-8 on p. 656 for the care of persons with chest tubes.

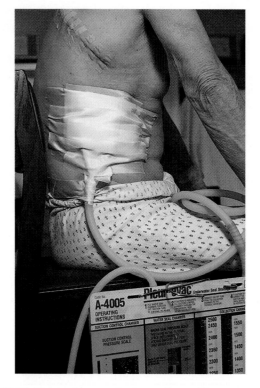

Fig. 27-30 Chest tubes attached to a disposable water-seal drainage system. *(From Elkin Mk, Perry AG, Potter PA: Nursing interventions and clinical skills, ed 2, St Louis, 2000, Mosby.)*

Fig. 27-31 Water-seal drainage system. *(From Potter PA, Perry AG: Fundamentals of nursing: concepts, process, and practice, ed 4, St Louis, 1997, Mosby.)*

Box 27-8	**Care of the Person With Chest Tubes**

When caring for persons with chest tubes, you need to:
- Keep the drainage system below the level of the person's chest.
- Measure the person's vital signs as directed by the nurse. Report any changes in vital signs immediately.
- Report signs and symptoms of hypoxia and respiratory distress to the nurse immediately. Also report patient complaints of pain or difficulty breathing.
- Keep connecting tubing coiled on the bed. Allow enough slack so the chest tubes are not dislodged when the person moves. If tubing hangs in loops, drainage collects in the loop.
- Make sure the tubing is not kinked. Kinking obstructs the chest tube, causing air, blood, or fluid to collect in pleural space.
- Observe chest drainage. Immediately report to the nurse any change in chest drainage. This includes increases in drainage or the appearance of bright red drainage.
- Record chest drainage according to agency policy.
- Turn and position the person as directed by the nurse. The person must be turned carefully and gently to prevent the chest tubes from dislodging.
- Assist the person with coughing and deep breathing as directed by the nurse. Also assist with incentive spirometry as directed.
- Note bubbling activity in the drainage system. Tell the nurse immediately if the bubbling increases, decreases, or stops.
- Tell the nurse immediately if any part of the system is loose or disconnected.
- Make sure petrolatum gauze is at the bedside in case a chest tube comes out.
- Call for help immediately if a chest tube comes out. Cover the insertion site with sterile petrolatum gauze. Stay with the person until a nurse arrives. Follow the nurse's directions.

CARDIOPULMONARY RESUSCITATION

Persons with respiratory injuries and problems are at risk for respiratory and cardiac arrest. Agency policy will require you to be certified in basic life support procedures (see Chapter 36).

Circle the **BEST** answer.

1. Alcohol and narcotics affect oxygen needs because they
   A. Depress the brain
   B. Are pollutants
   C. Cause allergies
   D. Cause a pneumothorax

2. Hypoxia is
   A. A deficiency of oxygen in the blood
   B. The amount of hemoglobin that contains oxygen
   C. A deficiency of oxygen in the cells
   D. The lack of carbon dioxide

3. One of the earliest signs of hypoxia is
   A. Cyanosis
   B. Increased pulse and respiratory rates
   C. Restlessness
   D. Dyspnea

4. A person can breathe deeply and comfortably only while sitting or standing. This is called
   A. Biot's respirations
   B. Orthopnea
   C. Bradypnea
   D. Kussmaul's respirations

5. The person will probably need to rest after
   A. A chest x-ray
   B. A lung scan
   C. Arterial blood gases
   D. Pulmonary function tests

6. A person has pulse oximetry. The person's SpO_2 is 98%. Which is *true?*
   A. The machine is not accurate.
   B. The person's pulse is 98 beats per minute.
   C. The measurement is within normal range.
   D. The person needs suctioning.

7. Which is not a site for a pulse oximetry sensor?
   A. Toe
   B. Finger
   C. Ear lobe
   D. Upper arm

8. The best time to collect a sputum specimen is
   A. On awakening
   B. After meals
   C. At bedtime
   D. After suctioning

9. Before collecting a sputum specimen, you should
   A. Ask the person to use mouthwash
   B. Ask the person to rinse the mouth with clear water
   C. Ask the person to brush the teeth
   D. Apply lubricant to the person's lips

10. You are assisting a person with coughing and deep breathing. Which is *false?*
    A. The person inhales through pursed lips.
    B. The person needs to be in a comfortable sitting position.
    C. The person inhales deeply through the nose.
    D. The person holds a small pillow over an incision.

11. Which is useful for deep breathing?
    A. Pulse oximeter
    B. Incentive spirometry
    C. Chest tubes
    D. Partial-rebreathing mask

12. You are assisting with oxygen therapy. You can
    A. Turn the oxygen on and off
    B. Start the oxygen
    C. Decide what device to use
    D. Make sure the connecting tubing is secure and free of kinks

13. A person has a tracheostomy. Which is *false?*
    A. A nondisposable inner cannula is removed for cleaning.
    B. The obturator is inserted after the outer cannula.
    C. The outer cannula must be secured in place.
    D. The person must be protected from aspiration.

14. A person has a tracheostomy. The person can do the following *except*
    A. Shampoo
    B. Shave
    C. Shower with a hand-held nozzle
    D. Swim

15. A person has a trachostomy. The old ties are removed after
    A. Removing the inner cannula
    B. Cleaning the flange and stoma
    C. Removing the dressing
    D. Securing the new ties

16. These statements are about oroharyngeal suctioning. Which is *true?*
    A. Suction is applied while inserting the catheter.
    B. Suctioning is done every 2 hours.
    C. A suction cycle is no more than 10 to 15 seconds.
    D. The mouth is considered sterile.

17. Oropharyngeal suctioning requires
    A. Following Standard Precautions and the Bloodborne Pathogen Standard
    B. Sterile technique
    C. An artificial airway
    D. All of the above

18. Which is used to hyperventilate the lungs before tracheostomy suctioning?
    A. Incentive spirometer
    B. Pulse oximeter
    C. Ambu bag
    D. Partial-rebreathing mask

19. Mr. Long requires mechanical ventilation. Which is *false?*
    A. He has an endotracheal tube or a tracheostomy tube.
    B. The signal light must always be within his reach.
    C. You should use touch to provide comfort and reassurance.
    D. You can reset alarms on the ventilator.

20. An alarm sounds on Mr. Long's ventilator. What should you do first?
    A. Reset the alarm.
    B. Check to see if his airway is attached to the ventilator.
    C. Call the nurse immediately.
    D. Ask him what is wrong.

21. A person has a pneumothorax. This is the collection of
    A. Fluid in the pleural space
    B. Blood in the pleural space
    C. Air in the pleural space
    D. Respiratory secretions in the pleural space

22. Chest tubes are attached to water-seal drainage. You should do the following *except*
    A. Notify the nurse if bubbling increases, decreases, or stops
    B. Make sure the tubing is not kinked
    C. Keep the drainage system below the person's chest
    D. Hang tubing in loops

Answers to these questions are on p. 838.

CHAPTER

28

REHABILITATION AND RESTORATIVE CARE

Define the key terms listed in this chapter

Describe how rehabilitation involves the whole person

Identify the complications that are prevented for successful rehabilitation

Identify how to help disabled persons perform activities of daily living

Identify the common reactions to rehabilitation

Describe how rehabilitation can help a person work

Identify the members of the rehabilitation team

List the common rehabilitation services

Explain your responsibilities and how to promote quality of life during the rehabilitation process

KEY TERMS

activities of daily living (ADL) Self-care activities a person performs daily to remain independent and to function in society

disability Any lost, absent, or impaired physical or mental function

prosthesis An artificial replacement for a missing body part

rehabilitation The process of restoring the person to his or her highest possible level of physical, psychological, social, and economic functioning; restorative care

restorative care Rehabilitation

Disease, injury, and surgery can result in loss of function or loss of a body part. So can birth injuries and birth defects. Often more than one function is lost. Daily activities such as eating, bathing, dressing, and walking are hard or seem impossible. Some persons cannot work. Others cannot care for children or family.

Disability is any lost, absent, or impaired physical or mental function. It is caused by an acute or chronic illness or problem. An acute problem has a short course. Recovery is complete. A fracture is an acute problem. A chronic problem has a long course. The problem is controlled—not cured—with treatment. Diabetes and coronary artery disease are chronic health problems. Disabilities are short term or long term. The disabled person may totally or partially depend on others for basic needs. The degree of disability affects how much function is possible.

Rehabilitation is the process of restoring the person to his or her highest possible level of physical, psychological, social, and economic functioning. The focus is on improving the person's abilities. For some persons, the goal is to return to work. For others, self-care is the goal. Sometimes improvement is not possible. Then the focus is on maintaining the highest possible level of function and preventing further disability. **Restorative care** is another term for rehabilitation. Box 28-1 lists some common health problems that require rehabilitation.

(See Focus on Long-Term Care box.)

REHABILITATION AND THE WHOLE PERSON

The rehabilitation process involves the whole person. An illness or injury has physical, psychological, and social effects. So does a disability. How would you feel if an illness left you paralyzed from the waist down? Would you be angry, afraid, or depressed? Would you deny it happened? Could you dance, shop, or go to school? Could you attend church services or visit family and friends in their homes? Could you drive a car? Could you return to work? Could you find another job with your remaining skills?

	Common Health Problems
Box 28-1	**Requiring Rehabilitation**

- Alcoholism
- Amputation
- Brain tumor
- Burns
- Cerebral palsy
- Chronic obstructive pulmonary disease
- Head injury
- Myocardial infarction (heart attack)
- Parkinson's disease
- Spinal cord injury
- Spinal cord tumor
- Stroke (brain attack)
- Substance abuse

 Focus On... **LONG-TERM CARE**

Persons admitted to nursing centers often have physical disabilities. Some residents have suffered strokes, fractures, amputations, or other injuries. Rehabilitation programs help them regain their former level of functioning or adjust to a long-term disability. Often these residents are able to return home.

Other residents have progressive illness—they become more and more disabled. Rehabilitation helps them maintain their highest level of functioning and prevents unnecessary decline in functioning.

Focus On... **CHILDREN**

Disabilities in children occur from birth defects or from illness, injury, or surgery. They can affect normal growth and development (see Chapter 7). Factors important for normal growth and development include hand skills, mobility, communication, play, and relationships with parents, family, and peers. A disability can affect one or more of these factors.

Focus On... **OLDER PERSONS**

Rehabilitation often takes longer in older persons than in other age-groups. Changes from aging affect healing, mobility, vision and hearing, and other functions (see Chapter 8). Older persons often have chronic health problems that interfere with or slow recovery. They also are at higher risk for injuries. Older people do not tolerate long or fast-paced rehabilitation programs. Therefore their rehabilitation programs usually proceed at a slower pace.

Rehabilitation helps a person adjust to the disability physically, psychologically, socially, and economically. Abilities—what the person can do—are stressed. *(See Focus on Children and Focus on Older Persons boxes.)*

PHYSICAL ASPECTS

Rehabilitation begins when the person seeks health care. It starts with preventing complications. Complications can occur from bedrest or from prolonged illness or recovery. Bowel and bladder problems are prevented. Contractures and pressure ulcers are prevented with good body alignment, turning and repositioning, range-of-motion exercises, and supportive devices (see Chapters 11 and 20). Good skin care also prevents pressure ulcers (see Chapters 14 and 25).

Bladder training is described in Chapter 16. The method used depends on the person's problems, abilities, and needs. Bowel training is described in Chapter 17. It involves gaining control of bowel movements and developing a regular elimination pattern. Fecal impaction, constipation, and fecal incontinence are prevented. The nurse explains the method planned for the person. You must follow the person's care plan.

Self-care is a major goal. **Activities of daily living (ADL)** refer to self-care activities. The person performs ADL daily to remain independent and to function in society. ADL include bathing, oral hygiene, eating, bowel and bladder elimination, and moving about. A person's ability to do ADL and the need for self-help devices are evaluated.

Disease, injury, and birth defects can affect the hands, wrists, and arms. Self-help devices are often needed. Special eating devices include glass holders, plate guards, and silverware with curved handles or cuffs (see Fig. 18-6). Some devices attach to a special splint (Fig. 28-1, p. 662). Electric toothbrushes are helpful for persons who cannot perform the back-and-forth motions needed for brushing teeth. Longer handles are attached to combs, brushes, and sponges (Fig. 28-2, p. 662). There also are self-help devices for preparing meals, dressing, writing, dialing telephones, and many other tasks (Fig. 28-3, p. 663).

Some persons have to learn how to walk with supportive devices. The person is taught to use crutches or a walker, cane, or brace (Fig. 28-4, p. 664). If both legs are paralyzed or amputated, a wheelchair is used. Persons with hemiplegia also need wheelchairs. If possible, the person learns how to transfer to and from the wheelchair using a transfer board (Fig. 28-5, p. 664). The person learns to transfer to and from the bed, toilet, bathtub, sofas and chairs, and cars (Fig. 28-6, pp. 665-666).

Text continued on p. 664

Fig. 28-1 Self-help device attached to a splint.

Fig. 28-2 **A,** A long-handled comb for hair care. **B,** The brush has a long handle for bathing. **C,** This brush has a curved handle. *(A and B Courtesy Northcoast Medical, Inc., Morgan Hill, Calif.; C, courtesy Sammons Preston; An AbilityOne Company, Bolingbrook, Ill.)*

Fig. 28-3 A, A button hook is used to button and zip clothing. **B,** A sock puller is used to put on socks and stockings. **C,** A long-handled shoehorn for putting on shoes. **D,** Reachers are helpful for those in wheelchairs. **E,** A toilet paper holder is used for wiping. **F,** The telephone holder is used by those who cannot hold a phone. *(A, B, and E, Courtesy Northcoast Medical, Inc., Morgan Hill, Calif.; C, D, and F courtesy Sammons Preston; An AbilityOne Company, Bolingbrook, Ill.)*

Fig. 28-4 The person learns to walk in physical therapy.

Fig. 28-5 A transfer board is used to transfer from one seat to another. *(Courtesy Northcoast Medical, Inc., Morgan Hill, Calif.)*

Prostheses are helpful for persons with missing body parts. A **prosthesis** is an artificial replacement for a missing body part (see Chapter 30). A person usually can be fitted with an artificial arm or leg. The person learns to use the prosthesis. Modern technology will result in more sophisticated prostheses. The goal is for the prosthesis to be like the missing body part in function and appearance.

Difficulty swallowing *(dysphagia)* may occur after a stroke. When possible, the person is taught special exercises to improve swallowing. A gastrostomy tube is needed if the person cannot swallow again (see Chapter 18). The tube is used to feed the person. Difficulty speaking *(aphasia)* may occur after a stroke (see Chapter 30). Speech therapy and special devices (see Chapter 5) can help the person communicate.

Some persons need mechanical ventilation (see Chapter 27). These people need respiratory rehabilitation. Some are weaned from the ventilator. Others need permanent mechanical ventilation. The respiratory rehabilitation team works with the person and family. *(See Focus on Long-Term Care box.)*

PSYCHOLOGICAL AND SOCIAL ASPECTS

A disability often affects self-esteem and relationships. Appearance and function changes may cause the person to feel unwhole, unattractive, unclean, or undesirable to others. At first the person may refuse to accept the disability. The person may be depressed, angry, and hostile.

The person's attitude, acceptance of limits, and motivation are important. The person must focus on remaining abilities. Discouragement and frustration are common. Progress may be slow. Learning each new task is a reminder of the disability. Old fears and emotions may surface. The person needs help accepting the disability and the resulting limits. Support, reassurance, encouragement, and sensitivity from the health team are needed.

ECONOMIC ASPECTS

Some persons cannot return to their jobs. The person is assessed for work skills, past work history, interests, and talents. A job skill may be restored or a new one learned. The goal is for the person to become gainfully employed. Assistance often is given in finding a job.

Fig. 28-6 A, The person transfers from the wheelchair to the bed. **B,** A transfer from the wheelchair to the bathtub. *(From Hoeman SP:* Rehabilitation/restorative care in the community, *St Louis, 1990, Mosby).*   *Continued*

Fig. 28-6, cont'd C, A transfer to the car. The person has left-side paralysis.

THE REHABILITATION TEAM

Rehabilitation is a team effort. The team includes the person, doctor, nursing team, other health team members (see Chapter 1), and the family. All help the person regain function and become independent.

The team meets often to discuss the person's progress. Goals are set for the person. The person helps in goal setting. Changes in the rehabilitation plan are made as needed. The person and family are encouraged to attend the meetings.

REHABILITATION SERVICES

The person may need extended hospital care. Some need subacute or long-term care. Others are treated as outpatients. Home care agencies and day care centers often provide rehabilitation services. Some people are transferred to rehabilitation centers. There are centers for persons who are blind, deaf, mentally retarded, physically disabled, or mentally ill or who have speech problems. *(See Focus on Children box, Focus on Home Care box, and Focus on Long-Term Care box.)*

 Focus On... CHILDREN

Federal laws require that schools provide needed therapies. In-school therapy is required to meet the child's learning needs.

 Focus On... HOME CARE

The rehabilitation team assesses the person's home setting (Box 28-2, p. 668). Changes in the home are made to meet the person's needs. Some individuals require personal attendants 24 hours a day.

 Focus On... LONG-TERM CARE

OBRA requires that nursing centers provide rehabilitation services. Services required by a resident's comprehensive care plan must be provided. If a resident requires physical therapy, it must be provided. If occupational therapy is required, it must be provided. The same holds for speech and other therapies. All services require a doctor's order.

QUALITY OF LIFE

Successful rehabilitation improves the person's quality of life. A hopeful and winning attitude helps motivate the person. However, the process can be slow and frustrating. Promoting quality of life helps the person's attitude.

The person's rights are protected. The right to privacy is important. The person relearns old skills or practices new skills in private. Other persons do not need to watch. They do not need to see mistakes, falls, spills, or clumsiness. Nor do they need to see the person's anger or tears. Privacy protects the person's dignity and promotes self-respect.

Personal choice gives the person control. Not being able to control body movements or functions is very frustrating. Persons are allowed and encouraged to control the other aspects of their lives to the extent possible. You need to allow personal choice whenever possible. Sad and depressed persons may not want to make choices. Encourage them to do so. Making choices helps them have control of those things that affect them.

The person is part of the rehabilitation team. The team plans and evaluates the person's program. Being part of the team allows the individual personal choice in planning care.

The person has the right to be free from abuse and mistreatment. Rehabilitation is often a slow process. Sometimes improvement is not seen for weeks. Learning how to use an assistive device takes time. Learning to speak again after a stroke can take a long time. So can learning how to dress when there is paralysis. What seems so simple to you can be very hard for the person. Repeated explanations and demonstrations may have no or little results. You may become impatient and short with the person. Or you may see such behavior from other team members or the family. You must protect the person from physical and mental abuse and mistreatment. No one can shout, scream, or yell at the person. Nor can they hit or strike the person. The person cannot be called names. Unkind remarks must not be made. You must report signs of abuse or mistreatment to the nurse.

You must deal with your own anger and frustration. Remember that the person wants to function and control movements. The person does not choose loss of function. If the process frustrates you, just think how the person must feel. Discuss your feelings with the nurse. The nurse can suggest ways to help you control your feelings. Perhaps you can be reassigned for a while.

Box 28-2	Home Assessment

OUTDOORS

- Where is parking located? What is the distance from the parking area to the door?
- Where is the mailbox?
- Where is the motor vehicle stored?
- What is the width of doors?
- Can the person turn a key?
- Can the person open and close doors?
- Are ramps needed?
- Are handrails needed?
- Are entrances lighted?
- Does the person have access to private or public transportation?
- Can the person operate a motor vehicle?
- What is the width and height of ramps and sidewalks?

INDOORS

- Are there floor obstructions?
- Are there steps in the home? Where are they located?
- How is furniture arranged?
- Can the person use the furniture?
- Where are telephones located?
- Can the person raise and lower windows?
- How are floors covered (wall-to-wall carpeting, tile, hardwood floors, throw rugs)?
- Can the person use a wheelchair throughout the home?
- Where is the fuse or circuit-breaker box located?
- Can the person control the heat?
- Are walkways, doors, and halls wide enough for the person to use a wheelchair?
- Is there an elevator in an apartment or condominium building?

KITCHEN

- Does the person have access to the stove, sink, cupboards, storage areas, work space, refrigerator, and other appliances?
- What is the height of the sink and countertops?
- Is there an opening under the sink for wheelchair access?
- Can the person turn faucets on and off?
- Can the person use the microwave?
- Can the person reach stove knobs?
- Are appliances arranged conveniently for the person?

BATHROOM

- What is the height of the sink, toilet, shower, and tub?
- Can the person reach the faucets?
- Can the person turn the faucets on and off?
- Is there space for using a wheelchair and other assistive devices?
- Can the person get into and out of the tub or shower?
- Are there grab bars by the toilet, shower, and tub?

BEDROOM

- What is the height of the person's bed?
- Can the person access the closet? Can the person reach rods and shelves?
- Can the person transfer in and out of bed safely? Is there enough space around the bed for the person to move?
- How is furniture arranged?
- Does the furniture arrangement allow for the use of a wheelchair or assistive devices?

SAFETY

- Is the house number clearly visible and readable during an emergency?
- Are deadbolts and locks secure? Can the person use the locks?
- Can the person see and talk to a visitor at the door without being seen?
- Are steps, porch, and front door lighted?
- Are the steps, porch, and front door protected from rain, sleet, and snow?
- Is there a nonslip doormat?
- Can the person use the telephone?
- Are emergency telephone numbers available?
- Can the person control water temperature?
- Do electrical outlets have childproof covers?
- Where are the smoke detectors? Are they working?
- Are rooms and hallways well lighted?
- Can the person control indoor and outdoor lighting?
- Can the person exit the home in an emergency?
- Is oxygen used in the home? Are safety measures for the use of oxygen in place?
- Does the person have access to the telephone, television, radio, and lights while in bed?
- Are space heaters used in the home? Are safety measures in place?
- Does the person have good judgment for cooking and stove use?
- Is there a safe play area for children?
- Can the person safely dispose of blood, body fluids, secretions, and excretions?
- Is there a pest-free method of trash storage?

Modified from Hoeman SP: *Rehabilitation nursing: process and application,* ed 2, St Louis, 1996, Mosby.

Taking part in activities promotes quality of life. The person is encouraged to join in group activities. Often persons are concerned about how others view the disability. Provide support and reassurance. Remind the person that others have disabilities. Other persons are likely to provide support and understanding because of their own disabilities. Allow personal choice in activities. The person usually chooses those that are of interest and that are the least threatening.

The environment promotes quality of life. It must be safe and meet the person's needs. The setting may need changes because of disabilities. Location of the overbed table or the bedside stand may need to be changed. The person may need a special chair. If the signal light cannot be used, another way is needed to communicate with the staff. These and other changes are suggested by all health team members. The nurse or therapist explains the need and purpose of the change to the person and family.

YOUR RESPONSIBILITIES

Your role as a member of the rehabilitation team has value. A nurse directs you in performing care activities. Box 28-3 lists your responsibilities. Many procedures and care measures already learned are part of the person's care. Safety, communication, legal, and ethical aspects apply in rehabilitation. The many rules described throughout this book also apply, regardless of the disability.

Box 28-3   Nursing Assistant Responsibilities in Rehabilitation

- Follow the nurse's instructions and directions very carefully.
- Know and follow the person's care plan.
- Report early signs and symptoms of complications such as pressure ulcers, contractures, and bowel and bladder problems.
- Keep the person in good body alignment at all times (see Chapter 11).
- Practice measures to prevent pressure ulcers (see Chapter 25).
- Turn and reposition the person as directed (see Chapter 11).
- Perform range-of-motion exercises as instructed (see Chapter 20).
- Encourage the person to perform as many ADL as possible and to the extent possible.
- Give praise when even a little progress is made.
- Provide emotional support and reassurance.
- Know how to apply self-care devices used by the person.
- Try to understand and appreciate the person's situation, feelings, and concerns.
- Do not pity the person or give sympathy.
- Focus on the person's abilities, not the disabilities.
- Remember that muscles atrophy if they are not used.
- Practice the task that the person must do. This helps you guide and direct the person.
- Know how to use and operate special equipment used in the person's rehabilitation program.
- Convey an attitude of hopefulness to the person and family.

REVIEW

Circle the BEST answer.

1. Rehabilitation is concerned with
   A. What the person cannot do
   B. What the person can do
   C. The whole person
   D. The person's rights

2. Mr. Olson's rehabilitation begins with preventing
   A. Angry feelings
   B. Contractures and pressure ulcers
   C. Illness and injury
   D. Loss of self-esteem

3. Mr. Olson has weakness on his right side. ADL are
   A. Done by him to the extent possible
   B. Done by the nursing staff
   C. Postponed until he can use his right side
   D. Supervised by a therapist

4. Which reaction is Mr. Olson likely to experience?
   A. Feelings of being undesirable
   B. Anger and hostility
   C. Depression
   D. All of the above

5. Which statement is *false?*
   A. Disabled people can never work again.
   B. Disabled people may need to learn a new job skill.
   C. The disabled person is evaluated to determine the ability to work.
   D. Disabled people often are given help in finding a job.

6. Which statement is *false?*
   A. Sympathy and pity help the person adjust to the disability.
   B. You should know how to apply self-care devices.
   C. You should know how to use equipment used in the person's care.
   D. An attitude of hopefulness must be conveyed to the person.

7. Mr. Olson requires speech therapy after a stroke. Therapy should be provided in private.
   A. True
   B. False

8. Mr. Olson is learning to use a walker. He asks to have music played. You should
   A. Tell him music is not allowed
   B. Choose some music
   C. Ask him to choose some music
   D. Ask a therapist to choose some music

9. Mr. Olson is told that he cannot have dessert until he does his exercises. This is abuse and mistreatment.
   A. True
   B. False

10. Mr. Olson's right side is weak. The signal light is on his right side. You move it to the left side of the bed. You have promoted his quality of life by
    A. Protecting him from abuse and mistreatment
    B. Allowing personal choice
    C. Providing for his safety
    D. All of the above

Answers to these questions are on p. 838.

CHAPTER

29

HEARING AND VISION PROBLEMS

OBJECTIVES

Define the key terms listed in this chapter

Explain otitis media and Ménière's disease

Describe the effects of hearing loss and vision loss

Describe how to communicate with the hearing-impaired person

Explain how to communicate with the speech-impaired person

Explain the purpose of a hearing aid

Describe how to care for a hearing aid

Explain the differences between glaucoma and cataracts

Explain why you should not insert or remove contact lenses

Describe how to protect an artificial eye from loss or damage

Explain how to care for a blind person

Perform the procedure described in this chapter

KEY TERMS

braille A method of writing for the blind; raised dots are arranged to represent each letter of the alphabet; the first ten letters represent the numbers 0 through 9

otitis media Infection *(itis)* of the middle *(media)* ear *(ot)*

tinnitus Ringing in the ears

vertigo Dizziness

Sight and hearing are valuable senses. They allow communication with others, learning, and moving about. They also are important for activities of daily living and countless other activities. Hearing and vision are important for safety and security needs. For example, hearing and seeing the warning signs of danger allow the person to seek safety.

Most people take hearing and vision for granted. However, hearing and vision problems are common among all age-groups. Common causes include birth defects, accidents, infections, diseases, and aging. You will care for many people who have some degree of hearing or vision loss.

EAR DISORDERS

The ear is important for hearing and balance. Middle ear infections, Ménière's disease, and hearing loss are presented in this section. See Box 29-1 for a review of the structure and function of the ear.

OTITIS MEDIA

Otitis media is infection *(itis)* of the middle *(media)* ear *(ot)*. The infection is acute or chronic. Chronic otitis media can damage the tympanic membrane (eardrum) or the ossicles (see Fig. 29-1). The eardrum and ossicles are needed for hearing. Permanent hearing loss can occur from chronic otitis media.

Fluid buildup occurs in the ear. It causes pain and hearing loss. Other signs and symptoms include fever and ringing in the ears **(tinnitus).** The doctor usually orders antibiotics.

MÉNIÈRE'S DISEASE

Ménière's disease involves increased fluid in the inner ear. The increased fluid causes pressure in the middle ear. There are three symptoms. Vertigo is the major symptom. **Vertigo** means dizziness. The person feels whirling and spinning sensations. The person must lie down. Severe dizziness can cause nausea and vomiting. The two other main symptoms of Ménière's disease are ringing in the ears (tinnitus) and hearing loss.

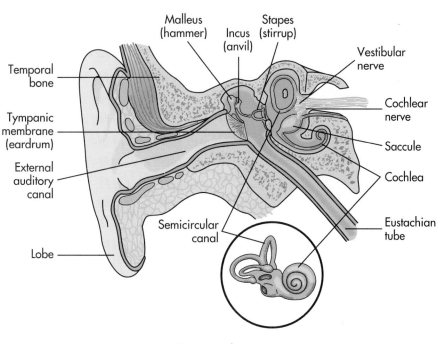

Fig. 29-1 The ear.

The ear is a sense organ that functions in hearing and balance. It is divided into the *external ear, middle ear,* and *inner ear.* Ear structures are shown in Figure 29-1.

The external ear (outer part) is called the *pinna* or *auricle.* Sound waves are guided through the external ear into the *auditory canal.* Glands in the auditory canal secrete a waxy substance called *cerumen.* The auditory canal extends about 1 inch to the *eardrum.* The eardrum *(tympanic membrane)* separates the external ear and middle ear.

The middle ear is a small space that contains the *eustachian tube* and three small bones called *ossicles.* The eustachian tube connects the middle ear and the throat. Air enters the eustachian tube so that there is equal pressure on both sides of the eardrum. The ossicles amplify sound received from the eardrum and transmit the sound to the inner ear. The three ossicles are:
- The *malleus,* which looks like a hammer
- The *incus,* which resembles an anvil
- The *stapes,* which is shaped like a stirrup

The inner ear consists of the *semicircular canals* and the *cochlea.* The cochlea, which looks like a snail shell, contains fluid. The fluid carries sound waves received from the middle ear to the *auditory nerve.* The auditory nerve then carries the message to the brain.

The three semicircular canals are involved with balance. They sense the head's position and changes in position and send messages to the brain.

The doctor can order different drugs for the person. Sometimes a low-salt diet decreases the amount of fluid in the ear. Safety is important during vertigo. The person must lie down. Falls are prevented. Bed rails usually are ordered. The head is kept still, and the person avoids turning the head. To talk to the person, stand directly in front of him or her. When movement is necessary, the person moves slowly. Bright or glaring lights are avoided. Assist with ambulation. The person should not walk alone in case vertigo occurs.

HEARING PROBLEMS

Hearing losses range from slight hearing impairments to complete deafness. Clear speech, responding to others, safety, and awareness of surroundings all require hearing. Many people deny having difficulty hearing. This is because hearing loss is often linked with aging. However, temporary hearing loss can occur when the ear canal is blocked with ear wax (cerumen). Hearing improves when the ear wax is removed. A doctor or nurse removes the wax.

Effects on the Person. A person may be unaware of gradual hearing loss. Others may see changes in the person's behavior or attitude. They may not know that the changes are caused by hearing difficulties. Symptoms and effects of hearing loss vary. They are not always obvious to the person or to others. *(See Focus on Children box, p. 674.)*

Focus On... **CHILDREN**

Infants with hearing impairments often fail to start talking. Lack of attention and failing grades are early signs of poor hearing in children.

Box 29-2	**Communicating With the Speech-Impaired Person**

- Listen, and give the person your full attention.
- Ask the person questions to which you know the answer. This helps you to become familiar with the person's speech.
- Determine the subject being discussed. This helps you to understand main points.
- Ask the person to repeat or rephrase statements if necessary.
- Repeat what the person has said. Ask if you have understood correctly.
- Ask the person to write down key words or the message.
- Watch the person's lip movements.
- Watch facial expressions, gestures, and body language for clues about what is being said.

There are some obvious signs of hearing impairment in children and adults. These include:

- Speaking too loudly
- Leaning forward to hear
- Turning and cupping the better ear toward the speaker
- Answering questions or responding inappropriately
- Asking for words to be repeated

Psychological and social effects are less obvious. People with hearing problems may give wrong answers or responses. Therefore they tend to avoid social situations. This is an attempt to avoid embarrassment. Loneliness, boredom, and feeling left out often result. Only parts of conversations are heard. People with hearing loss may become suspicious. They may think others are talking about them or talking softly on purpose. Some control conversations to avoid responding. Straining and working to hear can cause fatigue, frustration, and irritability.

Hearing loss may cause speech problems. You hear yourself as you talk. How you pronounce words and voice volume depend on how you hear yourself. Hearing loss may result in slurred speech and improper pronunciation. Monotone speech and dropping word endings also may occur. Understanding what the person is saying can be hard. Do not assume that you understand what the person says. Do not pretend to understand to avoid embarrassing the person. Serious problems can result if you assume or pretend to understand. The guidelines listed in Box 29-2 will help you communicate with the speech-impaired person.

Communicating With the Person. Hearing-impaired persons may wear hearing aids or read lips. They also watch facial expressions, gestures, and body language. Some people learn sign language (Figs. 29-2 at right and 29-3 on p. 676). Some hearing-impaired people have *hearing* dogs. The dog alerts the person to such things as ringing phones, doorbells, sirens, or oncoming cars. Certain measures are needed when communicating with the person. The measures listed in Box 29-3 on p. 677 can help the person hear or speech-read (lip-read).

Fig. 29-2 Manual alphabet. *(Courtesy National Association of the Deaf, Silver Spring, Md.)*

Wash

Eat, Food

Begin, Start

Help, Aid, Assist

Bath, Bathe

Good

Lie (lie down)

Sit, Seat, Chair

Hot

Thank you

Stand (arise)

Dress, Clothing

Cold, Winter

Tired

Walk

Permission, Privilege

Shower

Invite, Welcome

Thirsty

Better

Fig. 29-3 Sign language.

Box 29-3	Communicating With the Hearing-Impaired Person

- Gain attention and alert the person to your presence. Raise an arm or hand, or lightly touch the person's arm. Do not startle or approach the person from behind.
- Face the person directly when speaking. Do not turn or walk away while you are talking. Also, do not talk to the person from the doorway or another room.
- Make sure the person is wearing his or her hearing aid.
- Stand or sit in good light. Shadows and glares affect the person's ability to see your face clearly.
- Make sure the person is wearing needed eyeglasses or contact lenses. This helps the person see your face for speechreading.
- Speak clearly, distinctly, and slowly.
- Speak in a normal tone of voice. Do not shout.
- Do not cover your mouth, smoke, eat, or chew gum while talking. These things affect mouth movements.

- Stand or sit on the side of the better ear.
- State the topic of conversation first.
- Use short sentences and simple words.
- Use gestures as appropriate.
- Write out important names and words.
- Say things in a different way if the person does not seem to understand.
- Keep conversations and discussions short to avoid tiring the person.
- Repeat and rephrase statements as needed.
- Be alert to the messages sent by your facial expressions, gestures, and body language.
- Reduce or eliminate background noises. Examples include radios, stereos, televisions, air conditioners, and fans.

Fig. 29-4 Types of hearing aids. **A,** Behind-the-ear hearing aid. **B,** In-the-ear hearing aid. **C,** Eyeglass aid. **D,** Body-worn aid. *(Courtesy CLG Photographics, St Louis.)*

Hearing Aids. A *hearing aid* amplifies sound (Fig. 29-4). It does not correct or cure the hearing problem. The ability to hear is not improved. However, the person hears better with a hearing aid. This is because the hearing aid makes sounds louder. Both background noise and speech are amplified. Noise is minimized to help the person adjust to the hearing aid. Remember that the hearing aid does not make speech clearer—only louder. The measures for communicating with hearing-impaired persons apply to those with hearing aids (see Box 29-3).

Hearing aids operate on batteries. There is an *on* and *off* switch. Sometimes hearing aids do not seem to work properly. Often only simple measures are needed to get them to work:

- Check if the hearing aid is *on.*
- Check the battery position.
- Insert a new battery if needed.
- Clean the earmold if necessary.

Hearing aids are expensive. You must handle and care for them properly. Report lost or damaged hearing aids to the nurse immediately. *Check with the nurse before washing a hearing aid.* Also follow the manufacturer's instructions for proper care and use. Only the earmold is washed. It usually is washed daily with soap and water. Thoroughly dry the earmold before putting it back in place. The battery is removed at night. When not in use, the hearing aid is turned off.

Box 29-4	**Structures and Functions of the Eye**

Receptors for vision are in the eyes. The eye is a delicate organ that is easily injured. Bones of the skull, eyelids and eyelashes, and tears protect the eyes from injury. Eye structures are shown in Figure 29-5. The eye has three layers:

* The *sclera,* the white of the eye, is the outer layer. It is made of tough connective tissue.
* The *choroid* is the second layer. Blood vessels, the *ciliary muscle,* and the *iris* make up the choroid. The iris gives the eye its color. The opening in the middle of the iris is the *pupil.* Pupil size varies with the amount of light entering the eye. The pupil constricts (narrows) in bright light and dilates (widens) in dim or dark places.
* The *retina* is the inner layer of the eye. Receptors for vision and the nerve fibers of the optic nerve are contained in the retina.

Light enters the eye through the *cornea.* The cornea is the transparent part of the outer layer that lies over the eye. Light rays pass to the *lens,* which lies behind the pupil. The light is then reflected to the retina and carried to the brain by the optic nerve.

The *aqueous chamber* separates the cornea from the lens. The chamber is filled with a fluid called *aqueous humor.* The fluid helps the cornea keep its shape and position. The *vitreous body* is behind the lens. The vitreous body is a gelatin-like substance that supports the retina and maintains the eye's shape.

EYE DISORDERS

Vision problems occur at all ages. Problems range from very mild vision loss to complete blindness. Vision loss may be sudden or gradual in onset. One or both eyes are affected. Surgery, eyeglasses, or contact lenses are often necessary. (See Box 29-4 for a review of the structures and functions of the eye.)

GLAUCOMA

With glaucoma, pressure within the eye is increased. This damages the optic nerve. The result is visual loss with eventual blindness. The disease is gradual or sudden in onset. Signs and symptoms include tunnel vision (Fig. 29-6), blurred vision, and blue-green halos around lights. Eye discomfort and aching are common. With sudden onset, the person has severe eye pain, nausea, and vomiting. Glaucoma is a major cause of blindness. Persons over 40 years of age and blacks are at risk. The cause is unknown.

Treatment involves drug therapy and possibly surgery. The goal is to prevent further damage to the optic nerve. Damage that has already occurred cannot be reversed.

Fig. 29-5 The eye.

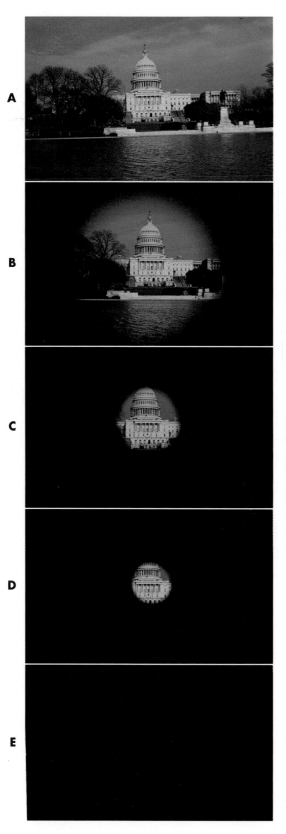

Fig. 29-6 A, Normal vision. **B,** Tunnel vision. **C, D, E,** Visual loss continues, with eventual blindness.

CATARACT

Cataract is an eye disorder in which the lens becomes cloudy (opaque). The cloudiness prevents light from entering the eye (Fig. 29-7). Cataract comes from the Greek word that means *waterfall*. Gradual blurring and dimming of vision occur. The person is sensitive to light and glares. Sight eventually is lost. A cataract can occur in one or both eyes. Aging is the most common cause. Persons age 60 and older are at risk.

Surgery is the only treatment. A tiny incision is made into the eye. The cloudy lens is removed. A plastic lens is implanted into the eye (Fig. 29-8). Vision returns to near normal.

Normal eye   Cataract

Fig. 29-7 There is a cataract in the left eye. *(From Phipps WJ, Cassmeyer VL, Sands JK, Lehman MK: Medical-surgical nursing: a nursing process approach, ed 5, St Louis, 1995, Mosby.)*

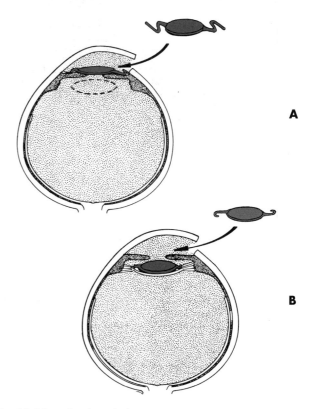

Fig. 29-8 Lens implant during cataract surgery. *(From Long BC, Phipps WJ, Cassmeyer VL: Medical-surgical nursing: a nursing process approach, ed 3, St Louis, 1993, Mosby.)*

The person may have to wear an eye shield or patch a day or two after surgery. The shield protects the eye from injury. One or both eyes may be covered. Measures for the blind person are practiced when an eye shield is worn. Even if only one shield is worn, the person may have vision loss in the other eye from cataract formation or other causes.

Postoperative care required after cataract surgery includes the following:

- Keep the eye shield in place as directed. Some doctors allow the shield to be off during the day if the person wears eyeglasses. The shield is worn for sleep, including napping.
- Remind the person not to rub the affected eye.
- Do not shower or shampoo the person without a doctor's order.
- Take care not to bump the eye.
- Eye drainage or complaints of pain are reported to the nurse immediately.

CORRECTIVE LENSES

Eyeglasses and contact lenses are prescribed to correct vision problems. Sometimes eyeglasses are worn only for certain activities, such as reading or seeing at a distance. Some people wear them all the time while awake. Contact lenses are usually worn continuously while awake.

Eyeglasses. People are often upset when glasses are first needed. However, adjustment is usually rapid. Most people know that glasses will be needed sooner or later. Appearance is often a concern. Frames are chosen that fit face shape, personality, and life-style. There are many styles and shapes.

Lenses are made of hardened glass or plastic. They are made to prevent shattering. Glass lenses are washed with warm water and dried with soft tissue. Plastic lenses are easily scratched. Special cleaning solutions, tissues, and cloths are used to clean and dry them.

Glasses are costly. They are protected from breakage or other damage. When not worn, they are put in their case. The case is put in the drawer of the bedside stand to prevent loss or damage to the glasses.

Fig. 29-9 A, Remove eyeglasses by holding the frames in front of both ears. **B,** Lift the frames from the ears, and bring the glasses down away from the face.

Caring for Eyeglasses

QUALITY OF LIFE

Remember to:
- Knock before entering the person's room
- Address the person by name
- Introduce yourself by name and title

Pre-Procedure

1 Explain the procedure to the person.
2 Wash your hands.
3 Collect the following:

- Eyeglass case
- Cleaning solution or warm water
- Tissues

Procedure

4 Remove the person's glasses.
  a Hold the frames in front of the ear on both sides (Fig. 29-9, *A*).
  b Lift the frames from the ears, and bring the glasses down away from the face (Fig. 29-9, *B*).
5 Clean the glass with the cleaning solution or warm water. Dry the lenses with tissues.
6 Open the eyeglass case.
7 Fold the glasses, and put them in the case. Do not touch the clean lenses.

8 Place the glass case in the top drawer of the bedside stand. Or put the glasses back on the person as follows:
  a Unfold the glasses.
  b Hold the frames at each side, and place them over the ears.
  c Adjust the glasses so the nosepiece rests on the nose.
  d Return the glass case to the drawer in the bedside stand.
9 Wash your hands.

Contact Lenses. Contact lenses fit directly on the eye. There are hard contacts and soft contacts. Many people like contacts because they cannot be seen. They do not break easily and can be worn for sports. However, contacts cost more than eyeglasses and are easily lost. Depending on the type of lens, contacts can be worn for 12 to 24 hours or for 1 week. Contacts are often removed for swimming and sleeping.

Contact lenses are removed and cleaned following the manufacturer's instructions and agency policy. Report any redness or eye drainage to the nurse. Also report complaints of eye pain or blurred vision.

ARTIFICIAL EYES

Removal of an eye is sometimes necessary because of injury or disease. The person is then fitted with an ocular prosthesis or artificial eye (Fig. 29-10, p. 682). The artificial eye is made of glass or plastic. It matches the other eye in color and shape. Some prostheses are permanent implants, and others are removable. If the prosthesis is removable, the person is taught to remove, clean, and insert it. The person performs routine prosthesis care.

Fig. 29-10 An artificial eye is inserted. *(From Lewis SM, Heitkemper MM, Dirkson SR: Medical-surgical nursing: assessment and management of clinical problems, ed 5, St Louis, 2000, Mosby.)*

The artificial eye is the person's property. Like dentures, eyeglasses, and other valuables, it is protected from loss or damage. The following measures are practiced if the eye is removed and will not be reinserted:

- Wash the eye with mild soap and warm water. Then rinse it well.
- Line a container with a soft cloth or 4 × 4 gauze. This prevents scratches and damage to the eye.
- Fill the container with water or a saline (salt) solution.
- Place the eye in the container. Close the container.
- Label the container with the person's name and room number.
- Place the labeled container in the drawer in the bedside stand.
- Wash the eye socket with warm water or saline. Use a washcloth or gauze square. Use a gauze square to remove excess moisture.
- Wash the eyelid with mild soap and warm water. Clean from the inner to the outer aspect of the eye (see Chapter 14). Dry the eyelid.

The person is blind on the side of the artificial eye. Vision in the other eye may be normal or impaired.

BLINDNESS

Birth defects, accidents, and eye diseases are among the many causes of blindness. It also is a complication of some diseases. The level of blindness varies. Some blind persons cannot sense light and have no usable vision. These persons are totally blind. Others sense some light but have no usable vision. Still others have some usable vision but cannot read newsprint. The legally blind person sees at 20 feet what a person with normal vision sees at 200 feet.

A person's life is seriously affected by the loss of sight. Physical and psychological adjustments are hard and long. Special education and training are needed. Moving about, activities of daily living, reading braille, and using a guide (seeing-eye) dog all require training.

Braille is a method of writing for the blind that uses raised dots. Dots are arranged to represent each letter of the alphabet. The first 10 letters also represent the numbers 0 through 9 (Fig. 29-11). The person feels the arrangement of dots with the fingers (Fig. 29-12). Many books, magazines, and newspapers are available in braille. So are typewriters and computer keyboards.

Braille is hard to learn, especially for many older people. Entire books and articles are available on compact disks and audiotapes. They are bought in bookstores or borrowed from libraries.

The blind person is taught to move about using a white cane with a red tip or a guide dog. Both are recognized worldwide as signs that the person is blind. The dog serves as the eyes of the blind person. The dog recognizes danger and guides the person through traffic.

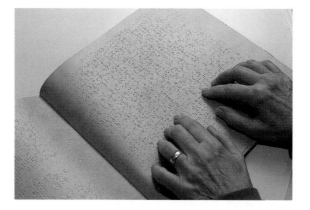

Fig. 29-11 Braille.

Fig. 29-12 Braille is "read" with the fingers.

You must treat the blind person with respect and dignity—not with pity. Most blind people have adjusted well. They lead independent lives. Some have been blind for a long time and others for a short time. The practices listed in Box 29-5 are necessary for all blind persons. (See Focus on Home Care box.)

Focus On... HOME CARE

The practices in Box 29-5 apply in the home setting. A safe environment is important. Outdoor walks and stairs must be free of toys, ice, and snow. Remember, furniture, closets, drawers, shelves, and other items are arranged to meet the person's needs. Always replace items where you found them. Avoid rearranging the person's belongings.

Box 29-5 Caring for the Blind Person

- Ask the person how much he or she can see. Do not assume the person is totally blind or that the person has some vision.
- Ask the person what type of lighting he or she prefers. Provide enough lighting. Tell the person when the lights are on or off.
- Adjust blinds and shades to adjust lighting for glares. Sunny days and bright snowy days cause glares.
- Face the person when speaking. Speak slowly and clearly.
- Use a normal tone of voice. Do not shout or speak loudly. Blindness does not mean the person is hearing impaired.
- Identify yourself when you enter the room. Give your name, title, and reason for being there. Do not touch the person until you have indicated your presence in the room.
- Identify others in the room. Explain where each person is located and what the person is doing.
- Address the person by name. This let's the person know that you are directing a comment or question to him or her.
- Do not avoid using the words "see," "look," or "read."
- Orient the person to the room. Describe the layout. Also identify the location and purpose of furniture and equipment.
- Let the person move about and touch and locate furniture and equipment if able.
- Do not let the person alone in the middle of a room. Make sure the person can reach a wall, chair, table, or sofa.
- Do not rearrange furniture and equipment.
- Keep doors open or shut—never partially open.
- Give step-by-step explanations of procedures as you perform them. Indicate when the procedure is over.
- Offer assistance. Simply say, "May I help you?" Respect the person's answer.
- Tell the person when you are leaving the room.
- Assist the person in ambulating by walking slightly ahead of him or her (Fig. 29-13). Offer your right or left arm. Tell the person which arm you are offering so he or she can take your arm. Never push, pull, or guide the person in front of you.
- Walk at a normal pace when guiding the person.
- Let the person know when you are coming to a curb or steps. Let the person know if you will step up or down.
- Inform the person of doors, turns, furniture, and other obstructions when assisting with ambulation.
- Give specific directions. For example, say "right behind you," "on your left," or "in front of you." Avoid phrases like "over here" or "over there."
- Keep hallways and walkways free of carts, equipment, toys, and other items.
- Assist in food selection by reading the menu to the person.
- Avoid plates, napkins, place mats, and tablecloths with patterns and designs. These items should be solid colors and provide contrast. For example, a white plate is placed on a dark place mat or tablecloth.
- Explain the location of food and beverages on the tray. Use the face of a clock (see Fig. 18-10), or guide the person's hand to each item on the tray.
- Cut meat, open containers, butter bread, and perform other similar activities if needed.
- Keep the signal light within the person's reach.
- Provide a radio, compact disks or audiotapes, television, and braille books for entertainment.
- Let the person perform self-care if able.

Fig. 29-13 The blind person walks slightly behind the nursing assistant and touches the assistant's arm lightly.

Circle the BEST answer.

1. Mr. Percy has Ménière's disease. Which is *true?*
   A. He has a middle ear infection.
   B. Vertigo is the major symptom.
   C. Hearing aids will correct the problem.
   D. He may develop a speech problem.

2. Nursing care for Mr. Percy includes preventing
   A. Infection
   B. Falls
   C. Pain
   D. All of the above

3. Mr. Percy is hearing impaired. He may
   A. Avoid social situations
   B. Become suspicious
   C. Control conversations
   D. All of the above

4. Which is *not* an obvious effect of hearing loss?
   A. Loneliness and boredom
   B. Speaking too loudly
   C. Asking to repeat things
   D. Answering questions inappropriately

5. You are talking to Mr. Percy. You should do the following *except*
   A. Speak clearly, distinctly, and slowly
   B. Sit or stand where there is good light
   C. Shout
   D. Stand or sit on the side of the better ear

6. You are talking to Mr. Percy. You can do the following *except*
   A. State the topic of discussion
   B. Chew gum while talking
   C. Use short sentences and simple words
   D. Write out important names and words

7. A person has a speech problem. You should
   A. Pretend to understand so the person is not embarrassed
   B. Have the person write out all messages
   C. Ask the person to repeat or rephrase statements when necessary
   D. All of the above

8. Mr. Percy has a hearing aid. The hearing aid
   A. Corrects the hearing problem
   B. Makes sounds louder
   C. Makes speech clearer
   D. All of the above

9. Mr. Percy's hearing aid does not seem to be working. First, you should
   A. See if it is turned on
   B. Wash the entire instrument with soap and water
   C. Have it repaired
   D. Change the batteries

10. Mr. Percy has a cataract. Which is true?
    A. Surgery is the only treatment.
    B. There is no cure.
    C. He will be blind eventually.
    D. There is pressure in the eye.

11. An eye shield is ordered for Mr. Percy. Which is *true?*
    A. The eye shield protects the eye from injury.
    B. The eye shield is worn at bedtime and when napping.
    C. Measures for the blind person are practiced.
    D. All of the above

12. Mr. Percy is not wearing his eyeglasses. They should be
    A. Soaked in a cleansing solution
    B. Kept within his reach
    C. Put in the case and in the top drawer of the bedside stand
    D. Placed on the overbed table

13. Braille involves
    A. A white cane with a red tip for walking
    B. Raised dots arranged to represent letters of the alphabet
    C. An artificial eye
    D. Books and articles on compact disks or audiotapes

14. Mrs. Hart is blind. You should do the following except
    A. Touch her to get her attention
    B. Move equipment and furniture to provide variety
    C. Explain procedures step by step
    D. Have her walk behind you

15. You can provide for Mrs. Hart's safety by
    A. Keeping doors partially open
    B. Informing her of steps and curbs
    C. Rearranging furniture
    D. All of the above

Answers to these questions are on p. 838.

CHAPTER
30

COMMON HEALTH PROBLEMS

OBJECTIVES

Define the key terms listed in this chapter

Describe cancer and its treatment

Explain how to maintain joint function in persons with arthritis

Explain how to care for persons in casts, in traction, and with hip pinnings

Describe osteoporosis and the care required

Describe the effects of amputation

Describe stroke, its signs and symptoms, and the care required

Describe Parkinson's disease and multiple sclerosis

Identify the causes and effects of head and spinal cord injuries and the care required

Describe common respiratory disorders and the care required

Identify the signs, symptoms, and treatment of hypertension

List the risk factors for coronary artery disease

Describe angina pectoris, myocardial infarction, heart failure, and the care required

Describe the care required by persons with urinary system disorders

Identify the signs, symptoms, and complications of diabetes

Explain how to help the person who is vomiting

Describe hepatitis and AIDS, their signs and symptoms, and necessary precautions

Identify the sexually transmitted diseases and the communicable diseases common in children

KEY TERMS

alopecia Loss of hair

amputation The removal of all or part of an extremity

aphasia The inability *(a)* to speak *(phasia)*

arthritis Joint *(arthr)* inflammation *(itis)*

arthroplasty The surgical replacement *(plasty)* of a joint *(arthro)*

benign tumor A tumor that grows slowly and within a localized area

cancer Malignant tumor

closed fracture The bone is broken but the skin is intact; simple fracture

compound fracture The bone is broken and has come through the skin; open fracture

dialysis Process of removing waste products from the blood

expressive aphasia Difficulty expressing or sending out thoughts

expressive-receptive aphasia Difficulty expressing or sending out thoughts and difficulty receiving information

fracture A broken bone

gangrene A condition in which there is death of tissue; tissues become black, cold, and shriveled

hemiplegia Paralysis on one side of the body

hyperglycemia High *(hyper)* sugar *(glyc)* in the blood *(emia)*

hypoglycemia Low *(hypo)* sugar *(glyc)* in the blood *(emia)*

malignant tumor A tumor that grows rapidly and invades other tissues; cancer

metastasis The spread of cancer to other parts of the body

open fracture Compound fracture

paraplegia Paralysis of the legs

KEY TERMS *continued*

quadriplegia Paralysis of the arms, legs, and trunk

receptive aphasia Difficulty receiving information

simple fracture Closed fracture

stomatitis Inflammation *(itis)* of the mouth *(stomat)*

tumor A new growth of cells; tumors are benign or malignant

ureterostomy The surgical creation of an artificial opening *(stomy)* between the ureter *(uretero)* and the abdomen

This chapter gives basic information about common health problems. The RN uses the nursing process to meet the needs of persons with these and other health problems. Understanding a disorder makes the required care meaningful. A nurse gives you more information as needed.

A review of Chapter 6 (Body Structure and Function) will help you study this chapter.

CANCER

A **tumor** is a new growth of abnormal cells. Tumors are benign or malignant (Fig. 30-1). **Benign** tumors grow slowly and within a localized area. They do not usually cause death. A malignant tumor is cancerous. A **malignant** tumor **(cancer)** grows rapidly and invades healthy tissues (Fig. 30-2). Death occurs if the cancer is not treated and controlled. **Metastasis** is the spread of cancer to other body parts (Fig. 30-3). It occurs if the cancer is not treated and controlled. Cancer can occur in almost any body part. The most common sites are the lung, colon and rectum, breast, prostate, uterus, and urinary tract. Cancer is the second leading cause of death in the United States. It occurs in people of all ages.

The exact causes of cancer are unknown. However, certain factors contribute to its development. They include:

- A family history of cancer
- Exposure to radiation (including the sun)
- Exposure to certain chemicals
- Smoking
- Alcohol
- High-fat, high-calorie diet
- Food additives
- Viruses
- Hormones

Cancer can be treated and controlled with early detection. The seven warning signs identified by the American Cancer Society (ACS) are listed in Box 30-1.

Treatment depends on the type of tumor, its site and size, and if it has spread. One or a combination of treatments is used. The three major cancer treatments are surgery, radiation therapy, and chemotherapy.

Surgery involves removing malignant tissue. Surgery is done to cure or control cancer. It is also done to relieve pain from advanced cancer. Some surgeries are very disfiguring. The person's self-esteem and body image are affected.

Radiation therapy destroys living cells. X-rays are directed at the tumor. Cancer cells and normal cells are exposed to radiation. Both are destroyed. Radiation therapy is used to cure certain cancers or to control the growth of cancer cells. Pain is relieved or prevented by controlling cell growth. Radiation therapy has side effects. Discomfort, nausea and vomiting, fatigue (tiredness), anorexia (loss of appetite), and diarrhea are common. Skin breakdown can occur in the exposed area. The doctor may order special skin care procedures.

Chemotherapy involves drugs that kill cells. Like radiation, chemotherapy affects normal cells and cancer cells. It is used to cure cancer or control the growth rate of cancer cells. Side effects can be severe. They are caused by the destruction of normal cells. The gastrointestinal tract is irritated. Nausea, vomiting, and diarrhea result. **Stomatitis,** an inflammation *(itis)* of the mouth *(stomat),* also may develop. Hair loss **(alopecia)** may occur. Decreased production of blood cells occurs. As a result, the person is at risk for bleeding and infection.

Box 30-1	Seven Warning Signs of Cancer

Change in bowel or bladder habits
A sore that does not heal
Unusual bleeding or discharge from a body opening
Thickening or lump in the breast or elsewhere in the body
Indigestion or difficulty swallowing
Obvious change in a wart or mole
Nagging cough or hoarseness

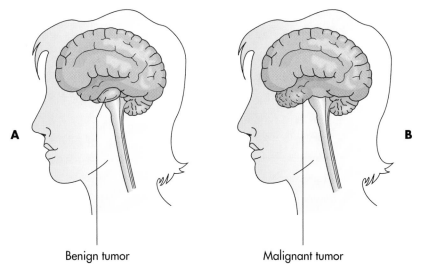

Benign tumor   Malignant tumor

Fig. 30-1 A, Benign tumors grow within a localized area. **B,** Malignant tumors invade other tissues.

Fig. 30-2 A malignant tumor on the skin. *(From Belcher AE:* Cancer nursing, *St Louis, 1992, Mosby.)*

Primary lesion

Fig. 30-3 A, A tumor in the lung. **B,** The tumor has metastasized to the other lung. *(From Belcher AE:* Cancer nursing, *St Louis, 1992, Mosby).*

Focus On... CHILDREN

Leukemia is the most common type of cancer in children. Leukemia means an increased number of white blood cells *(leuk)* in the blood *(emia)*. According to the ACS, other common sites are the bone, lymph nodes, brain, nervous system, and kidneys. The ACS has identified the following warning signs of cancer in children:
- An unusual mass or swelling
- Unexplained paleness and loss of energy
- Sudden tendency to bruise
- Persistent, localized pain or limping
- Prolonged, unexplained fever or illness
- Frequent headaches, often with vomiting
- Sudden eye or vision changes
- Excessive, rapid weight loss

Persons with cancer have many needs. They include:

- Pain relief or control
- Adequate rest and exercise
- Fluids and nutrition
- Preventing skin breakdown
- Preventing bowel elimination problems (constipation occurs from pain drugs; diarrhea occurs from chemotherapy)
- Dealing with the side effects of radiation therapy and chemotherapy
- Psychological, social, sexual, and spiritual needs

The person's psychological and social needs are great. Anger, fear, and depression are common. Disfigurement from surgery may cause the person to feel unwhole, unattractive, or unclean. The person and family need much emotional support. Talk to the person. Do not avoid the person because you are uncomfortable. Use touch to communicate that you care. Listen to the person. Often the person needs to talk and have someone listen. Being there when needed is important. You may not have to say anything. Just be there to listen.

The person's spiritual needs also are important. Some people get much comfort by talking to a spiritual leader. To many people, spiritual needs are as important as physical needs.

Persons with cancer often are referred to hospice programs (see Chapters 1 and 37). Hospice staff provide added support to the person and family.

(See Focus on Children box.)

MUSCULOSKELETAL DISORDERS

Musculoskeletal disorders affect the ability to move about. Some are caused by injury. Others result from aging.

ARTHRITIS

Arthritis means joint *(arth)* inflammation *(itis)*. It is the most common joint disease. Pain and decreased mobility occur in the affected joints. There are two basic types of arthritis.

Osteoarthritis. This type of arthritis, also called degenerative joint disease, occurs with aging. Joint injury and obesity are other causes. The hips, knees, and spine are commonly affected. These joints bear the body's weight. Joints in the fingers and thumbs also can be affected. Symptoms are joint stiffness and pain. Joint stiffness occurs with rest and lack of motion. Pain occurs with weight-bearing and joint motion. Severe pain can interfere with rest and sleep. Cold weather and dampness seem to increase the symptoms. Bony growths called *Heberden's nodes* (Fig. 30-4) are common in the fingers.

Osteoarthritis has no cure. Treatment involves relieving pain and stiffness. Doctors often order aspirin for pain. Local heat or local cold applications may be ordered. For obese persons, weight loss is stressed. A low-fat, low-calorie diet is often ordered. When the condition is advanced, the person may need a cane or walker. Measures to prevent falls are important. Assistance with daily activities is given as needed. Elevated toilet seats are helpful when there is limited range of motion in the hips and knees. Sometimes joint replacement surgery is necessary.

Rheumatoid Arthritis (RA). Rheumatoid arthritis is a chronic disease. It occurs at any age and is more common in women. Connective tissue throughout the body is affected. The disease affects the heart, lungs, eyes, kidneys, and skin. However, mainly the joints are affected. Smaller joints in the fingers, hands, and feet are affected first (Fig. 30-5). Eventually, larger

Fig. 30-4 Heberden's nodes occur in the finger joints. *(From Lewis SM, Heitkemper MM, Dirkson SR: Medical-surgical nursing: assessment and management of clinical problems, ed 5, St Louis, 2000, Mosby.)*

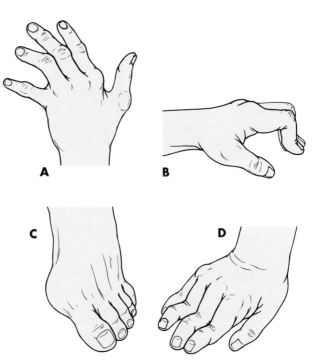

Fig. 30-5 Finger deformities caused by rheumatoid arthritis. *(From Lewis SM, Heitkemper MM, Dirkson SR: Medical-surgical nursing: assessment and management of clinical problems, ed 5, St Louis, 2000, Mosby.)*

joints are involved (wrists, elbows, and shoulders; ankles, knees, and hips). Joint inflammation usually occurs on both sides of the body. For example, if the right wrist is involved, so is the left wrist.

Severe inflammation causes very painful and swollen joints. The person restricts movement with severe pain. As the disease progresses, more and more joints become involved. Changes in other organs eventually occur.

Signs and symptoms of RA include:

- Pain, redness, warmth, and swelling in the joint area
- Joint stiffness upon awakening and after inactivity
- Limited joint motion
- Fever
- Fatigue
- Loss of appetite
- Weight loss
- Muscle aches

Treatment goals are to maintain joint motion, control pain, and prevent deformities. Rest is balanced with exercise. Bedrest is needed if several joints are involved and if fever is present. Turning and repositioning are done every 2 hours. Good body alignment is essential. Positioning to prevent contractures and deformities promotes comfort. Bed boards, a bed cradle, trochanter rolls, and pillows are used for alignment and positioning. Adequate sleep—8 to 10 hours—is needed each night. Morning and afternoon rest periods are also necessary.

Range-of-motion exercises are done. Walking aids may be needed. Splints may be applied to the affected body parts. Safety measures to prevent falls are practiced.

Focus On... CHILDREN

When RA occurs in children, it is called *juvenile rheumatoid arthritis (JRA)*. JRA can affect the child's growth and development. Eye inflammation is another complication.

The doctor orders drugs for pain. Local heat or local cold applications may be ordered. Back massages are relaxing. Joint replacement surgery may be indicated.

Emotional support and reassurance are needed. The disease is chronic. Death from other organ involvement is always possible. A good attitude is important. Being active is important. The more persons can do for themselves, the better off they are. A person may need someone to talk to. You must be a good listener when the person needs to talk.

(See Focus on Children box.)

Total Joint Replacement. Arthroplasty is the surgical replacement *(plasty)* of a joint *(arthro)*. Ankle, knee, hip, shoulder, wrist, finger, and toe joints can be replaced. The diseased joint is removed and replaced with a prosthesis (Fig. 30-6, p. 692). The surgery relieves pain and restores joint motion.

A **B** **C**

Fig. 30-6 A, Hip replacement prosthesis. **B,** Hip replacement prosthesis stems. C, Knee replacement prosthesis. *(Courtesy Zimmer, Inc. a Bristol-Myers Squibb Company, Warsaw, Ind.)*

OSTEOPOROSIS

Osteoporosis is a bone *(osteo)* disorder in which the bone becomes porous and brittle *(porosis)*. Bones are fragile and break easily. Bones of the spine, hips, and wrists are affected most often. It is common in older persons and in women after menopause. The ovaries do not produce the hormone *estrogen* after menopause. The lack of estrogen results in bone changes. Lack of dietary calcium is also a major cause of osteoporosis. Smoking, high alcohol intake, and lack of exercise also are risk factors. Bedrest and immobility are other causes because they do not allow for proper bone use. For bone to form properly, it must bear weight. If not, calcium is not absorbed and the bone becomes porous and brittle.

Signs and symptoms of osteoporosis include low back pain, gradual loss of height, and stooped posture. Fractures are a major threat. Sometimes bones are so brittle that the slightest stress can cause a fracture. Turning in bed or getting up from a chair can cause a fracture. Fractures are a great risk if the person falls or has an accident.

Prevention is important. Calcium, estrogen replacement therapy, and exercise are key. The diet must contain enough calcium. Often doctors order calcium and vitamin supplements. Estrogen is often ordered for women after menopause. Exercise that involves weight bearing is best. Walking, jogging, dancing, and stair climbing are examples. Good posture is also important. Some people wear a back brace or corset or need walking aids. Protect the person from falls and accidents (see Chapter 9). Always turn and reposition the person gently.

FRACTURES

A **fracture** is a broken bone. Tissues around the fracture (muscles, blood vessels, nerves, and tendons) are usually injured. Fractures are open or closed (Fig. 30-7). A **closed fracture (simple fracture)** means the bone is broken but the skin is intact. An **open fracture (compound fracture)** means the broken bone has come through the skin.

Fractures are caused by falls and accidents. Bone tumors, metastatic cancer, and osteoporosis are other causes. Signs and symptoms of a fracture are:

- Pain
- Swelling
- Limited movement and loss of function
- Bruising and color changes in the skin at the fracture site
- Bleeding (internal or external)

The bone has to heal. The bone ends are brought into normal position. This is called reduction. *Closed reduction* involves moving the bone back into place. The skin is not opened. *Open reduction* involves surgery. The bone is exposed and brought back into alignment. Nails, rods, pins, screws, plates, or wires are used to keep the bone in place (Fig. 30-8). After reduction, the fracture is immobilized. That is, movement of the bone ends is prevented. This is done with a cast or traction. *(See Focus on Children box.)*

Focus On... CHILDREN

Falls and accidents involving motor vehicles, bicycles, skate boards, and roller blades are common causes of fractures in children. Fractures in infants may be a sign of child abuse.

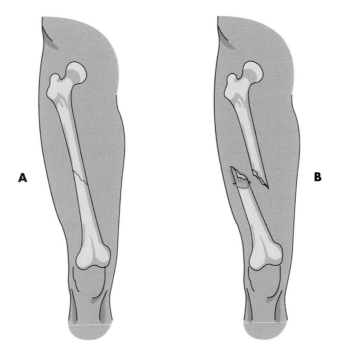

Fig. 30-7 A, Closed fracture. **B,** Open fracture. *(From Beare PG, Myers, JL: Principles and practice of adult health nursing, ed 3, St Louis, 1998, Mosby.)*

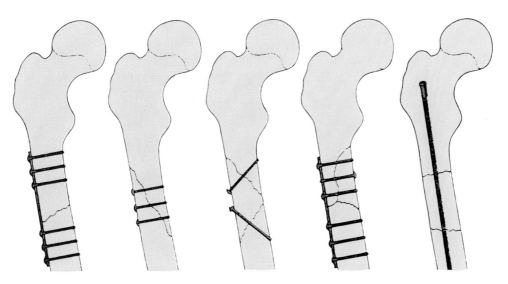

Fig. 30-8 Devices used to reduce a fracture. *(From Beare PG, Myers, JL: Principles and practice of adult health nursing, ed 3, St Louis, 1998, Mosby.)*

Cast Care. Casts are made of plaster of paris, plastic, or fiberglass. The cast covers all or part of an extremity (Fig. 30-9). Before the doctor applies a cast, the extremity is covered with stockinette. This protects the skin. Casting material comes in rolls. The rolls are moistened and wrapped around the part. Plastic and fiberglass casts dry quickly. A plaster of paris cast needs 24 to 48 hours to dry. It is odorless, white, and shiny when dry. When wet, it is gray and cool and has a musty smell. The rules listed in Box 30-2 are for cast care.

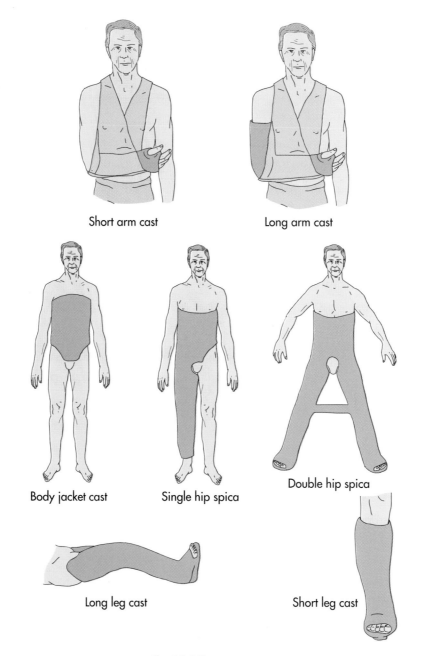

Short arm cast

Long arm cast

Body jacket cast

Single hip spica

Double hip spica

Long leg cast

Short leg cast

Fig. 30-9 Common casts.

Box 30-2   Rules for Cast Care

- Do not cover the cast with blankets, plastic, or other material. A plaster cast gives off heat as it dries. Covers prevent the escape of heat. Burns can occur if the heat cannot escape.
- Turn the person as directed by the nurse. All cast surfaces are exposed to the air at one time or another. Turning promotes even drying.
- Do not place a wet cast on a hard surface. A hard surface flattens the cast. The cast must maintain its shape. Use pillows to support the entire length of the cast (Fig. 30-10).
- Support a wet cast with your palms when turning and positioning the person (Fig. 30-11, p. 696). Fingers can dent the cast. The dents can cause pressure areas that can lead to skin breakdown.
- Protect the person from rough edges of the cast. Petaling involves covering the cast edges with tape (Fig. 30-12, p. 696). If stockinette is used, the doctor pulls it up over the cast. The stockinette is secured in place with a roll of cast material.
- Keep a plaster cast dry. A wet plaster cast loses its shape. It must be protected from moisture from the perineal area. The nurse may apply a waterproof material around the perineal area once the cast is dry.
- Do not let the person insert anything into the cast. Itching often occurs under the cast and causes an intense desire to scratch. Items used for scratching (pencils, coat hangers, knitting needles, back scratchers) can open the skin. An infection can develop. Items used for scratching can also wrinkle the stockinette. The object can be lost in the cast. Both can cause pressure and lead to skin breakdown.
- Elevate a casted arm or leg on pillows. This reduces swelling.
- Have enough help when turning and repositioning the person. Plaster casts are heavy and awkward. Balance is lost easily.
- Position the person as directed by the nurse and the care plan.
- Report these signs and symptoms immediately:
  - Pain—warns of a pressure ulcer, poor circulation, or nerve damage
  - Swelling and a tight cast—a sign of reduced blood flow to the part
  - Pale skin—a sign of reduced blood flow to the part
  - Cyanosis—a sign of reduced blood flow to the part
  - Odor—a sign of infection
  - Inability to move fingers or toes—a sign of pressure on a nerve
  - Numbness—a sign of pressure on a nerve or reduced blood flow to the part
  - Temperature changes—cool skin means poor circulation; hot skin means inflammation
  - Drainage on or under the cast—a sign of infection under the cast
  - Chills, fever, nausea, and vomiting—may signal an infection under the cast

Fig. 30-10 Pillows support the entire length of the wet cast. *(From Harkness GH, Dincher JR: Medical-surgical nursing: total patient care, ed 10, St Louis, 1999, Mosby.)*

Fig. 30-11 The cast is supported with the palms during lifting.

Fig. 30-12 A, The edges of the cast are petaled. **B,** Pieces of tape are used to make petals. The petal is placed inside the cast and then brought over the edge.

Traction. Traction is used to reduce and immobilize fractures. A steady pull from two directions keeps the fractured bone in place. Traction is also used for muscle spasms, to correct or prevent deformities, and for other musculoskeletal injuries. Weights, ropes, and pulleys are used (Fig. 30-13). Traction can be applied to the neck, arms, legs, or pelvis.

A doctor applies traction to the skin or to the bone. With *skin traction*, bandages and strips of material are applied to the skin. Weights are attached to the material or bandage (see Fig. 30-13). Traction applied directly to the bone is called *skeletal traction*. It is used for some arm and leg fractures. A pin, nail, or wire is inserted through the bone (Fig. 30-14). For traction to the cervical spine, tongs are applied to the skull (Fig. 30-15). Weights are attached to the device.

The rules listed in Box 30-3 on p. 698 apply when caring for a person in traction.

Fig. 30-13 Traction setup. Note the weights, pulleys, and ropes. *(From Phipps WJ, Sands JK, Marek JF: Medical-surgical nursing: concepts and clinical practice, ed 6, St Louis, 1999, Mosby.)*

Fig. 30-14 Skeletal traction is attached to the bone. *(From Phipps WJ, Cassmeyer VL, Sands JK, Lehman MK: Medical-surgical nursing: concepts and clinical practice, ed 5, St Louis, 1995, Mosby.)*

Fig. 30-15 Tongs are inserted into the skull for traction to the cervical spine. *(From Phipps WJ, Sands JK, Marek JF: Medical-surgical nursing: concepts and clinical practice, ed 6, St Louis, 1999, Mosby.)*

Box 30-3 Caring for Persons in Traction

- Keep the person in good body alignment.
- Do not remove the traction.
- Keep weights off the floor. Weights must hang freely from the traction setup (see Fig. 30-13).
- Do not remove weights from the traction setup.
- Do not add weights to the traction setup.
- Perform range-of-motion exercises for the uninvolved body parts as directed by the nurse.
- Position the person as directed by the nurse. Usually only the back-lying position is allowed. Slight turning is allowed with some types of traction.
- Provide the fracture pan for elimination.
- Give skin care often. Follow the care plan.
- Put bottom linens on the bed from the top down. The person uses the trapeze to raise the body off the bed.
- Check pin, nail, wire, or tong sites for redness, drainage, or odors. Report any observations to the nurse immediately.
- Observe for the signs and symptoms listed under cast care (see Box 30-2). Report these observations to the nurse immediately.

Hip Fractures. Fractured hips are common in older persons, especially older women (Fig. 30-16). They are especially serious because healing is slower in older people. The person may have other disorders. These disorders and slow healing may complicate the person's condition and care. The person is also at great risk for postoperative complications. These include pneumonia, atelectasis, urinary tract infections, and thrombi in the leg veins. The person can die from these complications. The person is also at risk for pressure ulcers, constipation, and confusion.

Open reduction is usually required. The fracture is fixed in position with a pin, nail, plate, screw, or prosthesis (Fig. 30-17). The person needs preoperative and postoperative care as described in Chapter 24. The person also requires the care described in Box 30-4. *(See Focus on Home Care box and Focus on Long-Term Care box.)*

Fig. 30-17 A, Hip fracture repaired with a prosthesis. **B,** Hip fracture repaired with a hip nail. *(From Thompson JM et al: Mosby's clinical nursing, ed 4, St Louis, 1997, Mosby.)*

Fig. 30-16 Hip fractures. *(From Phipps WJ, Sands JK, Marek JF: Medical-surgical nursing: concepts and clinical practice, ed 6, St Louis, 1999, Mosby.)*

Focus On... HOME CARE

The prosthesis can dislocate (move out of place) with adduction, internal rotation (turning inward), and severe hip flexion. Lying on the affected side, sitting in low seats, sitting with the legs crossed, bending from the waist, and putting on shoes and socks or stockings involve these movements. Therefore such movements are avoided for 6 to 8 weeks after surgery. An occupational therapist helps the person learn to do activities of daily living. Assistive devices are used for dressing (see Chapter 28). The person needs a raised toilet seat for elimination and a shower chair for bathing. The person uses a pillow or abductor splint between the legs when in bed. Muscle-strengthening exercises are also needed. A physical therapist helps the person with the exercises. A walker is usually needed for ambulation.

Focus On... LONG-TERM CARE

Older persons often require rehabilitation after a hip fracture. If home care is not possible, the person requires subacute or long-term care. Unless complications develop, the person usually returns home after successful rehabilitation. As in home care, adduction, internal rotation, and severe hip flexion are avoided.

Box 30-4   Caring for the Person With a Hip Fracture

- Give good skin care. Skin breakdown can occur rapidly.
- Encourage incentive spirometry and coughing and deep breathing exercises as directed by the nurse. See Chapter 27.
- Turn and reposition the person as directed by the nurse. The doctor's orders for turning and positioning depend on the type of fracture and the surgery performed. Usually the person is not positioned on the operative side.
- Keep the operated leg abducted at all times. The leg is abducted when the person is supine, being turned, or in a side-lying position (Fig. 30-18, *A*, p. 700). Pillows or abductor splints are used as directed (Fig. 30-18, *B*, p. 700).
- Prevent external rotation of the hip (turning outward). Use trochanter rolls, pillows, sandbags, or abductor splints as directed.
- Perform range-of-motion exercises as directed (see Chapter 20). Do not exercise the affected leg.
- Provide a straight-backed chair with armrests when the person is to be up. The person needs a high, firm seat. A low, soft chair is not used.
- Place the chair on the unaffected side.
- Assist the nurse in transferring the person from the bed to the chair as directed.
- Do not let the person stand on the operated leg unless allowed by the doctor.
- Support and elevate the leg as directed when the person is in the chair.
- Apply elastic stockings as directed (see Chapter 24).
- Remind the person not to cross his or her legs while seated.

Fig. 30-18 A, The hip is abducted when the person is turned. **B,** Pillows are used to maintain the hip in abduction. *(From Phipps WJ, Sands JK, Marek JF:* Medical-surgical nursing: concepts and clinical practice, *ed 6, St Louis, 1999, Mosby.)*

LOSS OF A LIMB

An **amputation** is the removal of all or part of an extremity. Usually the part is removed surgically. Traumatic amputations can occur from vehicle, workplace, and farming accidents. Severe injuries, bone tumors, severe infections, and circulatory disorders may require amputations.

Gangrene is a condition in which there is death of tissue. It can result from infection, injuries, and circulatory disorders. These conditions interfere with blood supply to the tissues. The tissues do not get enough oxygen and nutrients. Poisonous substances and waste products build up in the affected tissues. Tissue death results. The tissue becomes black, cold, and shriveled (Fig. 30-19) and eventually falls off. If untreated, gangrene spreads through the body and causes death.

All or part of an extremity may be amputated. Fingers, the hand, forearm, or entire arm may be removed. Toes, the foot, lower leg, upper leg, or entire leg may be amputated.

Much support is needed. A major psychological adjustment is necessary. The person's life is affected by the amputation. Appearance, activities of daily living, moving about, and work are some areas affected.

At some point most persons with amputations are fitted with a prosthesis. A prosthesis is an artificial replacement for a missing body part (Fig. 30-20). The stump is conditioned so the prosthesis fits. Stump conditioning involves shrinking and shaping the stump into a cone shape. An elastic stocking or bandage is used to shrink and shape the stump (Fig. 30-21). Exercises are ordered to strengthen the other limbs. Physical therapists help the person use the prosthesis. Occupational therapy is necessary if the stump or prosthesis is used for activities of daily living.

The person may feel that the limb is still there or may complain of pain in the amputated part. This is called *phantom limb pain.* The exact cause is unknown. However, it is a normal reaction. The sensation may occur only for a short time after surgery. However, some persons have phantom limb pain for many years.

Fig. 30-19 Gangrene.

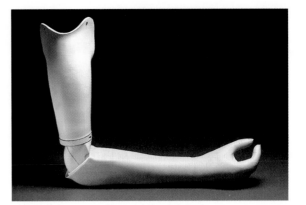

Fig. 30-20 Arm prosthesis. *(Courtesy Motion Control, Subsidiary of Fillauer, Salt Lake City, Utah.)*

Fig. 30-21 A midthigh amputation is bandaged to shrink and shape the stump. *(From Phipps WJ, Sands JK, Marek JF: Medical-surgical nursing: concepts and clinical practice, ed 6, St Louis, 1999, Mosby.)*

NERVOUS SYSTEM DISORDERS

Nervous system disorders can affect mental and physical functions. They can affect the ability to speak, understand, feel, see, hear, touch, think, control bowels and bladder, or move.

STROKE

The American Heart Association (AHA) defines stroke as a cardiovascular disease affecting the blood vessels that supply blood to the brain. Blood supply to a part of the brain is suddenly interrupted. Brain cells in the area affected do not get oxygen and nutrients. Brain damage occurs. Functions controlled by that part of the brain are lost or impaired. A ruptured blood vessel is one cause of stroke. This causes hemorrhage (excessive bleeding) into the brain. Blood clots are another cause. A blood clot obstructs blood flow to the brain. A stroke is also called a *cerebrovascular accident (CVA)* or *brain attack.*

Stroke is the third leading cause of death in the United States. It is the leading cause of disability in adults. Stroke is a medical emergency. The person needs immediate medical attention. (See Chapter 36 for emergency care.) Box 30-5 on p. 702 lists the warning signs of stroke. Sometimes the warning signs last a few minutes. This is called a *transient ischemic attack (TIA).* (*Transient* means temporary or short term. *Ischemic* means to hold back [ischein] blood [hemic].) Blood supply to the brain is interrupted for a short time. Sometimes a TIA occurs before a stroke. The person having a TIA needs medical attention. The TIA warns of a stroke.

Stroke is more common among persons over 65 years of age. However, it does occur in young and middle-age adults. A common cause of stroke is hypertension (high

Box 30-5	Warning Signs of a Stroke (CVA or Brain Attack)

- Sudden weakness or numbness of the face, arm, or leg on one side of the body
- Sudden dimness or loss of vision, particularly in one eye
- Loss of speech, or trouble talking or understanding speech
- Sudden, severe headaches with no known cause
- Unexplained dizziness, unsteadiness, or sudden falls (especially with any of the other signs)

From American Heart Association, 1999.

blood pressure). Other risk factors include diabetes, family history of stroke, hardening of the arteries, smoking, heart disease, and stress. Lack of exercise and high alcohol intake also are risk factors. So is race. Black men and women are at greater risk than white persons.

Signs and symptoms vary. Warning signs may occur (see Box 30-5). Dizziness, ringing in the ears, headache, nausea and vomiting, and memory loss also can occur. The stroke may occur suddenly. Unconsciousness, noisy breathing, high blood pressure, slow pulse, redness of the face, seizures, and paralysis on one side of the body (**hemiplegia**) may occur. The person may lose bowel and bladder control and the ability to speak. **Aphasia** is the inability (*a*) to speak (*phasia*).

If the person survives, some brain damage is likely. The functions lost depend on the area of brain damage (Fig. 30-22). The effects of a stroke include:

- Loss of hand, arm, leg, or body control
- Loss of face control
- Hemiplegia
- Changing emotions (the person can cry easily, sometimes for no reason)
- Difficulty swallowing (dysphagia)
- Dimmed vision
- Aphasia
- Slow or slurred speech
- Changes in perception (sight, touch, movement, and thought)
- Impaired memory
- Urinary frequency, urgency, or incontinence
- Depression
- Frustration

These effects change the person's behavior. The person may forget about or ignore the weaker side. This is from loss of movement and feeling on that side. If vision is affected, the person may not see that side of the body. The person may not recognize or know how to use familiar items. Activities of daily living and other tasks are difficult. The person may for-

Box 30-6	Care of the Person With a Stroke (CVA, Brain Attack)

- The lateral position is used to prevent aspiration.
- Coughing and deep breathing are encouraged.
- The bed is kept in a semi-Fowler's position.
- Turning and repositioning are done at least every 2 hours.
- Food and fluid needs are met.
- Elastic stockings are ordered to prevent thrombi (blood clots) in the legs.
- Range-of-motion exercises are performed to prevent contractures.
- A catheter must be inserted or a bladder training program started.
- A bowel training program may be necessary.
- Safety precautions are practiced. Check with the nurse about the use of bed rails.
- Assistance is given for self-care activities. The person is encouraged to do as much as possible.
- Communication methods are established. Magic Slates, pencil and paper, a picture board, or other methods are used. Questions are limited to those that have "yes" or "no" answers. Speak slowly. Allow the person time to respond. (See Chapter 5.)
- Good skin care is given to prevent pressure ulcers.
- Speech therapy, physical therapy, and occupational therapy are ordered. Assistive devices are used as necessary (see Chapter 28).
- Emotional support and encouragement are given. Praise is given for even the slightest accomplishment.

get what to do and how to do it. If the person does know, the body may not respond.

Rehabilitation starts immediately. The person may depend partially or totally on others for care. The RN uses the nursing process to meet the person's needs. Common care measures are listed in Box 30-6.

Aphasia. There are two basic types of aphasia. **Expressive aphasia** involves difficulty expressing or sending out thoughts. There are problems with speaking, spelling, counting, gesturing, or writing. The person thinks one thing but says another. For example, the person thinks about food but asks for a newspaper. People are called the wrong names even when correct names are known. Or the person thinks clearly but cannot speak. Some only produce sounds and no words. The person may cry or swear for no apparent reason.

Receptive aphasia relates to receiving information. The person has trouble understanding what is said or read. Everyday objects are not recognized. The person may not know how to use a fork, toilet, water glass, TV, telephone, or other items. The person may not recognize people.

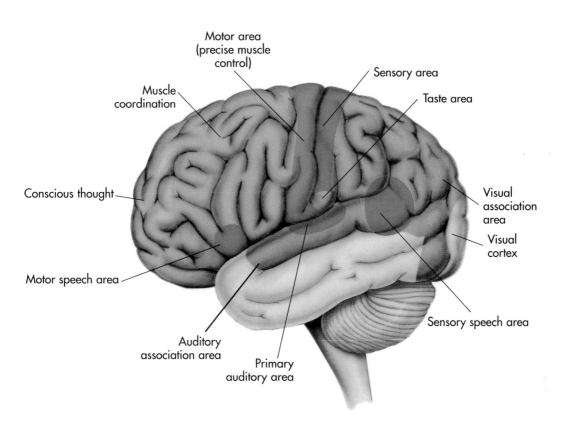

Fig. 30-22 Functions lost from a stroke depend on the area of brain damage. *(From Thibodeau GA, Patton KT: The human body in health & disease, ed 2, St Louis, 1997, Mosby.)*

Remember, for communication to occur, the message sent must be received and correctly interpreted. The person with *receptive* aphasia simply cannot interpret the message received. The person with *expressive* aphasia cannot send messages. Some people have both expressive and receptive aphasia. This is called **expressive-receptive aphasia.**

Persons with aphasia have many emotional needs. Frustration, depression, and anger are common. Communication is important for functioning and relationships with others. Remember, the person wants to communicate but cannot. You need to be patient and kind. *(See Focus on Home Care box and Focus on Long-Term Care box.)*

PARKINSON'S DISEASE

Parkinson's disease is a slow, progressive disorder with no cure. Degeneration of a part of the brain occurs. The disease is usually seen in persons over 50 years of age. Signs and symptoms are a masklike expression, tremors, pill-rolling movements of the fingers, a shuffling gait, stooped posture, impaired balance, stiff muscles (rigidity), slow movements, and drooling. Difficulty swallowing and chewing, bowel and bladder problems, sleep problems, and depression can occur. Some persons have memory loss, slow thinking, and emotional changes (fear and insecurity). Speech changes include slurred, monotone, and soft speech. Some patients talk too fast or repeat what they said.

 Focus On... **HOME CARE**

Many stroke survivors return home. A partner or family members assist with the person's care. Home nursing services are often needed. The care measures in Box 30-6 continue in the home. The nurse and therapists also recommend changes in the home setting to help the person function.

Focus On... **LONG-TERM CARE**

Some stroke survivors need subacute or long-term care. Some persons need rehabilitation and are able to return home. Long-term care is often permanent for survivors who totally depend on others for care. Many measures listed in Box 30-6 are part of the person's care.

The doctor orders drugs specific for Parkinson's disease. Exercise and physical therapy are ordered. These help the person improve strength, posture, balance, and mobility. The person may need help with eating and other self-care activities. Measures to promote normal elimination are practiced. Safety practices are followed to prevent injury. Remember, mental function may not be affected. Talk to and treat the person as an adult and with dignity and respect.

MULTIPLE SCLEROSIS

Multiple sclerosis (MS) is a progressive disease. The myelin sheath (which covers the nerves), the spinal cord, and the white matter in the brain are destroyed. Nerve impulses are not sent to and from the brain in a normal manner. Functions are impaired or lost.

Symptoms usually start between the ages of 20 and 40 years. Women are affected more often than men. The onset is gradual. Blurred or double vision occurs first. Muscle weakness and difficulty with balance and walking occur. Tremors, numbness and tingling, loss of feeling, speech impairment, dizziness, and poor co-ordination eventually occur. So do urinary inconti-nence, anal incontinence or constipation, and behav-ior changes. The person's condition worsens over many years. Blindness, contractures, paralysis of all extremities (quadriplegia), loss of bowel and bladder control, and respiratory muscle weakness are among the person's many problems. The person becomes to-tally dependent on others for care. Anger and depres-sion are common.

There is no known cure. Persons are kept active as long as possible. They need to do as much for them-selves as possible. Nursing care depends on the per-son's needs and condition. Skin care, hygiene, and range-of-motion exercises are important. Measures are taken to prevent injury and to promote bowel and blad-der elimination. Turning, positioning, coughing, and deep breathing are also important. Complications from bedrest are prevented. *(See Focus on Home Care box.)*

HEAD INJURIES

Injuries can occur to the scalp, skull, and brain tissue. Some injuries are minor. They cause only temporary loss of consciousness. Others are more serious. Brain tissue is bruised or torn. Bleeding can occur in the brain or surrounding structures. Permanent brain damage or death may result.

Head injuries are caused by falls, vehicle accidents, workplace accidents, and sports injuries. Other body parts are often injured. Spinal cord injuries are likely. If the person survives a severe head injury, some per-manent damage is likely. Paralysis, mental retarda-tion, personality changes, speech problems, breathing difficulties, and loss of bowel and bladder control may be permanent. Rehabilitation is required. Nursing care depends on the person's needs and remaining abilities. *(See Focus on Children box.)*

Focus On... HOME CARE

At first, the person may need help with housekeep-ing tasks to avoid fatigue. As mobility decreases, the person depends more on others. Eventually the per-son becomes bedridden and depends on others for basic needs. The nursing care plan reflects the per-son's changing needs. Occupational and physical therapists are often involved in the person's care. The National Multiple Sclerosis Society can provide resources for the person and family.

Focus On... CHILDREN

Birth injuries are a major cause of head trauma in newborns. As a child grows older, motor vehicle accidents, biking accidents, and falls are the major causes of brain damage. According to the National SAFE KIDS Campaign, falling is the greatest home danger for infants and toddlers. Falling down stairs and falling from windows are common accidents. See Chapter 9 for safety practices for infants and children and for how to prevent falls.

SPINAL CORD INJURIES

Spinal cord injuries can permanently damage the nervous system. Common causes are stab or bullet wounds, motor vehicle accidents, workplace accidents, falls, or sports injuries. Cervical traction is often neces-sary (see Fig. 30-15). The person in cervical traction is placed on a device that keeps the spine straight while the person is turned (Stryker frame or rotation bed).

The type of damage depends on the level of injury. The higher the level of injury, the greater the loss of function (Fig. 30-23). With lumbar injuries, muscle function in the legs is lost. Injuries at the thoracic level cause loss of muscle function below the chest. Persons with injuries at the lumbar or thoracic levels are para-plegics. **Paraplegia** is paralysis of the legs. Cervical in-juries cause loss of function to the arms, chest, and all muscles below the chest. Persons with these injuries are quadriplegics. **Quadriplegia** is paralysis of the arms, legs, and trunk.

Fig. 30-23 The *shaded areas* indicate the areas of paralysis.

Box 30-7 — Care of Persons With Paralysis

- Prevent falls. Keep the bed rails up, the bed in low position, and the signal light within reach. Check the person often if he or she cannot use the signal light.
- Prevent burns. Check bath water, heat applications, and food for the proper temperature.
- Turn and reposition the person at least every 2 hours.
- Give skin care and other measures to prevent pressure ulcers.
- Maintain good body alignment at all times. Use pillows, trochanter rolls, foot boards, and other devices as needed.
- Carry out bowel and bladder training programs.
- Perform range-of-motion exercises to maintain muscle function and prevent contractures. Assist with other exercises as ordered.
- Assist with food and fluids as needed. Provide self-help devices as ordered. Feed the person if necessary.
- Give emotional and psychological support. The person's care may involve psychiatrists or psychologists.
- Physical therapy, occupational therapy, and vocational rehabilitation are ordered. They help the person regain independent functioning to the extent possible.

Focus On... LONG-TERM CARE

Persons with spinal cord injuries often enter special rehabilitation centers. There they learn to function at their highest possible level. The person learns to use self-help and assistive devices and other special equipment. The person needs the care listed in Box 30-7.

Focus On... HOME CARE

Rehabilitation often continues when the person goes home. The RN, physical therapist, and occupational therapist suggest changes in the home to meet the person's needs. Ramps for wheelchair use usually are needed. So are changes in the kitchen, bathroom, and bedroom. For example, the refrigerator door may need to open from the other side. Kitchen shelves may need rearranging. A raised toilet seat, safety rails by the toilet and tub, bathtub seats, and tub transfer benches may help the person. The person may need a hospital bed, overbed trapeze, and a bedside commode. Furniture in all rooms may need rearranging to allow wheelchair access.

The person may need assistance with activities of daily living and with housekeeping tasks. The RN instructs you in the person's care and reviews the nursing care plan with you.

If the person survives, rehabilitation is necessary. The person's needs and the rehabilitation program depend on the functions lost and remaining abilities. Attention is given to emotional needs. These persons have severe emotional reactions to paralysis and the loss of function. Paralyzed persons generally need the care listed in Box 30-7. (*See Focus on Long-Term Care box and Focus on Home Care box.*)

RESPIRATORY DISORDERS

The respiratory system brings oxygen (O_2) into the lungs and removes carbon dioxide (CO_2) from the body. Respiratory disorders interfere with this function and threaten life.

CHRONIC OBSTRUCTIVE PULMONARY DISEASE

Three disorders are grouped under chronic obstructive pulmonary disease (COPD). They are chronic bronchitis, emphysema, and asthma. These disorders interfere with the exchange of O_2 and CO_2 in the lungs. They obstruct airflow.

Chronic Bronchitis. Chronic bronchitis occurs after repeated episodes of bronchitis (inflammation of the bronchi). Cigarette smoking is the major cause. Air pollution and industrial dusts are other causes. *Smoker's cough* in the morning is usually the first symptom. At first the cough is dry. Eventually the person coughs up mucus, which may contain pus. The cough becomes more frequent as the disease progresses. The person has difficulty breathing and tires easily. The mucus and inflamed breathing passages *obstruct* airflow into the lungs. Therefore the body cannot get normal amounts of oxygen.

The person must stop smoking. Oxygen therapy and breathing exercises often are ordered. Respiratory tract infections are prevented. If one occurs, prompt treatment is essential.

Emphysema. In emphysema, the alveoli enlarge. Walls of the alveoli are less elastic. They do not expand and shrink normally with inspiration and expiration. As a result, some air is trapped in the alveoli during expiration. Trapped air is not exhaled. As the disease progresses, more alveoli are involved. Therefore more air is trapped. The normal exchange of O_2 and CO_2 cannot occur in affected alveoli. Chronic bronchitis and emphysema often occur together.

Cigarette smoking is the most common cause. Signs and symptoms include shortness of breath and smoker's cough. At first, shortness of breath occurs with exertion. As the disease progresses, it occurs at rest. Sputum may contain pus. As more air is trapped in the lungs, the person develops a *barrel chest* (Fig. 30-24). Persons usually prefer to sit upright and slightly forward (see Chapter 27). Breathing is easier in this position.

The person must stop smoking. Respiratory therapy, breathing exercises, oxygen, and drug therapy are ordered.

Fig. 30-24 Barrel chest from emphysema.

Asthma Air passages narrow with asthma. Dyspnea results. Allergies and emotional stress are common causes. Episodes occur suddenly and are called *asthma attacks*. The person also has shortness of breath, wheezing, coughing, rapid pulse, perspiration, and cyanosis. The person is very frightened during the attack. Fear causes the attack to become worse.

Drugs are used to treat asthma. Emergency room treatment may be necessary for severe attacks. The person and family are taught how to prevent asthma attacks. Repeated attacks can damage the respiratory system.

PNEUMONIA

Pneumonia is an inflammation of lung tissue. Alveoli in the affected area fill with fluid. Because of fluid in the alveoli, O_2 and CO_2 are not exchanged normally.

Pneumonia is caused by bacteria, viruses, aspiration, or immobility. The person is very ill. Fever, chills, painful cough, chest pain on breathing, and a rapid pulse occur. Cyanosis may be present. Sputum is clear, green, yellowish, or rust colored. The color depends on the cause.

Focus On... CHILDREN

Pneumonia occurs in children of all ages. However, it is more common in infants and toddlers.

Focus On... OLDER PERSONS

The older person is at high risk for pneumonia. Changes from aging, other diseases, and decreased mobility increase the risk of pneumonia. Decreased mobility after surgery also is a risk factor. Other diseases and the drugs taken for them can mask the signs and symptoms of pneumonia. Pneumonia can lead to death.

Aspiration pneumonia is common in older persons. Decreased cough and gag reflexes and nervous system disorders increase the risk of aspiration. So do drugs that depress the brain. Such drugs include narcotics, sedatives, and the drugs given for general anesthesia. Alcohol also depresses the brain.

Drugs are ordered for infection and pain. Oral fluids are encouraged, and IV fluids may be ordered. Fluids are needed for fever and to help thin mucous secretions. Thin secretions are easier to cough up. Oxygen may be necessary. Most persons prefer semi-Fowler's position for breathing. Standard Precautions are followed. Transmission-Based Precautions may be necessary, depending on the cause. Mouth care is important. Frequent linen changes are needed because of fever. (*See Focus on Children box and Focus on Older Persons box.*)

TUBERCULOSIS

Tuberculosis (TB) is a bacterial infection. The lungs are affected. However, TB can also occur in the kidney and bones. TB was a major cause of death in the early 1900s. TB drug therapy was introduced in the 1940s and 1950s. A dramatic decline in the number of TB cases resulted. However, TB still occurs and is a major health problem. In the late 1980s the number of cases began to increase.

The bacteria causing TB are spread by airborne droplets (see Chapter 10). Bacteria are spread when the person coughs, sneezes, speaks, or sings. Others in the environment can inhale the bacteria. Persons who have close, frequent contact with an infected person are at risk. TB is more likely to occur in close, crowded areas such as inner-city neighborhoods. Persons with HIV infection are also at risk.

Sometimes bacteria do not cause an infection until many years later. The person may not have symptoms at first. The disease is found when routine chest x-rays are done or when a TB skin test is required for a job. Early signs and symptoms are tiredness, loss of appetite, weight loss, fever, and night sweats. Coughing occurs. The cough is more frequent as the disease progresses. Sputum production also increases. Chest pain occurs.

Treatment involves drugs for TB. Hospital care usually is not necessary. Persons with TB need to cover their noses and mouths with tissues when coughing or sneezing. Tissues are flushed down the toilet or placed in a paper bag and burned. In health care agencies, tissues are placed in a biohazard bag and disposed of following agency policy. Handwashing after contact with sputum is essential. Standard Precautions and Airborne Precautions are practiced.

CARDIOVASCULAR DISORDERS

Cardiovascular disorders are the leading causes of death in the United States. Problems occur in the heart or in the blood vessels.

HYPERTENSION

Hypertension *(high blood pressure)* is a condition in which the blood pressure is abnormally high. The systolic pressure is 140 mm Hg or higher. Or the diastolic pressure is 90 mm Hg or higher. Elevated measurements must occur on two different occasions. Risk factors are listed in Box 30-8 on p. 708. Narrowed blood vessels are a common cause. When vessels narrow, the heart pumps with more force to move blood through the vessels. Kidney disorders, head injuries, some complications of pregnancy, and adrenal gland tumors also can cause hypertension.

Hypertension can damage other body organs. The heart may enlarge so it can pump with more force. Blood vessels in the brain may burst and cause a stroke. Blood vessels in the eyes and kidneys may be damaged.

At first, hypertension may not cause signs or symptoms. Usually it is discovered when blood pressure is measured. Signs and symptoms develop as the disorder progresses. Headache, blurred vision, and dizziness may be reported. Complications of hypertension include stroke, heart attack, kidney (renal) failure, and blindness.

Certain drugs can lower blood pressure. The person needs to quit smoking, exercise, and get enough rest. A sodium-restricted diet may also be ordered. If the person is overweight, a low-calorie diet is ordered.

- *Age*—the risk increases with aging beginning at about age 35
- *Sex*—younger men are at greater risk than younger women; the risk increases for women after menopause
- *Race*—blacks are at greater risk than whites
- *Family history*—tends to run in families
- *Obesity*—related to lack of exercise and atherosclerosis
- *Stress*—increased sympathetic nervous system activity
- *Cigarette smoking*—nicotine narrows blood vessels
- *High-salt diet*—sodium causes fluid retention; increased fluid raises the blood volume
- *Alcohol*—increases chemical substances in the body that increase blood pressure
- *Lack of exercise*—leads to obesity
- *Atherosclerosis*—arteries narrow because of fatty buildup in the vessels

Fig. 30-25 A, Normal artery. **B,** Fatty deposits collect on the walls of arteries in atherosclerosis.

CORONARY ARTERY DISEASE

The coronary arteries are in the heart. They supply the heart with blood. In coronary artery disease (CAD), the coronary arteries narrow. One or all of the arteries may be affected. Because of narrowed vessels, the heart muscle gets less blood. The most common cause is atherosclerosis. In atherosclerosis, fatty material collects on the arterial walls (Fig. 30-25). The arteries narrow and obstruct blood flow. Blood flow through an artery may be totally blocked. Permanent damage occurs in the part of the heart receiving its blood supply from that artery.

CAD is the leading cause of death in the United States. Risk factors include:

- Sex (male gender)
- Age (more common in older persons)
- Obesity
- Cigarette smoking
- Lack of exercise
- A diet high in fat and cholesterol
- Hypertension
- Family history of CAD
- Uncontrolled diabetes

The major complications of CAD are angina pectoris and myocardial infarction (heart attack). Treatment involves reducing risk factors. Nothing can be done about the person's gender, age, and family history. However, efforts are directed at losing weight, regular exercise, no smoking, and eating a healthy diet. Controlling blood pressure and diabetes also is important.

Angina Pectoris. Angina *(pain)* pectoris *(chest)* means chest pain. The chest pain is from reduced blood flow to a part of the heart muscle (myocardium). Commonly called *angina*, it occurs when the heart needs more oxygen. Normally, blood flow to the heart increases when the heart's need for oxygen increases. Physical exertion, a heavy meal, emotional stress, and excitement increase the heart's need for oxygen. In CAD, narrowed vessels prevent increased blood flow.

Signs and symptoms include chest pain. The pain may be described as a tightness or discomfort in the left side of the chest. Pain may radiate to other sites (Fig. 30-26). Pain in the left jaw and down the inner aspect of the left arm is common. The person may be pale, feel faint, and perspire. Dyspnea is common. These signs and symptoms cause the person to stop activity and rest. Rest often relieves the symptoms in 3 to 15 minutes. Rest reduces the heart's need for oxygen. Therefore normal blood flow is achieved and heart damage is prevented.

Besides rest, a drug called *nitroglycerin* is taken to relieve angina. A nitroglycerin tablet is taken when an angina attack occurs. The tablet is put under the tongue. It dissolves under the tongue and is rapidly absorbed into the bloodstream. Most doctors want the tablets kept at the bedside. The person takes a tablet when one is needed and then tells the nurse. The person does not have to wait for someone to answer the signal light and then for a nurse to get the tablet. The person needs the tablets nearby at all times. This includes when the person goes to physical therapy, occupational therapy, the x-ray department, the dining room, the lounge, or other areas.

Persons are taught to avoid things likely to cause angina pectoris. These include overexertion, heavy meals and overeating, and emotional times. They need to stay indoors during cold weather and during hot, humid weather. Exercise programs supervised by doctors are helpful.

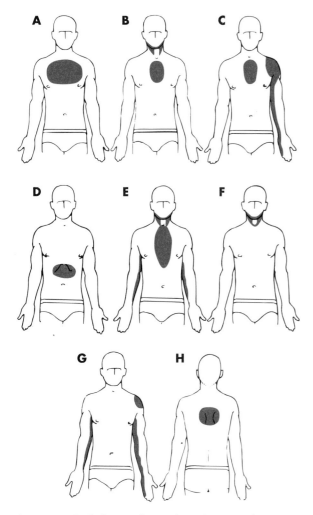

Fig. 30-26 *Shaded areas* show where the pain of angina pectoris is located. *(From Phipps WJ, Cassmeyer VL, Sands JK, Lehman MK: Medical-surgical nursing: concepts and clinical practice, ed 5, St Louis, 1995, Mosby.)*

Some people need coronary artery bypass surgery. The surgery bypasses the diseased part of the artery (Fig. 30-27) and increases blood flow to the heart. Many persons with angina pectoris eventually have heart attacks. Chest pain that is not relieved by rest and nitroglycerin may have a more serious cause.

Myocardial Infarction. A myocardial infarction (MI) is caused by lack of blood supply to the heart muscle (myocardium). Tissue death occurs (infarction). Common terms for MI are *heart attack, coronary, coronary thrombosis,* and *coronary occlusion.* Blood flow to the myocardium is suddenly interrupted. Atherosclerosis or a thrombus (blood clot) obstructs blood flow through an artery. The area of damage may be small or large (Fig. 30-28, p. 710). Sudden cardiac death *(cardiac arrest)* can occur (see Chapter 36).

The person has one or more signs and symptoms listed in Box 30-9 on p. 710. Myocardial infarction is an emergency. Efforts are directed at relieving pain, stabilizing vital signs, giving oxygen, and calming the person. Many drugs are given. The person is treated in a coronary care unit (CCU). The unit has emergency equipment and drugs needed during cardiac arrest. Measures are taken to prevent life-threatening complications.

The person is in the CCU for 2 to 3 days. When stable, the person is transferred. Activity is increased gradually. Drug therapy and measures to prevent complications are continued. Cardiac rehabilitation is planned. The goal is to prevent another heart attack. The program includes an exercise program and teaching about drugs, dietary changes, and sexual activity. Life-style changes may be necessary. *(See Focus on Home Care box, p. 710.)*

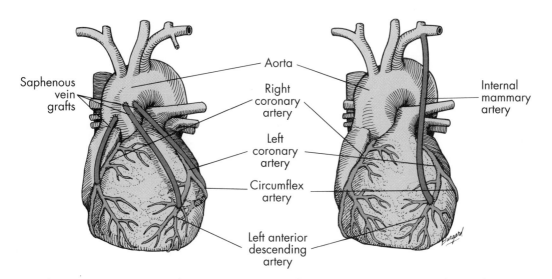

Fig. 30-27 Coronary artery bypass surgery. *(From Phipps WJ, Cassmeyer VL, Sands JK, Lehman MK: Medical-surgical nursing: concepts and clinical practice, ed 5, St Louis, 1995, Mosby.)*

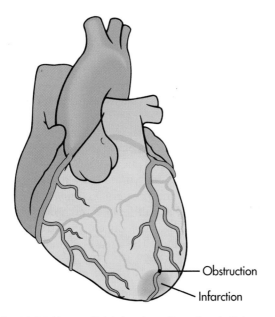

Obstruction

Infarction

Fig. 30-28 Myocardial infarction. *(From Lewis SM, Heitkemper MM, Dirkson SR:* Medical-surgical nursing: assessment and management of clinical problems, *ed 5, St Louis, 2000, Mosby.)*

Box 30-9	**Signs and Symptoms of Myocardial Infarction**

- Sudden, severe chest pain
- Pain is usually on the left side
- Pain is described as crushing, stabbing, or squeezing; some describe pain in terms of someone sitting on the chest
- Pain may radiate to the neck and jaw, and down the arm or to other sites
- Pain is more severe and lasts longer than angina pectoris
- Pain is not relieved by rest and nitroglycerin
- Indigestion
- Dyspnea
- Nausea
- Dizziness
- Perspiration
- Pallor
- Cyanosis
- Cold and clammy skin
- Low blood pressure
- Weak and irregular pulse
- Fear and apprehension
- A feeling of doom

Focus On... HOME CARE

Cardiac rehabilitation continues. The person may go to a fitness center for exercise. Many hospitals have fitness centers for cardiac rehabilitation. Some persons go to indoor malls for walking. Normal activities are increased slowly. Eventually the person returns to work with the doctor's approval.

HEART FAILURE

Heart failure or congestive heart failure (CHF) occurs when the heart cannot pump blood normally. Blood backs up and causes congestion of tissues. Left-sided heart failure, right-sided heart failure, or both can occur.

When the heart's left side fails to pump efficiently, blood backs up into the lungs. Signs and symptoms of respiratory congestion occur. These include dyspnea, increased sputum, cough, and gurgling sounds in the lungs. Also, blood is not pumped out of the heart to the rest of the body in adequate amounts. Organs do not get enough blood. Signs and symptoms occur from effects on the organs. Poor blood flow to the brain causes confusion, dizziness, and fainting. Poor blood flow to the kidneys causes reduced kidney function and decreased urinary output. The skin becomes pale or cyanotic. Blood pressure falls. A very severe form of left-sided failure is *pulmonary edema* (fluid in the lungs). Pulmonary edema is an emergency. Death can occur.

With right-sided failure, blood backs up into the venae cavae and into the venous system. Feet and ankles swell. Neck veins bulge. Liver congestion causes decreased liver function. The abdomen becomes congested with fluid. The right side of the heart cannot pump blood to the lungs efficiently. Normal blood flow does not occur from the lungs to the left side of the heart. Less blood than normal is pumped from the left side of the heart to the rest of the body. As with left-sided heart failure, the body's organs have a reduced blood supply. The signs and symptoms described in the previous paragraph eventually occur.

Heart failure is usually caused by a weakened heart. Myocardial infarction and hypertension are common causes. Damaged heart valves are another cause.

Heart failure can be treated and controlled. Drugs strengthen the heart and reduce the amount of fluid in the body. A sodium-restricted diet is ordered. Oxygen is given. Most persons prefer semi-Fowler's or Fowler's position for breathing. You may be involved in these aspects of the person's care:

- Maintaining bedrest or a limited activity program
- Measuring intake and output
- Measuring weight daily
- Restricting fluids as ordered by the doctor
- Giving good skin care to prevent skin breakdown
- Performing range-of-motion exercises
- Assisting with transfers or ambulation
- Assisting with self-care activities
- Maintaining good body alignment
- Applying elastic stockings

(*See Focus on Children and Focus on Older Persons boxes below.*)

DISORDERS OF THE URINARY SYSTEM

The kidneys, ureters, bladder, and urethra are the major urinary system structures. Disorders can occur in one or more of these structures.

URINARY TRACT INFECTIONS

Urinary tract infections (UTIs) are common. They can occur in the bladder or in a kidney. Infection in one area of the urinary tract can lead to infection of the entire urinary system. Normally the urinary system is sterile. It has no pathogens or nonpathogens. Microbes can enter the urinary system through the urethra. Catheterization, urological examinations, sexual intercourse, poor perineal hygiene, and poor fluid intake are common causes. UTI is a common nosocomial infection (see Chapter 10).

Women are at greater risk for UTIs than men. Women have a shorter urethra, which microbes can easily enter. In men, prostate gland secretions offer protection from UTIs. (*See Focus on Older Persons box at right.*)

Focus On... CHILDREN

Congenital heart defects can cause heart failure in children. (Congenital comes from the Latin work *congenitus*. It means to be *born with*.)

Focus On... OLDER PERSONS

Many older persons suffer from heart failure. They may need home care or long-term care.

The older person is at risk for skin breakdown. Tissue swelling, poor circulation, and fragile skin combine to increase the risk of pressure ulcers. Good skin care and regular position changes are essential.

Focus On... OLDER PERSONS

An enlarged prostate increases the risk of a UTI. Therefore older men are at risk.

Incomplete bladder emptying, perineal soiling from fecal incontinence, and poor nutrition increase the risk of UTI in older men and women.

Cystitis. Cystitis is inflammation (*itis*) of the bladder (*cyst*). It is caused by bacteria. The person may have one or more of the following:

- Urinary frequency
- Urgency
- Dysuria—difficult or painful (*dys*) urination (*uria*)
- Pain
- Foul-smelling urine
- Hematuria—blood (*hemat*) in the urine (*uria*)
- Pyuria—pus (*py*) in the urine (*uria*)

Antibiotics are the treatment of choice. Fluids are encouraged.

Pyelonephritis. Pyelonephritis is inflammation (*itis*) of the kidney (*nephr*) pelvis (*pyelo*). Infection is the most common cause. Chills, fever, back pain, and nausea and vomiting occur. So do the signs and symptoms of cystitis. Treatment consists of antibiotics and fluids.

URINARY DIVERSIONS

Sometimes it is necessary to surgically remove the urinary bladder. Cancer and bladder injuries are common. When the bladder is removed, a new pathway is necessary for urine to exit the body. The new pathway is called a *urinary diversion.*

There are many types of urinary diversions. Often an ostomy is involved. A **ureterostomy** is the surgical creation of an artificial opening (*stomy*) between the ureter (*uretero*) and the abdomen (Fig. 30-29, p. 712). The nurse provides stoma care in the early postoperative period. You may care for persons who have long-standing ureterostomies.

The person wears a ureterostomy pouch (Fig. 30-30, p. 712). The disposable, plastic pouch is applied over the stoma. Urine drains through the stoma into the pouch. The pouch is replaced anytime it leaks. Leakage can cause skin irritation, breakdown, and infection. Standard Precautions and the Bloodborne Pathogen Standard are followed when giving stoma care or emptying the pouch.

Fig. 30-29 Ureterostomies. **A,** Both ureters are brought through the skin onto the abdomen. The person has two stomas. **B,** The ileal conduit. A small section of the small intestine (ileum) is resected (removed) from the intestine. One end is sutured closed. The other end is brought through the skin onto the abdomen to form a stoma. The ureters are attached to the resected ileum. *(From Beare PG, Myers JL: Principles and practice of adult health nursing, ed 3, St Louis, 1998, Mosby.)*

Fig. 30-30 Ureterostomy pouch.

RENAL CALCULI

Renal calculi are kidney *(renal)* stones *(calculi)*. White men between the ages of 20 and 40 years have the greatest risk. Bedrest and immobility also are risk factors. Stones vary in size. Signs and symptoms include:

- Severe, cramping pain in the back and side; pain can also occur in the abdomen, thigh, and urethra
- Nausea and vomiting
- Fever and chills
- Dysuria—difficult or painful *(dys)* urination *(uria)*
- Urinary frequency and urgency
- Oliguria—scant *(olig)* urine *(uria)*
- Hematuria—blood *(hemat)* in the urine *(uria)*

Treatment involves pain relief and encouraging fluids. The person needs to drink about 4000 ml of fluid a day. Encouraging fluids helps promote passage of the stone through the urine. All urine is strained (see Chapter 16). Surgical removal of the stone may be necessary.

RENAL FAILURE

In renal failure (kidney failure) the kidneys do not function or are severely impaired. Waste products are not removed from the blood. Fluids are retained in the body. Heart failure and hypertension easily result. Renal failure may be acute or chronic. The person is very ill.

Acute Renal Failure. Acute renal failure occurs suddenly. Severe decreased blood flow to the kidneys is a common cause. The many causes of decreased blood flow to the kidneys include postoperative bleeding, bleeding from trauma, myocardial infarction (heart attack), severe congestive heart failure, burns, and severe allergic reactions.

At first the person has *oliguria* (scant amount of urine). Urine output is less than 400 ml in 24 hours. This is followed by *anuria* (absence of urine). It can last a few days to 2 weeks. Then diuresis occurs. *Diuresis* means the process *(esis)* of passing *(di)* the urine *(ur)*. Large amounts of urine are produced. Urine output ranges from 1000 to 5000 ml a day. Kidney function improves and returns to normal during the recovery phase. This phase can take from 1 month to 1 year. Some persons develop chronic renal failure.

Every system is affected by the buildup of waste products in the blood. Death can occur.

The doctor orders drug therapy, restricted fluids, and diet therapy. The person's diet is low in protein, high in carbohydrates, and low in potassium. The nurse plans for the person's physical and psychological needs. The person's care plan is likely to include:

- Measuring and recording urine output every hour; an output of less than 30 ml per hour is reported to the nurse immediately
- Measuring and recording intake and output
- Restricting fluid intake
- Daily weight measurements with the same scale
- Turning and repositioning at least every 2 hours
- Measures to prevent pressure ulcers
- Frequent oral hygiene
- Measures to prevent infection
- Coughing and deep-breathing exercises
- Measures to meet the person's emotional needs

Chronic Renal Failure. In chronic renal failure the kidneys cannot meet the body's needs. Nephrons of the kidney are slowly destroyed over many years. Hypertension and diabetes are the most common causes. Infections, urinary tract obstructions, and tumors are other causes.

Signs and symptoms appear when 80% to 90% of kidney function is lost. Every body system is affected by the buildup of waste products in the blood. Box 30-10 lists some of the signs and symptoms that occur.

Treatment includes fluid restriction, diet therapy, drugs, and dialysis. **Dialysis** is the process of removing waste products from the blood. It is a complex process. Specially trained nurses perform the procedure. Some persons have kidney transplants.

Nursing measures for the person in chronic renal failure are listed in Box 30-11.

THE ENDOCRINE SYSTEM

The endocrine system is made of glands. The endocrine glands secrete hormones that affect other organs and glands. The most common endocrine disorder is diabetes mellitus.

DIABETES MELLITUS

In this disorder the body cannot use sugar properly. Insulin is needed for the proper use of sugar. Insulin is secreted by the pancreas. In diabetes mellitus the pancreas does not secrete enough insulin. Sugar builds up in the blood. Cells do not have enough sugar for energy. Therefore cells cannot perform their functions.

Diabetes mellitus occurs in children and adults. Risk factors include obesity and a family history of diabetes. The risk increases after age 40.

There are three types of diabetes mellitus:

- *Immune-mediated diabetes (or type 1 diabetes)*—occurs most often in children and young adults. The body destroys the insulin producing cells in the pancreas. Therefore, the pancreas does not secrete insulin. The person needs daily insulin injections. Onset is rapid. This type of diabetes was formerly called insulin-dependent diabetes (IDDM).

Box 30-10	Signs and Symptoms of Chronic Renal Failure

- Yellow, tan, or dusky skin
- Dry, itchy skin
- Thin, brittle skin
- Bruises
- Bad breath (halitosis)
- Stomatitis (inflammation of the mouth)
- Nausea and vomiting
- Loss of appetite
- Diarrhea or constipation
- Bleeding tendencies
- Susceptibility to infection
- Hypertension
- Congestive heart failure
- Gastric ulcers
- Irregular pulse
- Abnormal breathing patterns
- Burning sensation in the legs and feet
- Muscle twitching
- Leg cramps at night
- Fatigue
- Headache
- Convulsions
- Confusion
- Coma

Box 30-11	Care of the Person in Chronic Renal Failure

- A diet low in protein, potassium, and sodium
- Fluid restriction
- Measuring blood pressure in the supine, sitting, and standing positions
- Measuring weight daily (with the same scale)
- Measuring and recording intake and output
- Turning and repositioning
- Measures to prevent pressure ulcers
- Range-of-motion exercises
- Measures to prevent itching (bath oils, lotions, and creams)
- Measures to prevent injury and bleeding
- Frequent oral hygiene
- Measures to prevent infection
- Measures to prevent diarrhea or constipation
- Measures to meet the person's emotional needs
- Measures to promote rest

- *Type 2 diabetes*—occurs in adults over 40 years of age. The pancreas secretes insulin. However, the body cannot use it effectively. Another form of type 2 diabetes is that the body does not make enough insulin. Onset of type 2 diabetes is slow. Type 2 diabetes was formerly called non-insulin dependent diabetes (NIDDM).
- *Gestational diabetes*—develops during pregnancy. (Gestation comes from the Latin word *gestare*, which means to *bear*.) It usually disappears after the baby is born. However, the woman is at risk for type 2 diabetes.

Signs and symptoms include increased urine production, increased thirst, hunger, weight loss, and extreme tiredness. Blurred vision is common. Frequent infections and slow healing of sores is common in persons with type 2 diabetes. In both types, blood tests show increased sugar levels.

If diabetes is not controlled, complications occur. These include blindness, renal failure, nerve damage, hypertension, and circulatory disorders. Circulatory disorders can lead to stroke, heart attack, and slow wound healing. Foot and leg wounds are very serious. Infection and gangrene can occur and require amputation of the part.

Risk factors include a family history of the disease. Obesity is also a risk factor. Blacks, Hispanics, and Native Americans are at risk. So are older persons.

Type 1 diabetes is treated with daily insulin therapy, diet, and exercise. Type 2 diabetes is treated with diet and exercise. Overweight persons need to lose weight. Oral drugs may be ordered. Some persons need insulin.

Both types require blood glucose monitoring. Good foot care is very important. Corns, blisters, and calluses on the feet can lead to an infection and amputation.

Hypoglycemia (insulin shock) occurs with too much insulin. **Hypoglycemia** means low *(hypo)* sugar *(glyc)* in the blood *(emia)*. Hyperglycemia (diabetic coma) develops if a person does not get enough insulin. **Hyperglycemia** means high *(hyper)* sugar *(glyc)* in the blood *(emia)*. Table 30-1 lists the causes, signs, and symptoms of hypoglycemia and hyperglycemia. Both can lead to death if not corrected. *(See Focus on Children box.)*

Focus On... CHILDREN

You may prepare meals for the child with diabetes. Follow the child's diet carefully. Also prepare snacks for the child to take to school. The snack is needed in case the child's blood sugar level drops.

Table 30-1 Hypoglycemia and Hyperglycemia	Causes	Signs and Symptoms
Hypoglycemia (insulin shock)	Too much insulin Omitting a meal Eating too little food Increased exercise Vomiting	Hunger Weakness Trembling Perspiration Headache Dizziness Rapid pulse Low blood pressure Confusion Cold, clammy skin Convulsions Unconsciousness
Hyperglycemia (diabetic coma)	Undiagnosed diabetes Not enough insulin Eating too much food Too little exercise Stress (e.g., from surgery, illness, emotional upset)	Weakness Drowsiness Thirst Hunger Frequent urination Flushed face Sweet breath odor Slow, deep, and labored respirations Rapid, weak pulse Low blood pressure Dry skin Headache Nausea and vomiting Coma

DIGESTIVE DISORDERS

The digestive system breaks down food for absorption by the body. It also eliminates solid wastes. Some digestive disorders are discussed in Chapter 17: diarrhea, constipation, flatulence, anal incontinence, and care of persons with colostomies and ileostomies.

VOMITING

Vomiting is the act of expelling stomach contents through the mouth. It is a sign of illness or injury. It can be life threatening. The vomitus (material vomited) can be aspirated and obstruct the airway. Shock can also occur if large amounts of blood are vomited. The following measures are practiced:

- Use Standard Precautions, and follow the Bloodborne Pathogen Standard.
- Turn the person's head well to one side. This prevents aspiration.
- Place a kidney basin under the person's chin.
- Remove the vomitus from the person's immediate environment.
- Provide for oral hygiene. This helps eliminate the taste of vomitus.
- Eliminate odors.
- Change linens as necessary.
- Observe vomitus for color, odor, and undigested food. Vomitus that looks like coffee grounds contains digested blood. This indicates bleeding.
- Measure the amount of vomitus. Report the amount to the nurse. Note the amount on the I&O record.
- Save a specimen for laboratory study.
- Do not discard vomitus until it is observed by the nurse.

COMMUNICABLE DISEASES

Communicable diseases (contagious or infectious diseases) can be transmitted from one person to another. They can be transmitted in the following ways:

- Direct—from the infected person
- Indirect—from dressings, linens, or surfaces
- Airborne—from the person through sneezing or coughing
- Vehicle—through ingestion of contaminated food, water, drugs, blood, or fluids
- Vector—from animals, fleas, and ticks

This section discusses hepatitis, AIDS, and sexually transmitted diseases. Table 30-2 on p. 716 outlines common childhood communicable diseases. Standard Precautions and Transmission-Based Precautions are followed.

HEPATITIS

Hepatitis is an inflammation of the liver. The major types of hepatitis are:

- *Hepatitis A*—is spread by the fecal-oral route. Food, water, or drinking or eating vessels can be contaminated with feces. The virus is ingested when eating or drinking contaminated food or water. It is also ingested when eating or drinking from a contaminated vessel. Causes include poor sanitation, crowded living conditions, poor nutrition, and poor hygiene. Handle bedpans, feces, and rectal thermometers carefully. Good handwashing is essential for everyone.
- *Heptatitis B*—is caused by the hepatitis B virus (HBV). The virus is present in blood and body fluids (saliva, semen, vaginal secretions) of infected persons. It is transmitted by needle sharing among IV drug users. The virus is also spread by sexual contact, especially anal sex. (The HBV vaccine is discussed in Chapter 10.)
- *Hepatitis C*—is caused by a virus spread through needle sharing and sexual contact.
- *Hepatitis D*—occurs in persons infected with HBV. Persons who receive frequent blood transfusions are at risk.
- *Hepatitis E*—occurs in countries with poor sanitation. It is spread by the fecal-oral route.

Hepatitis can be mild or can cause death. The signs and symptoms of hepatitis are listed in Box 30-12. Treatment involves bedrest and a healthy diet. The person is not allowed to drink alcohol. Full recovery takes about 8 weeks.

You must protect yourself and others from the hepatitis virus. Standard Precautions and the Bloodborne Pathogen Standard are followed. Transmission-Based Precautions are ordered as necessary (see Chapter 10). (*See Focus on Children box, p. 716.*)

Box 30-12 | Signs and Symptoms of Hepatitis

- Loss of appetite
- Weakness, fatigue, exhaustion
- Nausea and vomiting
- Fever
- Skin rash
- Dark urine
- Jaundice (yellowish color to the skin and whites of the eyes)
- Light-colored stools
- Headache
- Chills
- Abdominal pain
- Muscle aches

Table 30-2	Common Communicable Childhood Diseases	
Disease	**Transmission**	**Signs and Symptoms**
Chickenpox (varicella)	Direct contact and airborne contact with respiratory secretions; direct contact with skin lesions	Fever, rash, and skin lesions
Diphtheria	Direct or indirect contact with respiratory secretions and skin lesions from the person or a carrier	Sore throat, fever, nasal discharge, enlarged lymph glands in the neck, cough, hoarseness, patches (lesions) on the tonsils, pharynx, larynx, nasal membranes, and skin
Measles (rubeola)	Direct or indirect contact with nasal secretions	Fever, cough, rash, inflammation of the mucous membranes of the nose, nasal discharge; bronchitis
Mumps	Direct contact with saliva droplets	Fever, headache, swollen salivary glands, earache
Pertussis (whooping cough)	Airborne or direct contact with droplets from the respiratory tract	Fever, sneezing, severe cough at night, coughs are short and rapid followed by a "whoop" or crowing sound with inhalation
Poliomyelitis	Airborne or direct contact with respiratory secretions; direct contact with feces	Fever, sore throat, headache, nausea and vomiting, loss of appetite, abdominal pain, neck and spinal stiffness, paralysis
Rubella (German measles)	Airborne or direct contact with secretions from the nose and pharynx	Fever, headache, loss of appetite, nasal inflammation, sore throat, cough, rash
Scarlet fever	Airborne or direct contact with nasal and pharyngeal secretions	Fever, chills, headache, vomiting, abdominal pain, red and swollen tonsils and pharynx, rash

Focus On... CHILDREN

Hepatitis A is more common in preschool and school-age children. Poor hygiene practices after defecation lead to contamination of eating and drinking vessels. Also, young children often put their hands into their mouths.

ACQUIRED IMMUNODEFICIENCY SYNDROME

Acquired immunodeficiency syndrome (AIDS) is caused by a virus. The virus is called the *human immunodeficiency virus (HIV)*. The virus attacks the immune system. The person's ability to fight other diseases is affected. AIDS has no cure at present. It eventually leads to death.

The virus is spread through certain body fluids—blood, semen, vaginal secretions, and breast milk. HIV is not spread by saliva, tears, sweat, sneezing, coughing, insects, or casual contact. AIDS is transmitted mainly by:

- Unprotected anal, vaginal, or oral sex with an infected person ("unprotected" is without a latex condom)
- Needle-sharing among IV drug users
- HIV-infected mothers before or during childbirth
- HIV-infected mothers through breast-feeding

Box 30-13	**Signs and Symptoms of Acquired Immunodeficiency Syndrome (AIDS)**

- Loss of appetite
- Weight Loss
- Fever
- Night sweats
- Diarrhea
- Painful or difficulty swallowing
- Tiredness, extreme or constant
- Skin rashes
- Swollen glands in the neck, underarms, and groin
- Cough
- Sores or white patches in the mouth or on the tongue
- Purple blotches or bumps on the skin that look like bruises but do not disappear
- Confusion
- Forgetfulness
- Dementia (see Chapter 32)

Box 30-14	**Care of the Person with AIDS**

- Practice Standard Precautions.
- Follow the Bloodborne Pathogen Standard.
- Provide daily hygiene. Avoid harsh soaps that irritate the skin.
- Provide oral hygiene before meals and at bedtime. Make sure the person uses a toothbrush with soft bristles.
- Provide oral fluids as ordered.
- Measure and record intake and output.
- Measure weight daily.
- Have the person perform deep breathing exercises as ordered.
- Practice measures to prevent pressure ulcers.
- Assist with range-of-motion exercises and ambulation as ordered.
- Encourage the person to perform self-care as able. The person may need assistive devices (walkers, commode, eating devices).
- Encourage the person to be as active as possible.
- Change linens, gowns, or pajamas as often as needed when fever is present.
- Be a good listener and provide emotional support.

The virus enters the bloodstream through the rectum, vagina, penis, or mouth. Small breaks in the mucous membrane of the vagina or rectum may occur when the penis, finger, or other objects are inserted. Gum disease can cause breaks in the mucous membrane of the gums. The breaks in the mucous membrane of the mouth, vagina, or rectum provide a route for the virus to enter the bloodstream.

Intravenous drug users transmit AIDS through the use of contaminated needles and syringes. The virus is carried in the contaminated blood left in needles or syringes. When needles and syringes are used by others, contaminated blood enters their bloodstreams.

Infection can also occur when infected body fluids come in contact with open areas on the skin. Babies can become infected during pregnancy, shortly after birth, or from breast-feeding.

The virus is very fragile. It cannot live outside the body. Therefore HIV is not spread by casual, everyday contact. Such contact includes using public telephones, restrooms, or water fountains. Other forms of casual contact include talking to, hugging, or dancing with an infected person. HIV is not transmitted by food prepared by the infected person.

Signs and symptoms of AIDS are listed in Box 30-13. Some persons infected with HIV do not develop AIDS for as long as 10 to 15 years. They may not show signs or symptoms of the disease. However, they are carriers of the virus. They can spread the disease to others.

Persons with AIDS develop other diseases. Their bodies do not have the ability to fight disease. Their immune system, which fights diseases, is damaged. The person is at risk for pneumonia, Kaposi's sarcoma

Focus On... OLDER PERSONS

AIDS is often viewed as a young person's disease. Also, people often think that older persons are not sexually active and do not consider them to be at risk for AIDS. Except for childbirth and breast-feeding, older persons do get and spread AIDS in the same ways as younger persons.

The disease is often missed during diagnosis. Aging and other diseases can mask the signs and symptoms of AIDS. Often the person dies without the disease being diagnosed.

(a type of cancer), and central nervous system damage. The person with central nervous system damage may show memory loss, loss of coordination, paralysis, mental health disorders, and dementia.

You may care for persons with AIDS or who are HIV carriers (Box 30-14). You may have contact with the person's blood and body fluids. Mouth-to-mouth contact is possible during CPR. Certain precautions are necessary to protect yourself and others from the AIDS virus. Standard Precautions and the Bloodborne Pathogen Standard are followed. *These precautions apply when caring for all persons.* Remember, you may care for a person who has the HIV virus but shows no symptoms. You may also care for a person who is not yet diagnosed as having AIDS. *(See Focus on Older Persons box.)*

SEXUALLY TRANSMITTED DISEASES

Sexually transmitted diseases (STDs) are spread by sexual contact (Table 30-3). Some people are not aware of being infected. Others know but do not seek treatment. Embarrassment is a common reason for not seeking treatment.

The genital area is usually associated with STDs. However, other areas may be involved. These areas include the rectum, ears, mouth, nipples, throat, tongue, eyes, and nose. Most STDs are spread by sexual contact. The use of condoms helps prevent the spread of STDs. The use of condoms is very important for preventing the spread of HIV and AIDS. Some STDs are also spread through a break in the skin, by contact with infected body fluids (blood, semen, saliva), or by contaminated blood or needles.

Standard Precautions are necessary. The Bloodborne Pathogen Standard is also followed.

Table 30-3	Sexually Transmitted Diseases	
Disease	**Signs and Symptoms**	**Treatment**
Genital herpes	Painful, fluid-filled sores on or near the genitalia (Fig. 30–31) The sores may have a watery discharge Itching, burning, and tingling in the genital area Fever Swollen glands	No known cure Drugs can be given to control discomfort
Venereal warts	*Male*—Warts appear on the penis, anus, or genitalia *Female*—Warts appear near the vagina, cervix, and labia	Application of special ointment that causes the warts to dry up and fall off Surgical removal may be necessary if the ointment is not effective
AIDS (acquired immuno-deficiency syndrome)	See pp. 716-717	See pp. 716-717
Gonorrhea	Burning on urination Urinary frequency and urgency Vaginal discharge in the female Urethral discharge in the male	Antibiotic medications
Syphilis	*Stage 1*—10 to 90 days after exposure Painless chancre on the penis, in the vagina, or on genitalia; the chancre may also be on the lips or inside of the mouth, or anywhere else on the body *Stage 2*—About 2 months after the chancre General fatigue, loss of appetite, nausea, fever, headache, rash, sore throat, bone and joint pain, hair loss, lesions on the lips and genitalia *Stage 3*—3 to 15 years after infection Damage to the cardiovascular system and central nervous system, blindness	Antibiotic medications

Fig. 30-31 Genital herpes. **A,** Sores on the penis. **B,** Sores on the perineum. *(Courtesy USPHS, Washington, D.C.)*

REVIEW

Circle the BEST answer.

1. Which is *not* a warning sign of cancer?
   A. Painful, swollen joints
   B. A sore that does not heal
   C. Unusual bleeding or discharge from a body opening
   D. Nagging cough or hoarseness

2. Joan Martin has arthritis. Care includes the following *except*
   A. Measures to prevent contractures
   B. Range-of-motion exercises
   C. A cast or traction
   D. Assistance with activities of daily living

3. A cast needs to dry. Which is *false?*
   A. The cast is covered with blankets or plastic.
   B. The person is turned as directed so the cast dries evenly.
   C. The entire length of the cast is supported with pillows.
   D. The cast is supported by the palms when lifted.

4. A person has a cast. Which are reported immediately?
   A. Pain, numbness, or inability to move the fingers or toes
   B. Chills, fever, or nausea and vomiting
   C. Odor, cyanosis, or temperature changes of the skin
   D. All of the above

5. A person is in traction. You should do the following *except*
   A. Perform range-of-motion exercises as directed
   B. Keep the weights off the floor
   C. Remove the weights if the person is uncomfortable
   D. Give skin care at frequent intervals

6. After a hip pinning, the operated leg is
   A. Abducted at all times
   B. Adducted at all times
   C. Externally rotated at all times
   D. Flexed at all times

7. Joan Martin has osteoporosis. She is at risk for
   A. Fractures
   B. An amputation
   C. Phantom limb pain
   D. All of the above

8. A person had a stroke. The nurse tells you to do the following. Which should you question?
   A. Elevate the head of the bed to a semi-Fowler's position.
   B. Do range-of-motion exercises every 2 hours.
   C. Turn, reposition, and give skin care every 2 hours.
   D. Keep the bed in the highest horizontal position.

9. Receptive aphasia means that the person
   A. Cannot talk
   B. Cannot write
   C. Has trouble understanding messages
   D. All of the above

10. A person has Parkinson's disease. Which is *false?*
    A. Parkinson's disease affects part of the brain.
    B. The person's mental function is affected first.
    C. Signs and symptoms include stiff muscles, slow movements, and a shuffling gait.
    D. The person is protected from injury.

11. A person has multiple sclerosis. Which is *false?*
    A. Nerve impulses are sent to and from the brain in a normal manner.
    B. Symptoms usually begin in young adulthood.
    C. There is no cure.
    D. The person is eventually paralyzed and depends on others for care.

12. Persons with head or spinal cord injuries require
    A. Rehabilitation
    B. Speech therapy
    C. Long-term care
    D. Psychiatric care

13. A person has emphysema. Which is *false?*
    A. The person has dyspnea only with activity.
    B. Cigarette smoking is the most common cause.
    C. The person will probably breathe easier sitting upright and slightly forward.
    D. Sputum may contain pus.

14. A person has hypertension. Which complication can occur?
    A. Stroke
    B. Heart attack
    C. Renal failure
    D. All of the above

15. A person has hypertension. Treatment will probably include the following *except*
    A. No smoking and regular exercise
    B. A high-sodium diet
    C. A low-calorie diet if the person is obese
    D. Drugs to lower the blood pressure

16. A person has angina pectoris. Which is *true?*
    A. Damage to the heart muscle occurs.
    B. The pain is described as crushing, stabbing, or squeezing.
    C. The pain is relieved with rest and nitroglycerin.
    D. All of the above

17. A person is having a myocardial infarction. You know that
    A. The person is having a heart attack
    B. This is an emergency situation
    C. Cardiac arrest may occur
    D. All of the above

18. A person has heart failure. The following measures have been ordered. Which should you question?
    A. Encourage fluids
    B. Measure intake and output
    C. Measure weight daily
    D. Perform range-of-motion exercises

19. A person has cystitis. This is
    A. A kidney infection
    B. Kidney stones
    C. A urinary diversion
    D. An inflammation of the bladder

20. The person with a urinary diversion
    A. Wears a disposable pouch
    B. Needs dialysis
    C. Needs to have urine strained
    D. Has urine tested before meals and at bedtime

21. A person has chronic renal failure. Care will include all of the following *except*
    A. A diet low in protein, potassium, and sodium
    B. Measuring urinary output every hour
    C. Measures to prevent pressure ulcers
    D. Measuring weight daily

22. Which is not a sign of diabetes mellitus?
    A. Increased urine production
    B. Weight gain
    C. Hunger
    D. Increased thirst

23. Joan Martin has diabetes. She needs all of the following *except*
    A. Her meals served on time
    B. Good foot care
    C. Oral insulin
    D. Diet therapy

24. Vomiting is dangerous because of
    A. Aspiration   C. Fluid loss
    B. Cardiac arrest   D. Stroke

25. AIDS and hepatitis require
    A. Airborne Precautions   C. Standard Precautions
    B. Droplet Precautions   D. Contact Precautions

26. AIDS is usually spread by contact with infected
    A. Blood   C. Tears
    B. Urine   D. Saliva

27. These statements are about HIV and AIDS. Which is *false?*
    A. Standard Precautions are practiced, and the Blood Pathogen Standard is followed.
    B. There may be signs and symptoms of central nervous system damage.
    C. The person is at risk for infection.
    D. The person always shows some signs and symptoms.

28. Which statement is *false?*
    A. STDs are usually spread by sexual contact.
    B. STDs can affect the genital area and other parts of the body.
    C. Signs and symptoms of STDs are always obvious.
    D. Some STDs result in death.

Answers to these questions are on p. 838.

MENTAL HEALTH PROBLEMS

OBJECTIVES

Define the key terms listed in this chapter

Explain the difference between mental health and mental illness

List the causes of mental illness

Explain how personality develops

Describe three levels of awareness

Describe anxiety and three anxiety disorders

Understand the defense mechanisms used to relieve anxiety

Describe common phobias

Explain schizophrenia

Describe bipolar disorder and depression

Describe three personality disorders

Describe substance abuse, anorexia nervosa, and bulimia

Describe the care required by a person with a mental health disorder

KEY TERMS

affect Feelings and emotions

anxiety A vague, uneasy feeling that occurs in response to stress

compulsion The uncontrolled performance of an act

conscious Awareness of the environment and experiences; the person knows what is happening and can control thoughts and behaviors

defense mechanism An unconscious reaction that blocks unpleasant or threatening feelings

delusion A false belief

delusion of grandeur An exaggerated belief about one's own importance, wealth, power, or talents

delusion of persecution A false belief that one is being mistreated, abused, or harassed

ego The part of the personality dealing with reality; deals with thoughts, feelings, good sense, and problem solving

emotional illness Mental illness, mental disorder, psychiatric disorder

hallucination Seeing, hearing, or feeling something that is not real

id The part of the personality at the unconscious level; concerned with pleasure

mental Relating to the mind; something that exists in the mind or is performed by the mind

mental disorder Mental illness; emotional disorder, psychiatric disorder

mental health A state of mind in which the person copes with and adjusts to the stresses of everyday living in ways accepted by society

mental illness A disturbance in the person's ability to cope or adjust to stress; behavior and functioning are impaired; mental disorder, emotional illness, psychiatric disorder

obsession A persistent thought or idea

panic An intense and sudden feeling of fear, anxiety, terror, or dread

paranoia A disorder (para) of the mind (noia); false beliefs (delusions) and suspicion about a person or situation

personality The set of attitudes, values, behaviors, and traits of a particular person

phobia Fear, panic, or dread

psychiatric disorder Mental illness, mental disorder, emotional disorder

psychosis A serious mental disorder; the person does not view or interpret reality correctly

schizophrenia Split (schizo) mind (phrenia)

723

stress The response or change in the body caused by any emotional, physical, social, or economic factor

stressor Any emotional, physical, social, or economic factor that causes stress

subconscious Memory, past experiences, and thoughts of which the person is not aware; they are easily recalled

superego The part of the personality concerned with what is right and wrong

unconscious Experiences and feelings that cannot be remembered

The whole person has physical, social, psychological, and spiritual parts. Each part affects the other. A physical problem has social, mental, and spiritual effects. Likewise, mental health problems affect the person physically, socially, and spiritually. A social problem can have physical, mental health, and spiritual effects.

You will assist the nurse in caring for persons who have physical problems. In turn, emotional or mental health problems may develop. Mentally ill persons often have physical problems resulting from mental illness.

BASIC CONCEPTS

Mental health and mental illness are opposites. However, like physical health and illness, there are levels of seriousness. The common cold is at one extreme. The person has chills, fever, and respiratory congestion. At the other extreme is a life-threatening illness. Mental health has the same extremes.

MENTAL HEALTH

Mental relates to the mind. It is something that exists in the mind or is done by the mind. Therefore mental health involves the mind. Definitions of mental health and mental illness vary among textbooks and cultures. Most definitions include the concept of stress. In this textbook, these definitions are used:

- **Stress**—the response or change in the body caused by any emotional, physical, social, or economic factor.
- **Mental health**—a state of mind in which the person copes with and adjusts to the stresses of everyday living in ways accepted by society.
- **Mental illness**—a disturbance in the person's ability to cope or adjust to stress. The person's behavior and functioning are impaired. **Mental disorder, emotional illness**, and **psychiatric disorder** also mean mental illness.

Mental health disorders have many causes. Some result when the person cannot cope or adjust to stress. Others are caused by chemical imbalances in the body. Some are genetic in origin. (Genes are found in chromosomes. Characteristics from parents are passed on to children through genes contained in the chromosomes.) Other causes include drug or substance abuse. Social and cultural factors also can lead to mental illness.

PERSONALITY

Personality is the set of attitudes, values, behaviors, and traits of a person. Personality development starts at birth. It is affected by many factors. They include genes, culture, environment, parenting, and social experiences.

Maslow's theory of basic needs (see Chapter 5) affects personality development. Lower-level needs must be met before higher-level needs. Safety and security, love and belonging, esteem, and self-actualization needs cannot be met unless the physical needs are met. A child who grows up hungry, neglected, cold, or abused will not feel safe and secure. Higher-level needs cannot be met. Unmet needs at any age affect personality development.

The growth and development tasks presented in Chapter 7 also affect personality development. Remember, there is a sequence, order, and pattern to growth and development. Certain developmental tasks must be accomplished at each stage. Each stage lays the foundation for the next stage.

Sigmund Freud's theory of personality development involves the id, ego, and superego. To understand his theory, you need to understand three levels of awareness:

- **Conscious**—awareness of the environment and experiences. The person knows what is happening and can control thoughts and behavior.
- **Subconscious**—the memory, past experiences, and thoughts of which the person is not aware. Such thoughts, experiences, and memory are easily recalled.
- **Unconscious**—experiences and feelings that cannot be remembered.

The **id** part of the personality is at the unconscious level. The id is concerned with pleasure. The need for pleasure must be satisfied almost right away. The id deals with hunger, comfort, sex, and warmth. People are not aware that they behave and act in ways to satisfy the id.

The **ego** deals with reality—with what is happening in the person's world. Thoughts, feelings, reasoning, good sense, and problem solving occur in the ego. The ego decides what to do and when.

The **superego** is concerned with right and wrong. Morals and values are in the superego. The superego judges what the ego thinks and does. It is like a parent helping a child look at behaviors.

ANXIETY

Anxiety is a vague, uneasy feeling. It is a response to stress. The person may not know the source or cause of the uneasy feeling. The person has a sense of danger or harm. Danger or harm may be real or imagined. Anxiety is usually a normal emotion. The person acts to relieve the unpleasant feeling. Anxiety generally occurs when the person's needs are not met. Anxiety is seen in all mental health disorders.

The many signs and symptoms of anxiety are listed in Box 31-1. They depend on the degree of anxiety. Persons with mental health disorders have higher levels of anxiety.

Anxiety level depends on the stressor. A **stressor** is any emotional, physical, social, or economic factor that causes stress. Past experiences with the same or a similar stressor affect how a person reacts. The number of stressors also affects the person's reaction. A stressor at one time in a person's life may produce only mild anxiety. The same stressor may produce a higher level of anxiety at another time.

Coping and defense mechanisms are used to relieve anxiety. Common coping mechanisms include eating, drinking, smoking, exercising, talking about the problem, and fighting. Some people play music, go for a walk, take a hot bath, or want to be alone. Some coping mechanisms are healthier than others.

Defense mechanisms are unconscious reactions that block unpleasant or threatening feelings. Defense mechanisms protect the ego. They are used by everyone. Some use of defense mechanisms is normal. They relieve anxiety. Persons with mental health disorders use defense mechanisms poorly. Box 31-2 on p. 726 describes the common defense mechanisms.

MENTAL HEALTH DISORDERS

There are many types of mental health disorders. Some affect thinking; others affect mood. There are anxiety disorders and personality disorders. Substance abuse and eating disorders also are mental health problems. Changes in the brain are another cause. Dementia can occur (see Chapter 32).

ANXIETY DISORDERS

Persons with anxiety disorders have high degrees of anxiety. Signs and symptoms depend on the anxiety level.

Panic Disorder. Panic is the highest level of anxiety. **Panic** is an intense and sudden feeling of fear, anxiety, terror, or dread. It occurs suddenly with no obvious reason. The person cannot function and has severe signs and symptoms of anxiety. *Panic attacks* can last for a few minutes or for hours. They can occur several times a week.

Phobic Disorders. Phobia means fear, panic, or dread. The person with a phobia has an intense fear of an object or situation. Common phobias are described in Box 31-3 on p. 726.

Obsessive-Compulsive Disorder. An **obsession** is a persistent thought or idea. The thought or idea may be violent. **Compulsion** is the uncontrolled performance of an act. The person knows the act is wrong but has much anxiety if the act is not done. Some eating disorders are obsessive-compulsive. The person is obsessed with thoughts of food and eats constantly. Constant handwashing because of mysophobia (fear of dirt or contamination) is another. Some obsessive-compulsive disorders involve violent acts.

Box 31-1	Signs and Symptoms of Anxiety

- A "lump" in the throat
- "Butterflies" in the stomach
- Rapid pulse
- Rapid respirations
- Increased blood pressure
- Rapid speech
- Voice changes
- Dry mouth
- Perspiration
- Nausea
- Diarrhea
- Urinary frequency
- Urinary urgency
- Poor attention span
- Difficulty following directions
- Difficulty sleeping
- Loss of appetite

Box 31-2   Defense Mechanisms

Compensation—to compensate means to make up for, replace, or substitute. Compensation means to make up for or substitute a strength for a weakness.

Example: A boy is not good in sports. But he learns to play the guitar well.

Conversion—to convert means to change. Conversion is when an emotion is expressed or changed into a physical symptom.

Example: A girl knows she will have to read out loud in school today. She does not want to go to school. She complains of a stomachache.

Denial—to deny means to refuse to accept or believe something that is true or correct. Denial is when the person refuses to face or accept something that is unpleasant or threatening.

Example: A man had a heart attack. He is told to quit smoking and to eat a low-fat diet. He continues to smoke and eat fatty foods.

Displacement—to displace means to move or take the place of. Displacement is when an individual moves behaviors or emotions from one person, place, or thing to another person, place, or thing. The behavior or emotion is directed at a safe person, place, or thing.

Example: You are angry with your supervisor. Instead of yelling at your supervisor, you yell at a friend.

Identification—to identify means to relate or recognize. Identification is when a person assumes the ideas, behaviors, and traits of another person.

Example: A little girl admires her neighbor who is a high school cheerleader. The little girl practices cheerleading in her back yard.

Projection—to project means to blame or assign responsibility to another. Projection is blaming another person or object for one's own unacceptable behavior, emotions, ideas, or wishes.

Example: Two girls are in the same class. One fails a test. She blames the other girl for not helping her study.

Rationalization—to rationalize means to give some acceptable reason or excuse for one's behavior or actions. The real reason is not given. Rational means sensible, reasonable, or logical.

Example: A student does not study for a test and gets a poor grade. She says that the teacher is too hard and does not like her.

Reaction formation—a person acts in a way that is opposite to what he or she truly feels.

Example: A man does not like his boss. He buys the boss an expensive gift for Christmas.

Regression—to regress means to move back or to retreat. Regression means to retreat or move back to an earlier time or condition.

Example: A 3-year-old wants to drink from a baby bottle when a new baby comes into the family.

Repression—to repress means to hold down or keep back. Repression is keeping unpleasant or painful thoughts or experiences from the conscious mind. Such thoughts and experiences are in the unconscious mind and cannot be recalled or remembered.

Example: A little girl was sexually abused by her father. She is now 33 years old and has no memory of the event.

Box 31-3   Common Phobias

Agoraphobia—*agora* means marketplace. *Fear of being in an open, crowded, or public place.*

Algophobia—*algo* means pain. *Fear of being in pain or seeing others in pain.*

Aquaphobia—*aqua* means water. *Fear of water.*

Claustrophobia—*claustro* means closing. *Fear of being in or being trapped in an enclosed or narrow space.*

Gynephobia—*gyne* means woman. *Fear of women.*

Laliophobia—*lalio* means to talk or babble. *Fear of talking because of the fear of stuttering.*

Mysophobia—*myso* means anything that is disgusting. *Fear of the slightest uncleanliness; fear of dirt or contamination.*

Nyctophobia—*nycto* means night or darkness. *Fear of night or darkness.*

Photophobia—*photo* pertains to light. *Fear of light with the need to avoid light places.*

Pyrophobia—*pyro* means fire. *Fear of fire.*

Xenophobia—*xeno* means strange. *Fear of strangers.*

SCHIZOPHRENIA

Schizophrenia means split (*schizo*) mind (*phrenia*). You need to know the following terms to understand schizophrenia:

- **Psychosis** means a serious mental disorder. The person does not view or interpret reality correctly.
- **Delusion** is a false belief. A person believes he or she is God, a movie star, or some other person.
- **Hallucination** is seeing, hearing, or feeling something that is not real. A person may see animals, insects, or people that are not present.
- **Paranoia** means a disorder (*para*) of the mind (*noia*). The person has false beliefs (delusions) and is suspicious about a person or situation. For example, the person believes his or her food and drinks are poisoned.
- **Delusion of grandeur** is an exaggerated belief about one's own importance, wealth, power, or talents. For example, a man believes he is Superman or a woman believes she is the Queen of England.
- **Delusion of persecution** is the false belief that one is being mistreated, abused, or harassed. For example, a person believes that someone is "out to get" him or her.

The person with schizophrenia has a disorder of the mind (psychosis). Thinking and behavior are disturbed. The person has delusions (false beliefs) and hallucinations (seeing, hearing, or feeling things that are not real). The person has difficulty relating to others and may be paranoid (suspicion about a person or situation). The person's responses are inappropriate. Communication is disturbed. The person may ramble or repeat what another says. Sometimes speech cannot be understood. The person may withdraw from others and the world. That is, the person lacks interest in others and is not involved with people or society. The person may sit for hours alone without moving, speaking, or responding. Some persons *regress*. To regress means to retreat or move back to an earlier time or condition. For example, it is normal for a 5-year-old to regress back to bedwetting when a new baby comes into the family. It is not normal for an adult to have the behaviors of an infant or child. However, that is often seen in schizophrenia.

AFFECTIVE DISORDERS

Affect relates to feelings and emotions. Affective disorders involve feelings, emotions, and moods. There are two major affective disorders.

Bipolar Disorder. *Bipolar* means two (*bi*) poles or ends (*polar*). The person with bipolar disorder has extreme mood swings. Depression is at one extreme. Mania (elation) is at the other extreme. The person may:

- Be more depressed than manic
- Be more manic than depressed
- Alternate between depression and mania

When depressed, the person is very sad and feels lonely, worthless, empty, and hopeless. Self-esteem is low. The person may think about suicide.

In the manic phase, the person is excited, has much energy, and is very busy. The person cannot sleep and does not take time to eat or tend to self-care needs. Delusions of grandeur are common.

Major Depression. The person is very unhappy, lacks motivation, and feels unwanted. These feelings are extreme. Problems with concentration occur. Body functions are depressed. Sleeping problems and inactivity are common. Constipation can occur. (*See Focus on Older Persons box.*)

PERSONALITY DISORDERS

The individual with a personality disorder has rigid, inflexible, and maladaptive behaviors. To *adapt* means to change or adjust. *Mal* means bad, wrong, or ill. *Maladaptive* means to change or adjust in the wrong way. Because of their behaviors, individuals with personality disorders cannot function well in society. Personality disorders include:

Focus On... OLDER PERSONS

Depression is common in older persons. They experience many losses—death of family and friends, loss of health, loss of body functions, loss of independence. Loneliness and the side effects of some drugs also can cause depression. The signs and symptoms of depression in older persons are listed in Box 31-4.

Depression in older persons is often overlooked or misdiagnosed. Often the person is thought to have a cognitive disorder (see Chapter 32). Therefore the depression often goes untreated.

Box 31-4   Signs and Symptoms of Depression in Older Persons

- Fatigue
- Lack of interest
- Inability to experience pleasure
- Feelings of uselessness
- Feelings of hopelessness
- Feelings of helplessness
- Decreased sexual interest
- Increased dependency
- Anxiety
- Slow or unreliable memory
- Paranoia
- Agitation
- Focus on the past
- Thoughts of death
- Thoughts of suicide
- Difficulty completing activities of daily living
- Changes in sleep patterns
- Lower energy level
- Poor grooming
- Withdrawal from people and interests
- Muscle aches
- Abdominal pain
- Nausea and vomiting
- Dry mouth
- Headaches

From Lueckenotte AG: *Gerontologic nursing*, St Louis, 1996, Mosby.

- *Abusive personality*—the person copes with anxiety by abusing others. Behavior may be violent.
- *Paranoid personality*—the person is very suspicious. There is distrust of others.
- *Antisocial personality*—the person has poor judgment, lacks responsibility, and is hostile. The person has no loyalty to any person or group. Morals and ethics are lacking. The person blames others for actions and behaviors. The rights of others are not considered. The person feels no guilt and does not learn from past experiences or punishment. The person is often in trouble with law enforcement authorities.

SUBSTANCE ABUSE

Substance abuse occurs when a person physically or psychologically depends on drugs or alcohol. Alcohol is abused more than any other drug or substance. Both legal and illegal drugs are abused. Legal drugs are approved for use in the United States. Doctors prescribe them. Illegal drugs are not approved for use. They are obtained through illegal means. Commonly abused drugs are listed in Box 31-5. Abused substances affect the central nervous system. Some have a depressing effect. Others stimulate the nervous system. All affect the mind and thinking.

Box 31-5	Commonly Abused Substances

NARCOTICS
- Heroin (Horse; Smack)
- Morphine (Duramorph; MS-Contin; Roxanol; Oramorph SR)
- Codeine (Tylenol with Codeine; Empirin with Codeine; Robitussin A-C; Fiorinal with Codeine; APAP with Codeine)
- Hydrocodone (Tussionex; Vicodin; Hycodan; Lorcet)
- Hydromorphone (Dilaudid)
- Oxycodone (Percodan; Percocet; Tylox; Roxicet; Roxicodone)
- Methadone (Dolophine; Methadose)
- Fentanyl (Innovar, Sublimaze, Alfenta, Sufenta; Duragesic)
- Other narcotics (Opium, Darvon, Demerol)

DEPRESSANTS
- Chloral Hydrate (Noctec; Somnos; Felsules)
- Barbiturates (Amytal; Florinal; Nembutal; Seconal; Tuinal; Phenobarbital; Pentobarbital)
- Benzodiazepines (Ativan; Dalmane; Diazepam; Librium; Xanax; Serax; Valium; Tranxene; Verstran; Versed; Halcion; Paxipam; Restoril)
- Glutethimide (Doriden)
- Other depressants (Equanil; Miltown; Noludar; Placidyl; Valmid)

STIMULANTS
- Cocaine (Coke, Flake, Snow, Crack)
- Amphetamine/Methamphetamine (Biphetamine; Desoxyn; Dexedrine; Obetrol; Ice)
- Methylphenidate (Ritalin)
- Other stimulants (Adipex; Didrex; Ionamin; Melfiat; Plegine; Captagon; Sanorex; Tenuate; Tepanil; Prelu-2; Preludin)

CANNABIS
- Marijuana (Pot; Acapulco Gold; Grass; Reefer; Sinsemilla; Thai Sticks)
- Tetrahydrocannabinol (THC; Marinol)
- Hashish and hashish oil (Hash; Hash Oil)

HALLUCINOGENS
- LSD (Acid; Microdot)
- Mescaline and Peyote (Mescal; Buttons, Cactus)
- Amphetamine variants (2,5-DMA; STP; MDA; MDMA; Ecstasy; DOM; DOB)
- Phencyclidine (PCE; PCPy; TCP; PCP; Hog; Loveboat; Angel Dust)
- Other Hallucinogens (Bufotenin; Ibogaine; DMT; DET; Psilocybin; Psilocyn)

ANABOLIC STEROIDS
- Testosterone (Depo-Testosterone; Delatestryl)
- Nandrolene (Nortestosterone; Durabolin; Deca-Durobolin; Deca)
- Oxymetholone (Anadrol-50)

Modified from U.S. Department of Justice, Drug Enforcement Agency.

Eating Disorders

Eating disorders involve disturbances in eating behaviors. The two common eating disorders are anorexia nervosa and bulimia.

Anorexia Nervosa. *Anorexia* means no *(a)* appetite *(orexis)*. *Nervosa* relates to *nerves or emotions*. Anorexia nervosa occurs when a person has an abnormal fear of weight gain and obesity. The person refuses to eat. The disorder is more common in adolescent girls than boys. The person believes she is fat despite body weight and appearance. She has a poor self-image. Sleep problems, depression, and amenorrhea occur. *Amenorrhea* means lack of *(a)* monthly *(meno)* flow *(rrhea)*. In other words, she stops having monthly menstrual periods. There also may be suicidal thoughts. The person with anorexia nervosa is severely emaciated (Fig. 31-1). *Emaciation* means extreme leanness from disease or poor nutrition.

Fig. 31-1 Emaciation from anorexia nervosa. *(From Ezrin D, Godden JO, Volpe R:* Systematic endocrinology, *ed 2, New York, 1979, Harper & Row.)*

Bulimia. *Bulimia* comes from the Greek words that mean ox *(bous)* and hunger *(limos)*. The person with bulimia craves food. Constant eating or binge eating can occur. After eating, the person induces vomiting. That is, the body is purged (rid) of the food eaten. Some persons with bulimia take diuretics. Diuretics cause the kidneys to produce large amounts of urine. Extra fluid in the body is lost. This results in weight loss. Laxative abuse may occur. Laxatives are drugs that rid the intestines of feces through defecation.

Care of Persons With Mental Health Disorders

Treatment of mental health disorders involves having the person explore his or her thoughts and feelings. This is done through psychotherapy, group therapy, occupational therapy, art therapy, and family therapy. Often drugs are ordered for anxiety or depression.

The RN uses the nursing process to meet the person's needs. The needs of the total person must be met. This includes the person's physical, safety and security, and emotional needs.

Communication is important. Be alert to nonverbal communication. This includes the person's nonverbal communication and your own.

Circle the BEST answer.

1. Kathy has a mental health problem. The doctor says that she is under stress. Stress is
   A. The way she copes with and adjusts to everyday living
   B. A response or change in the body caused by some factor
   C. A mental or emotional disorder
   D. A thought or idea

2. The doctor asks Kathy's parents about her personality development. Personality is
   A. The id and the ego
   B. A person's attitudes, values, behaviors, and traits
   C. The coping and defense mechanisms used by a person
   D. All of the above

3. The doctor says that Kathy has many unpleasant experiences in her subconscious. You know that Kathy
   A. Can remember those experiences
   B. Cannot remember those experiences
   C. Is aware of those experiences
   D. Is projecting those experiences to others

4. Which part of Kathy's personality is concerned with right and wrong?
   A. The id
   B. The ego
   C. The superego
   D. The conscious

5. Kathy uses defense mechanisms. Defense mechanisms are used to
   A. Blame others
   B. Make excuses for behavior
   C. Return to an earlier time
   D. Block unpleasant feelings

6. These statements are about defense mechanisms. Which is *false*?
   A. Mentally healthy persons do not use defense mechanisms.
   B. Defense mechanisms protect the ego.
   C. Defense mechanisms relieve anxiety.
   D. All of the above

7. Kathy also has phobias. A phobia is
   A. A serious mental disorder
   B. A false belief
   C. An intense fear of an object or situation
   D. Feelings and emotions

8. Kathy believes she is married to a rock singer. She is constantly trying to telephone him. This behavior is a
   A. Delusion
   B. Hallucination
   C. Compulsion
   D. Obsession

9. Kathy's belief that she is married to a rock singer is called a
   A. Fantasy
   B. Delusion of grandeur
   C. Delusion of persecution
   D. Hallucination

10. Kathy believes that her parents are against her marriage. This belief is called
    A. Fantasy
    B. Delusion of grandeur
    C. Delusion of persecution
    D. Hallucination

11. Kathy's roommate has bipolar disorder. This means that the person
    A. Is very suspicious
    B. Has poor judgment, lacks responsibility, and is hostile
    C. Is very unhappy and feels unwanted
    D. Has severe mood swings

12. A person has an abusive personality. You know that the person
    A. Abuses drugs or alcohol
    B. Has an eating disorder
    C. Has bulimia
    D. May have violent behavior

Answers to these questions are on p. 838.

CHAPTER

32

CONFUSION AND DEMENTIA

Define the key terms listed in this chapter

Describe confusion and its causes

List the measures that help confused persons

Explain the difference between delirium, depression, and dementia

Describe Alzheimer's disease

Describe the signs, symptoms, and behaviors associated with Alzheimer's disease

Explain the care required by persons with Alzheimer's disease and other dementias

Describe the effects of Alzheimer's disease on the family

KEY TERMS

delirium A state of temporary but acute mental confusion that comes on suddenly

delusion A false belief

dementia The term used to describe the loss of cognitive function (thinking, remembering, and reasoning) caused by changes in the brain

hallucination Seeing, hearing, or feeling something that is not real

pseudodementia False (*pseudo*) disorder of the mind (*dementia*)

sundowning Increased signs, symptoms, and behaviors of Alzheimer's disease during hours of darkness

Some changes in the brain and nervous system occur normally with aging (Box 32-1). Certain diseases also can cause changes in the brain. No matter the cause, changes in the brain can affect the person's cognitive function. (*Cognitive* relates to knowledge.) Cognitive functioning relates to memory, thinking, reasoning, ability to understand, judgment, and behavior.

CONFUSION

Confusion has many causes. Diseases, infections, losses of hearing and sight, and drug reactions are major causes. Brain injury and changes from aging are other causes. With aging, there is reduced blood supply to the brain and progressive loss of brain cells. Sometimes personality and mental changes result. Memory and the ability to make good judgments are lost. A person may not know people, the time, or the place. Gradual loss in the ability to perform activities of daily living is common. So are behavior changes. Anger, restlessness, depression, and irritability may occur.

Acute confusion (delirium) occurs suddenly. It usually is caused by infection, illness, injury, or drugs. It can occur after surgery. Treatment is aimed at the cause of the confusion. Usually acute confusion is temporary.

Confusion caused by physical changes cannot be cured. Some measures help to improve the person's functioning (Box 32-2). The person's physical and safety needs must be met.

DEMENTIA

Dementia is the term used to describe the loss of cognitive function (thinking, remembering, and reasoning) caused by changes in the brain. The prefix *de* means *opposite, away, off of, out of, to remove, down,* or *from. Mentia* comes from the Latin word for *mind.* Alzheimer's disease is the most common type of dementia. Other types and causes of dementia are listed in Box 32-3.

Box 32-1 Changes in the Nervous System From Aging

- Loss of brain cells
- Slower nerve conduction
- Slower response and reaction times
- Slower reflexes
- Decreased vision and hearing
- Decreased senses of taste and smell
- Reduced sense of touch and sensitivity to pain
- Reduced blood flow to the brain
- Changes in sleep patterns
- Shorter memory
- Forgetfulness
- Confusion
- Dizziness

Box 32-2 Caring for the Confused Person

- Follow the person's care plan to meet basic needs.
- Provide for the person's safety.
- Face the person, and speak clearly and slowly.
- Call the person by name every time you are in contact with him or her.
- State your name, and show your name tag.
- Tell the person the date and time each morning. Repeat the information as often as necessary during the day or evening.
- Explain what you are going to do and why.
- Give clear and simple answers to questions.
- Ask clear and simple questions. Allow enough time for the person to respond.
- Give short, simple instructions.
- Keep calendars and clocks with large numbers in the person's room and in nursing areas (Fig. 32-1).
- Encourage the person to wear glasses and a hearing aid if needed.
- Use touch to communicate (see Chapter 5).
- Allow the person to place familiar objects and pictures within view.
- Provide newspapers and magazines. Read to the person if appropriate.
- Discuss current events with the person.
- Provide access to television and radios.
- Maintain the day-night cycle. Open curtains, shades, and drapes during the day, and close them at night. Use a night-light at night. Encourage the person to wear regular clothes during the day rather than gowns or pajamas.
- Maintain a calm, relaxed, and peaceful atmosphere. Prevent loud noises, rushing, and congested hallways and dining rooms.
- Maintain the person's routine. Meals, bathing, exercise, television programs, and other activities are on a schedule. This promotes a sense of order and anticipation of what to expect.
- Do not rearrange furniture or the person's belongings.
- Encourage the person to participate in self-care activities.
- Be consistent.
- Remind the person of holidays, birthdays, and other special events.

Box 32-3 Types and Causes of Dementia

- Alcohol-related dementia and Korsokoff's disease—alcohol depresses the brain and has a toxic effect on brain cells
- AIDS-related dementia—see Chapter 30
- Brain tumors—see Chapter 30
- Cerebrovascular disease—diseased blood vessels *(vascular)* in the brain *(cerebro)*
- Delirium—a temporary state of acute confusion
- Depression—see p. 734
- Drugs—some drugs affect how the brain functions
- Huntington's disease—a nervous system disease
- Infection—see Chapter 10
- Multi-infarct dementia—many *(multi)* strokes leave areas of damage *(infarct)*
- Multiple sclerosis—see Chapter 30
- Parkinson's disease—see Chapter 30
- Stroke—see Chapter 30
- Syphilis—see Chapter 30
- Trauma and head injury—see Chapter 30

Fig. 32-1 A large calendar can help confused persons.

Dementia is not a normal part of aging. Most older people do not show signs of dementia. Some early warning signs of dementia include:

- Recent memory loss that affects job skills
- Difficulty with familiar tasks (dressing, cooking, driving)
- Problems with language; forgetting simple words
- Getting lost in familiar places
- Misplacing things and putting things in unusual places (putting a watch in a washing machine)
- Personality changes
- Poor or decreased judgment (going out in the snow without a coat or shoes)
- Loss of interest in life

Persons with signs and symptoms of dementia need to see a doctor. To determine the cause and type of problem, the doctor orders many tests. Treatment depends on the cause and problem. Some dementias can be reversed. When the cause is removed, so are the signs and symptoms of dementia. Treatable causes include:

- Drugs
- Alcohol
- Delirium
- Depression
- Tumors
- Heart, lung, and blood vessel problems
- Head injuries
- Infections
- Vision and hearing problems

Permanent dementias result from changes in the brain. Parkinson's disease and cerebrovascular disease cause permanent changes in the brain. Multi-infarct dementia (MID) is caused by many *(multi)* strokes. The stroke leaves an area of damage called an *infarct.* Alzheimer's disease is the most common type of permanent dementia.

Permanent dementias have no cure. The loss of cognitive function becomes progressively worse. The rate of progression varies.

Pseudodementia means false *(pseudo)* dementia. The person has the signs and symptoms of dementia. However, changes in the brain do not occur. This can occur with delirium and depression.

DELIRIUM AND DEPRESSION

Delirium and depression can be mistaken for dementia. They can occur alone or with dementia. Or the person with dementia can also suffer from delirium and depression.

Delirium. **Delirium** is a state of temporary but acute mental confusion. It comes on suddenly. Delirium is common in older persons with acute or chronic

illnesses. Infections, heart and lung diseases, poor nutrition, and hormone disorders are common causes. Hypoglycemia is also a cause (see Chapter 30). Alcohol can cause delirium. So can many types of drugs. Delirium is an emergency. The cause must be identified and treated. Signs and symptoms of delirium include:

- Anxiety
- Disorientation
- Tremors
- Hallucinations
- Delusions
- Disturbances in attention
- Decline in level of consciousness

Depression. Depression is the most common mental health problem in older persons. It is often overlooked when the person has physical problems. A correct diagnosis is important. Otherwise the person does not receive proper treatment. The person and family both experience unnecessary emotional, physical, social, and financial discomfort.

Some signs and symptoms of depression are also signs of aging. They also are the side effects of some drugs. Signs and symptoms of depression include:

- Sadness
- Inactivity
- Difficulty thinking
- Problems concentrating
- Feelings of despair
- Problems sleeping
- Changes in appetite
- Fatigue
- Agitation
- Withdrawal

ALZHEIMER'S DISEASE

Alzheimer's disease (AD) is a brain disease. Brain cells that control intellectual function are damaged. Memory, thinking, judgment, and behavior are affected. Mood and personality changes are seen. The person has difficulty with work and everyday functions. The person also has problems with family and social relationships.

Gradual in onset, the disease progresses over 3 to 20 years. It gets worse and worse. AD occurs in both men and women. Though more common in older persons, it occurs also in younger people. Some people in their 40s and 50s have AD. The risk increases after the age of 65. The cause is unknown. However, a family history of AD and Down syndrome are risk factors. (Down syndrome is a congenital disease [*congenital* means to be born with]. The child has mental retardation and many physical defects. See Chapter 33.)

SIGNS OF AD

According to the Agency for Health Care Policy and Research, the classic sign of AD is gradual loss of short-term memory. Other early signs include:

- Problems finding or speaking the right word
- Not recognizing objects
- Forgetting how to use simple, everyday things (like using a pencil)
- Forgetting to turn off the stove, close windows, or lock doors
- Mood and personality changes
- Agitation
- Poor judgment

AD affects the person's ability to perform complex and simple tasks. Problems with complex tasks appear first. The person has problems using the telephone, driving a car, managing money, planning meals, and working. As the disease progresses, problems occur with simple tasks. The person has problems with bathing, dressing, eating, using the toilet, and walking.

STAGES OF AD

The stages of AD are described in Box 32-4. Signs and symptoms are more severe with each stage. The following problems are common. The disease ends in death.

Wandering. Persons with AD are disoriented to person, time, and place. They may wander from home or the agency and not find their way back. They may be with caregivers one moment and gone the next. Judgment is poor. They cannot tell what is safe or dangerous. They are in danger of accidents. A person may walk into traffic or into a nearby river, lake, or forest. If they are not properly dressed, exposure is a risk in cold climates.

Sundowning. Sundowning occurs in the late afternoon and evening hours. As daylight ends and darkness occurs, confusion, restlessness, and other symptoms increase. Behavior is worse after the sun goes down. Sundowning may relate to fatigue or hunger. Inadequate light may cause the person to see things that are not there. Persons with AD may be afraid of the dark.

Box 32-4	Stages of Alzheimer's Disease

STAGE 1
- Memory loss—forgetfulness; forgets recent events
- Difficulty finding words, finishing thoughts, following directions, and remembering names
- Poor judgment; bad decisions (including when driving motor vehicles)
- Disoriented to time and place
- Lack of spontaneity—less outgoing or interested in things
- Blames others for mistakes, forgetfulness, and other problems
- Moodiness
- Difficulty performing everyday tasks

STAGE 2
- Restlessness; increases during the evening hours
- Sleep disturbances
- Memory loss increases—may not know family and friends
- Dulled senses—cannot tell the difference between hot and cold; cannot recognize dangers
- Bowel and bladder incontinence
- Needs assistance with activities of daily living—problems with bathing, feeding, and dressing self; afraid of bathing; will not change clothes
- Loses impulse control—may use foul language, have poor table manners, be sexually aggressive, or be rude

- Movement and gait disturbances—walks slowly; has a shuffling gait
- Communication problems—cannot follow directions; has problems with reading, writing, and math; speaks in short sentences or single words; statements may not make sense
- Repeats motions and statements—may move things back and forth constantly; may say the same thing over and over again
- Agitation—behavior may be violent

STAGE 3
- Seizures (see Chapter 36)
- Cannot communicate—may groan, grunt, or scream
- Does not recognize self or family members
- Depends totally on others for all activities of daily living
- Disoriented to person, time, and place
- Totally incontinent of urine and feces
- Cannot swallow—choking and aspiration are risks
- Sleep disturbances increase
- Becomes bed bound—cannot sit or walk
- Coma
- Death

Hallucinations. A **hallucination** is seeing, hearing, or feeling something that is not really there. Senses are dulled. Affected persons see animals, insects, or people that are not present. Some hear voices. They may feel bugs crawling on their bodies or feel that they are being touched.

Delusions. **Delusions** are false beliefs. People with AD may think they are God, movie stars, or some other person. Some believe they are in jail, are going to be murdered, or are being attacked. A person may believe that the caregiver is actually someone else. Many other false beliefs can occur.

Catastrophic Reactions. Catastrophic reactions are extreme responses. The person reacts as if a disaster or tragedy has occurred. The person may scream, cry, or be agitated or combative. These reactions often occur when there is too much stimuli at one time. Eating, music or television playing, and being asked questions all at one time can overwhelm the person.

Agitation and Restlessness. The agitated and restless person may pace, hit, or yell. Such behaviors may be caused by pain or discomfort, anxiety, lack of sleep, too much or too little stimuli, hunger, or the need to eliminate. A calm, quiet setting and meeting basic needs help calm the person.

Caregivers can cause agitation and restlessness. A caregiver may rush the person or be impatient. Or a caregiver's communication may give mixed verbal and nonverbal messages. Caregivers always need to look at how their behaviors affect other persons.

Aggression and Combativeness. Aggressive and combative behaviors occur in some persons. They may result from agitation and restlessness. Examples include hitting, pinching, grabbing, biting, or swearing. Such behaviors are frightening to caregivers, to others in the home, or to patients and residents. Sometimes aggressive and combative behaviors are part of the person's personality. See Chapter 5 for dealing with the angry person and Chapter 9 for workplace violence.

Screaming. Persons with AD have communication problems. At first, the person has difficulty finding the right words. As the AD progresses, the person may speak only short sentences or one word. Often the person's speech is not understandable.

The person may scream to communicate. Screaming is seen in persons who are very confused and have poor communication skills. The person may scream a word or a name. Or the person may just make screaming sounds.

Screaming has many causes. Possible causes include hearing and vision problems, pain or discomfort, fear, and fatigue. Too much or not enough stimulation can cause the person to scream. Sometimes the person reacts to a caregiver or family member by screaming.

A calm, quiet setting is helpful. Soft music can calm the person. If it is safe for the person to have them, make sure hearing aids and eyeglasses are worn. Sometimes the person is comforted by a family member. Many patients and residents have favorite caregivers. They may have a calming effect on the person. If the person responds to touch, use touch to calm him or her.

Abnormal Sexual Behaviors. Sexual behaviors are labeled abnormal because of how and when they occur. Remember, persons with AD are disoriented to person, time, and place. Therefore sexual behaviors may involve the wrong person, the wrong place, and the wrong time. They also have lost the ability to control behavior. Normally they would know not to undress or expose themselves in front of others. They would know not to masturbate or engage in sexual pleasures in public. Normally they would know their sexual partners. Persons with AD often mistake a sexual partner for someone else. The person kisses and hugs the other person.

Sexual behaviors may mean that the person's sexual needs are not being met. Touching, scratching, and rubbing the genitals can signal infection, pain, or discomfort involving the urinary or reproductive system. Poor hygiene is another cause. So is being wet or soiled from urine or feces.

The nurse encourages the person's sexual partner to show affection. The couple's normal practices are encouraged. Examples include hand holding, hugging, kissing, and touching. When a person masturbates in public, lead the person to his or her room. Provide privacy, and make sure the person is safe. Good hygiene is important to prevent itching. If the person urinates or has a bowel movement, make sure the person is cleaned quickly and thoroughly. Do not let the person stay wet or soiled.

The RN needs to assess the person for urinary or reproductive system problems. The doctor is contacted as necessary.

Repetitive Behaviors. Repetitive means to repeat over and over again. Persons with AD repeat the same motions over and over again. For example, the person folds the same napkin over and over. Or the person says the same words or asks the same question over and over. Such behaviors are usually harmless. They do not hurt the person. However, they can annoy the caregivers and the family.

The person is allowed to continue harmless acts. Music and TV can distract the person. Taking the person for a walk can help. Such measures also are useful when the person repeats words or questions.

CARE OF THE PERSON WITH AD AND OTHER DEMENTIAS

Alzheimer's disease and other dementias are frustrating to the person, family, and caregivers. Usually the person is cared for at home until symptoms are severe. Adult day care may help. Care in a nursing center is often required. The person may develop other illnesses and need hospital care. Thus you may care for a person with AD in an adult day care setting or in a hospital, nursing center, or private home. The person needs your support and understanding. So does the family.

Remember, people with AD do not choose to be forgetful, incontinent, agitated, or rude. Nor do they choose to have all of the other behaviors, signs, and symptoms of the disease. They have no control over what is happening to them. The disease causes the be-

haviors. The person may do something that a healthy individual would not do. When this happens, remember that the disease is responsible, not the person.

There is no effective treatment for AD. Signs and symptoms worsen over many years. The disease progresses at a different rate for each person. Eventually persons with AD depend on others for care. They develop bowel and bladder incontinence. They are fed, bathed, groomed, and dressed. Persons in stage 3 of the disease cannot ask for help or tell you what they need.

The RN uses the nursing process to plan measures to meet the person's specific needs. The person's safety, personal hygiene, nutrition and fluids, elimination, and activity needs must be met. So must the need for comfort and sleep. Many of the measures listed in Box 32-5 are part of the person's care plan.

Box 32-5 Care of the Person With Alzheimer's Disease

ENVIRONMENT
- Follow established routines.
- Avoid changing rooms or roommates.
- Place picture signs on rooms, bathrooms, dining rooms, and other areas (Fig. 32-2, p. 738).
- Keep personal items where the person can see them.
- Stay within the person's sight to the extent possible.
- Place memory aids (large clocks and calendars) where the person can see them.
- Keep noise levels low.
- Play music and show movies from the person's past.
- Keep tasks and activities simple.

COMMUNICATION
- Approach the person in a calm, quiet manner.
- Follow the rules of communication described in Chapter 5.
- Practice measures to promote communication (see Chapter 5).
- Provide simple explanations of all procedures and activities.
- Give consistent responses.

SAFETY
- Remove harmful, sharp, and breakable objects from the environment. This includes knives, scissors, glass, dishes, razors, and tools.
- Provide plastic eating and drinking utensils. This helps prevent breakage and cuts.
- Place safety plugs in electrical outlets.
- Keep cords and electrical equipment out of reach.
- Store personal care items in a safe place (shampoo, deodorant, lotion, and others).
- Keep childproof caps on medicine containers and household cleaners.
- Store household cleaners and medicines in locked storage areas.
- Store dangerous equipment and tools in a safe place.

- Remove knobs from stoves, or place childproof covers on the knobs.
- Remove dangerous appliances and power tools from the home.
- Remove firearms from the home.
- Store keys to the car or other motor vehicle in a safe place.
- Supervise the person who smokes.
- Store cigarettes, cigars, pipes, matches and other smoking materials in a safe place.
- Practice safety measures to prevent falls (see Chapter 9).
- Practice safety measures to prevent fires (see Chapter 9).
- Practice safety measures to prevent burns (see Chapter 9).
- Practice safety measures to prevent poisoning (see Chapter 9).

WANDERING
- Make sure doors and windows are securely locked. Locks often are placed at the top and bottom of doors (Fig. 32-3, p. 738). The person is not likely to look for a lock at the top or bottom of the door.
- Make sure door alarms are turned on. The alarm goes off when the door is opened. These are common in nursing centers.
- Make sure the person wears an ID bracelet at all times.
- Exercise the person as ordered. Adequate exercise often reduces wandering.
- Do not restrain the person. Restraints require a doctor's order. They also tend to increase confusion and disorientation.
- Do not argue with the person who wants to leave. Remember, the person does not understand what you are saying.
- Go with the person who insists on going outside. Make sure he or she is properly dressed. Guide the person inside after a few minutes (Fig. 32-4, p. 739).

Continued

| Box 32-5 | **Care of the Person With Alzheimer's Disease—cont'd** |

WANDERING—cont'd

- Let the person wander in enclosed areas if provided. Many nursing centers have enclosed areas where residents can walk about (Fig. 32-5). These areas provide a safe place for the person to wander.

SUNDOWNING

- Provide a calm, quiet setting late in the day. Treatments and activities are done early in the day.
- Do not restrain the person.
- Encourage exercise and activity early in the day.
- Make sure the person has eaten. Hunger can increase restlessness.
- Promote urinary and bowel elimination. A full bladder or constipation can increase restlessness.
- Do not try to reason with the person. Remember, he or she cannot understand what you are saying.
- Do not ask the person to tell you what is bothering him or her. The person's ability to communicate is impaired. He or she does not understand what you are asking. The person cannot think or speak clearly.
- Dim lights and play soft music to help calm the person.

HALLUCINATIONS AND DELUSIONS

- Do not argue with the person. He or she does not understand what you are saying.
- Reassure the person. Tell him or her that you will provide protection from harm.
- Distract the person with some item or activity.
- Use touch to calm and reassure the person (Fig. 32-6).

BASIC NEEDS

- Provide for the person's food and fluid needs (see Chapter 18). Provide finger foods. Cut food and pour liquids as needed.
- Provide good skin care (see Chapter 14). Keep the person's skin free of urine and feces.
- Promote urinary and bowel elimination (see Chapters 16 and 17).
- Promote exercise and activity during the day (see Chapter 20). This helps reduce wandering and sundowning behaviors. The person may also sleep better.
- Reduce the person's intake of coffee, tea, and cola drinks. These contain caffeine. Caffeine is a stimulant. It can increase the person's restlessness, confusion, and agitation.
- Provide a quiet, restful setting (see Chapter 21). Soft music is better in the evening than loud television programs. Play music during care activities such as bathing and during meals.
- Promote personal hygiene (see Chapter 14). Do not force the person into a shower or tub. People with AD are often afraid of bathing. Try bathing the person when he or she is calm. Use the bathing method preferred by the person (tub bath, shower, bed bath). Provide for privacy, and keep the person warm. Do not rush the person.
- Provide oral hygiene (see Chapter 14).
- Have equipment ready for any procedure ahead of time. This reduces the amount of time the person is involved in care measures.
- Observe for signs and symptoms of other disorders or diseases (see Chapter 30).
- Protect the person from infection (see Chapter 10).

Fig. 32-2 Signs provide cues to the person with dementia.

Fig. 32-3 A slide lock is at the top of the door. The person tries to open the lock on the knob.

Fig. 32-4 Walk outside with the person who wanders. Then guide her back inside.

Fig. 32-5 An enclosed garden allows persons with AD to wander in a safe setting.

Fig. 32-6 Use touch to calm a person with Alzheimer's disease.

Focus On... LONG-TERM CARE

Many nursing centers provide hospice care as the person nears death (see Chapter 37).

You must keep the person comfortable and safe. Good skin care and proper body alignment are needed to prevent skin breakdown and contractures. You must take special care to treat the person with dignity and respect. The person has the same rights as alert and active patients and residents. You must talk to the person in a calm voice. Always explain what you are going to do. Massage, soothing touch, music, and aroma therapy can promote comfort and relaxation. *(See Focus on Long-Term Care box.)*

Your observations are important. The person can develop other health problems. Injuries can occur. However, the person may not know there is pain, fever, constipation, incontinence, or other signs and symptoms. You need to carefully observe the person. Report any change in the person's usual behavior to the nurse.

Infection is a major risk. Remember, the person's ability to give full attention to activities of daily living is greatly reduced. Infection can occur from poor hygiene. This includes poor skin care, oral hygiene, and perineal care after bowel and bladder elimination. Inactivity and immobility can lead to pneumonia and pressure ulcers.

Besides the measures listed in Box 32-5, other activities and therapies are ordered. These are intended to make the person feel useful, worthwhile, and active. They help the person's self-esteem. The therapist may work with one person, a small group, or a large group. Therapies and activities focus on the person's strengths and past successes. For example:

- A person used to cook. The person is given the task of cleaning vegetables.
- A person was a good dancer. Activities are planned so the person can dance.
- A person likes to clean. The person helps dust furniture.

Activities are planned to meet the person's needs. They are based on the person's likes and dislikes. All activities are supervised. They include crafts, exercise, gardening activities, and listening and moving to music. Sing-alongs, reminiscing, and board games are other activities appropriate for some people. Others respond well to repeated tasks such as stringing beads, folding towels, or rolling dough. Massage, range-of-motion exercises, and touch also are important activities.

(See Focus on Long-Term Care box, p. 740.)

> ### Focus On... LONG-TERM CARE
>
> Many long-term care centers have special nursing units for persons with AD and other dementias. The setting is designed to meet the special needs of these persons. Some units are secured. Entrances and exits to the unit are blocked. This prevents the confused person from wandering away. Some residents have aggressive, disruptive, or unsafe behaviors. They also may need a secured unit.
>
> The person is transferred to another nursing unit when a secured unit is no longer needed. For example, a person progresses from stage 2 to stage 3. The person cannot sit or walk. Wandering is no longer a concern.

> ### Focus On... HOME CARE
>
> Home care is an option for many families. Sometimes the family needs someone to prepare the person's meals. Help often is needed with bathing and elimination. The family may need someone to supervise the person while family members work, do errands, or need time to themselves. The amount and kind of care depends on the person's needs and the family's ability to provide care.

THE FAMILY

Persons with AD or other dementias may live at home or with children or other family members. Care is given by family members in the household. Or arrangements are made for a family member or someone else to stay with the person. Health professionals can help family members cope with the situation or help meet the person's needs. Home health care may help for awhile. Adult day care is another option. The decision for long-term care is usually made when:

- Family members can no longer meet the person's needs
- The person no longer knows the caregiver
- Family members have health problems
- Money problems occur
- The person has behaviors that are dangerous to self or others

Diagnostic tests, doctor's visits, drugs, and home care are costly. So is long-term care. The person's medical care can drain family finances.

The family has special needs. Care of the person at home or in a nursing center is stressful. There are physical, emotional, social, and financial stresses. Children find themselves in the *sandwich generation.* They are in the middle—between their own children who need to be taken care of and an ill parent who needs care. The stress of caring for two families is great. Often caregiving children have jobs too.

Caring for loved ones can be exhausting. Caregivers need much support and encouragement. Many join AD support groups. These groups are sponsored by hospitals, nursing centers, and the Alzheimer's Association. The Alzheimer's Association has chapters in cities and towns across the country. Support groups offer encouragement, advice, and ideas about care. Group members share their feelings, anger, frustration, guilt, and other emotions.

The family often feels helpless. No matter what is done for the loved one, the person only gets worse. Much time, money, energy, and emotion are needed to care for the person. Anger and resentment may result. Then the family feels guilty because of their anger and resentment. They know that the person did not choose to develop the disease. The family also knows that the person does not choose to have the signs, symptoms, and behaviors of the disease. They may be frustrated and angry that the loved one can no longer show love or affection. How would you feel if your mother, father, or partner did not know you? Sometimes the person's behavior is embarrassing.

The family has to learn some of the same care measures and procedures that you learn. They need to learn how to bathe, feed, dress, and give oral hygiene to the person. They also need to learn how to provide a safe setting. The RN and support group will help them learn to give necessary care. *(See Focus on Home Care box and Focus on Long-Term Care box on p. 741.)*

Focus On ... LONG-TERM CARE

Quality of life is important for all persons with confusion and dementia. Those in nursing centers have the same rights under OBRA as other residents. Residents with confusion and dementia may not know or be able to exercise their rights. However, the family is aware of the resident's rights. They need to know that their loved one's rights are protected. The family also needs to know that the loved one is treated with respect and dignity.

Residents with confusion and dementia have the right to privacy and confidentiality. You must protect the person from exposure. Only those involved in the person's care are present for care and procedures. The resident is allowed to visit with others in private. When family and friends visit, they are given space for a private visit. Confidentiality is also important. The resident's care and condition are not shared with others.

Personal choice is important. Some residents can still make simple choices. For example, a person may be able to choose between wearing a dress or slacks. Choosing to watch or not watch television may be a simple choice. Others cannot make choices themselves. The family may do so. The family chooses bath times, menus, clothing, activities, and other aspects of care.

The resident has the right to keep and use personal possessions. Some items comfort the resident. A pillow, blanket, afghan, or sweater may be important to the person. The resident may not be able to tell you why or even recognize the item. Still, it is important. The resident's personal items are kept safe. You must also protect the person's property from loss or damage.

The person must be kept free from abuse, mistreatment, and neglect. Caring for persons with confusion and dementia can be very frustrating. The person's behaviors may be difficult to deal with. Family and staff can become short-tempered and angry. The resident must be protected from abuse (see Chapter 2). Report any signs of abuse to the nurse right away. You need to be patient and calm when caring for these residents. Talk with the nurse if you find yourself becoming frustrated. Sometimes an assignment change is needed for a while.

All residents have the right to be free from restraints. Remember, restraints require a doctor's order. They are used only when it is the best way to protect the resident. They are not used for staff convenience. Restraints can make confusion and demented behaviors worse. The nurse tells you when to use restraints.

Activity and a safe setting promote quality of life. Box 32-5 identifies safety measures for persons with confusion and dementia. These residents also need activities that are safe, calm, and quiet. The recreation therapist and other health team members will find activities that are best for each person. These are part of the person's care plan.

REVIEW

Circle the BEST answer.

1. Cognitive impairment
   A. Occurs in all older people
   B. Refers to a decrease in intellectual functioning
   C. Refers to memory loss
   D. Is always permanent

2. A person is confused after surgery. The confusion is like to be
   A. Permanent
   B. Temporary
   C. Caused by an infection
   D. Caused by brain injury

3. The confused person is
   A. Restrained in bed at night
   B. Given many tasks to keep busy
   C. Easily distracted
   D. Never a danger to self or others

4. Joe Dunn has dementia. Dementia describes
   A. A false belief
   B. An illness caused by changes in the brain
   C. Seeing, hearing, or feeling something that is not real
   D. Alzheimer's disease

5. Joe Dunn was diagnosed with AD. Which is *true?*
   A. AD occurs only in older persons.
   B. Diet and drugs can control the disease.
   C. AD and delirium are the same.
   D. AD ends in death.

6. Which are common in persons with AD?
   A. Memory loss, poor judgment, and sleep disturbances
   B. Loss of impulse control and the ability to communicate
   C. Wandering, delusions, and hallucinations
   D. All of the above

7. Sundowning means that
   A. The person becomes sleepy when the sun sets
   B. Behaviors become worse in the late afternoon and evening hours
   C. Behavior improves at night
   D. The person is in stage 3 of the disease

8. Joe Dunn is screaming. You know that this is
   A. An agitated reaction
   B. His way of communicating
   C. Caused by a delusion
   D. A repetitive behavior

9. AD support groups do the following *except*
   A. Provide care
   B. Offer encouragement and care ideas
   C. Provide support for the family
   D. Promote the sharing of feelings and frustrations

10. Joe Dunn tends to wander. You should do the following *except*
    A. Make sure doors and windows are locked
    B. Make sure he wears an ID bracelet
    C. Help him with exercise as ordered
    D. Restrain him

11. Safety is important for Joe Dunn. Which is *false?*
    A. Safety plugs are placed in electrical outlets.
    B. Cleaners and drugs are kept out of his reach.
    C. He can keep smoking materials.
    D. Sharp and breakable objects are removed from his environment.

12. You are caring for Joe Dunn. Which is *false?*
    A. It is possible to reason with him.
    B. Touch can calm and reassure him.
    C. A calm, quiet setting is important.
    D. Assistance is needed with ADL.

Answers to these questions are on p. 839.

DEVELOPMENTAL DISABILITIES

Define the key terms listed in this chapter

Identify the areas of function limited by a developmental disability

Explain how a developmental disability affects the child and family across the life span

Explain when developmental disabilities occur

Describe the causes of developmental disabilities

Explain how mental retardation, Down syndrome, cerebral palsy, autism, epilepsy, spina bifida, and hydrocephalus affect a person's functioning

KEY TERMS

cerebral palsy (CP) A term applied to a group of disorders characterized by paralysis *(palsy)* that is caused by a defect in the motor region of the brain *(cerebral)*

convulsion A seizure

developmental disability A severe, permanent physical or mental disability that occurs before 22 years of age

diplegia Similar body parts are affected on both sides of the body; paralysis of both arms or both legs

epilepsy A condition the produces brief disturbances in the brain's normal electrical functions

seizure The violent and sudden contractions or tremors of muscles; convulsion

spastic Uncontrolled contractions of skeletal muscles

Many diseases, illnesses, and injuries that cause permanent disability occur in adulthood. However, some infants are born with defects that result in disabilities. Childhood illnesses and injuries also can result in disabilities. If a disability occurs before 22 years of age, it is called a **developmental disability.** The disability is severe and permanent. It may be a physical impairment, intellectual impairment, or both. The disability limits the person's ability to function in at least three of the following areas:

- Self-care
- Understanding or expressing language
- Learning
- Mobility
- Self-direction
- The ability to live independently
- Economic self-sufficiency (supporting oneself financially)

Developmentally disabled children become developmentally disabled adults. They do not remain children forever. The person needs lifelong assistance, support, and special services. The health care team is involved in the person's care.

Some parents care for the child at home. Family and community agencies often provide needed support and services. However, as the child and parents grow older, caring for the child is often more difficult. Some parents cannot lift or move an adolescent or adult child. A parent may become ill, injured, or disabled. A parent may die. Yet the person with a developmental disability still needs care.

Some severely disabled children require long-term care in special centers for those who are developmentally disabled. Some nursing centers admit developmentally disabled children and adults. OBRA requires that centers provide age-appropriate activities for these residents. Staff must also receive special training to prepare them to meet the special care needs of developmentally disabled persons.

The causes of developmental disabilities occur before, during, and after birth. Conditions that commonly involve developmental disabilities include:

- Mental retardation
- Down syndrome
- Cerebral palsy
- Autism
- Epilepsy
- Spina bifida

MENTAL RETARDATION

Mental retardation is a disorder involving low intellectual functioning and impaired adaptive behavior. (*Intellectual function* relates to learning, thinking, and reasoning. *Adapt* means to change or adjust.) According to the American Association on Mental Retardation (AAMR), the person with mental retardation:

- *Has an IQ score below 70 to 75.* The person learns at a slower rate than normal. The ability to learn also is less than normal.
- *Is limited in 2 or more adaptive skills.* Adaptive skills are those skills needed to live, work, and play. They involve communication, self-care, home living, social skills, leisure, health and safety, self-direction, basic academics, community use, and work. The person has difficulty with activities of daily living. Understanding the behavior of others is limited. So is the person's ability to respond in socially appropriate ways.
- *Shows signs of the disorder before 18 years of age.*

In mental retardation, brain development is impaired. It can occur before birth, during birth, or before the age of 18. The many causes of mental retardation are listed in Box 33-1.

Mental retardation ranges from mild to severe. Mildly affected persons are slow to learn in school. As adults, they can function in society with some support. For example, the person needs help finding a job. However, the person does not need support every day. Some persons need extensive support every day at home or at work. Still others need constant support in all adaptive skill areas.

The Arc of the United States is a national organization on mental retardation. (It was formerly called the Association of Retarded Citizens of the United States.) The Arc believes that children with mental retardation should live in a family. They should also learn and play with children who do and do not have disabilities. Adults with mental retardation should control their lives to the extent possible. That is, they should speak, make choices, and act for themselves. They should live in a home, have friends, work, and enjoy adult activities. Some have life partners. Others marry and have children.

The Arc also recognizes the sexuality of persons with mental retardation. This includes their physical, emotional, and social needs and desires. Reproduc-

Box 33-1	Causes of Mental Retardation

- Genetic conditions
  - Abnormal genes from one or both parents
  - Down syndrome
  - Fragile X syndrome
- During pregnancy
  - Alcohol use (fetal alcohol syndrome)
  - Drug use
  - Poor nutrition
  - Rubella (German measles)
  - Diabetes mellitus
  - HIV infection
  - Lack of oxygen to the brain
- During birth
  - Head injury
  - Prematurity
  - Low birth weight
  - Lack of oxygen to the brain
- After birth
  - Childhood diseases (whooping cough, chickenpox, measles)
  - Head injuries
  - Near drowning
  - Mercury poisoning
  - Lead poisoning
  - Poor nutrition
  - Child abuse (including shaken baby syndrome)

tive organs develop in persons with mental retardation. Remember, adaptive skills vary from mild to severe. Some persons cannot control their sexual urges. The type and location of their sexual responses may be inappropriate. Also, some adults sexually abuse persons with mental retardation. The Arc believes that persons with mental retardation have the right to privacy and to love and be loved. The Arc also believes that persons with mental retardation should learn about sex, sexual abuse, safe sex, and other sex and sexuality issues.

DOWN SYNDROME

Down syndrome (DS) is named for a British doctor who first identified the syndrome. Down syndrome is most commonly caused by an extra 21st chromosome. Remember, at fertilization, a male sex cell (sperm) unites with a female sex cell (ovum). The sperm and the ovum each have 23 chromosomes. When they unite, the fertilized cell has 46 chromosomes. In Down syndrome, an extra chromosome is present. Thus Down syndrome occurs at fertilization.

Down syndrome causes some degree of mental retardation. The child also has certain physical characteristics caused by the extra chromosome (Fig. 33-1, p. 746):

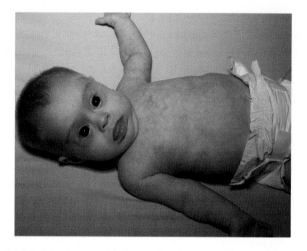

Fig. 33-1 An infant with Down Syndrome. *(From Wong DL: Whaley and Wong's nursing care of infants and children, ed 6, St Louis, 1999, Mosby.)*

- Oval-shaped eyes
- Short, wide neck
- Large tongue
- Wide, flat nose
- Small ears
- Short stature
- Short, wide hands with stubby fingers

Many children with Down syndrome are born with heart defects. They tend to have vision and hearing problems. They also are at risk for ear infections, respiratory infections, and thyroid gland problems.

Children and adults with DS need speech, language, physical, and occupational therapies. Most can learn self-care skills. They also need health and sex education. Because weight gain and constipation are problems, they need a well-balanced diet and regular exercise.

CEREBRAL PALSY

Cerebral palsy (CP) is a term applied to a group of disorders characterized by paralysis *(palsy)*. It is caused by a defect in the motor region of the brain *(cerebral)*. The defect results from brain damage that occurs before, during, or shortly after birth. Lack of oxygen to the brain is the usual cause. Congenital brain defects also can result in cerebral palsy.

Infants at risk for cerebral palsy include:

- Premature infants
- Low-birth-weight infants
- Infants who do not cry in the first 5 minutes after delivery
- Infants who require mechanical ventilation
- Infants who have bleeding in the brain
- Infants with congenital heart, kidney, or spinal cord defects

- Infants with seizure activity
- Infants with fetal alcohol syndrome

Brain damage in early childhood also can result in cerebral palsy. Lack of oxygen to the brain can occur from:

- Choking (see Chapter 36)
- Poisoning
- Near drowning
- Head injuries from accidents or child abuse (including shaken baby syndrome)
- Meningitis (inflammation of the covering around the brain and spinal cord)
- Encephalitis (inflammation of the brain)

Cerebral palsy affects body movements and body parts. Two types of CP affect body movements: spastic and athetoid cerebral palsy. *Spastic* comes from the Greek word *spastikos* that means to draw in. **Spastic** means uncontrolled contractions of skeletal muscles. That is, the muscles contract or shorten. The muscles cannot relax. One or both sides of the body may be involved. Posture, balance, and movement are affected. So are hand skills. Therefore eating, writing, dressing, and other activities of daily living are affected.

In the athetoid type, the person cannot control muscle movements. *Athetoid* comes from the Greek word *athetos, which* means not fixed. The person has continuous, slow, weaving or writhing motions of the trunk, arms, and legs. The tongue and face and neck muscles also may be involved.

Hemiplegia, diplegia, and quadriplegia are used to describe the body parts involved:

- *Hemiplegia*—the arm and leg on one side of the body are affected.
- *Diplegia*—di comes from the Greek word meaning twice. Therefore **diplegia** means that similar body parts are affected on both sides of the body. The person has paralysis of both arms or both legs. The legs are commonly involved.
- *Quadriplegia*—both arms and both legs are paralyzed. So are the trunk and neck muscles.

The person with CP can have many other impairments. They include:

- Mental retardation
- Learning disabilities
- Hearing impairments
- Vision impairments
- Drooling
- Constipation
- Epilepsy
- Difficulty swallowing (dysphagia)
- Attention deficit hyperactivity disorder (short attention span, poor concentration, and increased activity)

AUTISM

Autism begins in early childhood. This mental disorder comes from the Greek word *autos*, which means self. Brain function is affected. Reasoning, social interaction, verbal and nonverbal communication skills, and play activities are impaired. The child has difficulty relating to people.

Children are severely to mildly affected. The following behaviors are common:

- Slow language development
- Repeats words or phrases
- Uses gestures to communicate
- Short attention span
- Spends time alone
- Little or no eye contact
- Overly reacts to touch; does not like to cuddle
- Little reaction to pain
- Frequent tantrums for no apparent reason
- Strong attachment to a single item
- Needs routines; does not like change
- No fear of danger
- Does not respond to others; may act deaf
- Very active or very quiet
- Aggressive or violent behavior; may injure self

Autism has no cure. With appropriate therapy, the person can learn to change or control behaviors. Many therapies are used to help the person. They include behavior modification, speech and language therapy, music therapy, auditory training, sensory therapies, physical therapy, occupational therapy, drugs, and diet therapy. Communication therapy and developing social and work skills also are very important.

Children with autism become adults. Some adults work and live independently. Others continue to need support and assistance from family and other services. Some live in group homes or residential care centers.

Persons with autism may have other disorders and disabilities. Mental retardation and epilepsy are common.

EPILEPSY

The Epilepsy Foundation of America describes **epilepsy** as a condition that produces brief disturbances in the brain's normal electrical functions. These disturbances occur from time to time. They involve bursts of electrical energy that cause seizures. (Epilepsy comes from the Greek word *epilepsia*, which means seizure.)

A **seizure** (or **convulsion**) involves violent and sudden contractions or tremors of muscles. The person has uncontrolled body movements and may lose consciousness. Seizures can occur in one part of the brain. These are called *partial seizures*. Some seizures involve the whole brain. They are called *generalized seizures*.

Illnesses that cause high fever or lack of oxygen to the brain can cause seizures. So can head injuries. However, having a single seizure does not mean the person has epilepsy. In epilepsy, seizures recur. The person with epilepsy has a permanent brain injury or defect. Often there are no known causes. The known causes of epilepsy include:

- Brain injury before, during, or after birth
- Maternal injury or infection during pregnancy
- Lack of oxygen during birth
- Head trauma (vehicle accidents, gunshot wounds, sports accidents, falls, blows to the head)
- Chemical imbalance
- Poor nutrition
- Brain tumor
- Childhood fever
- Poison—such as lead and alcohol poisoning
- Infection—such as meningitis and encephalitis
- Stroke

Children and young adults are commonly affected. However, epilepsy can develop at any time. It also occurs with other problems affecting the brain. Such problems include cerebral palsy, mental retardation, autism, Alzheimer's disease, and traumatic brain injury.

Epilepsy has no known cure at this time. Many drugs are available to prevent seizures. However, some persons do not have complete seizure control with drugs. For other persons, drug therapy does not work.

When controlled, epilepsy usually does not interfere with learning and activities of daily living. In severe cases, persons may have activity and job limits. For example, because seizures can occur at any time, the person may not be allowed to drive a vehicle. Not being able to drive may limit job choices.

Persons with epilepsy have an increased risk of death. Prolonged seizures can result in brain damage. The Epilepsy Foundation of America reports that persons with epilepsy have higher rates for suicide and sudden unexplained death syndrome. They also have higher rates of accidental death, especially drowning.

See Chapter 36 for the emergency care of persons having seizures.

SPINA BIFIDA

Spina bifida is a congenital defect of the spinal column. (It comes from the Latin words *spina*, which means backbone, and *bifid*, which means split in two parts.) The defect occurs during the first 29 days of pregnancy. Hydrocephalus often occurs with spina bifida.

Bones of the spinal column are called *vertebrae*. The vertebrae protect the spinal cord. In spina bifida, bones of the vertebrae do not form properly. This leaves a split in the vertebrae. The split leaves the spinal cord unprotected. Only a membrane covers the spinal cord. Remember, the spinal cord contains nerves that send messages to and from the brain. If the spinal cord is unprotected, nerve damage occurs. Affected body parts do not function properly. Paralysis may occur. Bowel and bladder problems are common. Infection also is a threat.

Spina bifida can occur anywhere in the spine. However, the lower back is the most common site. The different types of spina bifida include:

- *Spina bifida occulta*—occult means hidden. The vertebrae are closed but there is a defect in the vertebrae closure. The spinal cord and nerves are normal. The person has a dimple or tuft of hair on the back (Fig. 33-2). Often the person has no symptoms. Foot weaknesses and bowel and bladder problems can occur.
- *Spina bifida cystica*—*cystica* comes from the Greek word meaning bag, pouch, or sac. Part of the spinal column is contained in the pouch or sac. A membrane or a thin layer of skin covers the sac. It looks like a large blister on the person's back. The pouch is easily injured. Infection is a threat. There are two types of spinal bifida cystica (Fig. 33-3):
  - *Meningocele*—meningo comes from the Greek word *meninx*, which means membrane, and the suffix *cele*, which means hernia or swelling. Remember, meninges is the connective tissue that covers and protects the brain and spinal cord. Cerebrospinal fluid also protects the brain and spinal cord. In meningocele the sac contains meninges and cerebrospinal fluid (see Fig. 33-3, *A* and Fig. 33-4). The sac does not contain nerve tissue. The spinal cord and nerves are usually normal. Therefore nerve damage is not usually a problem. The defect is corrected with surgery.
  - *Myelomeningocele (or meningomyelocele)*—*myelo* comes from the prefix meaning spinal cord. In myelomeningocele, the pouch contains nerves and spinal cord, meninges, and cerebrospinal fluid (see Fig. 33-3, *B*). Nerve damage occurs. Loss of function occurs below the level of damage. Leg paralysis, lack of sensation, and lack of bowel and bladder control are common problems. The defect is closed with surgery. Some children learn to walk using braces or crutches. Others use wheelchairs.

Fig. 33-2 Spina bifida occulta.

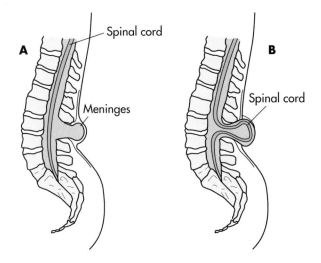

Fig. 33-3 A, Meningocele. **B,** Myelomeningocele.

Fig. 33-4 Meningocele. *(From Zitelli BJ, Davis HW: Atlas of pediatric physical diagnosis, St Louis, 1987, Gower Medical Publishing.)*

Fig. 33-5 Hydrocephalus. *(From Hart CA, Broadhead RL: Color atlas of pediatric infectious diseases, London 1992, Mosby-Wolfe.)*

Fig. 33-6 A shunt drains cerebrospinal fluid from the brain. *(From Wong DL: Whaley & Wong's nursing care of infants and children, ed 6, St Louis, 1999, Mosby.)*

HYDROCEPHALUS

Hydrocephalus is a condition in which cerebrospinal fluid collects in and around the brain. (It comes from the Greek words *hydro,* meaning water, and root *cephalo,* meaning head.) A spinal defect prevents the cerebrospinal fluid from draining properly. Therefore the head enlarges (Fig. 33-5). Pressure inside the head increases. Mental retardation and neurological damage occur without treatment.

To allow draining of the cerebrospinal fluids, a shunt is placed in the brain. The shunt is a long flexible tube that goes from the brain to a body cavity (Fig. 33-6). Fluid drains from the brain through the tube. Usually it drains into the abdominal cavity or a heart chamber. The shunt must remain patent (open). If blockage occurs, the cerebrospinal fluid cannot drain from the brain.

The person with hydrocephalus can have various problems. Visual impairment, seizures, and learning disabilities can occur.

QUALITY OF LIFE

Persons with developmental disabilities have the same rights as every citizen in the United States. They have the right to live, learn, work, and enjoy life. The Americans With Disabilities Act of 1990 (ADA) further protects their rights. For those requiring care in a nursing center, the Omnibus Budget Reconciliation Act of 1987 (OBRA) offers additional protection.

Independence to the extent possible is the goal for persons with developmental disabilities. This includes having a job and living in the community. A variety of federal, state, and community resources are available to assist the person and family. Such support includes needed assistive devices, education, job training, personal assistance services, home and vehicle changes, financial assistance, and therapy services. Therapy services include physical, occupational, speech and language, respiratory, hearing, vision, and other therapies.

The disability affects the child and the family throughout the life span. Remember, the person with a developmental disability does not remain an infant or a child. The person grows older, becoming an adolescent, young adult, middle-age adult, and older adult. Changes from aging occur (see Chapter 8). However, the onset of such changes may occur earlier than normal in persons with severe developmental disabilities. Older parents may not have the energy or means to care for the aging child. Then long-term care may be required.

REVIEW

Circle the BEST answer.

1. All developmental disabilities occur
   A. At birth
   B. From trauma
   C. During pregnancy
   D. Before 22 years of age

2. These statements are about developmental disabilities. Which is *true?*
   A. Self-care, learning, and mobility are always affected.
   B. The disability is severe and permanent.
   C. Both physical and intellectual impairment occur together.
   D. The person cannot live independently or hold a job.

3. The person with mental retardation
   A. Has delayed development of sexual organs
   B. Does not have the skills to live, work, and play
   C. Requires care in a special setting
   D. Learns at a slower rate than normal

4. Mental retardation
   A. Is always severe
   B. Can occur before, during, or after birth
   C. Is caused by an extra chromosome
   D. Affects the motor region in the brain

5. Down syndrome occurs
   A. At fertilization
   B. During the first 29 days of pregnancy
   C. Any time before, during, or after birth
   D. From trauma

6. The person with Down syndrome always has some degree of
   A. Cerebral palsy
   B. Autism
   C. Impaired mobility
   D. Mental retardation

7. Cerebral palsy is usually caused by
   A. An extra chromosome
   B. High fever
   C. Lack of oxygen to the brain
   D. Infection during pregnancy

8. The person with the spastic type of cerebral palsy has problems with
   A. Learning
   B. Drooling
   C. Posture, balance, and movement
   D. Weaving motions of the trunk, arms, and legs

9. Autism begins
   A. At fertilization
   B. During pregnancy
   C. At birth
   D. In early childhood

10. The person with autism has
    A. Impaired movement
    B. Difficulty relating to people
    C. Diplegia
    D. Mental retardation

11. The person with epilepsy has
    A. Seizures
    B. Diplegia
    C. Athetoid
    D. Spastic movements

12. Which is used to control epilepsy?
    A. Physical therapy
    B. Occupational therapy
    C. Drugs
    D. A shunt

13. Spina bifida involves
    A. Nerve damage
    B. Cerebrospinal fluid collecting in the head
    C. Seizures
    D. Mental retardation

14. Which is common in spina bifida?
    A. Short attention span
    B. Hearing and vision problems
    C. Learning problems
    D. Bowel and bladder problems

15. Hydrocephalus often occurs with
    A. Down syndrome
    B. Mental retardation
    C. Spina bifida
    D. Autism

Answers to these questions are on p. 839.

CHAPTER

34

SEXUALITY

Define the key terms listed in this chapter

Describe the differences between sex and sexuality

Explain the importance of sexuality throughout life

Describe five types of sexual relationships

Explain how injury and illness can affect sexuality

Explain how aging affects sexuality in older persons

Explain how the nursing team can promote a person's sexuality

Explain why some persons become sexually aggressive

Describe how to deal with sexually aggressive persons

KEY TERMS

bisexual A person who is attracted to both sexes

heterosexual A person who is attracted to people of the other sex

homosexual A person who is attracted to members of the same sex

impotence The inability of the male to have an erection

menopause The time when menstruation stops; it marks the end of the woman's reproductive years

sex The physical activities involving the organs of reproduction; the activities are done for pleasure or to produce children

sexuality The physical, psychological, social, cultural, and spiritual factors that affect a person's feelings and attitudes about his or her sex

transsexual A person who believes that he or she is really a member of the other sex

transvestite A person who becomes sexually excited by dressing in the clothes of the other sex

Another part of the person involves the physical, psychological, social, and spiritual. That part is sexuality. Illness and injury can affect a person's sexuality. This chapter describes the effects of illness, injury, and aging on sexuality. You must view patients and residents, young and old, as total persons. Total persons have sexuality. (See Box 34-1 for a review of the structures and functions of the reproductive system.)

SEX AND SEXUALITY

Sex and sexuality are different. **Sex** is the physical activities involving the reproductive organs. The activities are done for pleasure or to produce children. **Sexuality** involves the personality and the body. A person's attitudes and feelings are involved. Physical, psychological, social, cultural, and spiritual factors influence sexuality. It affects how a person behaves, thinks, dresses, and responds to others.

Sexuality is present when a baby's sex is known. Names, colors, and toys reflect sexuality. Blue is used

Box 34-1 Review of the Structure and Function of the Reproductive System

THE MALE REPRODUCTIVE SYSTEM

The structures of the male reproductive system are shown in Figure 34-1 on p. 754. The testes *(testicles)* are the male sex glands *(gonads)*. Male sex cells *(sperm cells)* are produced in the testes. So is *testosterone*, the male hormone. This hormone is needed for reproductive organ function and for the development of male secondary sex characteristics (see Chapter 7). The testes are suspended between the thighs in a sac called the *scrotum*.

Sperm travel from the testis to the *epididymis*. The epididymis is a coiled tube on top and to the side of the testis. From the epididymis, sperm travel through a tube called the *vas deferens*. Eventually each vas deferens joins a *seminal vesicle*. The two seminal vesicles store sperm and produce *semen*. Semen is a fluid that carries sperm from the male reproductive tract. The ducts of the seminal vesicles join to form the *ejaculatory duct*. The ejaculatory duct passes through the prostate gland.

The *prostate gland*, shaped like a doughnut, lies just below the bladder. The gland secretes fluid into the semen. As the ejaculatory ducts leave the prostate they join the *urethra*, which also runs through the prostate. The urethra is the outlet for urine and semen. The penis contains the urethra.

The *penis* is outside the body and has *erectile* tissue. When the man is sexually aroused, blood fills the erectile tissue. The penis becomes enlarged, hard, and erect. The erect penis can enter the vagina of the female reproductive tract. The semen, which contains sperm, is released into the vagina.

THE FEMALE REPRODUCTIVE SYSTEM

The structures of the female reproductive system are shown in Figure 34-2, p. 754. The female gonads are two almond-shaped glands called *ovaries*. There is an ovary on each side of the uterus in the abdominal cavity. The ovaries contain *ova* (eggs). Ova are female sex cells. One ovum (egg) is released monthly during the woman's reproductive years. Release of an ovum from an ovary is called *ovulation*. The ovaries also secrete the female hormones *estrogen* and *progesterone*. These hormones are needed for reproductive system function and the development of female secondary sex characteristics (see Chapter 7).

When an ovum is released from an ovary, it travels through a *fallopian tube*. There are two fallopian tubes, one on each side. The tubes are attached at one end to the uterus. The ovum travels through a fallopian tube to the *uterus*. The uterus is a hollow, muscular organ shaped like a pear. The uterus is in the center of the pelvic cavity behind the bladder and in front of the rectum. The main part of the uterus is the *fundus*. The neck or narrow section of the uterus is the *cervix*. Tissue lining the uterus is called the *endometrium*. The endometrium has many blood vessels. If sex cells from the male and female unite into one cell, that cell implants into the endometrium. There it grows into a baby. The uterus serves as a place for the unborn baby to grow and receive nourishment.

The cervix projects into a muscular canal called the *vagina*. The vagina opens to the outside of the body and is located just behind the urethra. The vagina receives the penis during sexual intercourse and is part of the birth canal. Glands in the vaginal wall keep it moistened with secretions.

The external genitalia of the female are called the *vulva* (Fig. 34-3, p. 755). The *mons pubis* is covered with hair in the adult female. The *labia majora* and *labia minora* are two folds of tissue on each side of the vaginal opening. The *clitoris* is a small organ composed of erectile tissue. The clitoris becomes enlarged and hard when sexually stimulated.

Menstruation

The endometrium is rich in blood to nourish the cell that grows into an unborn baby *(fetus)*. If pregnancy does not occur, the endometrium breaks up and is discharged through the vagina to the outside of the body. This process is called *menstruation*. Menstruation occurs about every 28 days. Therefore it is also called the *menstrual cycle*.

The first day of the cycle starts with menstruation. Blood flows from the uterus through the vaginal opening. Menstrual flow lasts 3 to 7 days. Ovulation occurs during the next phase. An ovum is released from the ovary. Ovulation usually occurs on or about day 14 of the cycle. Meanwhile, the ovaries secrete estrogen and progesterone (female hormones). These hormones cause the endometrium to thicken for possible pregnancy. If pregnancy does not occur, the hormones decrease in amount. Blood supply to the endometrium decreases because of the decrease in hormones. The endometrium breaks up and is discharged through the vagina. Another menstrual cycle begins.

FERTILIZATION

For reproduction to occur, a male sex cell (sperm) must unite with a female sex cell (ovum). The uniting of the sperm and ovum into one cell is called *fertilization*. A sperm and an ovum each have 23 chromosomes. When the two cells unite, the fertilized cell has 46 chromosomes.

During intercourse, millions of sperm are deposited in the vagina. Sperm travel up the cervix, through the uterus, and into the fallopian tubes. If a sperm and an ovum unite in a fallopian tube, fertilization occurs and pregnancy results. The fertilized cell travels down the fallopian tube to the uterus. After a short time, the fertilized cell implants in the thick endometrium and grows during pregnancy.

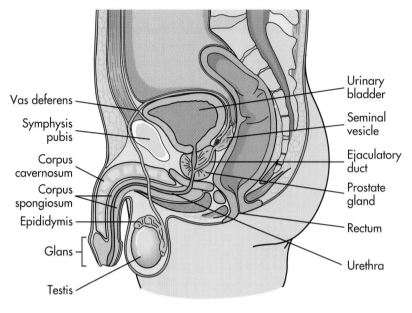

Fig. 34-1 Male reproductive system.

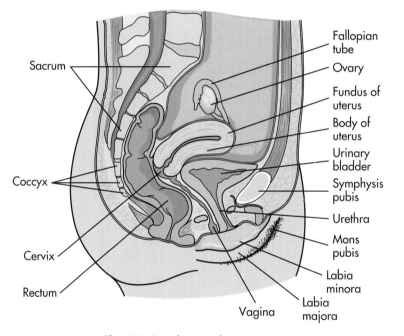

Fig. 34-2 Female reproductive system.

for boys and pink for girls. Dolls are for girls. Trains are for boys. By the age of 2, children know their own sex. Three-year-olds know the sex of other children. Children learn male and female roles from their parents (Fig. 34-4). Children learn early that there are certain behaviors for boys and certain ones for girls.

As children grow older, interest increases about the human body and how it works. Body changes during adolescence bring more interest about sex and the body. Their bodies respond to stimulation. Teenagers engage in sexual behaviors. They kiss, embrace, pet,

or have intercourse. Pregnancy and sexually transmitted diseases are great risks for sexually active teenagers.

Sex has more meaning as young adults mature. Attitudes and feelings are important. Sexual partners are selected. Sex before marriage and birth control are other decisions.

Sexuality is important into adulthood and old age. Attitudes and sex needs change as a person grows older. Life circumstances change. These include divorce, death of a partner, injury, and illness.

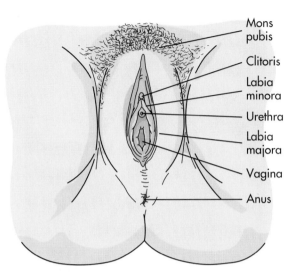

Fig. 34-3 External female genitalia.

Fig. 34-4 This little girl is learning female roles from her mother.

SEXUAL RELATIONSHIPS

Sex and sexuality usually involve a partner. A **heterosexual** is a person who is attracted to people of the other sex. Men are attracted to women, and women are attracted to men. Sexual behavior is male-female.

A **homosexual** is attracted to members of the same sex. Men are attracted to men, and women are attracted to women. *Gay* refers to homosexuality. Homosexual men are referred to as *gay men*. *Lesbian* refers to a female homosexual.

Homosexuality has existed for centuries. Before the 1960s and 1970s, many gay persons were secret about their sexual orientation. Now many gay men and lesbians are more open about their sexual preference and relationships.

Bisexuals are attracted to both sexes. Some alternate between same-gender and male-female behaviors. Bisexuals often are married and have children. They may seek a same-gender relationship or experience outside of marriage.

Some people believe that they are really members of the other sex. These people are **transsexuals**. A male believes he is really a female in a man's body. A female believes she is really a male in a woman's body. Transsexual persons often describe feeling "trapped" in the wrong body. Most have had these feelings for as long as they can remember. As children they usually show behaviors of the other sex. Many seek psychiatric treatment. Some have sex-change operations. Psychiatric treatment and sex-change operations do not always help these people.

Transvestites become sexually excited by dressing in clothes of the other sex. Most are male. They are usually married and heterosexual. They dress normally as men most of the time. Dressing as a woman is usually done in private. Some dress completely as women. Others focus on bras and panties. The sex partner may not know about the practice. Some partners take part in transvestite activities. Some transvestites have same-gender friends with similar interests.

INJURY AND ILLNESS

Sexuality and sex involve the mind and body. Injury and illness can affect sexual function. A person may feel unclean, unwhole, unattractive, or mutilated after surgery or injury. Attitudes about sex may change. The person may feel unfit for closeness and love. Therefore the person may develop sexual problems that are psychological. Time, understanding, and a caring partner are very helpful. Counseling or psychiatric help may be needed.

Many illnesses, injuries, and surgeries affect the nervous, circulatory, and reproductive systems. If one or more of these systems are involved, the person's sexual ability may change. Most chronic illnesses affect sexual function.

Impotence is the inability of the male to have an erection. Diabetes mellitus, spinal cord injuries, multiple sclerosis, and alcoholism are common causes. Circulatory disorders and drugs can interfere with achieving an erection. Impotence is a side effect of some drugs that control high blood pressure. Today new drugs are available for impotence.

Heart disease, stroke, chronic obstructive pulmonary disease, and nervous system disorders can affect sexual ability. Some reproductive system surgeries have physical and psychological effects. Prostate or testes removal affects erections. Removal of the uterus, ovaries, or a breast may affect a woman.

Changes in sexual functioning greatly impact the person. Fear, anger, worry, and depression are common. You see these in the person's behavior and comments. The person's feelings are very normal and expected.

AGE-RELATED CHANGES

Reproductive organs change with aging. In men, the hormone *testosterone* decreases. The hormone affects strength, sperm production, and reproductive tissues. These changes affect sexual activity. It takes longer for an erection to occur. The phase between erection and orgasm is also longer. Orgasm is less forceful than in the younger years. After orgasm, the erection is lost quickly. The time between erections is also longer. Older men may need the penis stimulated for sexual arousal. These changes result in decreased frequency of sexual activity.

Mental and physical fatigue, overeating, and excessive drinking affect erections. Some men fear performance problems. Therefore they may avoid sexual activity.

Physical changes occur in women. Menopause occurs around 50 years of age. **Menopause** is when a woman stops menstruating. Her reproductive years end. Female hormones (*estrogen* and *progesterone*) decrease. Reduced hormone levels affect reproductive tissues. The uterus, vagina, and external genitalia atrophy (shrink). Intercourse may be uncomfortable or painful. This is from thin vaginal walls and vaginal dryness. Older women also have changes in sexual excitement. Arousal takes longer. The time between excitement and orgasm is longer. Orgasm is less intense. The pre-excitement state returns more quickly.

Frequency of sexual activity decreases for many men and women. Reasons relate to weakness, mental and physical fatigue, pain, and reduced mobility. The normal aging process and chronic illness are common causes. Pain and reduced mobility from illness and aging can affect frequency. One or both partners may have a chronic illness. It may lead to decreased frequency or no sexual activity.

Some people cannot have sexual intercourse. This does not mean sexual needs or desires are lost. They can express their needs in other ways. Hand holding, touching, caressing, and embracing bring closeness and intimacy.

Having a sexual partner is also important. Death and divorce result in loss of a sexual partner. The partner may also be in a hospital or nursing center. These situations occur in adults of all ages. *(See Focus on Older Persons box.)*

Fig. 34-5 Love and affection are important to older persons.

Focus On... OLDER PERSONS

Sexual relationships are important to older persons (Fig. 34-5). They fall in love, hold hands, embrace, and have sex. They need sex, love, and affection. Many have sexual intercourse.

Love, affection, and intimacy are needed throughout life. As other losses occur, feeling close to another person is more important. Children leave home. Friends and relatives die. People retire. Health problems may develop. Decreasing strength and a changing appearance add to these losses.

MEETING THE PERSON'S SEXUAL NEEDS

Sexuality is part of the total person. Some people are so ill that sexual activity is impossible. Others want and are capable of sexual activity. Sexual activity does not always mean intercourse. It may be expressed in other ways. The nursing team has an important role in sexuality. They allow and promote the meeting of sexual needs. Patients and residents appreciate the measures listed in Box 34-2. They are carried out in cooperation with the nurse supervising your work. *(See Focus on Long-Term Care box and Focus on Older Persons box.)*

Box 34-2   Promoting Sexuality

- Let the person practice grooming routines. This includes applying makeup, nail polish, body lotion, and cologne. Hair care is important. Women may want to shave their legs and underarms and pluck eyebrows. Men may use after-shave lotion. The person may need help with these activities.
- Let the person choose clothing. Hospital gowns embarrass both men and women. Street clothes are worn if the person's condition permits.
- Protect the right to privacy. Avoid exposing the person. Drape and screen the person appropriately.
- Accept the person's sexual relationships. The person may not share your sexual attitudes, values, or practices. Do not expect the person to follow your standards. The person may have a homosexual, premarital, or extramarital relationship. Do not judge or gossip about relationships.

- Allow privacy. You can usually tell when two people want to be alone. If the person has a private room, close the door for privacy. Some agencies have *Do Not Disturb* signs for doors. Let the person and partner know how much time they have alone. For example, remind them about meal times, medications, or treatments. Tell other staff members that the person wants time alone.
- Knock before you enter any room. This is a simple courtesy that shows respect for privacy.
- Consider the person's roommate. Privacy curtains provide little privacy. Arrange for privacy when the roommate is out of the room. Sometimes roommates volunteer to leave for a while. If the roommate cannot leave, other areas on the nursing unit are used for privacy.
- Allow privacy for masturbation. It is a normal form of sexual expression and release. Close the privacy curtain and the door. Knock before you enter any room to save you and the person embarrassment. Sometimes confused persons masturbate in public areas. Lead the person to a private area or engage his or her interest in some other activity.

 Focus On... **LONG-TERM CARE**

Married couples in nursing centers are allowed to share the same room. This is an OBRA requirement. The couple has lived together for many years. Long-term care is no reason to keep them apart in rooms for men and women. They can share the same bed if their conditions permit. A double, queen-size, or king-size bed is provided by the couple or the center.

Sexual partners are lost through death and divorce. A single resident may develop a relationship with another single resident. Instead of keeping them apart, they should be allowed time together (Fig. 34-6).

Fig. 34-6 Relationships occur in nursing centers.

Focus On... **OLDER PERSONS**

Older persons have the right to be sexual. The measures described in Box 34-2 apply to older persons.

THE SEXUALLY AGGRESSIVE PERSON

Some persons want their sexual needs met by the health team. They flirt, make sexual advances or comments, expose themselves, masturbate, or touch staff. The staff member is usually angry or embarrassed when this happens. These reactions are normal. Often there are reasons for the person's behavior. Understanding this helps you deal with the situation.

Illness, injury, surgery, or aging often threaten a male's sense of manhood. He tries to prove to himself that he is still attractive and able to perform sexually. Therefore he may behave sexually toward a staff member.

Some sexually aggressive behaviors are from confusion or disorientation. Common causes are nervous system disorders, drugs, fever, dementia (see Chapter 32), and poor vision. The person may confuse a staff member with his or her partner. Or the person cannot control behavior because of changes in mental function. The healthy person is able to control sexual urges. However, changes in the brain can make control difficult. Sexual behavior in these cases is usually innocent on the person's part.

Some persons do touch workers inappropriately. Their purpose is sexual. However, sometimes touch is the only way the person can get someone's attention. For example, Mr. Olson had a stroke. His right side is paralyzed, and he cannot speak. Your back is to him, and you are bending over. Your buttocks are the closest part of your body to him. To get your attention, he touches your buttocks. You should not consider his behavior as sexual.

Often masturbation is viewed as a sexually aggressive behavior. It could indeed be touching and manipulating the genitals for sexual pleasure. However, urinary or reproductive system disorders can cause genital soreness or itching. Poor hygiene is another cause of itching. So is being wet or soiled from urine or a bowel movement. The nursing team must remember that touching the genitals could be a sign of a health problem.

Sexual advances may be intentional. You need to be professional about the matter. These suggestions may help:

- Ask the person not to touch you. State the places where you were touched.
- Tell the person that you will not do what he or she wants.
- Tell the person that those behaviors make you uncomfortable. Politely ask the person not to act in that way.
- Allow privacy if the person is becoming sexually aroused. Provide for safety; for example, raise bed rails if ordered for the person, place the signal light within reach (see Chapter 9). Tell the person when you will return.
- Discuss the situation with the nurse. The nurse can help you understand the person's behavior.

SEXUALLY TRANSMITTED DISEASES

Some diseases are spread by sexual contact. They are grouped under the heading of sexually transmitted diseases (STDs). STDs are presented in Chapter 30.

REVIEW

Circle the BEST answer.

1. Sex involves
   A. The organs of reproduction
   B. Attitudes and feelings
   C. Cultural and spiritual factors
   D. All of the above

2. Sexuality is important to
   A. Small children
   B. Teenagers and young adults
   C. Middle-age adults
   D. Persons of all ages

3. Impotence is
   A. When menstruation stops
   B. A psychological reaction to disfigurement
   C. The inability of the male to achieve an erection
   D. The complete absence of sexual activity

4. Reproductive organs change with aging.
   A. True
   B. False

5. Mr. and Mrs. Green live in the same nursing center. Which will *not* promote their sexuality?
   A. Allowing their normal grooming routines
   B. Assigning them to separate rooms
   C. Allowing them privacy
   D. Accepting their relationship

6. An older lady and an older gentleman live in a nursing center. They are holding hands. Nursing staff should keep them apart.
   A. True
   B. False

7. Mr. Green wants time alone with his wife. The nurse tells you this is okay. You should
   A. Close the door to the room
   B. Put a *Do Not Disturb* sign on the door
   C. Tell other staff that Mr. and Mrs. Green want some time alone
   D. All of the above

8. Mr. Cole is masturbating in the dining room. You should do the following *except*
   A. Cover him and take him quietly to his room
   B. Scold him for his bad behavior
   C. Provide privacy and respect his rights
   D. Report the behavior to the nurse

9. Mr. Dawson is being sexually aggressive. The behavior may be
   A. An attempt to prove he is still attractive and able to perform sexually
   B. Caused by confusion or disorientation
   C. Done on purpose
   D. All of the above

10. A person makes sexual advances to you. You should do the following *except*
    A. Discuss the situation with the nurse
    B. Do what the person asks
    C. Explain to the person that the behaviors make you uncomfortable
    D. Ask the person not to touch you in places where you were touched

Answers to these questions are on p. 839.

CARING FOR MOTHERS AND NEWBORNS

OBJECTIVES

Define the key terms listed in this chapter

Describe how to meet an infant's safety and security needs

Identify the signs and symptoms of illness in infants

Explain how to help mothers with breast-feeding

Describe three forms of baby formulas

Explain how to bottle-feed babies

Explain how to burp a baby

Describe how to give cord care

Describe the purposes of circumcision, the necessary observations, and the required care

Explain how to bathe infants

Explain why infants are weighed

Describe the care needed by mothers during the postpartum period

Perform the procedures described in this chapter

KEY TERMS

circumcision The surgical removal of foreskin

episiotomy Incision *(otomy)* into the perineum

lochia The vaginal discharge that occurs during the postpartum period

postpartum After *(post)* childbirth *(partum)*

umbilical cord The structure that carries blood, oxygen, and nutrients from the mother to the fetus

You may care for new mothers and newborns. They usually stay in the hospital only a short while. Some need home care after discharge. *(See Focus on Home Care box.)*

Babies are helpless. They depend on others for their basic needs. Besides physical needs, babies have safety and security and love and belonging needs. A review of growth and development will help you care for newborns and infants (see Chapter 7).

INFANT SAFETY AND SECURITY

Babies cannot protect themselves. Like everyone else, babies need to feel safe and secure. They feel secure when warm and when wrapped and held snugly. Babies cry to communicate. They cry when wet, hungry, hot or cold, tired, uncomfortable, or in pain. Responding to their cries and feeding them when hungry promote safety and security. Infant safety is discussed in

---

Focus On... HOME CARE

Common reasons for home care include:
- Complications in the mother before or after childbirth
- Help with childcare when other young children are in the home
- Multiple births (e.g., twins, triplets)
- Help with meals and housekeeping

Chapter 9. The measures listed in Box 35-1 on p. 762 are also important for hospital or home care.

Nursery equipment must be safe and in good repair. The Consumer Product Safety Commission has issued a safety guide for buying new or used nursery equipment (Box 35-2, pp. 763-765). You can use the guide when checking nursing equipment in an agency or home setting.

Text continued on p. 766

Box 35-1 Infant Safety

- Follow the safety measures listed in Chapter 9.
- Keep the baby warm. Check windows for drafts. Close windows securely.
- Keep your fingernails short. Do not wear rings or bracelets. Long nails and jewelry can scratch the baby.
- Use both hands to lift a newborn.
- Hold the baby securely. Use the cradle hold, football hold, or shoulder hold (Fig. 35-1).
- Support the baby's head and neck when lifting or holding the baby (see Fig. 35-1). Neck support is necessary for the first 3 months after birth.
- Handle the baby with gentle, smooth movements. Avoid sudden or jerking movements. Do not startle the baby.
- Hold and cuddle infants. This is comforting and helps them learn to feel love and security.
- Talk, sing, or play with the baby often. Be sure to talk to the baby during the bath, dressing, and diapering.
- Respond to the baby's crying. Babies cry when they are hungry, uncomfortable, wet, frightened, or tired or when they want attention. Crying is how they communicate. Responding to their cries helps them feel safe and secure.
- Tighten all nuts, bolts, and screws on cribs, highchairs, and other infant furniture. Do this periodically.
- Check mattress hooks to make sure none are bent or broken.
- Do not leave a baby unattended on a table, bed, sofa, highchair, or other high surface. Keep one hand on the baby if you must look away (see Fig. 9-1).
- Use safety straps for babies in infant seats or highchairs. Do not use safety straps on changing tables. The baby can roll off the table and strangle on the straps.
- Make sure the crib is within hearing distance of the caregivers.
- Keep crib rails up at all times.
- Do not put a pillow, quilts, or soft toys in the crib. They can cause suffocation.
- Do not lay an infant on soft bedding products. This includes fluffy, plush products such as sheepskin, quilts, comforters, pillows, and toys. These soft products can cover the baby's nose and mouth and cause suffocation.
- Lay babies on their backs or in a side-lying position for sleep. The back-lying position is preferred. *Do not lay babies on their stomachs for sleep. This can interfere with chest expansion and breathing. The baby can suffocate.* If the side-lying position is used, bring the baby's lower arm forward (Fig. 35-2). This prevents the baby from rolling onto the stomach. Infants can lie on their stomachs when awake.
- Keep pins and small objects out of the baby's reach.
- Do not shake powders directly over the baby. The powder can get into the baby's eyes and lungs. Shake some on your hand away from the baby.

A **B** **C**

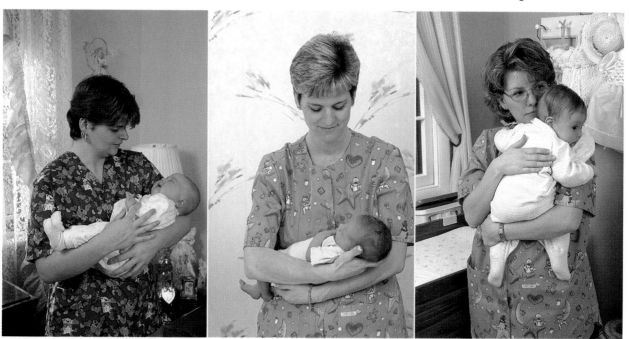

Fig. 35-1 Holding a baby. **A,** The cradle hold. **B,** The football hold. **C,** The shoulder hold.

Fig. 35-2 The baby's lower arm is brought forward in the side-lying position. This prevents the baby from rolling onto her stomach.

Box 35-2	**Consumer Product Safety Commission's Safety Guide for New or Used Nursery Equipment**		
		YES	**NO**

BACK CARRIERS
- Carrier has a restraining strap to secure the child.   ____ ____
- Leg openings are small enough to prevent the child from slipping out.   ____ ____
- Leg openings are large enough to prevent chafing.   ____ ____
- Frames have no pinch points in the folding mechanism.   ____ ____
- There is a padded covering over the metal frame near the baby's face.   ____ ____

COMMISSION RECOMMENDATION: *Do not use a back carrier until the baby is 4 or 5 months old. By then the baby's neck is able to withstand jolts and not sustain injury.*

BASSINETS AND CRADLES
- The item has a sturdy bottom and a wide base for stability.   ____ ____
- The item has smooth surfaces—no protruding staples or other hardware that could injure the baby.   ____ ____
- Legs have strong, effective locks to prevent folding while in use.   ____ ____
- The mattress is firm and fits snugly.   ____ ____

COMMISSION RECOMMENDATION: *Follow the manufacturer's guidelines on the weight and size of a baby who can safely use these products.*

BABY BATH RINGS OR SEATS
- Suction cups are securely fastened to the product.   ____ ____
- Suction cups are securely attached to the smooth surface of the tub.   ____ ____
- The tub is filled only with enough water to cover the baby's legs.   ____ ____
- The baby is *NEVER* left alone or with a sibling while in a bath ring or seat for even a moment.   ____ ____

COMMISSION RECOMMENDATION: *NEVER leave a baby unattended or with a sibling in a tub of water. Do not rely on the bath ring or seat to keep the baby safe.*

CARRIER SEATS
- The item has a wide, sturdy base for stability.   ____ ____
- The item has non-skid feet to prevent slipping.   ____ ____
- Supporting devices lock securely.   ____ ____
- The seat has a crotch and waist strap.   ____ ____
- The buckle or strap is easy to use.   ____ ____

COMMISSION RECOMMENDATION: *Never use the carrier as a car seat.*

Modified from the Consumer Product Safety Commission: *Tips for your baby's safety,* CPSC document #4200, Washington DC.

Continued

	Box 35-2	Consumer Product Safety Commission's Safety Guide for New or Used Nursery Equipment—cont'd

	YES	NO

CHANGING TABLES
- The table has drawers or shelves that are easy to reach without leaving the baby unattended.

COMMISSION RECOMMENDATION: *Do not leave the baby on the table unattended.*

CRIBS
- Slats are spaced no more than $2\frac{3}{8}$ inches (60 mm) apart.
- No slats are missing or cracked.
- The mattress fits snugly—less than a 2 finger width between the edge of mattress and crib side.
- The mattress support is securely attached to the head and footboards.
- Corner posts are no higher than $\frac{1}{16}$ inch (1.5 mm) to prevent entanglement of clothing or other objects worn by the child.
- There are no cutouts in the headboard and footboard to allow head entrapment.
- Drop-side latches cannot be easily released by the baby.
- Drop-side latches securely hold the side rails in the raised position.
- All screws or bolts that secure parts of the crib are present and tight.

COMMISSION RECOMMENDATION: *Do not place the crib near drapes or blinds where the child could become entangled and strangle on the cords. When the child reaches 35 inches in height or can climb or fall over the sides, replace the crib with a bed.*

CRIB TOYS
- No strings or loops with openings greater than 14 inches (356 mm).
- No strings or cords longer than 7 inches (178 mm) should dangle into the crib.
- A crib gym has a label warning to remove the device from the crib when the child can push on the hands and knees or reaches 5 months of age, whichever comes first.
- Toy parts are not small enough to be a choking hazard.

COMMISSION RECOMMENDATION: *Avoid hanging toys across the crib or on crib corner posts with strings long enough to cause strangulation. Remove crib gyms when the child can pull or push up on the hands and knees.*

GATES AND ENCLOSURES
- Gate openings are too small to entrap a child's head.
- The gate has a pressure bar or other fastener that will resist forces exerted by a child.

COMMISSION RECOMMENDATION: *To avoid head entrapment, do not use accordion-style gates or expandable enclosures with large v-shaped openings along the top edge, or diamond-shaped openings within.*

HIGHCHAIRS
- The highchair has waist and crotch restraining straps that are not part of the tray.
- The tray locks securely.
- The buckle on the waist strap is easy to use.
- The highchair has a wide, stable base.
- Caps or plugs on tubing are firmly attached and cannot be pulled off and choke a child.
- A folding highchair has an effective locking device to keep the chair from collapsing.

COMMISSION RECOMMENDATION: *Always use restraining straps. Otherwise the child can slide under the tray and strangle.*

HOOK-ON CHAIRS
- The chair has a restraining strap to secure the child.
- The chair has a clamp that locks onto the table for added security.
- Caps or plugs on tubing are firmly attached and cannot be pulled off and choke a child.
- The hook-on chair has a warning never to place the chair where the child can push off with the feet.

COMMISSION RECOMMENDATION: *Do not leave a child unattended in a hook-on chair.*

Modified from the Consumer Product Safety Commission: *Tips for your baby's safety,* CPSC document #4200, Washington DC.

		YES	NO

Box 35-2 | Consumer Product Safety Commission's Safety Guide for New or Used Nursery Equipment—cont'd

	YES	NO
PACIFIERS		
• No ribbons, strings, cords, or yarn are attached to a pacifier.	____	____
• The shield is large enough and firm enough to not fit in the child's mouth.	____	____
• The guard or shield has ventilation holes so the baby can breath if the shield does get into the mouth.	____	____
• The pacifier nipple has no holes or tears that might cause it to break off in the baby's mouth.	____	____

COMMISSION RECOMMENDATION: *To prevent strangulation, never hang a pacifier or other items on a string around a baby's neck.*

	YES	NO
PLAYPENS		
• A drop-mesh playpen or crib has a label warning never to leave the side in the down position.	____	____
• The mesh has small weave (less than $1/4$ inch openings).	____	____
• The mesh has no tears, holes, or loose threads.	____	____
• The mesh is securely attached to the top rail and floorplate.	____	____
• The top rail cover has no tears or holes.	____	____
• A wooden playpen has slats spaced no more than 2 inches (60 mm) apart.	____	____
• If staples are used in construction, they are firmly installed and none are missing or loose.	____	____

COMMISSION RECOMMENDATION: *Never leave an infant in a mesh playpen or crib with the drop-side down. Even a young infant can suffocate by rolling into the space between the mattress and loose mesh side.*

	YES	NO
RATTLES, SQUEEZE TOYS, AND TEETHERS		
• Rattles, squeeze toys, and teethers are too large to lodge in the baby's throat.	____	____
• Rattles are of study construction that will not break apart in use.	____	____
• Squeeze toys do not contain a squeaker that could detach and choke a baby.	____	____

COMMISSION RECOMMENDATION: *Remove rattles, squeeze toys, teethers, and other toys out of the crib or playpen when the baby sleeps to prevent suffocation.*

	YES	NO
STROLLER AND CARRIAGES		
• There is a wide base to prevent tipping.	____	____
• The seat belt and crotch strap securely attach to the frame.	____	____
• The seat buckle is easy to use.		
• Brakes securely lock the wheels.		
• The shopping basket is low on the back and directly over or in front of the rear wheels for stability.	____	____
• When used in the carriage position, the leg openings can be closed.	____	____

COMMISSION RECOMMENDATION: *Always secure seat belts. Never leave a child unattended in a stroller or carriage. Keep the child's hands away from pinching areas when folding or unfolding the stroller or when reclining the seat back.*

	YES	NO
TOY CHESTS		
• There is no lid latch which could entrap the child inside the chest.		
• The hinged lid has a spring-loaded lid support that will support the lid in any position. It will not require periodic adjustments.	____	____
• The chest has ventilation holes or spaces in the front and sides or under the lid in case the child gets caught inside.	____	____

COMMISSION RECOMMENDATION: *If a toy chest has a freely falling lid, remove the lid to avoid head injury to a small child. Install a spring-loaded lid support.*

	YES	NO
WALKERS		
• There is a wide wheel base for stability.		
• There are covers over coil springs to avoid finger pinching.		
• The seat is securely attached to the frame or walker.	____	____
• There are no x-frames that could pinch or amputate the fingers.	____	____

COMMISSION RECOMMENDATION: *Place gate guards at the top of all stairways. Or keep stairway doors closed to prevent falls. Do not use the walker as a baby sitter.*

SIGNS AND SYMPTOMS OF ILLNESS

Your observations are important for the infant's safety and well-being. Babies can become ill quickly. Signs and symptoms may be sudden. Therefore you must be very alert. Box 35-3 lists the signs and symptoms that are reported to the nurse immediately.

Tell the nurse when a sign or symptom began. You may need to take an infant's or child's temperature, pulse, and respirations (see Chapter 19). Axillary temperatures are taken on infants. Tympanic, rectal, or axillary temperatures are taken on children younger than 5 years. The nurse tells you which method to use for the child. Apical pulses are taken on infants and young children.

Box 35-3	Signs and Symptoms of Illness in Babies

- The baby has jaundice—a yellowish color to the skin and whites of the eyes.
- The baby looks sick.
- The baby has redness or drainage around the cord stump or circumcision.
- The baby has a high temperature (see Chapter 19).
- The baby is limp and slow to respond.
- The baby cries all the time or does not stop crying.
- The baby is flushed, pale, or perspiring.
- The baby has noisy, rapid, difficult, or slow respirations.
- The baby is coughing or sneezing.
- The baby has reddened or irritated eyes.
- The baby turns his or her head to one side or puts a hand to one ear (signs of an earache).
- The baby screams for a long time.
- The baby has skipped feedings.
- The baby has vomited most of the feeding or vomits between feedings.
- The baby has hard, formed stools or watery stools.
- The baby has a rash.

HELPING MOTHERS BREAST-FEED

Many mothers breast-feed their babies. Breast-fed babies usually nurse every 2 to 3 hours. They are fed on demand. In other words, they are fed when hungry, not on a schedule. At first, babies nurse for a short time (5 minutes at each breast). Eventually, nursing time takes up to 30 minutes.

Nurses help new mothers learn to breast-feed. They also teach breast care. Mothers and babies learn how to nurse in a very short time. If the mother or baby is having problems breast-feeding, you must tell the nurse.

Mothers may need help getting ready to breast-feed. They may need help with positioning. You may be responsible for bringing babies to mothers. You must help as needed. When you leave the room, make sure the signal light is within reach. The mother and baby need privacy during breast-feeding. Box 35-4 describes how you can help with breast-feeding. *(See Focus on Home Care box.)*

Focus On... HOME CARE

When the mother is nursing, stay within hearing distance in case she needs help.

The nursing mother needs good nutrition. If you are providing home care, you may need to plan meals and grocery shop. Remember the following when planning meals or grocery shopping:
- Calorie intake may be increased. The nurse tells you how much to increase the mother's calorie intake.
- The mother should have 3 servings a day from the milk, yogurt, and cheese group. She can drink whole, 2%, or skim milk. The nurse will tell you if more servings are needed.
- Include foods high in calcium in the diet.
- The mother should avoid spicy and gas-forming foods. They can cause cramping and diarrhea in the infant. She should avoid onions, garlic, spices, cabbage, brussels sprouts, asparagus, and beans. Chocolate, cola beverages, and coffee also can cause cramping and diarrhea.

Box 35-4   Helping With Breast-Feeding

- Practice Standard Precautions. Remember, HIV can be transmitted through breast milk (see Chapter 30).
- Help the mother wash her hands. Handwashing is necessary before she handles her breasts.
- Help the mother to a comfortable position. She may want to nurse sitting up in bed, in a chair, or in the side-lying position (Fig. 35-3).
- Change the baby's diaper if necessary. Bring the baby to the mother.
- Make sure the mother holds the baby close to her breast.
- Have the mother stroke the baby's cheek closest to the breast (Fig. 35-4). This stimulates the *rooting reflex*. The baby turns his or her head when the cheek or mouth is stroked. The head is turned toward the direction of the stimulus, and the baby starts to suck. If the right cheek is stroked, the baby turns the head to the right.
- Have the mother keep breast tissue away from the baby's nose with her thumb (Fig. 35-5).
- Give her a baby blanket to cover the baby and her breast. This promotes privacy during the feeding.
- Encourage nursing from both breasts at each feeding. If the baby finished the last feeding at the right breast, the baby starts the next feeding at the left breast.
- Remind her how to remove the baby from the breast. She needs to break the seal or suction between the baby and the breast. She can press a finger down on her breast close to the baby's mouth. Or she can insert a finger into a corner of the baby's mouth (Fig. 35-6).
- Help the mother burp the baby if necessary. The baby is burped after nursing at each breast.
- Have the mother put a diaper pin on the bra strap of the breast last used. This reminds her which breast to use at the next feeding.
- Change the baby's diaper after the feeding.
- Lay the baby in the crib if he or she has fallen asleep. *Remember to lay the baby on his or her back or in the side-lying position. Do not lay the baby on his or her stomach.*
- Encourage the mother to wear a nursing bra day and night. The bra supports the breasts and promotes comfort.
- Encourage the mother to place cotton pads in the bra. The pads absorb leaking milk.
- Have the mother apply cream (if prescribed) to her nipples after each feeding. The cream prevents nipples from drying and cracking. Remind her to wash her breasts before a feeding to remove the cream.
- Help the mother straighten clothing after the feeding if necessary.
- Remind the mother to wash her breasts with a clean washcloth and warm water. Soap is not used. It can cause the nipples to dry and crack.

Fig. 35-3 A mother nursing in the side-lying position.

Fig. 35-4 The mother strokes the baby's cheek with her breast. This stimulates the rooting reflex.

Fig. 35-5 The thumb is used to keep breast tissue away from the baby's nose.

Fig. 35-6 The mother inserts a finger in the baby's mouth to remove the baby from the breast.

▶ BOTTLE-FEEDING BABIES

Formula is given to babies who are not breast-fed. The doctor prescribes the formula. It provides the essential nutrients needed by the infant.

Formula comes in three forms. The *ready-to-feed* form is ready to use. It is poured directly from the can into the baby bottle (Fig. 35-7). Water is added to *powdered* and *concentrated* formula. Container directions tell how much formula to use and how much water to add. Bottles are prepared one at a time or in batches for the whole day. Extra bottles are capped (Fig. 35-8) and stored in the refrigerator. These bottles are used within 24 hours.

Babies must be protected from infection. Therefore baby bottles, caps, and nipples must be as clean as possible. Disposable equipment is used in hospitals. Reusable equipment may be used in homes. Reusable bottle-feeding equipment is carefully washed in hot, soapy water or in a dishwasher. Complete rinsing is needed to remove all soap. Some mothers use plastic nursers. They require plastic liners that are used once and then discarded.

Fig. 35-7 Ready-to-feed formula is poured from the can into the bottle. A funnel is used to prevent spilling.

Fig. 35-8 Bottles are capped for storage in the refrigerator.

Cleaning Baby Bottles

Pre-Procedure

1 Wash your hands.
2 Collect the following:
   • Bottles, nipples, and caps
   • Funnel
   • Can opener
   • Bottle brush
   • Dishwashing soap
   • Other items used to prepare formula
   • Towel

Procedure

3 Wash the bottles, nipples, caps, funnel, and can opener in hot, soapy water. Wash other items used to prepare formula.
4 Clean inside baby bottles with the bottle brush (Fig. 35-9).
5 Squeeze hot, soapy water through the nipples (Fig. 35-10). This removes formula from them.
6 Rinse all items thoroughly in hot water. Squeeze hot water through the nipples to remove soap.
7 Lay a clean towel on the countertop.
8 Stand the bottles upside down to drain. Place the nipples, caps, and other items on the towel. Let the items dry.

Fig. 35-9 A bottle brush is used to clean the inside of the bottle.

Fig. 35-10 Water is squeezed through the nipples during cleaning.

FEEDING THE BABY

Babies want to be fed every 3 to 4 hours. The amount of formula taken increases as they grow older. The nurse or the mother tells you how much formula a baby needs at each feeding. Babies usually take as much formula as they need. The baby stops sucking and turns away from the bottle when satisfied.

Babies are not given cold formula out of the refrigerator. A bottle is warmed before the feeding. You can warm the bottle in a pan of water. The formula should feel warm. Test the temperature by sprinkling a few drops on the inside of your wrist (Fig. 35-11). Do not set the bottle out to warm at room temperature. This takes too long and allows the growth of microbes. Do not heat formula in microwave ovens. The formula can heat unevenly and burn the baby's mouth.

The guidelines in Box 35-5 will help you bottle-feed babies.

Fig. 35-11 Formula should feel warm on the wrist.

Box 35-5   Bottle-Feeding Babies

- Warm the bottle so the formula feels warm to your wrist.
- Assume a comfortable position for the feeding.
- Hold the baby close to you. Relax and snuggle the baby.
- Tilt the bottle so that the neck of the bottle and the nipple are always filled (Fig. 35-12). Otherwise some air is in the neck or nipple. The baby sucks air into the stomach. The air causes cramping and discomfort.
- Do not prop the bottle and lay the baby down for the feeding (Fig. 35-13).
- Burp the baby when he or she has taken half the formula. Also burp the baby at the end of the feeding.
- Do not leave the baby alone with a bottle.
- Discard remaining formula.
- Wash the bottle, cap, and nipple after the feeding (see *Cleaning Baby Bottles*).

Fig. 35-12 The bottle is tilted so that formula fills the bottle neck and nipple.

Fig. 35-13 Do not prop the bottle to feed the baby.

BURPING THE BABY

Babies take in air when they nurse. Bottle-fed babies take in more air than breast-fed babies. Air in the stomach and intestines causes cramping and discomfort. This can lead to vomiting. Burping helps to get rid of the air. Most babies burp in the middle and after the feeding.

Burping a baby is sometimes called *bubbling*. There are two ways to position the baby for burping (Fig. 35-14). One way is to hold the infant over your shoulder. First place a clean diaper or towel over your shoulder. This protects your clothing if the baby "spits up." You can also support the baby in a sitting position on your lap. The towel or diaper is held in front of the baby. To burp the baby, gently pat or rub the baby's back with circular motions. Do this for 2 to 3 minutes.

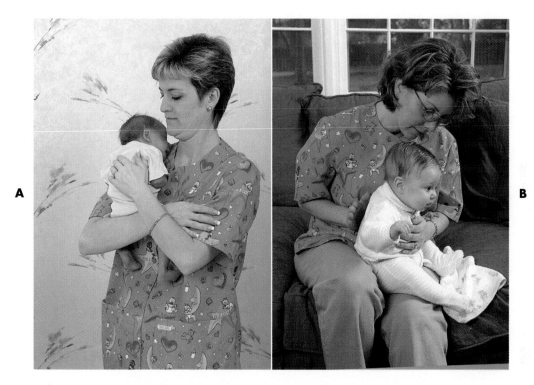

Fig. 35-14 Burping a baby. **A,** The baby is held over the shoulder for burping. **B,** The baby is supported in the sitting position for burping.

▶ DIAPERING

Babies urinate several times a day. Breast-fed babies usually have bowel movements after feedings. Bottle-fed babies may have 3 bowel movements a day. Stools are usually soft and unformed. Hard, formed stools mean the baby is constipated. This is reported to the nurse immediately. Watery stools mean diarrhea. Diarrhea is very serious in infants. Their water balance can be upset quickly (see Chapter 18). Tell the nurse immediately if you suspect a baby has diarrhea.

Diapers are changed when wet or soiled. Changing the diaper after a feeding is usually a good idea. Cloth and disposable diapers are available. Cloth diapers are washed, dried, and folded for reuse. They are washed daily or every 2 days with a laundry deter-gent made especially for baby clothes. Putting them through the wash cycle a second time without detergent helps remove all soap. If possible, hang diapers outside to dry. This gives them a fresh, clean smell. Cloth diapers are available with Velcro fasteners. Diaper pins are not needed. The danger of sticking the baby or yourself with a diaper pin is avoided.

Disposable diapers are placed in the trash. They are not flushed down the toilet. The use of disposable diapers is more costly.

Changing diapers often helps prevent diaper rash. Moisture, feces, and chemicals from urine irritate the baby's skin. When changing diapers, make sure the baby is clean and dry before applying a clean diaper. If a diaper rash develops, tell the nurse immediately. The nurse will tell you what to do.

Diapering a Baby

Pre-Procedure

1 Wash your hands.
2 Collect the following:
   - Gloves
   - Clean diaper
   - Waterproof changing pad
   - Washcloth
   - Disposable wipes or cotton balls
   - Basin of warm water
   - Baby soap
   - Baby lotion or cream
3 Place the changing pad under the baby.

Procedure

4 Put on the gloves.
5 Unfasten the dirty diaper. Place diaper pins out of the baby's reach.
6 Wipe the genital area with the front of the diaper (Fig. 35-15). Wipe from the front to the back.
7 Fold the diaper so urine and feces are well inside. Set the diaper aside.
8 Clean the genital area from front to back. Use a wet washcloth, disposable wipes, or cotton balls. Wash with mild soap and water if there is a lot of feces or if the baby has a rash. Rinse thoroughly, and pat the area dry.
9 Give cord care and clean the circumcision at this time.
10 Apply cream or lotion to the genital area and buttocks. Do not use too much. Caking can occur.
11 Raise the baby's legs. Slide a clean diaper under the buttocks.

12 Fold a cloth diaper so extra thickness is in the front for a boy (Fig. 35-16, A). For girls, fold the diaper so the extra thickness is in the back (Fig. 35-16, B).
13 Bring the diaper between the baby's legs.
14 Make sure the diaper is snug around the hips and abdomen. It should be loose near the penis if the circumcision has not healed. The diaper should be below the umbilicus if the cord stump has not healed.
15 Secure the diaper in place. Use the plastic tabs on disposable diapers (Fig. 35-17, A, p. 774). Make sure the tabs stick in place. Use diaper pins or Velcro strips for cloth diapers. Pins should point away from the abdomen (Fig. 35-17, B, p. 774).
16 Apply plastic pants if cloth diapers are worn. Do not use plastic pants with disposable diapers. They already have waterproof protection.
17 Put the baby in the crib, infant seat, or other safe location.

Diapering a Baby—cont'd

Post-Procedure

18 Rinse feces from the cloth diaper in the toilet.

19 Store used cloth diapers in a covered pail or plastic bag. Take the disposable diaper to the trash.

20 Remove the gloves, and wash your hands.

21 Note and report your observations.

Fig. 35-15 The front of the diaper is used to clean the genital area.

Fig. 35-16 A, A cloth diaper is folded in front for boys. **B,** The diaper has a fold in the back for girls.

Fig. 35-17 Securing a diaper. **A,** A disposable diaper is secured in place with plastic tabs. **B,** Diaper pins are used to secure cloth diapers. Pins point away from the abdomen.

CARE OF THE UMBILICAL CORD

The **umbilical cord** connects the mother and the fetus (unborn baby). It carries blood, oxygen, and nutrients from the mother to the fetus (Fig. 35-18). The umbilical cord is not needed after birth. Shortly after delivery, the doctor clamps and cuts the cord. A stump of cord is left on the baby. The stump dries up and falls off in 7 to 10 days. Slight bleeding can occur when the cord comes off.

The cord provides an area for the growth of microbes. You need to keep it clean and dry. Cord care is done at each diaper change. Cord care is continued for 1 or 2 days after the cord comes off. It consists of the following:

- Keep the stump dry. Do not get the stump wet.
- Wipe the base of the stump with alcohol (Fig. 35-19). Use an alcohol wipe or a cotton ball moistened with alcohol. The alcohol promotes drying.
- Keep the diaper below the cord as in Figure 35-17. This prevents the diaper from irritating the stump. It also keeps the cord from becoming wet from urine.
- Report any signs of infection. These include redness or odor or drainage from the stump.
- Give sponge baths until the cord falls off. Then the baby can have a tub bath.
- Do not pull the cord off—even if looks ready to fall off.

Fig. 35-18 The umbilical cord connects the mother and fetus.

Fig. 35-19 The cord stump is wiped at the base with alcohol.

CIRCUMCISION

Boys are born with foreskin on the penis. The surgical removal of foreskin is called a **circumcision** (see Fig. 16-12). The procedure allows good hygiene and is thought to prevent cancer of the penis. It is usually done in the hospital before the baby goes home. Circumcision is a religious ceremony in the Jewish faith.

The penis will look red, swollen, and sore. However, the circumcision should not interfere with urination. You must carefully check for signs of bleeding and infection. There should be no odor or drainage. You should check the diaper for bleeding. The area should completely heal in 10 to 14 days.

The penis is thoroughly cleaned at each diaper change. Cleaning is especially important if the baby had a bowel movement. Mild soap and water or commercial wipes are used. The diaper is loosely applied. This prevents the diaper from irritating the penis. Some doctors advise applying petroleum jelly to the penis. This protects the penis from urine and feces. It also prevents the penis from sticking to the diaper. A cotton swab is used to apply the petroleum jelly (Fig. 35-20). The nurse tells you if other measures are needed.

Fig. 35-20 Petroleum jelly is applied to the circumcised penis.

► BATHING AN INFANT

A bath is important for cleanliness. Though babies do not get very dirty, they need good skin care. Baths comfort and relax babies. They also provide a wonderful time to hold, touch, and talk to babies. Stimulation is important for development. Being touched and held helps babies learn safety, security, and love and belonging.

Planning is an important part of the bath. You cannot leave the baby alone if you forget something. Therefore you need to gather equipment, supplies, and the baby's clothes before you start the bath. Everything you need must be within your reach.

Safety measures are also very important:

- Never leave the baby alone on a table or in the bathtub.
- Always keep one hand on the baby if you must look away for a moment.
- Hold the baby securely throughout the bath. Babies are very slippery when they are wet. A wet, squirming baby is hard to hold.
- Room temperature should be 75° to 80° F for the bath. Turn up the thermostat and close windows and doors about 20 minutes before the bath. The room temperature may be uncomfortable for you. You may want to remove a sweater or lab coat or roll up your sleeves before starting the bath.
- Water temperature needs special attention. Babies have delicate skin and are easily burned. Bath water temperature should be 100° to 105° F (37.7° to 40.5° C). Bath water temperature is measured with a bath thermometer. If one is not available, test the water temperature with the inside of your wrist (Fig. 35-21). The water should feel warm and comfortable to your wrist. *(See Focus on Home Care box.)*

There are two bath procedures for babies. Sponge baths are given until the baby is about 2 weeks old. They are given until the cord stump falls off and the umbilicus and circumcision heal. *The cord must not get wet.* The tub bath is given after the cord site and circumcision heal (Fig. 35-22).

Focus On... HOME CARE

Bath time should be part of the baby's daily routine. Some mothers like to bathe their babies in the morning. Others prefer the evening. Evening baths have two important advantages. The bath is comforting and relaxing. This helps some babies sleep longer at night. Working fathers are usually home in the evening. The evening bath lets them be involved. Sometimes fathers bathe babies to give mothers time to rest or tend to other children. You must follow the family's routine when working in the home.

Fig. 35-21 The wrist is used to test the temperature of the bath water.

Fig. 35-22 The baby is given a tub bath.

Giving a Baby a Sponge Bath

Pre-Procedure

1 Wash your hands.
2 Place the following items in your work area:
   - Bath basin
   - Bath thermometer
   - Bath towel
   - Two hand towels
   - Receiving blanket
   - Washcloth
   - Clean diaper
   - Clean clothing for the baby
   - Cotton balls
   - Baby soap
   - Baby shampoo
   - Baby lotion
   - Gloves

Procedure

3 Fill the bath basin with warm water. Water temperature should be 100° to 105° F (37.7° to 40.5° C). Measure water temperature with the bath thermometer or use the inside of your wrist. The water should feel warm and comfortable on your wrist.
4 Provide for privacy.
5 Identify the baby. Check the ID bracelet against the assignment sheet.
6 Undress the baby. Leave the diaper on.
7 Wash the baby's eyelids (Fig. 35-23, p. 778):
   a Dip a cotton ball into the water.
   b Squeeze out excess water.
   c Wash one eyelid from the inner part to the outer part.
   d Repeat this step for the other eye with a new cotton ball.
8 Moisten the washcloth. Clean the outside of the ear and then behind the ear. Repeat this step for the other ear. Be gentle.
9 Rinse and squeeze the washcloth. Make a mitt with the washcloth (see Fig. 14-10).
10 Wash the baby's face (Fig. 35-24, p. 778). Clean inside the nostrils with the washcloth. *Do not use cotton swabs to clean inside the ears.* Pat the face dry.
11 Pick up the baby. Hold the baby over the bath basin using the football hold. Support the baby's head and neck with your wrist and hand.
12 Wash the baby's head (Fig. 35-25, p. 778):
   a Squeeze a small amount of water from the washcloth onto the baby's head.
   b Apply a small amount of baby shampoo to the head.
   c Wash the head with circular motions.
   d Rinse the head by squeezing water from a washcloth over the baby's head. Be sure to rinse thoroughly. Avoid getting soap in the baby's eyes.
   e Use a small hand towel to dry the head.
13 Lay the baby on the table.
14 Put on the gloves.
15 Remove the diaper.
16 Wash the front of the body. Use a soapy washcloth. You may also apply soap to your hands and wash the baby with your hands (Fig. 35-26, p. 778). Do not get the cord wet. Rinse thoroughly. Pat dry. Be sure to wash and dry all creases and folds.
17 Turn the baby to the prone position. Repeat step 16 for the back and buttocks.
18 Give cord care, and clean the circumcision.
19 Apply baby lotion to the baby's body as directed by the nurse.
20 Put a clean diaper and clean clothes on the baby.
21 Remove the gloves.
22 Wrap the baby in the receiving blanket. Put the baby in the crib or other safe location.

Post-Procedure

23 Clean and return equipment and supplies to the proper place. Do this step when the baby is settled.
24 Wash your hands.
25 Note and report your observations.

Fig. 35-23 The baby's eyelids are washed with cotton balls. The eyelid is cleaned from the inner to the outer part.

Fig. 35-24 The baby's face is washed with a mitted washcloth.

Fig. 35-25 The baby's head is washed over the basin.

Fig. 35-26 The hands are used to wash the baby.

Giving a Baby a Tub Bath

Procedure

1 Follow steps 1 through 15 in *Giving a Baby a Sponge Bath, p. 777*.

2 Hold the baby as in Figure 35-27:

   a Place your right hand* under the baby's shoulders. Your thumb should be over the baby's right shoulder. Your fingers should be under the right arm.

   b Use your left hand to support the baby's buttocks. Slide your left hand under the thighs. Hold the right thigh with your left hand.

3 Lower the baby into the water feet first.

4 Wash the front of the baby's body. Be sure to wash all folds and creases. Rinse thoroughly.

5 Reverse your hold. Use your left hand to hold the baby.

6 Wash the baby's back as in Figure 35-22. Rinse thoroughly.

7 Reverse your hold again. Use your right hand to hold the baby.

8 Wash the genital area.

9 Lift the baby out of the water and onto a towel.

10 Wrap the baby in the towel. Also cover the baby's head.

11 Pat the baby dry. Be sure to dry all folds and creases.

12 Follow steps 19-25 of the *Sponge Bath* procedure.

*This procedure was written for right-handed persons. Reverse the hand position if you are left-handed.

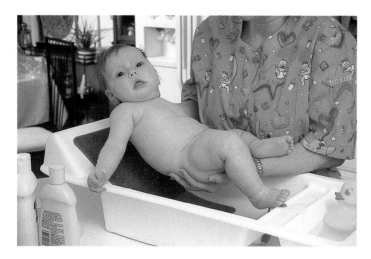

Fig. 35-27 The baby is held for the tub bath.

NAIL CARE

The baby's fingernails and toenails are kept short. Otherwise, the baby can scratch himself or herself and others. Nails are best cut when the baby is sleeping. The baby is quiet and will not squirm or fuss. Use nail clippers or file nails with an emery board. If using nail clippers, clip nails straight across as for an adult (see Fig. 15-7).

▶ WEIGHING INFANTS

Infants are weighed at birth. The birth weight is the baseline for measuring the infant's growth. The RN uses weight measurements in the assessment step of the nursing process. It is also used to evaluate how much breast milk was taken during breast-feeding. The baby is weighed before and after breast-feeding. The difference in the weights is the amount of milk taken in during breast-feeding. The nurse uses this information to determine if the baby is getting enough milk.

The nurse tells you when to weigh the baby. You must meet the baby's safety needs. Protect the baby from chills. Keep the room warm and free of drafts. Also protect the baby from falling. Always keep a hand over the baby when taking the weight measurement. Remember to keep one hand on the baby if you need to look away. Breast-fed babies wear the same diaper, clothes, and blanket for each weight measurement before and after the feeding.

Weighing an Infant

Pre-Procedure

1 Wash your hands.
2 Collect the following:
   • Baby scale

   • Paper for the scale
   • Items for diaper changing (see *Diapering a Baby*, p. 772)

Procedure

3 Identify the baby.
4 Place the paper on the scale. Adjust the scale to zero (0).
5 Put on the gloves.
6 Undress the baby, and remove the diaper. Clean the genital area.

7 Lay the baby on the scale. Keep one hand over the baby to prevent falling.
8 Read the digital display (Fig. 35-28), or move the pointer until the scale is balanced.
9 Diaper and dress the baby. Lay the baby in the crib.
10 Remove and discard the gloves.

Post-Procedure

11 Return the scale to its proper place.
12 Wash your hands.

13 Report your observations to the nurse.
14 Record the weight according to agency policy.

Fig. 35-28 Digital infant scale.

CARE OF THE MOTHER

Postpartum means after (*post*) childbirth (*partum*). The postpartum period starts with birth of the baby. It ends 6 weeks later. The mother's body returns to its normal state during this time. The mother adjusts physically and emotionally to childbirth.

The uterus returns almost to its pre-pregnant size. This is called *involution of the uterus*. If the mother does not breast-feed, she can expect a menstrual period within 3 to 8 weeks. The mother can get pregnant again unless she practices birth control measures.

A vaginal discharge occurs during the postpartum period. It is called **lochia.** (Lochia comes from the Greek word *lochos*, which means childbirth.) Lochia consists of blood and other substances left in the uterus from childbirth. The lochia changes color and decreases in amount during the postpartum period:

- *Lochia rubra*—is dark or bright red (*rubra*) discharge. It is mainly blood and is seen during the first 3 to 4 days.
- *Lochia serosa*—is pinkish brown (*serosa*) drainage. It lasts until about 10 days after birth.
- *Lochia alba*—is whitish (*alba*) drainage. It continues for 2 to 6 weeks after birth.

Lochia increases with breast-feeding and activity. When she stands after lying or sitting, the mother may feel a gush of lochia. The mother wears a sanitary napkin to absorb the lochia. Normally, lochia smells like menstrual flow. Foul-smelling lochia is a sign of infection.

Good perineal care is important. Sanitary pads are changed often. When wiping after elimination, the mother wipes from front to back. Sanitary napkins are applied and removed from front to back. Good hand-washing is essential after perineal care, changing sanitary napkins, and elimination. Standard Precautions and the Bloodborne Pathogen Standard are followed.

Some mothers have episiotomies. An **episiotomy** is an incision (*otomy*) into the perineum. (*Episeion* is from the Greek word meaning pubic region.) The doctor performs this procedure during childbirth. The incision increases the size of the vaginal opening for delivery of the baby. The incision is sutured after the delivery. The doctor may order sitz baths for comfort and hygiene (see Chapter 26). Practice Standard Precautions and the Bloodborne Pathogen Standard when helping the mother with sitz baths. As with other incisions, complications can develop. These include infection and wound separation (dehiscence). Tell the nurse immediately if the mother complains of pain, discomfort, or a discharge.

If the mother delivered the baby by *cesarean section* (*C-section*), she has an abdominal incision. With a cesarean section, the doctor makes an incision into the abdominal wall. The baby is delivered through the incision. This is done:

- When the baby must be delivered to save the baby's or mother's life
- When the baby is too large to pass through the birth canal
- When the mother has a vaginal infection that could be transmitted to the baby
- When a normal vaginal delivery will be difficult for the baby or mother

The C-section incision needs to heal. See Chapter 25 for wound healing and wound care.

The mother has emotional reactions after childbirth. Hormone changes, life-style changes, and lack of sleep can cause her to have mood swings. So can frequent visits and telephone calls from friends and family. This is especially true if they interfere or offer advice and opinions about parenting. The mother can help herself by resting when the baby is sleeping. She needs to take time for herself and her partner. She is likely to feel better after pampering herself with a shower, washing and styling her hair, and getting dressed. These can be done while the baby is sleeping.

Complications can occur at any time during pregnancy, labor, and delivery. They also can occur during the postpartum period. Box 35-6 lists the signs and symptoms of postpartum complications. Report any sign or symptom to the nurse immediately.

Box 35-6	**Signs and Symptoms of Postpartum Complications**

- Fever of 100.4° F or higher
- Abdominal or perineal pain
- Foul-smelling vaginal discharge
- Bleeding from an episiotomy or C-section incision
- Redness, swelling, or drainage from an episiotomy or C-section incision
- Saturating a sanitary napkin within 1 hour of application
- Red lochia after lochia has changed color to pinkish-brown or white
- Burning on urination
- Leg pain, tenderness, or swelling
- Sadness or feelings of depression
- Breast pain, tenderness, or swelling

Circle the BEST answer.

1. A newborn's head is supported for the first
   A. 7 to 10 days
   B. Month
   C. 3 months
   D. 6 months

2. Zach is a newborn. When holding him you should do the following *except*
   A. Hold him securely
   B. Cuddle him
   C. Sing and talk to him
   D. Hold him on his stomach

3. Which is *false?*
   A. Zach's crib should be within hearing distance of caregivers.
   B. Zach should have a pillow for sleep.
   C. Zach should be positioned on his back for sleep.
   D. Crib rails should be up at all times.

4. Report the following to the nurse *except*
   A. Zach looks flushed and is perspiring
   B. Zach has watery stools
   C. Zach's eyes are red and irritated
   D. Zach spits up a small amount when burped

5. Zach is breast-fed. The mother should do the following *except*
   A. Wash her hands
   B. Hold Zach close to her breast
   C. Stimulate the rooting reflex
   D. Clean her breasts with soap and water

6. A breast-fed baby is burped
   A. Every 5 minutes
   B. After nursing from one breast
   C. After nursing from both breasts
   D. After the feeding

7. Zach is being switched to bottle-feedings. You do the grocery shopping. Which formula should you buy?
   A. The one that is on sale
   B. The ready-to-feed type
   C. The one ordered by the doctor
   D. The powdered form

8. You are to warm Zach's bottle. Which is *true?*
   A. The bottle is warmed for 5 minutes in the microwave.
   B. The formula should warm at room temperature.
   C. The formula should feel warm on your wrist.
   D. The formula is warmed in a pan for 5 minutes.

9. When bottle-feeding Zach, you should
   A. Burp him every 5 minutes
   B. Save remaining formula for the next feeding
   C. Tilt the bottle so that formula fills the neck of the bottle and the nipple
   D. Leave him alone with the bottle

10. Zach's cord has not yet healed. His diaper should be
    A. Loose over the cord
    B. Snug over the cord
    C. Below the cord
    D. Disposable

11. Zach's cord stump is cleaned with
    A. Soap and water
    B. Baby shampoo
    C. Plain water
    D. Alcohol

12. Zach's cord and the circumcision are cleaned
    A. Once a day
    B. When he has a bowel movement
    C. Three times a day
    D. At every diaper change

13. Bath water for Zach should be
    A. 85° to 90° F
    B. 90° to 95° F
    C. 95° to 100° F
    D. 100° to 105° F

14. Which should you use to wash Zach's nose?
    A. A mitted washcloth
    B. Alcohol wipes
    C. A cotton swab
    D. Cotton balls

15. A mother has a red vaginal discharge the first few days after childbirth. This
    A. Is her menstrual flow
    B. Signals a postpartum complication
    C. Is lochia rubra
    D. Is from her episiotomy

16. A cesarean delivery involves
    A. A vaginal incision
    B. A perineal incision
    C. An abdominal incision
    D. A normal delivery through the birth canal

Circle T if the answer is true and F if it is false.

17. T F Zach's diapers are changed whenever he is wet.

18. T F Zach's cord and circumcision have not healed. He should have a sponge bath.

19. T F Cotton swabs are used to clean inside Zach's ears.

20. T F Zach is being breast-fed. He is weighed with his diaper on.

Answers to these questions are on p. 839.

CHAPTER

36

BASIC

EMERGENCY

CARE

Define the key terms listed in this chapter

Describe the general rules of emergency care

Identify the signs of cardiac arrest and obstructed airway

Describe basic life support and basic life support procedures

Explain the difference between internal and external hemorrhage

Explain how to control hemorrhage

Identify the signs of and emergency care for shock

Describe different types of seizures and how to care for a person during a seizure

Describe burns, their causes, and emergency care

Identify the common causes of and emergency care for fainting

Describe the signs of and emergency care for stroke

Perform the procedures described in this chapter

KEY TERMS

anaphylaxis A life-threatening sensitivity to an antigen

cardiac arrest The heart and breathing stop suddenly and without warning

convulsion A seizure

fainting The sudden loss of consciousness from an inadequate blood supply to the brain

first aid Emergency care given to an ill or injured person before medical help arrives

hemorrhage The excessive loss of blood in a short period of time

respiratory arrest Breathing stops but the heart still pumps blood for several minutes

seizure Violent and sudden contractions or tremors of muscles; convulsion

shock A condition that results when there is not enough blood supply to organs and tissues

Emergencies can occur anywhere. They happen in health care agencies, homes, and public places and on highways. Knowing what to do can mean the difference between life and death. This chapter describes some common emergencies and the basic care that is given. You are encouraged to take a first aid course from the National Safety Council or the American Red Cross. A basic life support course given by the American Heart Association, National Safety Council, or the American Red Cross also is recommended. These courses prepare you to give care in emergency situations.

GENERAL RULES OF EMERGENCY CARE

First aid is the emergency care given to an ill or injured person before medical help arrives. The goals of first aid are to:

- Prevent death
- Prevent injuries from becoming worse

When an emergency occurs, the local emergency medical services (EMS) system is activated. The system involves emergency personnel (paramedics, emergency medical technicians) who are trained and educated to give emergency care. They know how to treat, stabilize, and transport persons with life-threatening conditions. Their emergency vehicles have the equipment, supplies, and drugs used in emergencies. Emergency personnel communicate by telephone or two-way radio with doctors based in hospital emergency rooms. The doctors tell them what to do. In many areas the EMS system is activated by dialing 911. Calling the local fire or police department or the telephone operator also activates the system.

Box 36-1	General Rules of Emergency Care

- Know your limits. Do not do more than you are able. Do not perform an unfamiliar procedure. Do what you can under the circumstances.
- Stay calm. This helps the person feel more secure.
- Practice Standard Precautions, and follow the Bloodborne Pathogen Standard to the extent possible.
- Check for signs of life-threatening problems. Check for breathing, a pulse, and bleeding.
- Keep the person lying down or in the position in which he or she was found. Moving the person could make an injury worse.
- Perform necessary emergency measures.
- Call for help, or tell someone to activate the EMS system. An operator will send emergency vehicles and personnel to the scene. *Do not hang up until the operator has hung up.* Give the operator the following information:
  - Your location—street address and city or town you are in; names of cross streets or roads and landmarks if possible
  - Telephone number you are calling from

- What happened (e.g., heart attack, accident)—police, fire equipment, and ambulances may be needed
- How many people need help
- Condition of victims, any obvious injuries, and any life-threatening situations
- What aid is being given
- Do not remove the person's clothing unless you have to. If you must remove clothing, tear or cut garments along the seams.
- Keep the person warm. Cover the person with a blanket. Or use coats and sweaters.
- Reassure those who are conscious. Explain what is happening and that you called for help.
- Do not give the person any food or fluids.
- Do not move the person. Emergency personnel are trained to do so.
- Keep bystanders away from the person. Bystanders tend to stare, give advice, and comment about the person's condition. The person may think the situation is worse than it really is. Also, the person's privacy is invaded by onlookers.

Each emergency is different. However, the rules in Box 36-1 apply to any emergency. *(See Focus on Long-Term Care box.)*

BASIC LIFE SUPPORT

When the heart and breathing stop, the person is clinically dead. Blood is not circulated through the body. Body cells do not get oxygen. Permanent brain damage and other organ damage occur within minutes. Sometimes death is expected. Death is expected in persons suffering from terminal illnesses. However, the heart and breathing can stop suddenly and without warning. This is a state of **cardiac arrest**.

Cardiac arrest is a sudden, unexpected, and dramatic event. It can occur while driving, shoveling snow, playing golf or tennis, watching television, eating, and sleeping. Cardiac arrest can occur anywhere and at any time. Common causes include heart disease, drowning, electrical shock, severe injury, airway obstruction, and drug overdose. The person suffers permanent brain damage unless breathing and circulation are restored.

Respiratory arrest is when breathing stops but the heart still pumps blood for several minutes. Causes of respiratory arrest include drowning, stroke, obstructed airway, drug overdose, electrocution, lightning strike, smoke inhalation, suffocation, heart attack (myocardial infarction), coma, and other injuries. If breathing is not

Focus On... LONG-TERM CARE

In nursing centers, a nurse decides when to activate the EMS system. The nurse tells you what to do to help in the situation. If a resident has stopped breathing or is in cardiac arrest, the nurse may start cardiopulmonary resuscitation (CPR). Center policies vary about nursing assistants starting CPR. Some allow nursing assistants to start CPR and others do not. You need to know your center's policy about CPR.

Some residents are not resuscitated. The resident, family, and doctor have decided that the person should be allowed to die with peace and dignity. If so, the doctor writes a "do not resuscitate" (DNR) order (see Chapter 37). You need to know your center's policy about DNR orders. The nurse tells you which residents have DNR orders. This information is also in the care plan.

restored, cardiac arrest occurs. If the person still has a pulse, rescue breathing can prevent cardiac arrest.

Basic life support (BLS) involves preventing or promptly recognizing cardiac arrest or respiratory arrest. BLS procedures support breathing and circulation. These life-saving measures require speed, skill, and efficiency. Prompt activation of the EMS system is also part of BLS.

The American Heart Association, National Safety Council, and American Red Cross certify individuals to perform basic life support procedures. The basic life support procedures that follow are presented as information. They do not replace certification training. You are encouraged to take a basic life support course offered by one of these organizations.

CARDIOPULMONARY RESUSCITATION

There are three major signs of cardiac arrest—no pulse, no breathing, and unconsciousness. The person's skin is cool, pale, and gray. The person has no blood pressure.

Cardiopulmonary resuscitation (CPR) must be started as soon as cardiac arrest occurs. CPR provides oxygen to the brain, heart, kidneys, and other organs until more advanced emergency care can be given. CPR has three basic parts (the ABCs of CPR):

- **A**irway
- **B**reathing
- **C**irculation

The person must be supine on a hard, flat surface. The arms are positioned at the sides. If turning is necessary, use the logrolling procedure (see Chapter 11). The person may have other injuries. Therefore the person is turned as a unit to prevent twisting of the spinal cord.

Airway. The respiratory passages (airway) must be open to restore breathing. The airway is often blocked or obstructed during cardiac arrest. The person's tongue falls toward the back of the throat and blocks the airway. The *head-tilt/chin-lift maneuver* is used to open the airway (Fig. 36-1):

- Place one hand on the person's forehead.
- Apply pressure on the forehead with the palm to tilt the head back.
- Place the fingers of the other hand under the bony part of the chin.
- Lift the chin forward as the head is tilted backward with the other hand.

When the airway is open, check for vomitus, loose dentures, or other foreign bodies. These can obstruct the airway during rescue breathing. Remove dentures and wipe vomitus away with your index and middle fingers. Wear disposable gloves, or cover your fingers with a cloth. Although you must not waste time, try to protect the dentures from loss or damage.

Breathing. Air is not inhaled when breathing stops. The person must get oxygen. Otherwise, permanent brain and organ damage occur. Breathing is done for the person. This is called *rescue breathing*.

Before you start rescue breathing, determine breathlessness (Fig. 36-2). It should take 3 to 5 seconds to do the following:

- Maintain an open airway.
- Place your ear over the person's mouth and nose.
- Observe the person's chest.
- *Look* to see if the chest rises and falls.
- *Listen* for the escape of air.
- *Feel* for the flow of air on your cheek

Mouth-to-mouth resuscitation (Fig. 36-3) is the most common method of rescue breathing. The airway is kept open to give mouth-to-mouth resuscitation. Pinch the person's nostrils shut with the thumb and index finger of the hand on the forehead. Shutting the nostrils prevents the escape of air from the nose. After taking a deep breath, place your mouth tightly over the person's mouth. Slowly blow air into the person's mouth. You should see the person's chest rise as the lungs fill with air. You should also hear air escape when the person exhales. After giving a ventilation, remove your mouth from the person's mouth. Then take in a quick, deep breath.

Fig. 36-1 The head-tilt/chin-lift maneuver is used to open the airway. One hand is on the person's forehead, and pressure is applied to tilt the head back. The fingers of the other hand are placed under the chin. The chin is lifted forward with the fingers.

Fig. 36-2 Determine breathlessness by *looking* to see if the chest rises and falls, *listening* for the escape of air, and *feeling* for the flow of air.

Fig. 36-3 Mouth-to-mouth resuscitation. **A,** The person's airway is opened, and the nostrils are pinched shut. **B,** The person's mouth is sealed by the rescuer's mouth.

Fig. 36-4 Mouth-to-nose resuscitation.

Fig. 36-5 A stoma in the neck. The person breathes air in and out of the stoma.

Mouth-to-mouth resuscitation is not always indicated or possible. The *mouth-to-nose* technique is used when:

- You cannot ventilate the victim's mouth
- You cannot open the mouth
- You cannot make a tight seal for mouth-to-mouth resuscitation
- The mouth is severely injured

The mouth is closed for mouth-to-nose resuscitation. The head-tilt/chin-lift method is used to open the airway. Pressure is placed on the chin to close the mouth. To give the ventilation, place your mouth over the person's nose and blow air into the nose (Fig. 36-4). After the ventilation, remove your mouth from the person's nose.

Some people breathe through openings *(stomas)* in their necks (Fig. 36-5). They need *mouth-to-stoma* ventilation during cardiac or respiratory arrest. You will seal your mouth around the stoma and blow air into the stoma (Fig. 36-6, p. 780). Before giving mouth-to-mouth or mouth-to-nose resuscitation, always check to see if a person has a stoma. Other methods of rescue breathing are not effective if the person has a stoma.

Barrier devices prevent contact with the person's mouth and blood, body fluids, secretions, or excretions. Mask devices are available (Fig. 36-7, p. 780). *Mouth-to-barrier device* is another method of rescue breathing. The barrier device is placed over the person's mouth and nose. Make sure you have a tight seal. Then breathe into the barrier device.

Fig. 36-6 Mouth-to-stoma resuscitation.

Fig. 36-7 A, Mask device. **B,** Mask device placed over the person's mouth and nose.

When CPR is started, give 2 breaths at first. Exhale after each breath. Then give breaths at a rate of 10 to 12 breaths per minute. During one-rescuer CPR, give 2 breaths after every 15 chest compressions. During two-rescuer CPR, give a breath after every 5 chest compressions.

Circulation. Blood flow to the brain and other organs must be maintained. Otherwise, permanent damage results. The heart has stopped beating in cardiac arrest. Therefore blood must be pumped through the body in some other way. Artificial circulation is accomplished by chest compression. Each chest compression forces blood through the circulatory system.

Before starting chest compressions, determine pulselessness. Use the carotid artery on the side near you to check for pulselessness. To find the carotid pulse, place the tips of your index and middle fingers on the person's trachea (windpipe). Then slide your fingertips down off the trachea to the groove of the neck (Fig. 36-8).

Fig. 36-8 Locating the carotid pulse. Index and middle fingers are placed on the trachea. The fingers are moved down into the groove of the neck where the carotid pulse is located.

Fig. 36-9 The heart lies between the sternum and spinal column. The heart is compressed when pressure is applied to the sternum.

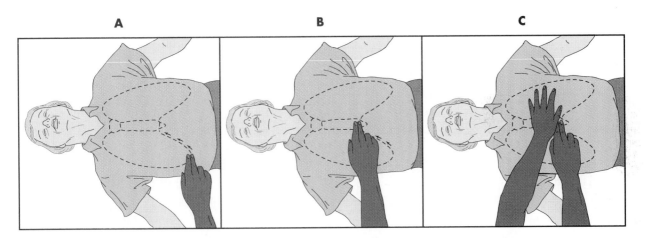

Fig. 36-10 Proper hand position for CPR. **A,** Locate the rib cage. **B,** Run the fingers along the rib cage to the notch. **C,** Place the heel of your other hand next to your index finger.

The heart lies between the sternum (breastbone) and the spinal column. When pressure is applied to the sternum, the sternum is depressed. This compresses the heart between the sternum and spinal column (Fig. 36-9). For effective chest compressions, the person must be supine and on a hard, flat surface.

Proper hand position is important for chest compressions. The process for locating hand position for adults is shown in Figure 36-10:

- Use your index and middle fingers to locate the lower part of the person's rib cage on the side near you.
- Then run your fingers up along the rib cage to the notch at the center of the chest. The notch is where the ribs and sternum meet.
- Place the heel of your other hand on the lower half of the sternum next to your index finger.
- Remove your index and middle fingers from the notch.
- Place that hand on the hand already on the sternum.
- Extend or interlace your fingers. Keep your fingers off the chest.

Fig. 36-11 Position of the shoulders for CPR.

You must be positioned properly for chest compressions. Your elbows are straight. Your shoulders are directly over the person's chest (Fig. 36-11). Exert firm downward pressure to depress the sternum about 1½ to 2 inches in the adult. Then release pressure without removing your hands from the chest. Give compressions in a regular rhythm.

▶ **Performing CPR.** CPR is done only for cardiac arrest. You must determine if cardiac arrest or fainting has occurred. *CPR is done when there is unresponsiveness, breathlessness, and pulselessness.* That is, the person does not respond, is not breathing, and has no pulse. Basic life support for the adult involves the following sequence:

1. Determine unresponsiveness. Tap or gently shake the person, and shout "Are you OK?" If there is no response, the person is unconscious.
2. *Activate the EMS system immediately if the person is unresponsive.*
3. Determine breathlessness. *Look* at the person's chest to see if it rises and falls. *Listen* for the escape of air during expiration. *Feel* for the flow of air. To feel for air, place your cheek near the person's nose.
4. Open the airway and give 2 breaths if the person is not breathing.
5. Determine pulselessness.
6. Start chest compressions if the person has no pulse.

You can do CPR alone or with another person. *Never practice CPR on another person.* You can cause serious damage. Mannequins are used to learn CPR.

Adult CPR—One Rescuer

Procedure

1 Check for unresponsiveness.

2 Activate the EMS system.

3 Position the person supine. Logroll the person so there is no twisting of the spine. The person must be on a hard, flat surface. Place the person's arms alongside the body.

4 Open the airway. Use the head-tilt/chin-lift maneuver.

5 Check for breathlessness.

6 Give 2 breaths. Each should be 1½ to 2 seconds long. Let the person's chest deflate between breaths.

7 Check for pulselessness. Check the carotid pulse for 5 to 10 seconds. Use your other hand to keep the airway open with the head-tilt maneuver.

8 Give chest compressions if the person has no pulse. Give compressions at a rate of 80 to 100 per minute. Give 15 compressions and then 2 breaths:

   a Establish a rhythm and count out loud (try: "1 and, 2 and, 3 and, 4 and, 5 and, 6 and, 7 and, 8 and, 9 and, 10 and, 11 and, 12 and, 13 and, 14 and, 15").

   b Open the airway, and give 2 breaths.

   c Repeat this step until you have given 4 cycles of 15 compressions and 2 breaths.

9 Check for a carotid pulse (3 to 5 seconds).

10 Continue CPR if the person has no pulse. Begin with chest compressions.

11 Continue the cycle of 15 compressions and 2 breaths. Check for a pulse every few minutes.

12 Repeat steps 10 and 11 as long as necessary.

Adult CPR—Two Rescuers

Procedure

1. Perform one-person CPR until a helper arrives.
2. Continue chest compressions. The helper says, "I know CPR. Can I help?"
3. Indicate that you want help. Ask that the EMS system be activated, if not already done.
4. Do not stop chest compressions. The helper kneels on the other side of the person. The two-rescuer procedure starts after you complete a cycle of 15 compressions and 2 breaths.
5. Stop compressions for 3 to 5 seconds. The helper checks for a carotid pulse. The helper states, "No pulse."
6. Perform two-person CPR (Fig. 36-12) as follows:
   a. The helper gives 2 breaths.
   b. Give chest compressions at a rate of 80 to 100 per minute. Count out loud in a rhythm (try: "1 and, 2 and, 3 and, 4 and, 5").
   c. The helper gives a breath immediately after the fifth compression. Pause for the breath. Continue chest compressions after the breath.
   d. A breath is given after every fifth compression.
7. Stop compressions after 1 minute. Your helper checks for a carotid pulse. After the first minute, compressions are stopped every few minutes to check for breathing and circulation. Compressions are stopped for only 5 seconds.
8. Call for a switch in positions when you are tired.
9. Change positions quickly:
   a. Helper gives a breath after you give the fifth compression.
   b. Helper moves down to kneel at the person's shoulder and finds the proper hand position.
   c. You move to the person's head after giving the fifth compression.
   d. Check for a carotid pulse (3 to 5 seconds).
   e. Say, "No pulse."
   f. Give 1 breath before your helper starts chest compressions.
10. Give 1 breath after every fifth compression.
11. Switch positions when the person giving the compressions is tired. Check for a pulse and breathing at every position change.

Fig. 36-12 Two people performing CPR.

▶ BASIC LIFE SUPPORT FOR INFANTS AND CHILDREN

Cardiac arrest caused by heart disease is rare in children. More common causes involve diseases and injuries that lead to respiratory arrest or circulatory failure. Sudden infant death syndrome (SIDS), respiratory diseases, airway obstruction, drowning, infection, and nervous system diseases are the most common causes of cardiac arrest in children under 1 year of age. Injuries are the most common cause in children older than 1 year. They include motor vehicle injuries, street injuries, bicycle injuries, drowning, burns, and firearm injuries.

Sequence of BLS. Basic life support for infants and young children (1 to 8 years) also involves determining unresponsiveness, activating the EMS system, and determining breathlessness and pulselessness. However, there are some important differences from the adult procedures:

- Injuries are a likely cause of respiratory or cardiac arrest. Head, neck, and spinal cord injuries are possible. Therefore do not move or shake the child to determine responsiveness. Check unresponsiveness by tapping or shouting to get a response.
- Shout for help, or send a second rescuer to activate the EMS system.
- If you are alone, provide basic life support for 1 minute before activating the EMS system. This can prevent respiratory arrest from advancing to cardiac arrest.
- If there are no injuries and if the person is small, carry the person to the telephone. This makes calling the EMS system easier.
- Move any person from a dangerous location. Also move the person if you cannot perform CPR where the person is lying.
- If you must move the person, make sure the head does not roll, twist, or tilt. Hold the head and body straight without twisting. Use the logrolling procedure to turn the person.
- Use the head-tilt/chin-lift maneuver for infants and children. Do not hyperextend the head as in the adult. Rather tilt the head to a normal (neutral) or *sniffing* position (Fig. 36-13).
- If neck injury is suspected, use the jaw-thrust maneuver (Fig. 36-14):
  1 Place 2 or 3 fingers under each side of the lower jaw at the angle of the jaw.
  2 Use your other finger to lift the jaw upward and outward.
  3 Rest your elbows on the surface on which the infant or child is lying.

Fig. 36-13 The head-tilt/chin-lift maneuver is used for infants. The infant's head is not tilted as far back as that of the adult. The infant's head is in a neutral or "sniffing" position.

Fig. 36-14 The jaw-thrust maneuver. Place 2 or 3 fingers on the lower jaw. Use your other fingers to lift the jaw upward and outward.

- Keep the airway open throughout CPR. Only use one hand for chest compressions. Keep the other hand on the forehead to maintain the head tilt. For children, use both hands for the head-tilt/chin-lift maneuver when giving breaths.
- In children under 1 year of age, use the brachial pulse to determine pulselessness.
- Give 20 breaths and 100 chest compressions per minute.

CPR for Infants and Children (Under 8 Years of Age)

Procedure

1 Check for unresponsiveness.
2 Activate the EMS system if help is available. Otherwise, activate the EMS system after 1 minute of CPR.
3 Logroll the child onto his or her back. Support the head and neck when turning the child. Position the child supine on a hard, flat surface.
4 Open the airway. Use the head-tilt/chin-lift maneuver. Do not hyperextend the head. Extension of the head usually opens an infant's or child's airway (see Fig. 36-13).
5 Check for breathlessness.
6 Give 2 slow breaths. Use enough force to make the chest rise. Take 1 to $1^1/2$ seconds for each breath. Cover an infant's nose and mouth with your mouth when giving a breath (Fig. 36-15, p. 796). Let the chest deflate between breaths.
7 Check for pulselessness. Use the brachial artery for infants and the carotid artery for children. Keep the airway open.
8 Give chest compressions to an *infant*:
  a Locate hand position (Fig. 36-16, p. 796):
    (1) Draw an imaginary line between the nipples.
    (2) Place your index finger just under the imaginary line.
    (3) Place your middle and ring fingers next to your index finger. The area for chest compression is below your middle and ring fingers.
  b Give compressions using your middle and ring fingers. Compress the sternum $1/2$ to 1 inch at least 100 times per minute. Release pressure after each compression. Do not remove your fingers from the chest.
  c Count out loud in a rhythm (try: "1, 2, 3, 4, 5").

  d Give 1 breath after every fifth compression.
  e Check for a brachial pulse after 20 cycles of 5 compressions and 1 breath (about 1 minute).
  f Activate the EMS system if there is no pulse.
  g Continue chest compressions and ventilation if there is no pulse.
  h Check for a pulse every few minutes.
9 Give chest compressions to a *child* (use the adult method if the child is large or older than age 8):
  a Locate proper hand position (Fig. 36-17, p. 796):
    (1) Run your middle finger up along the rib cage to the notch at the center of the chest.
    (2) Mark the notch with your middle finger.
    (3) Place your index finger next to your middle finger.
    (4) Place the heel of the same hand next to where the index finger was located.
  b Depress the sternum 1 to $1^1/2$ inches with the heel of your hand. Keep your fingers off the chest. Keep the airway open with your other hand.
  c Give 80 to 100 compressions per minute. Count out loud in a rhythm (try: "1 and 2 and 3 and 4 and 5").
  d Give a breath after every fifth compression.
  e Check for a carotid pulse after 20 cycles of 5 compressions and 1 breath.
  f Activate the EMS system if there is no pulse.
  g Continue chest compressions and breaths if there is no pulse.
  h Check for a pulse every few minutes.

Fig. 36-15 Cover the infant's mouth and nose during mouth-to-mouth resuscitation.

Fig. 36-17 The heel of one hand is used for CPR on a child. The heel is placed over the lower end of the sternum as for an adult.

Fig. 36-16 Locating hand position for infant chest compressions. **A,** Draw an imaginary line between the nipples. **B,** The index finger is placed just under the line. **C,** The middle and ring fingers are placed next to the index finger. **D,** The area for chest compressions is under the middle and ring fingers.

➤ OBSTRUCTED AIRWAY IN ADULTS

Airway obstruction (choking) can lead to cardiac arrest. Air cannot pass through the air passages to the lungs. The body does not get oxygen.

Foreign bodies can cause airway obstruction. This often occurs during eating. Meat is the most common food causing airway obstruction. Choking often occurs on large, poorly chewed pieces of meat. Laughing and talking while eating also can cause choking. Adults can choke on dentures. Excessive alcohol intake is another cause.

Airway obstruction can occur in unconscious persons. Common causes are aspiration of vomitus and the tongue falling back into the airway. These can occur during cardiac arrest.

Foreign bodies can cause partial or complete airway obstruction. With *partial obstruction*, the person moves some air into and out of the lungs. The person is conscious. Forceful coughing often removes the object. The EMS system is activated if the partial obstruction is not relieved.

With *complete airway obstruction*, the person clutches at the throat (Fig. 36-18). The person cannot breathe, speak, or cough. The person is pale and cyanotic. Air does not move into and out of the lungs. If conscious, the person is very apprehensive. The obstruction must be removed immediately before cardiac arrest occurs. Obstructed airway is an emergency. The EMS system must be activated.

The *Heimlich maneuver* is used to relieve an obstructed airway caused by a foreign body. It involves abdominal thrusts. The maneuver is performed with the person standing, sitting, or lying down. The *finger sweep* is used with the Heimlich maneuver when an adult becomes unconscious.

The Heimlich maneuver is not effective in extremely obese persons and in pregnant women. Chest thrusts are used for them (Box 36-2).

Fig. 36-18 A choking person will usually clutch the throat.

Box 36-2	Obstructed Airway: Chest Thrusts for Obese or Pregnant Persons

THE VICTIM IS SITTING OR STANDING
1 Stand behind the victim.
2 Place your arms under the victim's underarms. Wrap your arms around the victim's chest.
3 Make a fist. Place the thumb side of the fist on the middle of the sternum (breastbone).
4 Grasp the fist with your other hand.
5 Give backward chest thrusts until the object is expelled or the victim becomes unconscious.

THE VICTIM IS LYING DOWN OR UNCONSCIOUS
1 Position the victim supine.
2 Kneel next to the victim's body.
3 Position your hands as for external chest compression.
4 Give chest thrusts until the object is expelled or the victim becomes unconscious.

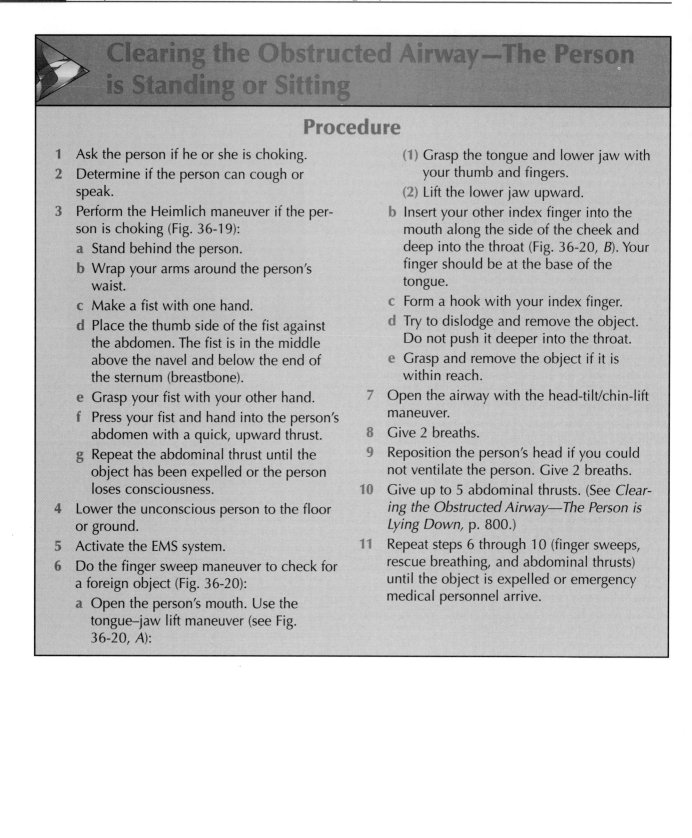

Clearing the Obstructed Airway—The Person is Standing or Sitting

Procedure

1 Ask the person if he or she is choking.

2 Determine if the person can cough or speak.

3 Perform the Heimlich maneuver if the person is choking (Fig. 36-19):

  a Stand behind the person.

  b Wrap your arms around the person's waist.

  c Make a fist with one hand.

  d Place the thumb side of the fist against the abdomen. The fist is in the middle above the navel and below the end of the sternum (breastbone).

  e Grasp your fist with your other hand.

  f Press your fist and hand into the person's abdomen with a quick, upward thrust.

  g Repeat the abdominal thrust until the object has been expelled or the person loses consciousness.

4 Lower the unconscious person to the floor or ground.

5 Activate the EMS system.

6 Do the finger sweep maneuver to check for a foreign object (Fig. 36-20):

  a Open the person's mouth. Use the tongue–jaw lift maneuver (see Fig. 36-20, A):

    (1) Grasp the tongue and lower jaw with your thumb and fingers.

    (2) Lift the lower jaw upward.

  b Insert your other index finger into the mouth along the side of the cheek and deep into the throat (Fig. 36-20, B). Your finger should be at the base of the tongue.

  c Form a hook with your index finger.

  d Try to dislodge and remove the object. Do not push it deeper into the throat.

  e Grasp and remove the object if it is within reach.

7 Open the airway with the head-tilt/chin-lift maneuver.

8 Give 2 breaths.

9 Reposition the person's head if you could not ventilate the person. Give 2 breaths.

10 Give up to 5 abdominal thrusts. (See *Clearing the Obstructed Airway—The Person is Lying Down,* p. 800.)

11 Repeat steps 6 through 10 (finger sweeps, rescue breathing, and abdominal thrusts) until the object is expelled or emergency medical personnel arrive.

Fig. 36-19 Abdominal thrusts with the person standing.

Fig. 36-20 Tongue–jaw lift maneuver. **A,** The person's tongue is grasped, and the jaw is lifted forward with one hand. **B,** The index finger of the other hand is used to check for a foreign object.

Clearing the Obstructed Airway—The Person is Lying Down

Procedure

1 Ask the person if he or she is choking.
2 Determine if the person can cough or speak.
3 Perform the Heimlich maneuver if the person is choking (Fig. 36-21):
   a Position the person supine.
   b Kneel next to the person's thighs.
   c Place the heel of one hand against the abdomen. It should be in the middle above the navel and below the end of the sternum (breastbone).
   d Place your second hand on top of your first.
   e Press your fist and hand into the abdomen with a quick, upward thrust.
   f Repeat abdominal thrusts until the object has been expelled or the person loses consciousness.

4 Activate the EMS system if the person becomes unconscious.
5 Do the finger sweep maneuver to check for a foreign object. See step 6 in *Clearing the Obstructed Airway—The Person Is Standing or Sitting*, p. 798.
6 Open the airway with the head-tilt/chin-lift maneuver.
7 Give 2 breaths.
8 Reposition the person's head if you could not ventilate the person. Give 2 breaths.
9 Give up to 5 abdominal thrusts.
10 Repeat steps 5 through 10 (finger sweeps, rescue breathing, abdominal thrusts) until the object is expelled or emergency medical personnel arrive.

Fig. 36-21 Abdominal thrusts with the victim lying down.

▶ **Finding an Unconscious Adult.** You may find an adult unconscious. You did not see the person lose consciousness, and you do not know the cause. You cannot assume the cause is choking. Therefore you need to establish unresponsiveness and attempt rescue breathing. Abdominal thrusts are done if you cannot ventilate the person. Then the finger sweep maneuver is used.

Clearing the Obstructed Airway— The Unconscious Adult

Procedure

1 Check for unresponsiveness.

2 Call for help. Have someone activate the EMS system.

3 Logroll the person to the supine position with his or her face up. The person's arms should be at the sides.

4 Open the airway. Use the head-tilt/chin-lift maneuver.

5 Give 2 breaths. Reposition the person's head and open the airway if you could not ventilate. Give 2 breaths.

6 Do the Heimlich maneuver if you could not ventilate the person. See *Clearing the Obstructed Airway—The Person Is Lying Down,* p. 800.

7 Do the finger sweep maneuver to check for a foreign object. See step 6 in *Clearing the Obstructed Airway—The Person Is Standing or Sitting,* p. 798.

8 Repeat steps 4 through 7 until the object is expelled or emergency personnel arrive.

▶ OBSTRUCTED AIRWAY IN CHILDREN

Children have choked on small objects such as pieces of hot dogs, marbles, hard candy, peanuts, and grapes. Peanut butter and popcorn also can cause choking. So can coins and small toys and toy parts.

As with the adult, airway obstruction may be partial or complete. If the child has a strong cough, encourage the child to continue coughing. Try to relieve the obstruction if the cough weakens or when respiratory difficulty increases. Loss of consciousness is another reason to relieve the obstruction. Activate the EMS system if the child is in distress or loses consciousness.

As with adults, you may find a child or infant unconscious. You cannot assume the cause is choking on a foreign object.

Fig. 36-22 The Heimlich maneuver performed on an unconscious child.

▶ Clearing an Obstructed Airway— The Conscious Child (Under 8 Years of Age)

Procedure

1 Stand behind the child.

2 Wrap your arms under the child's underarms and around the chest.

3 Make a fist with one hand. Place the thumb side of the fist against the child's abdomen. The fist should be in the middle, above the navel and below the end of the sternum (breastbone).

4 Grab the fist with the other hand.

5 Give a quick inward and upward thrust.

6 Repeat the abdominal thrusts until the object is expelled or the child loses consciousness.

7 Lay the child down if he or she loses consciousness.

8 Call for help, and ask someone to activate the EMS system.

9 Use the tongue–jaw lift maneuver to lift the chin.

10 Look for a foreign object.

11 Remove the foreign object with the finger sweep maneuver *only if you can see the object.*

12 Open the airway. Use the head-tilt/chin-lift maneuver.

13 Give 2 breaths. Reposition the child's head if you could not ventilate the child. Give 2 more breaths.

14 Do the Heimlich maneuver if you could not ventilate the child (Fig. 36-22):

   a Kneel beside the child or straddle the hips if he or she is on the floor.

   b Place the heel of one hand against the child's abdomen. The hand is in the middle and slightly above the navel and below the end of the sternum (breastbone).

   c Place your other hand directly on top of your fist.

   d Give up to 5 quick, upward abdominal thrusts.

15 Repeat steps 9 through 14 for 1 minute. *Activate the EMS system after 1 minute if you are alone.*

16 Continue steps 9 through 14 until the object is expelled or emergency personnel arrive.

Clearing an Obstructed Airway— The Unconscious Child (Under 8 Years of Age)

Procedure

1 Establish unresponsiveness.

2 Ask someone to activate the EMS system.

3 Open the airway. Use the head-tilt/chin-lift maneuver.

4 Give 2 breaths. Reposition the child's head if you could not ventilate the child. Give 2 more breaths.

5 Give up to 5 abdominal thrusts (see Fig. 36-22).

6 Use the tongue–jaw lift maneuver to lift the chin.

7 Look for a foreign object.

8 Remove the foreign object with the finger sweep maneuver *only if you can see the object.*

9 Repeat steps 3 through 8 for 1 minute. *Activate the EMS system after 1 minute if you are alone.*

10 Continue steps 3 through 8 until the object is expelled or emergency personnel arrive.

Clearing an Obstructed Airway— The Conscious Infant

Procedure

1 Determine if the infant has an airway obstruction.

2 Hold the infant face down over your forearm. Support your arm on your thigh. The infant's head should be lower than the trunk. Hold the infant's jaw to support the head.

3 Give up to 5 back blows with the heel of one hand. Give the blows between the infant's shoulder blades (Fig. 36-23, p. 804).

4 Turn the infant. Support the infant's head, neck, jaw, and chest with one hand. Support the back with your other hand.

5 Place the infant over your thigh. The baby's head is lower than the trunk.

6 Give chest thrusts (Fig. 36-24, p. 804):

   a Locate hand position as for chest compressions.

   b Give up to 5 downward chest thrusts (chest compressions).

7 Repeat steps 2 through 6 until the object is expelled or the child loses consciousness.

8 Call out for help if the child loses consciousness. Ask someone to activate the EMS system.

9 Use the tongue–jaw lift maneuver to lift the chin.

10 Look for a foreign object. Remove the foreign object with the finger sweep maneuver *only if you see the object.*

11 Open the airway. Use the head-tilt/chin-lift maneuver.

12 Give 2 breaths.

13 Reposition the head if you could not ventilate. Give 2 breaths.

14 Repeat up to 5 back blows and up to 5 chest thrusts.

15 Use the tongue–jaw lift maneuver to lift the chin. Look for a foreign object. Remove the object with the finger sweep maneuver *only if you see the object.*

16 Repeat steps 11 through 15 for 1 minute. Activate the EMS system.

17 Continue steps 11 through 15 until the object is expelled or emergency personnel arrive.

18 Check for breathing and a pulse when the object is expelled.

19 Do the following if the infant has a pulse after the object is expelled:

   a Keep the airway open.

   b Give 20 breaths per minute if the infant is not breathing.

20 Start CPR if the infant has no pulse.

Fig. 36-23 The infant is held face down and supported with one hand. The rescuer supports her arm on her thigh. Back blows are given with the heel of one hand. The blows are given between the infant's shoulder blades.

Fig. 36-24 The infant is positioned on the rescuer's thigh for chest thrusts. Hand position for chest thrusts in the infant is the same as for chest compressions.

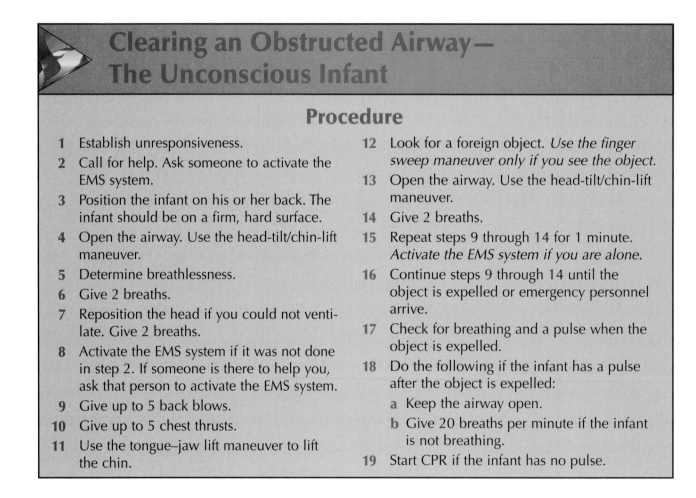

Clearing an Obstructed Airway— The Unconscious Infant

Procedure

1 Establish unresponsiveness.

2 Call for help. Ask someone to activate the EMS system.

3 Position the infant on his or her back. The infant should be on a firm, hard surface.

4 Open the airway. Use the head-tilt/chin-lift maneuver.

5 Determine breathlessness.

6 Give 2 breaths.

7 Reposition the head if you could not ventilate. Give 2 breaths.

8 Activate the EMS system if it was not done in step 2. If someone is there to help you, ask that person to activate the EMS system.

9 Give up to 5 back blows.

10 Give up to 5 chest thrusts.

11 Use the tongue–jaw lift maneuver to lift the chin.

12 Look for a foreign object. *Use the finger sweep maneuver only if you see the object.*

13 Open the airway. Use the head-tilt/chin-lift maneuver.

14 Give 2 breaths.

15 Repeat steps 9 through 14 for 1 minute. *Activate the EMS system if you are alone.*

16 Continue steps 9 through 14 until the object is expelled or emergency personnel arrive.

17 Check for breathing and a pulse when the object is expelled.

18 Do the following if the infant has a pulse after the object is expelled:

a Keep the airway open.

b Give 20 breaths per minute if the infant is not breathing.

19 Start CPR if the infant has no pulse.

Fig. 36-25 Recovery position.

RECOVERY POSITION

The recovery position is a side-lying position (Fig. 36-25). It is used when the person is breathing and has a pulse. Logroll the person into the recovery position, keeping the head, neck, and spine straight. Then keep the person in good alignment. An arm supports the head. This position keeps the airway open and prevents aspiration. *Do not use this position if the person might have neck injuries or other trauma.*

SELF-ADMINISTERED HEIMLICH MANEUVER

You yourself may choke. You can perform the Heimlich maneuver to relieve the obstructed airway. To do so:

- Make a fist with one hand.
- Place the thumb side of the fist above your navel and below the lower end of the sternum.
- Grasp your fist with your other hand.
- Press inward and upward quickly.
- Press the upper abdomen against a hard surface if the thrust did not relieve the obstruction. Use the back of a chair, a table, or a railing.
- Use as many thrusts as needed.

HEMORRHAGE

Life and body functions require an adequate blood supply. Blood must circulate through the body. If a blood vessel is torn or cut, bleeding occurs. The larger the blood vessel, the greater the bleeding and blood loss. **Hemorrhage** is the excessive loss of blood in a short period of time. If the bleeding is not stopped, death results.

Hemorrhage may be internal or external. You cannot see internal hemorrhage. Bleeding occurs inside the body into tissues and body cavities. Pain, shock, vomiting blood, coughing up blood, and loss of consciousness are signs of internal hemorrhage. There is little you can do for internal bleeding. Activate the EMS system. Then keep the person warm, flat, and quiet until medical help arrives. Do not give fluids. Follow Standard Precautions and the Bloodborne Pathogen Standard in case the person vomits or coughs up blood.

External bleeding is usually seen. However, it may be hidden by clothing. Hemorrhage may be from an injured artery or vein. Bleeding from an artery is bright red and occurs in spurts. There is a steady flow of blood from a vein. External bleeding must be stopped. You can do the following to control external hemorrhage:

- Activate the EMS system.
- Practice Standard Precautions, and follow the Bloodborne Pathogen Standard. Wear gloves if possible.
- Place a sterile dressing directly over the wound. Use any clean material (handkerchief, towel, cloth, or sanitary napkin) if you do not have a sterile dressing.
- Apply pressure with your hand directly over the bleeding site (Fig. 36-26, p. 806). Do not release the pressure until the bleeding is controlled.
- If direct pressure does not control bleeding, apply pressure over the artery above the bleeding site (Fig. 36-27, p. 806). For example, if bleeding is from the lower arm, apply pressure over the brachial artery. The brachial artery supplies blood to the lower arm. Use your first three fingers to apply pressure on the artery.

Fig. 36-26 Direct pressure is applied to the wound to stop bleeding. The hand is placed over the wound.

Fig. 36-27 Pressure points to control bleeding.

SHOCK

Shock results when there is not enough blood supply to organs and tissues. Blood loss, heart attack (myocardial infarction), burns, and severe infection can cause shock. Signs and symptoms include:

- Low or falling blood pressure
- Rapid and weak pulse
- Rapid respirations
- Cold, moist, and pale skin
- Thirst
- Restlessness
- Confusion and loss of consciousness as shock worsens

Shock is possible in any person who is acutely ill or injured. Do the following to prevent and treat shock:

- Keep the person lying down.
- Maintain an open airway.
- Control hemorrhage.
- Keep the person warm. Place a blanket over and under the person if possible.
- Reassure the person.
- Activate the EMS system.
- Follow Standard Precautions and the Bloodborne Pathogen Standard.

ANAPHYLACTIC SHOCK

Some people are allergic or sensitive to various substances such as foods, insects, chemicals, and drugs. Many people are allergic to penicillin. An antigen is a substance that the body reacts to. The body fights or attacks the antigen by releasing chemicals. The reaction may be a local area of redness, swelling, or itching. Or the reaction can involve the entire body.

Anaphylaxis is life-threatening sensitivity to an antigen. It comes from the Greek words that mean without *(ana)* protection *(phylaxis)*. In severe cases, anaphylactic shock can occur within seconds. Signs and symptoms include:

- Sweating
- Shortness of breath
- Low blood pressure
- Irregular pulse
- Respiratory congestion
- Swelling of the larynx (laryngeal edema)
- Hoarseness
- Dyspnea

Anaphylactic shock is an emergency. The EMS system must be activated. The person needs special drugs to reverse the allergic reaction. Until emergency help arrives, keep the person lying down. Also keep the airway open. CPR is necessary if cardiac arrest occurs.

> **Focus On... CHILDREN**
>
> Generalized absence (petit mal) seizures are more common in children than in the other age-groups. They usually disappear by adolescence.

SEIZURES

Seizures (convulsions) are violent and sudden contractions of muscles. The muscle contractions are involuntary. Seizures are caused by an abnormality in the brain. Causes include head injury during birth or from trauma, high fever, brain tumors, poisoning, seizure disorders, and central nervous system infections. Lack of blood flow to the brain also can cause seizures.

The major types of seizures are *partial seizures* and *generalized seizures.* Only a part of the brain is involved with a partial seizure. A body part may jerk. Or the person has hearing or vision problems or stomach discomfort. The person does not lose consciousness.

With generalized seizures, the whole brain is involved. The *generalized tonic-clonic seizure (grand mal seizure)* has two phases. The tonic phase is first. The person loses consciousness. If standing or sitting, the person falls to the floor. The body is rigid because all muscles contract at once. The clonic phase is next. Muscle groups contract and relax. This causes jerking and twitching movements of the body. Urinary and fecal incontinence may occur. After the seizure, the person usually falls into a deep sleep. The person may have confusion and headache on awakening.

The *generalized absence (petit mal) seizure* usually lasts a few seconds. There is loss of consciousness, twitching of the eyelids, and staring. No first aid is necessary. *(See Focus on Children box above.)*

You cannot stop a seizure. However, you can protect the person from injury during a seizure. The following measures are performed for a generalized tonic-clonic seizure:

- Call for help.
- Lower the person to the floor. This protects the person from falling.
- Place a folded blanket, towel, cushion, pillow, or other soft item under the person's head (Fig. 36-28, p. 808). Cradle the person's head in your lap if a soft item is not available. This prevents the person's head from striking the hard surface of the floor.
- Turn the person onto his or her side. Make sure the head is turned to the side.

Fig. 36-28 Protect the head during a seizure.

Fig. 36-29 Full-thickness burn from flames. (Courtesy St. Johns Mercy Hospital, St Louis.)

- Loosen tight clothing around the person's neck. This includes ties, scarves, or collars. Also loosen tight neck jewelry.
- Move furniture, equipment, and sharp objects away from the person. The person may strike these objects during the uncontrolled body movements.
- Do not try to restrain body movements during the seizure.
- Summon medical help. Do not leave the person during the seizure.
- Do not put your fingers between the person's teeth. The person can bite down on your fingers during the seizure.

BURNS

Burns can severely disable a person (Fig. 36-29). They can also cause death. Most burn injuries occur in the home. Common causes of burns and fires are:

- Scalds from hot liquids
- Playing with matches and lighters
- Electrical injuries (Fig. 36-30)
- Cooking accidents (barbecues, microwaves, stoves, ovens)
- Falling asleep while smoking
- Fireplaces
- Space heaters
- No smoke detectors or nonfunctioning smoke detectors
- Sunburn
- Chemicals

The skin has two layers: the dermis and the epidermis. Burns are described as partial thickness or full thickness. *Partial-thickness burns* involve the dermis and part of the epidermis. These burns are very painful. Nerve endings are exposed. *Full-thickness burns* involve the dermis and the entire epidermis.

Fig. 36-30 An electrical burn. **A,** The electrical current enters through the hand. **B,** The electrical current exits through the foot. *(From Sanders M: Mosby's paramedic textbook, St Louis, 1994, Mosby.)*

The fat layer, muscle, and bone may be injured or destroyed. Full-thickness burns are not painful. Nerve endings are destroyed.

Burns vary in seriousness. Burn size and depth, the body part involved, and the person's age affect the severity of the burn. Burns to the face, eyes, ears, hands, and feet are more serious than burns to an arm or leg.

Activate the EMS system as soon as possible. Emergency care of burns includes the following:

- Do not touch the person if he or she is in contact with an electrical source. Have the power source turned off or remove the electrical source first. Use an object that does not conduct electricity (rope or wood) to remove the electrical source.
- Remove the person from the fire or burn source.
- Stop the burning process. Extinguish flames with water, or roll the person in a blanket. Or use a coat, sheet, or towel.
- Remove hot clothing that is not sticking to the skin. Also remove jewelry and any tight clothing. If you cannot remove hot clothing, cool the clothing with water.
- Provide basic life support as needed. This includes activating the EMS system.
- Cover the burn wounds with a clean, moist covering. You can use towels, sheets, or any other clean cloth. Keep the covering wet.
- Do not put oil, butter, salve, or ointments on the burns.
- Cover the person with a blanket or coat to prevent heat loss.

(See Focus on Children box and Focus on Older Persons box.)

FAINTING

Fainting is the sudden loss of consciousness from an inadequate blood supply to the brain. Hunger, fatigue, fear, and pain are common causes. Some people faint at the sight of blood or injury. Standing in one position for a long time or being in a warm, crowded room can lead to fainting. Dizziness, perspiration, and blackness before the eyes are warning signals. The

Fig. 36-31 The person bends forward and places the head between the knees to prevent fainting.

person looks pale. The pulse is weak. Respirations are shallow if consciousness is lost. Emergency care for fainting includes the following:

- Have the person sit or lie down before fainting occurs.
- If sitting, the person bends forward and places his or her head between the knees (Fig. 36-31).
- If the person is lying down, elevate the legs.
- Loosen tight clothing.
- Keep the person lying down if fainting has occurred.
- Do not let the person get up until symptoms have subsided for about 5 minutes.
- Help the person to a sitting position after recovery from fainting. Observe for symptoms of fainting.

STROKE

Stroke (cerebrovascular accident, brain attack) is described in Chapter 30. A stroke occurs when the brain is suddenly deprived of its blood supply. Usually only part of the brain is affected. A stroke may be caused by a thrombus, an embolus, or cerebral hemorrhage. Cerebral hemorrhage is caused by the rupture of a blood vessel in the brain.

The signs of stroke vary. They depend on the size and location of brain injury. Loss of consciousness or semiconsciousness, rapid pulse, labored respirations, elevated blood pressure, vomiting, and hemiplegia are signs of stroke. The person may have aphasia (the inability to speak). Seizures may occur.

Emergency care includes the following:

- Turn the person onto the affected side. The affected side is limp, and the cheek appears puffy.
- Elevate the head without flexing the neck.
- Loosen tight clothing.
- Keep the person quiet and warm.
- Reassure the person.
- Activate the EMS system.

Focus On... CHILDREN

Infants and children are at risk for burns. Severe burns can be fatal. Remember, infants and young children do not know the difference between safety and danger. They cannot protect themselves. They rely on adults for protection.

Focus On... OLDER PERSONS

Older persons are at risk for burns. Severe burns can be fatal. Spilling hot liquids is a common cause of burns in older persons. Weakness and poor coordination put some older persons at risk. They need to be careful when handling hot liquids and when cooking.

QUALITY OF LIFE

Quality of life must be protected during emergencies. The victim is a person. He or she must be treated with dignity and respect.

The right to privacy and confidentiality are protected. Do not expose the person unnecessarily. You may be in a place where you cannot close doors, shades, and curtains. The victim may be in a lounge, dining area, or public place. Do what you can to protect the person's privacy.

Onlookers are major threats to privacy and confidentiality. If you are giving emergency care, your main concern is the person's illness or injuries. It is hard to give care and manage onlookers at the same time. Ask someone else to deal with the onlookers. If another person is giving care, you can help by keeping onlookers away from the victim.

People are naturally curious. They want to know what happened, the extent of injuries or illness, and if the person will be okay. You must be careful not to discuss the situation. Information about the person's care, treatment, and condition is confidential. Also, only doctors can make diagnoses. You can make observations about signs and symptoms. Only the doctor can determine what is wrong with the person.

The right to personal choice must be protected. It is often hard to give choices in emergencies. They are given when possible. Hospital care may be required. The person has the right to choose which hospital to be taken to.

Personal possessions are protected from loss and damage. Dentures and eyeglasses often are lost or broken in emergencies. Watches and other jewelry are easily lost. Clothing may be torn or cut. You must be very careful to protect the person's property. In public places, personal items are given to family members, police, or EMS personnel.

Physical and psychological safety are important. The person is protected from further injury. For example, a person is protected from falls after a stroke. The person having a seizure is protected from head injuries. The person needs to feel safe and secure. Reassurance, explanations about care, and a calm approach are important. They help the person feel safe and secure.

Circle the BEST answer.

1. The goals of first aid are to
   A. Call for help and keep the person warm
   B. Prevent death and prevent injuries from becoming worse
   C. Stay calm and perform emergency measures
   D. Reassure the person and keep bystanders away

2. When giving first aid, you should
   A. Be aware of your own limits
   B. Move the person
   C. Give the person fluids
   D. Perform any necessary emergency measures

3. The person is in cardiac arrest. Cardiac arrest is
   A. The same as stroke
   B. The sudden stopping of heart action and breathing
   C. The sudden loss of consciousness
   D. The condition that results when organs and tissues do not get enough blood

4. Which is *not* a sign of cardiac arrest?
   A. No pulse
   B. No breathing
   C. A sudden drop in blood pressure
   D. Unconsciousness

5. You are going to give rescue breathing. You should do the following *except*
   A. Pinch the person's nostrils shut
   B. Place your mouth tightly over the person's mouth
   C. Blow air into the person's mouth as you exhale
   D. Cover the person's nose with your mouth

6. External chest compressions are performed on an adult. The chest is compressed
   A. $^1/_2$ to 1 inch with the index and middle fingers
   B. 1 to $1^1/_2$ inches with the heel of one hand
   C. $1^1/_2$ to 2 inches with two hands
   D. With one hand in the middle of the sternum

7. Which does *not* determine breathlessness?
   A. Looking to see if the chest rises and falls
   B. Counting respirations for 30 seconds
   C. Listening for the escape of air
   D. Feeling for the flow of air

8. Which is used to feel for a pulse during adult CPR?
   A. The apical pulse
   B. The brachial pulse
   C. The carotid pulse
   D. The dorsalis pedis pulse

9. How many breaths are given at the beginning of CPR?
   A. 1
   B. 2
   C. 3
   D. 4

10. You are performing adult CPR alone. Which is *false*?
    A. Give 2 breaths after every 15 compressions
    B. Check for a pulse after 1 minute
    C. Give 1 breath after every fifth compression
    D. Count out loud

11. Adult CPR is being given by 2 people. Breaths are given
    A. After every fifth compression
    B. After every fifteenth compression
    C. After every compression
    D. Only when the positions are changed

12. External cardiac compressions are given to an infant at a rate of
    A. 60 per minute
    B. 75 per minute
    C. 80 per minute
    D. 100 per minute

13. The most common cause of obstructed airway in adults is
    A. A loose denture
    B. Meat
    C. Marbles
    D. Candy

14. If airway obstruction occurs, the person usually
    A. Clutches at the throat
    B. Can speak, cough, and breathe
    C. Is calm
    D. Has a seizure

15. The Heimlich maneuver is used to relieve an obstructed airway. Which is *false?*
    A. The person can be standing, sitting, or lying down.
    B. A fist is made with one hand.
    C. The thrusts are given inward and upward at the lower end of the sternum.
    D. The hands are positioned in the middle between the waist and lower end of the sternum.

16. An adult has an obstructed airway. Poking motions are used with the finger sweep maneuver.
    A. True
    B. False

17. Arterial bleeding is suspected. Arterial bleeding
    A. Cannot be seen
    B. Occurs in spurts
    C. Is dark red
    D. Oozes from the wound

18. A person is hemorrhaging from the left forearm. The first action is to
    A. Lower the body part
    B. Apply pressure to the brachial artery
    C. Apply direct pressure to the wound
    D. Cover the person

19. A person is in shock. The signs of shock are
    A. Rising blood pressure, rapid pulse, and slow respirations
    B. Rapid pulse, rapid respirations, and warm skin
    C. Falling blood pressure; rapid pulse and respirations; and skin that is cold, moist, and pale
    D. Falling blood pressure; slow pulse and respirations; thirst; restlessness; and warm, flushed skin

20. A person in shock needs
    A. Mouth-to-mouth resuscitation
    B. To be kept lying down
    C. Clothes removed
    D. To be placed in Trendelenburg's position

21. These statements relate to generalized tonic-clonic seizures. Which is *false?*
    A. There is contraction of all muscles at once.
    B. Lowering the person to the floor stops the seizure.
    C. The person's head is protected during the seizure.
    D. There is loss of consciousness during the seizure.

22. A person was burned. There are no complaints or signs of pain. You know that
    A. The burn is minor
    B. The burn is partial thickness
    C. The burn is full thickness
    D. The dermis was destroyed

23. Burns are covered with
    A. A clean, moist cloth or dressing
    B. Butter, oil, or salve
    C. Water
    D. Nothing

24. A person is about to faint. Which is *false?*
    A. Take the person outside for some fresh air.
    B. Have the person sit or lie down.
    C. Loosen tight clothing.
    D. Elevate the legs if the person is lying down.

25. Emergency care of the person having a stroke includes the following *except*
    A. Positioning the person on the affected side
    B. Giving the person sips of water
    C. Loosening tight clothing
    D. Keeping the person quiet and warm

Answers to these questions are on p. 839.

THE DYING PERSON

Define the key terms listed in this chapter

Describe terminal illness

Identify the psychological forces that influence living and dying

Explain how culture and religion influence attitudes about death

Describe how different age-groups view death

Describe the five stages of dying

Explain how to meet the dying person's psychological, social, and spiritual needs

Explain how you can help meet the physical needs of the dying person

Describe the needs of the family during the dying process

Describe hospice care

Explain the importance of the Patient Self-Determination Act

Explain what is meant by a *do not resuscitate* order

Explain how to promote quality of life for the dying person

Identify the signs of approaching death and the signs of death

Perform the procedure described in this chapter

KEY TERMS

advance directive A written document stating a person's wishes about health care when that person can no longer make his or her own decisions

postmortem After *(post)* death *(mortem)*

reincarnation The belief that the spirit or soul is reborn in another human body or in another form of life

rigor mortis The stiffness or rigidity *(rigor)* of skeletal muscles that occurs after death *(mortis)*

terminal illness An illness or injury for which there is no reasonable expectation of recovery

Dying people are cared for in hospitals or nursing centers or at home. Many are in hospice programs (see Chapter 1). Death can occur suddenly and without warning. Often it is expected.

Health team members see death often. Many are unsure of their feelings about death. They are uncomfortable with dying persons and the subject of death. Dying persons represent helplessness and failure to cure. They also remind us of our own eventual death or the death of loved ones.

You must examine your feelings about death. Your attitudes about death and dying affect the care you give. You will help meet the dying person's physical, psychological, social, and spiritual needs. Therefore you need to understand the dying process. Then you can approach the dying person with care, kindness, and respect.

TERMINAL ILLNESS

Many illnesses and diseases can be cured or controlled. Others have no cure. Many injuries can be repaired. Others are so serious that the body cannot function. Recovery is not expected. The disease or injury ends in death. An illness or injury for which there is no reasonable expectation of recovery is a **terminal illness.**

Doctors cannot predict the exact time of death. A person may have days, months, weeks, or years to live. Predictions can be wrong. People expected to live for only a short time have lived for years. Others were expected to live for a longer time. They died sooner than expected.

Modern medicine has found cures or has prolonged life in many cases. Future research will bring new cures. However, two very powerful psychological forces influence living and dying. They are hope and the will to live. People have died sooner than expected or for no apparent reason when they have lost hope or the will to live.

ATTITUDES ABOUT DEATH

Experiences, culture, religion, and age influence a person's attitude about death. Many people fear death. Others do not believe they will die. Some look forward to and accept death. Attitudes and beliefs about death often change as a person grows older. They are also affected by changing circumstances.

Dying people are usually cared for in health agencies or at home. The family is often involved in the person's care. Family members usually gather at the bedside to comfort the person and to say their last farewells. The family also comforts each other. When death occurs, the funeral director is called to take the body to the funeral home. There the body is prepared for funeral practices.

Many adults and children never have had contact with a dying person. Nor were they present when death occurred. Some have not attended a visitation (wake) or funeral. They have not seen the process of dying and death. Therefore it is frightening, morbid, and a mystery.

CULTURE AND RELIGION

American practices and attitudes are different from those of other cultures *(See Caring About Culture [Death Rites] box.)* In some cultures, dying people are cared for at home by the family. Some families care for the body after death and prepare it for burial.

Attitudes about death are closely related to culture and religion. Some believe that life after death is free of suffering and hardship. They also believe in future reunion with family and loved ones. Many believe there is punishment and suffering in the afterlife for sins and misdeeds. Others do not believe in the afterlife. They believe death is the end of life. There are also religious beliefs about the form of the human body after death. Some believe the body keeps its physical form. Others believe that only the spirit or soul is present in the afterlife. **Reincarnation** is the belief that the spirit or soul is reborn in another human body or in another form of life. Many people strengthen their religious beliefs when dying. Religion also provides comfort for the dying person and the family.

Many religions have rites and rituals that are practiced during the dying process and at the time of

Caring About Culture

DEATH RITES

In Vietnam, quality of life is more important than length of life because of beliefs in reincarnation. There is also the expectation of less suffering in the next life. Therefore the dying are helped to recall their past good deeds and to achieve a fitting mental state. Death at home is preferred over death in the hospital. Upon death, the body is washed and wrapped in clean white sheets. In some areas a coin or jewels (a wealthier family) and rice (a poorer family) are put in the dead person's mouth. This is from the belief that they will help the soul go through the encounters with gods and devils and the soul will be born rich in the next life. Relatives sew small pillows to place under the neck, feet, and wrists of the body. The body is placed in a coffin, and burial is in the ground.

The Chinese have an aversion to death and to anything concerning death. Autopsy and disposal of the body are individual preferences and are not prescribed by religion. Euthanasia is allowed. Donation of body parts is encouraged. The eldest son is responsible for all arrangements for the deceased. The deceased is initially buried in a coffin. After 7 years the body is exhumed and cremated. The urn is reburied in the tomb. White clothing is worn for mourning.

In India, Hindu persons may make indirect references to their own deaths, often accepting God's will. The person's desire to be clearheaded as death approaches must be assessed in planning medical treatment. Providing a time and place for prayer is essential for the family and the person. Prayer helps them deal with anxiety and conflict. The Hindu priest or anyone present may read from the Holy Sanskrit books. Some priests tie strings (signifying a blessing) around the neck or wrist. After death the priest pours water into the mouth of the deceased. Families may prefer that only Hindus touch the body and may wash the body themselves. Blood transfusions, organ transplants, and autopsies are allowed. Cremation is preferred. Reincarnation is a Hindu belief.

Modified from Geissler EM: *Pocket guide to cultural assessment*, ed 2, St Louis, 1998, Mosby.

death. Prayers, blessings, and scripture readings are common in many religions.

BELIEFS ABOUT DEATH

Adults fear pain and suffering, dying alone, and the invasion of privacy. They also fear loneliness and separation from family and loved ones. They worry about who will care for and support those left behind. Adults often resent death. This is particularly true when it interferes with plans, hopes, dreams, and ambitions. *(See Focus on Children and Focus on Older Persons boxes on p. 816.)*

Ideas about death change as people grow older. Infants and toddlers have no concept of death. Children between the ages of 3 and 5 start to be curious and have ideas about death. They recognize the death of family members or pets and notice dead birds or bugs. They think death is temporary. Children often blame themselves when someone or something dies. They see the death as punishment for being bad. When children ask questions about death, adults often give answers that cause fear and confusion. Children who are told, "He is sleeping," may be afraid to go to sleep.

Children between the ages of 5 and 7 years know death is final. They do not think that they will die. Death happens to other people. They also think death can be avoided. Children associate death with punishment and body mutilation. It is also associated with witches, ghosts, goblins, and monsters. These ideas come from fairy tales, cartoons, movies, video games, and television.

Older persons usually have fewer fears than younger adults. They accept that death will occur. They have had more experiences with dying and death. Many have lost family members and friends. Some welcome death as freedom from pain, suffering, and disability. Death also means reunion with those who have died first. Like younger adults, older persons often fear dying alone.

THE STAGES OF DYING

Dr. Elisabeth Kübler-Ross described five stages of dying. They are denial, anger, bargaining, depression, and acceptance:

- *Denial* is the first stage. Persons refuse to believe they are dying. "No, not me" is a common response. The person believes a mistake was made. Information about the illness or injury is not heard. The person cannot deal with any problem or decision about the illness or injury. This stage can last for a few hours, days, or much longer. Some people are still in denial when they die.
- *Anger* is the second stage of dying. The person thinks "Why me?" People in this stage feel anger and rage. They envy and resent those who have life and health. Family, friends, and the health team are usually targets of anger. They blame others. Fault is found with those who are loved and needed the most. The health team and family may have a hard time dealing with persons during this stage. Remember that anger is a normal, healthy reaction. Do not take the person's anger personally. You must control any urge to attack back or avoid the person.
- *Bargaining* is the third stage. Anger has passed. The person now says, "Yes, me, but. . . . " Often there is bargaining with God for more time. Promises are made in exchange for more time. The person may want to see a child marry, see a grandchild, have one more Christmas, or live for an important event. Usually more promises are made as the person makes "just one more" request. This stage may not be obvious to you. Bargaining is usually done privately and on a spiritual level.
- *Depression* is the fourth stage. The person thinks "Yes, me" and is very sad. There is mourning over things that were lost and the future loss of life. The person may cry or say little. Sometimes the person talks about people and things that will be left behind.
- *Acceptance* of death is the fifth and final stage of dying. The person is calm and at peace. The person has said what needs to be said. Unfinished business is completed. The person is ready to accept death. A person may be in this stage for many months or years. Reaching the acceptance stage does not mean death is near.

Dying persons do not always pass through all five stages. A person may never get beyond a certain stage. Some people move back and forth between stages. For example, a person who has reached acceptance may move back to bargaining. Then the person may move forward to acceptance. Some people are in one stage until death.

PSYCHOLOGICAL, SOCIAL, AND SPIRITUAL NEEDS

Dying people continue to have psychological, social, and spiritual needs. They may want family and friends present. They may want to talk about the fears, worries, and anxieties of dying. Some want to be alone. Often they want to talk to a nursing team member. Persons often need to talk during the night. Things are quiet, distractions are few, and there is more time to think.

Listening and touch are two very important aspects of communication when dealing with the dying person:

- *Listening.* The dying person is the one who needs to talk, express feelings, and share worries and concerns. Just being there and listening helps to meet the person's psychological and social needs. Do not worry about saying the wrong thing. Nor should you worry about finding the right words to comfort and cheer the person. Nothing really must be said. Being there for the person is what counts.
- *Touch.* Touch can convey caring and concern when words cannot. Sometimes a person does not want to talk but needs you nearby. Do not feel that you need to talk. Silence, along with touch, is a powerful and meaningful way to communicate.

Spiritual needs are important. The person may wish to see a priest, rabbi, minister, or other cleric. The person may also want to take part in religious practices. Privacy is provided during prayer and spiritual moments. Courtesy is given to the clergy. The person is allowed to have religious objects nearby (medals, pictures, statues, or religious books and writings). You must handle these items like other valuables.

PHYSICAL NEEDS

Dying may take a few minutes, hours, days, or weeks. There is general slowing of body processes, weakness, and changes in levels of consciousness. The person is allowed to be as independent as possible. As the person weakens, the nursing team helps meet basic needs. The person may totally depend on others for basic needs and activities of daily living. Every effort is made to promote the person's physical and psychological comfort. The person is allowed to die in peace and with dignity.

VISION, HEARING, AND SPEECH

Vision blurs and gradually fails. The person naturally turns toward light. A darkened room may frighten the person. The eyes may be half open. Secretions often collect in the corners of the eyes. Because of failing vision, explain what you are doing to the person or in the room. The room should be well lit. However, avoid bright lights and glares. Good eye care is essential (see Chapter 14). If the eyes stay open, a nurse may apply a protective ointment. Then the eyes are covered with moistened pads to prevent injury.

Hearing is one of the last functions lost. Many people hear until the moment of death. Even if unconscious, the person may hear. Always assume that the dying person, or any unconscious person, can hear. Speak in a normal voice, and provide reassurance and explanations about care. Offer words of comfort. Avoid topics that could upset the person.

Speech becomes difficult. It may be hard to understand the person. Sometimes the person cannot speak. The nursing team needs to anticipate the person's needs. Do not ask questions that have long answers. Ask "yes" or "no" questions. These are kept to a minimum. Although speech may be hard or impossible, you must still talk to the person.

MOUTH, NOSE, AND SKIN

Oral hygiene is essential for comfort. Routine mouth care is given if the person can eat and drink. Frequent oral hygiene is given as death approaches and when taking oral fluids is difficult. Oral hygiene is also important if mucus collects in the mouth and the person cannot swallow.

Crusting and irritation of the nostrils can occur. Common causes are increased nasal secretions, an oxygen cannula, or an NG tube. The nose is carefully cleaned. The nurse may have you apply a lubricant to the nostrils.

Circulation fails and body temperature rises as death approaches. Though body temperature rises, the skin is cool, pale, and mottled (blotchy). Perspiration increases. Good skin care, bathing, and the prevention of pressure ulcers are necessary. Linens and gowns are changed whenever needed because of perspiration. Although the skin feels cool, only light bed coverings are needed. Blankets may make the person feel warm and cause restlessness.

ELIMINATION

Dying persons may have urinary and fecal incontinence. Bed protectors or incontinent briefs are used. Perineal care is given as necessary. Some persons are constipated and have urinary retention. Doctors may order enemas and Foley catheters.

COMFORT AND POSITIONING

Measures are taken to promote comfort. Good skin care, personal hygiene, back massages, and oral hygiene help to increase comfort. Some persons have severe pain. The nurse gives pain medications ordered by the doctor. Frequent position changes promote comfort. So does good body alignment using supportive devices. Care is taken when turning the person. You may need help to turn the person slowly and gently. Persons with breathing difficulties usually prefer semi-Fowler's position.

THE PERSON'S ROOM

The person's room should be as pleasant as possible. It should be well lit and well ventilated. Unnecessary equipment is removed. Some equipment is upsetting to look at (suction machines, drainage containers). If possible, these items are kept out of the person's sight. The room should be near the nurse's station. The person can be watched more carefully.

Mementos, pictures, cards, flowers, religious objects, and other significant items comfort and reassure the person. Arranging them within the person's view is appreciated. The person and family are allowed to arrange the room as they wish. This helps meet the needs of love, belonging, and self-esteem. The room should be comfortable and pleasant and reflect the person's choices. This promotes physical and mental comfort.

THE FAMILY

The family is going through a hard time. It may be very hard to find the right words to comfort them. You can show your feelings to the family by being available, courteous, and considerate. Also use touch to show your concern.

The family usually spends a lot of time with their loved one. Normal visiting hours do not apply if the person is dying. You must respect the person's and family's right to privacy. They need as much time together as possible. However, you cannot neglect the person's care just because the family is present. Most agencies let family members help give care. If they do not want to help, you can suggest that they take a break for a beverage or meal.

The family may be very tired, sad, and tearful. They need support and understanding. Watching a loved one die is very painful. So is dealing with the eventual loss of that person. The family is given every possible courtesy and respect. They may find comfort in a visit from a member of the clergy. You need to communicate this request to the nurse immediately.

HOSPICE CARE

Hospice care is an option for the terminally ill (see Chapter 1). Hospices focus on the physical, emotional, social, and spiritual needs of dying persons and their families. Care does not focus on cures or with life-saving procedures. Rather, pain relief and comfort measures are stressed. The goal of hospice care is to improve the dying person's quality of life.

A hospice may be part of a hospital or nursing center or a separate agency. Many hospices offer home care. Follow-up care and support groups for survivors are other hospice services.

LEGAL ISSUES AND QUALITY OF LIFE

Much attention is given to the right to die. Many people do not want to be kept alive by machines or other measures. Consent must be given for any treatment. People make their own decisions when they are able. Some make their wishes known about prolonging death before the time comes.

THE PATIENT SELF-DETERMINATION ACT

The Patient Self-Determination Act and OBRA give persons the right to accept or refuse medical treatment. They also have the right to make advance directives. An **advance directive** is a written document stating a person's wishes about health care when that person can no longer make his or her own decisions. Advance directives usually forbid certain types of care if there is no hope of recovery. Living wills and durable power of attorney are common advance directives.

All health care agencies must inform all persons of the right to advance directives on admission. This information must be in writing. The person's medical record must document whether the person has made advance directives. The law also protects the person's quality of care. Quality of care cannot be less because the person has made advance directives.

Living Wills. A living will is a person's written statement about the use of life-sustaining measures. Life-sustaining measures are those that support or maintain life. Tube feedings, ventilators, and CPR are some examples. These measures and other machines keep the person alive when death is likely. A living will instructs doctors:

- Not to start measures that prolong dying
- To remove measures that prolong dying

Durable Power of Attorney. Durable power of attorney for health care is another type of advance directive. The power to make decisions about health care is given to another person. Usually this is a family member or friend. Sometimes it is a lawyer. A person may no longer be able to make decisions about his or her own health care. Then the person with durable power of attorney has the legal authority to do so.

"DO NOT RESUSCITATE" ORDERS

When death is sudden and unexpected, every effort is made to save the person's life. CPR is started (see Chapter 36), and an emergency *code* is called. Nurses, doctors, and emergency staff rush to the person's bedside. They bring emergency and life-saving equipment with them. CPR and other life-support measures are continued until the person is resuscitated or until the doctor declares the person dead.

Doctors often write *do not resuscitate (DNR)* or *no code* orders for terminally ill persons. This means that no attempts will be made to resuscitate the person. The person is allowed to die in peace and with dignity. The orders are often written after consulting with the person or family. Some advance directives address resuscitation.

QUALITY OF LIFE

A person has the right to die in peace and with dignity. Box 37-1 contains the dying person's bill of rights. (*See Focus on Long-Term Care box.*)

Focus On... LONG-TERM CARE

The dying person also has rights under OBRA. You must protect the person's right to privacy and confidentiality. Remember, do not expose the person unnecessarily. The person has the right not to have his or her body seen by others. Proper draping and screening procedures are important.

The person and family or other visitors have the right to visit in private. The dying person may be too weak to leave the bed or room. Therefore the roommate may have to leave the room. The nurse tries to work out a plan that satisfies both roommates. The dying person may need a private room. This gives the person and family privacy. The family can also stay as long as they like.

The right to confidentiality is important. This right is protected before and after death. The person's condition and diagnoses are shared only with those involved with the person's care. The person's final moments and cause of death are also kept confidential. So are statements, conversations, and family reactions.

The dying person has the right to be free from abuse, mistreatment, and neglect. Some health team members avoid the dying person. They are uncomfortable with death and dying. Others have superstitions or religious beliefs about being near dying people. Abuse and mistreatment may occur. Family members or health team members may be the sources of such actions. The person may be too weak to report the abuse or mistreatment. Or the person may feel that punishment is deserved for needing so much care. The person has the right to receive kind and respectful care

before and after death. Be sure to report signs of abuse, mistreatment, or neglect to the nurse.

Freedom of restraint applies to the dying person. Restraints are used only if ordered by the doctor. Dying persons are often too weak to be dangerous to themselves or others.

You must protect the individual's personal possessions. The person may want certain photos and religious items nearby. Religious items may include medals, a rosary, religious books or writings, a crucifix, and candles. Such items are provided if possible. The person's property is protected from loss or damage before and after death. They may be passed on as family treasures or mementos.

Nursing center residents have the right to a safe and homelike setting. They usually depend on others for safety. The health team must keep the environment safe and homelike. Remember, the center is the person's home. Try to keep equipment and supplies out of view. Also try to keep the room free of unpleasant odors and noises. Do your best to keep the room neat and clean.

The right to personal choice is especially important. Remember, the person has the right to be involved in treatment and care. The dying person may refuse treatment. The person may also have a living will. The person may not be mentally able to be involved in treatment decisions. The family or legal representative will act on the person's behalf. The decision may be to allow the person to die with peace and dignity. The health team needs to respect choices to refuse treatment or not prolong life.

Box 37-1   The Dying Person's Bill of Rights

- I have the right to be treated as a living human being until I die.
- I have the right to maintain a sense of hopefulness, however changing its focus may be.
- I have the right to be cared for by those who can maintain a sense of hopefulness, however changing this might be.
- I have the right to express my feelings and emotions about my approaching death, in my own way.
- I have the right to participate in decisions concerning my care.
- I have the right to expect continuing medical and nursing attention even though "cure" goals must be changed to "comfort" goals.
- I have the right not to die alone.
- I have the right to be free from pain.
- I have the right to have my questions answered honestly.
- I have the right not to be deceived.
- I have the right to have help from and for my family accepting my death.
- I have the right to die in peace and dignity.
- I have the right to retain my individuality and not be judged for my decisions, which may be contrary to the beliefs of others.
- I have the right to discuss and enlarge my religious and/or spiritual experiences, regardless of what they may mean to others.
- I have the right to expect that the sanctity of the human body will be respected after death.
- I have the right to be cared for by caring, sensitive, knowledgeable people who will attempt to understand my needs and will be able to gain some satisfaction in helping me face my death.

Modified from Barbus AJ: *Am J Nurs* 75(1):99, 1975.

SIGNS OF DEATH

There are signs of approaching death. They may occur rapidly or slowly:

- Movement, muscle tone, and sensation are lost. This usually starts in the feet and legs. It eventually spreads to the rest of the body. When the mouth muscles relax, the jaw drops. The mouth may stay open. There is often a peaceful facial expression.
- Peristalsis and other gastrointestinal functions slow down. There may be abdominal distention, fecal incontinence, impaction, nausea, and vomiting.
- Circulation fails, and body temperature rises. The person feels cool or cold, looks pale, and perspires heavily. The pulse is fast, weak, and irregular. Blood pressure starts to fall.
- The respiratory system fails. Cheyne-Stokes, slow, or rapid and shallow respirations are observed. Mucus collects in the respiratory tract. This causes the *death rattle* that is heard.
- Pain decreases as the person loses consciousness. However, some people are conscious until the moment of death.

The signs of death include no pulse, respirations, or blood pressure. The pupils are fixed and dilated. A doctor determines that death has occurred and pronounces the person dead. *(See Focus on Home Care box.)*

Focus On... HOME CARE

Death often occurs in the home setting. Before the body is taken to the funeral home, the person must be pronounced dead. This is a legal requirement. So is contacting the coroner or medical examiner. State laws and agency policies vary. If a person dies at home, the nurse will tell you what to do.

► CARE OF THE BODY AFTER DEATH

Care of the body after *(post)* death *(mortem)* is called **postmortem** care. A nurse gives postmortem care. You may be asked to assist. The care begins as soon as the doctor pronounces the person dead. Standard Precautions and the Bloodborne Pathogen Standard are followed. You may have contact with infected blood, body fluids, secretions, or excretions.

Postmortem care is done to maintain the body's appearance. Discoloration and skin damage are prevented. Postmortem care also includes gathering valuables and personal items for the family. The right to privacy and the right to be treated with dignity and respect apply after death.

Within 2 to 4 hours after death, rigor mortis develops. **Rigor mortis** is the stiffness or rigidity *(rigor)* of skeletal muscles. It occurs after death *(mortis)*. Postmortem care involves positioning the body in normal alignment before rigor mortis sets in. The family may want to see the body before it is taken to the morgue or funeral home. The body is placed in a comfortable and natural position for this viewing.

In some agencies the body is prepared only for viewing. Postmortem care is completed later by the funeral director.

Repositioning of the body is often required during postmortem care. The repositioning is done to bathe soiled areas and to put the body in good alignment. Movement of the body can cause remaining air in the lungs, stomach, and intestines to be expelled. When air is expelled, the body produces sounds. Do not be alarmed or frightened by these sounds. They are normal and expected.

Assisting With Postmortem Care

Pre-Procedure

1. Wash your hands.
2. Collect the following:
   - Postmortem kit if used in your agency (shroud or body bag, gown, two tags, gauze squares, and safety pins)
   - Valuables list
   - Waterproof bed protectors
   - Wash basin
   - Bath towels
   - Washcloth
   - Tape
   - Dressings
   - Gloves
   - Cotton balls
3. Provide for privacy.
4. Raise the bed to its highest level.
5. Make sure the bed is flat.

Procedure

6. Put on the gloves.
7. Position the body supine. Arms and legs are straight. Put a pillow under the head and shoulders (Fig. 37-1, p. 822).
8. Close the eyes. Gently pull the eyelids over the eyes. Apply a moistened cotton ball gently over the eyelids if the eyes will not stay closed.
9. Insert dentures if it is agency policy. If not, put them in a labeled denture container.
10. Close the mouth. Place a rolled towel under the chin to support the mouth in the closed position if necessary.
11. Follow agency policy about jewelry. Remove all jewelry except for wedding rings if this is agency policy. List the jewelry that was removed. Place the jewelry and the list in an envelope for the family.
12. Place a cotton ball over the wedding ring. Secure it in place with tape.
13. Remove drainage bottles, bags, and containers. Leave tubes and catheters in place if an autopsy is to be performed. Ask the nurse about removal of tubes.
14. Bathe soiled areas with plain water. Dry thoroughly.
15. Place a bed protector under the buttocks.
16. Remove soiled dressings, and replace them with clean ones.
17. Put a clean gown on the body. Make sure the body is positioned as in step 7.
18. Brush and comb the hair if necessary.
19. Fill out the ID tags. Tie one to an ankle or to the right big toe.
20. Cover the body to the shoulders with a sheet if the family will view the body.
21. Gather all of the person's belongings. Put them in a bag labeled with the person's name.
22. Remove all used supplies, equipment, and linens except the shroud and the other ID tag. Make sure the room is neat. Adjust lighting so it is soft.
23. Remove the gloves, and wash your hands.
24. Let the family view the body. Provide for privacy. Give the person's belongings to the family.
25. Get a stretcher if the body will be taken to the morgue.
26. Put on another pair of gloves.
27. Place the body on the shroud or in the body bag or cover the body with a sheet after the family has left the room. Apply the shroud as in Figure 37-2, p. 823:
   a. Bring the top down over the head.
   b. Fold the bottom up over the feet.
   c. Fold the sides over the body.
28. Secure the shroud in place with safety pins or tape.
29. Attach the second ID tag to the shroud or body bag.
30. Take the body to the morgue:
   a. Move the body onto the stretcher with the help of co-workers.

Continued

Assisting With Postmortem Care—cont'd

Procedure—cont'd

b Have the doors closed to other rooms along the hallway.

c Transport the body to the morgue. Leave the denture cup with the body.

d Return the stretcher to its proper place.

31 Leave the body on the bed if it will be taken directly to the funeral home. Leave the denture cup with the body. Close the door, or pull the privacy curtain around the bed.

Post-Procedure

32 Remove the gloves, and wash your hands.

33 Strip the person's unit after the body is removed. Wear gloves for this step.

34 Wash your hands.

35 Report the following to the nurse:

a The time the body was taken by the funeral director or the time the body was taken to the morgue

b What was done with jewelry and personal items

c What was done with dentures

Fig. 37-1 The body is in the dorsal recumbent position. Arms are straight at the sides. There is a pillow under the head and shoulders.

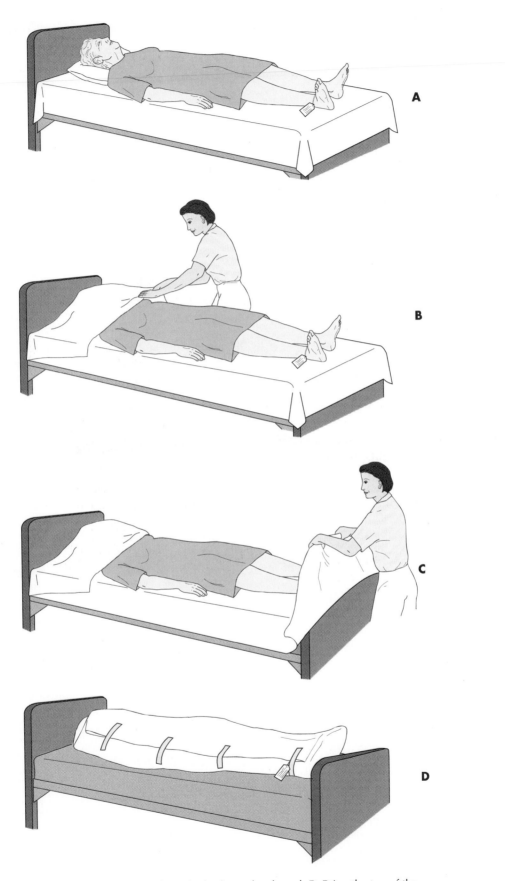

Fig. 37-2 Applying a shroud. **A,** Place the body on the shroud. **B,** Bring the top of the shroud down over the head. **C,** Fold the bottom over the feet. **D,** Fold the sides over the body, tape or pin the sides together, and attach the ID tag.

Circle the BEST answer.

1. Which is *true?*
   A. Death from terminal illness is sudden and unexpected.
   B. Doctors know when death will occur.
   C. An illness is terminal when there is no reasonable hope of recovery.
   D. All severe injuries result in death.

2. Which psychological forces influence living and dying?
   A. Hope and the will to live
   B. Reincarnation and belief in the afterlife
   C. Denial and anger
   D. Bargaining and depression

3. These statements relate to attitudes about death. Which is *false?*
   A. Dying people are often cared for in health agencies.
   B. Attitudes about death are influenced by religion.
   C. Infants and toddlers understand death.
   D. Young children often blame themselves when someone dies.

4. Reincarnation is the belief that
   A. There is no afterlife
   B. The spirit or soul is reborn into another human body or another form of life
   C. The body keeps its physical form in the afterlife
   D. Only the spirit or soul is present in the afterlife

5. Children between the ages of 5 and 7 view death as
   A. Temporary   C. Adults do
   B. Final   D. Going to sleep

6. Adults and the older persons usually fear
   A. Dying alone
   B. Reincarnation
   C. The five stages of dying
   D. All of the above

7. Persons in the stage of denial
   A. Are angry
   B. Make "deals" with God
   C. Are sad and quiet
   D. Refuse to believe they are dying

8. A dying person tries to gain more time during the stage of
   A. Anger   C. Depression
   B. Bargaining   D. Acceptance

9. When caring for a dying person, you should
   A. Use touch and listen   C. Keep the room d
   B. Do most of the talking   D. Speak in a loud v

10. As death nears, the last sense lost is
    A. Sight   C. Smell
    B. Taste   D. Hearing

11. The dying person's care includes the following *excep*
    A. Eye care   C. Active range-of-▸
    B. Mouth care   exercises
                        D. Position changes

12. The dying person is positioned in
    A. The supine position
    B. The Fowler's position
    C. Good body alignment
    D. The dorsal recumbent position

13. A "do not resuscitate" order was written. This means
    A. CPR will not be done
    B. The person has a living will
    C. Life-prolonging measures will be carried out
    D. The person is kept alive as long as possible

14. Which are *not* signs of approaching death?
    A. Rapid pulse and slowing of gastrointestinal func
    B. Loss of movement and muscle tone
    C. Increased pain and blood pressure
    D. Cheyne-Stokes respirations and the death rattle

15. The signs of death are
    A. Convulsions and incontinence
    B. No pulse, respirations, or blood pressure
    C. Loss of consciousness and convulsions
    D. The eyes stay open, no muscle movements, and the body is rigid

16. Postmortem care is done
    A. After rigor mortis sets in
    B. After the doctor pronounces the person dead
    C. When the funeral director arrives for the body
    D. After the family has viewed the body

Answers to these questions are on p. 839.

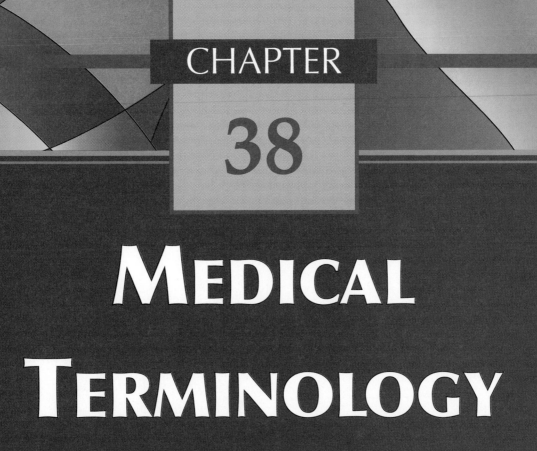

CHAPTER 38

MEDICAL TERMINOLOGY

Define the key terms listed in this chapter

Identify three word elements used in medical terms

Translate Greek and Latin prefixes, roots, and suffixes into English

Combine word elements into medical terms

Translate medical terms into English

Identify the four abdominal regions

Define the directional terms that describe the positions of the body in relation to other body parts

Identify the abbreviations used in health care and their meanings

KEY TERMS

abbreviation A shortened form of a word or phrase

anterior Located at or toward the front of the body or body part; ventral

combining vowel A vowel added between two roots or a root and a suffix to make pronunciation easier

distal The part farthest from the center or from the point of attachment

dorsal Located at or toward the back of the body or body part; posterior

lateral Relating to or located at the side of the body or body part

medial Relating to or located at or near the middle or midline of the body or body part

posterior Dorsal

prefix A word element placed at the beginning of a word to change the meaning of the word

proximal The part nearest to the center or to the point of origin

root A word element containing the basic meaning of the word

suffix A word element placed at the end of a root to change the meaning of the word

ventral Anterior

word element A part of a word

Many people find medical language mysterious and secretive—the private code of doctors and nurses. Yet people use medical terms every day. Examples are *flu, diarrhea, cancer, appendectomy, cardiac,* and *pneumonia.* Health and medicine get a lot of attention on television and the internet and in newspapers and magazines. Because of such great news coverage, many medical terms are commonly understood.

Knowing medical terminology is important in your work. As you gain more knowledge and experience, you will understand and use medical terms often and with ease. Learning medical terms for illnesses, diseases, and common things like bruises, baldness, and a "runny nose" can be fun and educational. This chapter introduces medical terminology and the common abbreviations used in health care.

WORD ELEMENTS

Like all words, medical terms are made up of parts or **word elements.** These elements are combined in various ways to form medical terms. A term is translated by separating the word into its elements. Important word elements are prefixes, roots, and suffixes.

PREFIXES

A **prefix** is a word element placed at the beginning of a word. A prefix changes the meaning of the word. The prefix *olig* (scant, small amount) is placed before the word *uria* (urine) to make *oliguria.* It means a scant amount of urine. Prefixes are always combined with other word elements. They are never used alone. Most prefixes are Greek or Latin. You need to learn the following prefixes to begin understanding medical terminology:

Prefix	Meaning
a-, an-	without, not, lack of
ab-	away from
ad-	to, toward, near
ante-	before, forward, in front of
anti-	against
auto-	self
bi-	double, two, twice
brady-	slow
circum-	around
contra-	against, opposite
de-	down, from
dia-	across, through, apart
dis-	apart, free from
dys-	bad, difficult, abnormal
ecto-	outer, outside
en-	in, into, within
endo-	inner, inside
epi-	over, on, upon
eryth-	red
eu-	normal, good, well, healthy
ex-	out, out of, from, away from
hemi-	half
hyper-	excessive, too much, high
hypo-	under, decreased, less than normal
in-	in, into, within, not
infra-	within
inter-	between
intro-	into, within
leuk-	white
macro-	large
mal-	bad, illness, disease
meg-	large
micro-	small
mono-	one, single
neo-	new
non-	not
olig-	small, scant
para-	beside, beyond, after
per-	by, through
peri-	around
poly-	many, much
post-	after, behind
pre-	before, in front of, prior to
pro-	before, in front of
re-	again, backward
retro-	backward, behind
semi-	half
sub-	under, beneath
super-	above, over, excess
supra-	above, over
tachy-	fast, rapid
trans-	across
uni-	one

ROOTS

The **root** contains the basic meaning of the word. It is combined with another root, with prefixes, and with suffixes in various combinations to form a medical term. Roots are mainly from Greek and Latin.

A vowel is added when two roots are combined or when a suffix is added to a root. The vowel is called a **combining vowel** and is usually an *o*. An *i* is sometimes used. An *i* is used when there is no vowel between the two combined roots or between the root and the suffix. A combining vowel makes pronunciation easier.

The most common roots and their combining vowels are listed here:

Root (combining vowel)	Meaning
abdomin (o)	abdomen
aden (o)	gland
adren (o)	adrenal gland
angi (o)	vessel
arterio	artery
arthr (o)	joint
broncho	bronchus, bronchi
card, cardi (o)	heart
cephal (o)	head
chole, chol(o)	bile
chondr (o)	cartilage
colo	colon, large intestine
cost (o)	rib
crani (o)	skull
cyan (o)	blue
cyst (o)	bladder, cyst
cyt (o)	cell
dent (o)	tooth
derma	skin
duoden (o)	duodenum
encephal (o)	brain
enter (o)	intestines
fibr (o)	fiber, fibrous
gastr (o)	stomach
gloss (o)	tongue
gluc (o)	sweetness, glucose
glyc (o)	sugar
gyn, gyne, gyneco	woman
hem, hema, hemo, hemat (o)	blood
hepat (o)	liver
hydr (o)	water
hyster (o)	uterus
ile (o), ili (o)	ileum
laparo	abdomen, loin, or flank
laryng (o)	larynx
lith (o)	stone
mamm (o)	breast, mammary gland

Prefix	Meaning
mast (o)	mammary gland, breast
meno	menstruation
my (o)	muscle
myel (o)	spinal cord, bone marrow
necro	death
nephr (o)	kidney
neur (o)	nerve
ocul (o)	eye
oophor (o)	ovary
ophthalm (o)	eye
orth (o)	straight, normal, correct
oste (o)	bone
ot (o)	ear
ped (o)	child, foot
pharyng (o)	pharynx
phleb (o)	vein
pnea	breathing, respiration
pneum (o)	lung, air, gas
proct (o)	rectum
psych (o)	mind
pulmo	lung
py (o)	pus
rect (o)	rectum
rhin (o)	nose
salping (o)	eustachian tube, uterine tube
splen (o)	spleen
sten (o)	narrow, constriction
stern (o)	sternum
stomat (o)	mouth
therm (o)	heat
thoraco	chest
thromb (o)	clot, thrombus
thyr (o)	thyroid
toxic (o)	poison, poisonous
toxo	poison
trache (o)	trachea
urethr (o)	urethra
urin (o)	urine
uro	urine, urinary tract, urination
uter (o)	uterus
vas (o)	blood vessel, vas deferens
ven (o)	vein
vertebr (o)	spine, vertebrae

SUFFIXES

A **suffix** is placed at the end of a root to change the meaning of the word. Suffixes are not used alone. Like prefixes and roots, they are from Greek and Latin. When translating medical terms, begin with the suffix. For example, *nephritis* means inflammation of the kidney. It is formed by combining *nephro* (kidney) and *itis* (inflammation).

You need to learn the suffixes listed in this chapter:

Suffix	Meaning
-algia	pain
-asis	condition, usually abnormal
-cele	hernia, herniation, pouching
-centesis	puncture and aspiration of
-cyte	cell
-ectasis	dilation, stretching
-ectomy	excision, removal of
-emia	blood condition
-genesis	development, production, creation
-genic	producing, causing
-gram	record
-graph	a diagram, a recording instrument
-graphy	making a recording
-iasis	condition of
-ism	a condition
-itis	inflammation
-logy	the study of
-lysis	destruction of, decomposition
-megaly	enlargement
-meter	measuring instrument
-metry	measurement
-oma	tumor
-osis	condition
-pathy	disease
-penia	lack, deficiency
-phasia	speaking
-phobia	an exaggerated fear
-plasty	surgical repair or reshaping
-plegia	paralysis
-ptosis	falling, sagging, dropping, down
-rrhage, -rrhagia	excessive flow
-rrhaphy	stitching, suturing
-rrhea	profuse flow, discharge
-scope	examination instrument
-scopy	examination using a scope
-stasis	maintenance, maintaining a constant level
-stomy, -ostomy	creation of an opening
-tomy, -otomy	incision, cutting into
-uria	condition of the urine

COMBINING WORD ELEMENTS

Medical terms are formed by combining word elements. A root can be combined with prefixes, roots, or suffixes. The prefix *dys* (difficult) can be combined with the root *pnea* (breathing). This forms the term *dyspnea,* meaning difficulty in breathing.

Roots can be combined with suffixes. The root *mast* (breast) combined with the suffix *ectomy* (excision or removal) forms the term *mastectomy.* It means the removal of a breast.

Combining a prefix, root, and suffix is another way to form medical terms. *Endocarditis* consists of the prefix *endo* (inner), the root *card* (heart), and the suffix *itis* (inflammation). *Endocarditis* means inflammation of the inner part of the heart.

There are more complex combinations of prefixes, roots, and suffixes:

- Two prefixes, a root, and a suffix
- A prefix, two roots, and a suffix
- Two roots and a suffix

The important things to remember are that prefixes always come before roots and suffixes always come after roots. You can practice forming medical terms by combining the word elements listed in this chapter.

ABDOMINAL REGIONS

The abdomen is divided into regions (Fig. 38-1) in order to help describe the location of body structures, pain, or discomfort. The regions are the:

- Right upper quadrant (RUQ)
- Left upper quadrant (LUQ)
- Right lower quadrant (RLQ)
- Left lower quadrant (LLQ)

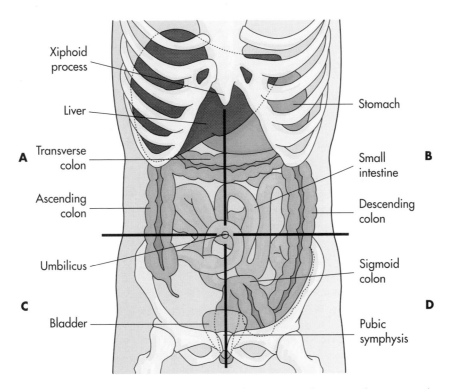

Fig. 38-1 The four regions of the abdomen. **A,** Right upper quadrant. **B,** Left upper quadrant. **C,** Right lower quadrant. **D,** Left lower quadrant.

DIRECTIONAL TERMS

Certain terms describe the position of one body part in relation to another. These terms give the direction of the body part when a person is standing and facing forward. The following directional terms come from some of the prefixes listed in this chapter:

- **Anterior (ventral)**—located at or toward the front of the body or body part
- **Distal**—the part farthest from the center or from the point of attachment
- **Lateral**—relating to or located at the side of the body or body part
- **Medial**—relating to or located at or near the middle or midline of the body or body part
- **Posterior (dorsal)**—located at or toward the back of the body or body part
- **Proximal**—the part nearest to the center or to the point of origin

ABBREVIATIONS

Abbreviations are shortened forms of words or phrases. They save time and space in written communication. Each agency has a list of accepted abbreviations. Obtain the list when you are hired, and use only the abbreviations accepted by the agency. If you are unsure an abbreviation is acceptable, write the term out in full to communicate accurately.

Common abbreviations are listed on the inside of the back cover for easy reference.

REVIEW

Fill in the blanks.

1 Word elements used in medical terminology are

   a _____

   b _____

   c _____

2 A _____ is placed at the beginning of a word to change the meaning of the word.

3 A _____ is placed at the end of a word to change the meaning of the word.

4 The four regions of the abdomen are

   a _____

   b _____

   c _____

   d _____

Match the item in column A with the item in column B.

Column A	Column B
5 Distal	a The part nearest to the center or point of origin
6 Proximal	b Relating to or located at the side of the body or body part
7 Anterior (ventral)	c Located at or toward the front part of the body or body part
8 Medial	d The part farthest from the center or point of attachment
9 Posterior (dorsal)	e Located at or toward the back of the body or body part
10 Lateral	f Relating to or located at or near the middle or the midline of the body or body part

Write the definition of the following prefixes.

11 a- _____

12 dys- _____

13 bi- _____

14 ab- _____

15 trans- _____

16 post- _____

17 olig- _____

18 hyper- _____

19 per- _____

20 hemi- _____

21 hypo- _____

22 ad- _____

Write the definition of the following suffixes.

23 -algia _____

24 -itis _____

25 -ostomy _____

26 -ectomy _____

27 -emia _____

28 -osis _____

29 -rrhage _____

30 -penia _____

31 -pathy _____

32 -otomy _____

33 -rrhea _____

34 -plasty _____

Write the definition of the following roots.

35 cranio _____

36 cardio _____

37 mammo _____

38 veno _____

39 urino _____

40 pnea _____

41 cyano _____

42 arterio _____

43 colo _____

44 arthro _____

45 litho _____

46 gastro _____

47 encephalo _____

48 gluco _____

49 hemo _____

50 hystero _____

51 hepato _____

52 myo _____

53 nephro _____

54 phlebo _____
55 oculo _____
56 osteo _____
57 neuro _____

58 pneumo _____
59 toxico _____
60 psycho _____
61 thoraco _____

Match the item in column A with the item in column B.

Column A	Column B
62 Intravenous	a Inflammation of a joint
63 Apnea	b Blood in the urine
64 Hemiplegia	c Excessive flow of blood
65 Thoracotomy	d Paralysis on one side
66 Arthritis	e Surgical removal of the uterus
67 Bronchitis	f No breathing
68 Anuria	g Inflammation of the bronchi
69 Hematuria	h Incision into the chest
70 Hysterectomy	i No urine
71 Hemorrhage	j Within a vein

Write the abbreviation for the following terms.

72 Bathroom privileges _____
73 As desired _____
74 Complains of _____
75 Twice a day _____
76 Hour of sleep _____
77 Intake and output _____
78 Nothing by mouth _____
79 When necessary _____
80 Postoperative _____
81 Every _____
83 Wheelchair _____
83 At once, immediately _____

Answers to these questions are on p. 840.

ANSWERS TO REVIEW QUESTIONS

Chapter 1
Introduction to Health Care Agencies
1. C
2. C
3. B
4. A
5. B
6. D
7. A
8. C

Chapter 2
The Nursing Assistant
1. D
2. C
3. A
4. B
5. A
6. A
7. A
8. B
9. A
10. C
11. B
12. C
13. A
14. A
15. D
16. A
17. D
18. C
19. A
20. B
21. A
22. A
23. A
24. C
25. C

Chapter 3
Work Ethics
1. C
2. D
3. C
4. D
5. B
6. D
7. C
8. B
9. C

10. D
11. C
12. B
13. A
14. A
15. B
16. C
17. D
18. A
19. D
20. C

Chapter 4
Communicating With the Health Team
1. A
2. C
3. D
4. B
5. B
6. C
7. C
8. C
9. B
10. C
11. D
12. D
13. C
14. D
15. B

Chapter 5
Understanding the Person
1. C
2. D
3. C
4. B
5. A
6. C
7. A
8. D
9. A
10. B
11. D
12. C
13. A
14. C
15. A
16. D
17. D
18. D

Chapter 6
Body Structure and Function
1. A
2. B
3. D
4. C
5. C
6. A
7. B
8. C
9. D
10. D
11. B
12. A
13. B
14. B
15. B
16. C
17. D
18. A
19. D
20. A
21. B

Chapter 7
Growth and Development
1. B
2. C
3. D
4. B
5. D
6. A
7. B
8. A
9. C
10. C
11. C
12. C
13. A
14. B
15. C
16. A
17. D
18. C

Chapter 8
Care of the Older Person
1. A
2. D
3. C
4. D
5. C
6. A
7. B
8. C
9. C
10. C
11. D
12. C
13. A
14. D
15. A
16. C
17. A
18. B

Chapter 9
Safety
1. False
2. True
3. True
4. True
5. True
6. False
7. True
8. True
9. False
10. True
11. True
12. True
13. True
14. True
15. True
16. False
17. True
18. True
19. True
20. False
21. True
22. True
23. True
24. True
25. D
26. D
27. C
28. A
29. A
30. D
31. D
32. B
33. C
34. A
35. A
36. C
37. D
38. D
39. B
40. B
41. C
42. C

Chapter 10
Preventing Infection
1. False
2. True
3. False
4. False
5. False
6. False
7. True
8. True
9. True
10. B
11. D
12. D
13. B
14. D
15. C
16. A
17. D
18. C
19. A
20. D
21. D
22. C
23. B
24. A

Chapter 11
Body Mechanics
1. False
2. True
3. False
4. True
5. False
6. True
7. True
8. False
9. True
10. True
11. False
12. True
13. False
14. True
15. False
16. True
17. False
18. True
19. False
20. True

Chapter 12
The Person's Unit
1. B
2. D
3. A
4. D
5. A
6. C
7. True
8. False
9. True
10. False
11. True
12. True
13. True
14. False

Chapter 13
Bedmaking
1. D
2. D
3. B
4. A
5. B
6. A
7. D
8. C

Chapter 14
Personal Hygiene
1. True
2. False
3. False
4. False
5. False
6. False
7. False
8. True
9. False
10. False
11. False
12. False
13. True
14. True
15. D
16. B
17. B
18. C
19. C
20. D

Chapter 15
Personal Care and Grooming
1. D
2. C
3. A
4. D
5. C
6. B
7. D
8. B
9. False
10. False
11. True
12. True

Chapter 16
Urinary Elimination
1. B
2. D
3. A
4. B
5. B
6. A
7. A
8. D
9. C
10. D
11. B
12. A
13. C
14. D
15. B

Chapter 17
Bowel Elimination
1. A
2. B
3. D
4. A
5. C
6. D
7. B
8. C
9. B
10. D
11. D
12. A

Chapter 18
Nutrition and Fluids
1. B
2. A
3. A
4. D
5. D
6. C
7. A
8. C
9. A
10. C
11. C
12. B
13. B
14. C
15. C
16. C
17. B
18. A
19. C
20. C

Chapter 19
Measuring Vital Signs
1. C
2. B
3. D
4. C
5. A
6. A
7. C
8. D
9. B
10. C
11. A
12. B

Chapter 20
Exercise and Activity
1. A
2. B
3. C
4. C
5. B
6. C
7. A
8. B
9. C
10. B
11. False
12. False
13. True
14. False
15. True

Chapter 21
Comfort, Rest, and Sleep
1. A
2. C
3. D
4. C
5. A
6. B
7. C
8. D
9. B
10. A
11. C
12. A
13. B
14. B

Chapter 22
Admissions, Transfers, and Discharges
1. False
2. True
3. True
4. True
5. False
6. True
7. True
8. False
9. True
10. True
11. True
12. False

Chapter 23
Assisting With the Physical Examination
1. B
2. D
3. C
4. B
5. C

Chapter 24
The Person Having Surgery
1. C
2. D
3. B
4. A
5. A
6. C
7. C
8. A
9. B
10. C
11. D
12. A
13. A

14. A
15. False
16. True
17. False
18. False
19. True
20. True
21. True
22. False
23. True
24. True

Chapter 25
Wound Care
1. B
2. C
3. A
4. C
5. B
6. C
7. A
8. D
9. A
10. A
11. B
12. A
13. D
14. C
15. C

Chapter 26
Heat and Cold Applications
1. D
2. B
3. D
4. B
5. C
6. B
7. D
8. A
9. D
10. C
11. A
12. B

Chapter 27
Oxygen Needs
1. A
2. C
3. C
4. B
5. D
6. C
7. D
8. A
9. B
10. A
11. B
12. D
13. B
14. D
15. D
16. C
17. A
18. C
19. D
20. B
21. C
22. D

Chapter 28
Rehabilitation and Restorative Care
1. C
2. B
3. A
4. D
5. A
6. A
7. A
8. C
9. A
10. C

Chapter 29
Hearing and Vision Problems
1. B
2. B
3. D
4. A
5. C
6. B
7. C
8. B
9. A
10. A
11. D
12. C
13. B
14. B
15. B

Chapter 30
Common Health Problems
1. A
2. C
3. A
4. D
5. C
6. A
7. A
8. D
9. C
10. B
11. A
12. A
13. A
14. D
15. B
16. C
17. D
18. A
19. D
20. A
21. B
22. B
23. C
24. A
25. C
26. A
27. D
28. C

Chapter 31
Mental Health Problems
1. B
2. B
3. A
4. C
5. D
6. A
7. C
8. C
9. B
10. C
11. D
12. D

Chapter 32
Confusion and Dementia
1. B
2. B
3. C
4. B
5. D
6. D
7. B
8. B
9. A
10. D
11. C
12. A

Chapter 33
Developmental Disabilities
1. D
2. B
3. D
4. B
5. A
6. D
7. C
8. C
9. D
10. B
11. A
12. C
13. A
14. D
15. C

Chapter 34
Sexuality
1. A
2. D
3. C
4. A
5. B
6. B
7. D
8. B
9. D
10. B

Chapter 35
Caring for Mothers and Newborns
1. C
2. D
3. B
4. D
5. D
6. B
7. C
8. C
9. C

10. C
11. D
12. D
13. D
14. A
15. C
16. C
17. True
18. True
19. False
20. True

Chapter 36
Basic Emergency Care
1. B
2. A
3. B
4. C
5. D
6. C
7. B
8. C
9. B
10. C
11. A
12. D
13. B
14. A
15. C
16. B
17. B
18. C
19. C
20. B
21. B
22. C
23. A
24. A
25. B

Chapter 37
The Dying Person
1. C
2. A
3. C
4. B
5. B
6. A
7. D
8. B
9. A
10. D
11. C
12. C
13. A
14. C
15. B
16. B

Chapter 38

Medical Terminology

1. A Prefix
    B Root
    C Suffix
2. Prefix
3. Suffix
4. A Right upper quadrant
    B Left upper quadrant
    C Right lower quadrant
    D Left lower quadrant
5. D
6. A
7. C
8. F
9. E
10. B
11. Without or not
12. Bad, difficult, abnormal
13. Double, two, twice
14. Away from
15. Across, over
16. After, behind
17. Scant, small
18. Excessive, too much
19. By, through
20. Half
21. Decreased, less than normal
22. Toward
23. Pain
24. Inflammation
25. Creation of an opening
26. Removal of, excision
27. Blood condition
28. Condition
29. Excessive flow
30. Lack, deficiency
31. Disease
32. Incision, cutting into
33. Profuse flow, discharge
34. Surgical repair or reshaping
35. Skull
36. Heart
37. Breast
38. Vein
39. Urine
40. Breathing, respiration
41. Blue
42. Artery
43. Colon, large intestine
44. Joint
45. Stone
46. Stomach
47. Brain
48. Glucose, sweetness
49. Blood
50. Uterus
51. Liver
52. Muscle
53. Kidney
54. Vein
55. Eye
56. Bone
57. Nerve
58. Lung
59. Poison
60. Mind
61. Chest
62. J
63. F
64. D
65. H
66. A
67. G
68. I
69. B
70. E
71. C
72. BRP
73. Ad lib
74. C/o
75. Bid
76. HS (hs)
77. I&O
78. NPO (npo)
79. prn
80. postop (post op)
81. q
82. w/c
83. stat

APPENDIX

National Nurse Aide Assessment Program (NNAAP™)
Written Examination Content Outline

The NNAAP Written Examination is comprised of seventy (70) multiple choice questions. Ten (10) of these questions are pre-test (non-scored) questions on which statistical information will be collected.

I. Physical Care Skills
A. Activities of Daily Living . . . . . . *12% of exam*
1. Hygiene
2. Dressing and Grooming
3. Nutrition and Hydration
4. Elimination
5. Rest/Sleep/Comfort

B. Basic Nursing Skills . . . . *29% of exam*
1. Infection Control
2. Safety/Emergency
3. Therapeutic/Technical Procedures
4. Data Collection and Reporting

C. Restorative Skills . . . . *6% of exam*
1. Prevention
2. Self Care/Independence

II. Psychosocial Care Skills
A. Emotional and Mental Health Needs . . . . *20% of exam*
B. Spiritual and Cultural Needs . . . . *2% of exam*

III. Role of the Nurse Aide
A. Communication . . . . *6% of exam*
B. Client Rights . . . . *14% of exam*
C. Legal and Ethical Behavior . . . . . . *3% of exam*
D. Member of the Health Care Team . . . . *8% of exam*

National Nurse Aide Assessment Program (NNAAP™)
Skills Evaluation*

LIST OF SKILLS
1. Washes hands
2. Measures and records weight of ambulatory client
3. Provides mouth care
4. Dresses client with affected right arm
5. Transfers client from bed to wheelchair
6. Assists client to ambulate
7. Cleans and stores dentures
8. Performs passive range of motion on one shoulder
9. Performs passive range of motion on one knee and one ankle
10. Measures and records urinary output
11. Assists client with use of bedpan
12. Provides perineal care for incontinent client
13. Provides catheter care
14. Takes and records oral temperature
15. Takes and records radial pulse and counts and records respirations
16. Takes and records client's blood pressure (one-step procedure)
17. Takes and records client's blood pressure (two-step procedure)
18. Puts one knee-high elastic stocking on client
19. Makes an occupied bed
20. Provides foot care
21. Provides fingernail care
22. Feeds client who cannot feed self
23. Positions client on side
24. Gives modified bed bath (face, and one arm, hand, and underarm)
25. Shampoos client's hair in bed

Reprinted with permission of the National Council of State Boards of Nursing, Chicago, Ill and ASI, Bala Cynwyd, Pa.
Prepared by ASI for the National Nurse Aid Assessment Program (NNAAP™) © 1998 by ASI Suite 300, Three Bala Plaza West • Bala Cynwyd, PA 19004-3481 • (610) 617-9300
*All states do not participate in the program. Such states have other arrangements for nurse aide competency and evaluation program. The NNAAP™ skills identified in this textbook may be evaluated in part, or in full, on the NNAAP™ Skills Evaluation.

GLOSSARY

abbreviation A shortened form of a word or phrase

abduction Moving a body part away from the midline of the body

abrasion A partial-thickness wound caused by the scraping away or rubbing of the skin

accountable Being responsible for one's actions and the actions of others who perform delegated tasks; answering questions about and explaining one's actions and the actions of others

acetone Ketone bodies that appear in the urine because of the rapid breakdown of fat for energy

active physical restraint A restraint attached to the person's body and to a stationary (nonmovable) object; movement and access to one's body are restricted

activities of daily living (ADL) Self-care activities a person performs daily to remain independent and to function in society

acute illness A sudden illness from which a person is expected to recover

acute pain Pain that is felt suddenly from injury, disease, trauma, or surgery; it generally lasts less than 6 months

adduction Moving a body part toward the midline of the body

admission Official entry of a person into an agency or nursing unit

adolescence A time of rapid growth and psychological and social maturity

advance directive A written document stating a person's wishes about health care when that person can no longer make his or her own decisions

affect Feelings and emotions

allergy A sensitivity to a substance that causes the body to react with signs and symptoms

alopecia Hair loss

ambulation The act of walking

AM care Routine care performed before breakfast; early morning care

amputation The removal of all or part of an extremity

anal incontinence The inability to control the passage of feces and gas through the anus; fecal incontinence

anaphylaxis A life-threatening sensitivity to an antigen

anesthesia The loss of feeling or sensation produced by a drug

anorexia The loss of appetite

anterior Located at or toward the front of the body or body part; ventral

anxiety A vague, uneasy feeling that occurs in response to stress

aphasia The inability (a) to speak (phasia)

apical-radial pulse Taking the apical and radial pulses at the same time

apnea The lack or absence (a) of breathing (pnea)

arterial ulcer An open wound on the lower legs and feet caused by decreased blood flow through the arteries

artery A blood vessel that carries blood away from the heart

arthritis Joint (arthr) inflammation (itis)

arthroplasty The surgical replacement (plasty) of a joint (arthro)

asepsis Being free of disease-producing microbes

aspiration Breathing fluid or an object into the lungs

assault Intentionally attempting or threatening to touch a person's body without the person's consent

assessment Collecting information about the person; a step in the nursing process

assistive personnel A broad term applied to nursing staff who assist nurses in giving care

atrophy A decrease in size or a wasting away of tissue

autoclave A pressure steam sterilizer

base of support The area on which an object rests

battery Unauthorized touching of a person's body without the person's consent

bedsore A pressure ulcer, pressure sore, or decubitus ulcer

benign tumor A tumor that grows slowly and within a localized area

biohazardous waste Items contaminated with blood, body fluids, secretions, and excretions and that may be harmful to others; *bio* means life, and *hazardous* means dangerous or harmful

Biot's respirations Irregular breathing with periods of apnea; respirations may be slow and deep or rapid and shallow

bisexual A person who is attracted to both sexes

blood pressure The amount of force exerted against the walls of an artery by the blood

body alignment The way in which body parts are aligned with one another; posture

body language Facial expressions, gestures, posture, and body movements that send messages to others

body mechanics Using the body in an efficient and careful way

body temperature The amount of heat in the body that is a balance between the amount of heat produced and the amount lost by the body

bradycardia A slow *(brady)* heart rate *(cardia)*; the rate is less than 60 beats per minute

bradypnea Slow *(brady)* breathing *(pnea)*; respirations are fewer than 10 per minute

braille A method of writing for the blind; raised dots are arranged to represent each letter of the alphabet; the first ten letters represent the numbers 0 through 9

calorie The amount of energy produced from the burning of food by the body

cancer Malignant tumor

capillary A tiny blood vessel; food, oxygen, and other substances pass from the capillaries to the cells

cardiac arrest The heart and breathing stop suddenly and without warning

carrier A human or animal that is a reservoir for microbes but does not have signs and symptoms of infection

case management A nursing care pattern; a case manager (an RN) coordinates a person's care from admission through discharge and into the home setting

catheter A tube used to drain or inject fluid through a body opening

catheterization The process of inserting a catheter

cell The basic unit of body structure

cerebral palsy (CP) A term applied to a group of disorders characterized by paralysis *(palsy)* that is caused by a defect in the motor region of the brain *(cerebral)*

chart Another term for the medical record

Cheyne-Stokes Respirations gradually increase in rate and depth and then become shallow and slow; breathing may stop *(apnea)* for 10 to 20 seconds

chronic illness An on-going illness, slow or gradual in onset, for which there is no known cure; the illness can be controlled and complications prevented

chronic pain Pain lasting longer than 6 months; it may be constant or occur off and on

chronic wound A wound that does not heal easily

circadian rhythm A daily rhythm based on a 24-hour cycle; the day-night cycle or body rhythm

circulatory ulcer An open wound on the lower legs and feet caused by a decrease in blood flow through the arteries and veins; vascular ulcer

circumcision The surgical removal of foreskin

civil law Laws concerned with relationships between people; private law

clean-contaminated wound A wound occurring from the surgical entry of the urinary, reproductive, respiratory, or gastrointestinal system

clean technique Medical asepsis

clean wound A wound that is not infected; microbes have not entered the wound

closed fracture The bone is broken but the skin is intact; simple fracture

closed wound A wound in which tissues are injured but the skin is not broken

colostomy An artificial opening *(stomy)* between the colon *(colo)* and abdominal wall

coma A state of being unaware of one's surroundings and being unable to react or respond to people, places, or things

combining vowel A vowel added between two roots or a root and a suffix to make pronunciation easier

comfort A state of well-being; the person has no physical or emotional pain and is calm and at peace

communicable disease A disease caused by pathogens that spread easily; a contagious disease

communication The exchange of information—a message sent is received and interpreted by the intended person

compound fracture The bone is broken and has come through the skin; open fracture

compulsion The uncontrolled performance of an act

confidentiality To trust others with personal and private information

conflict A clash between opposing interests or ideas

conscious Awareness of the environment and experiences; the person knows what is happening and can control thoughts and behaviors

constipation The passage of a hard, dry stool

constrict To narrow

contagious disease Communicable disease

contaminated wound A wound with a high risk of infection

contamination The process of becoming unclean

contracture The lack of joint mobility caused by abnormal shortening of a muscle

contusion A closed wound caused by a blow to the body

convulsion A seizure

courtesy A polite, considerate, or helpful comment or act

crime An act that violates a criminal law

criminal law Laws concerned with offenses against the public and society in general; public law

culture The language, values, beliefs, habits, likes, dislikes, customs, and characteristics of a group that are passed from one generation to the next

cyanosis Bluish skin color

Daily Reference Values (DRVs) The maximum daily intake values for total fat, saturated fat, cholesterol, sodium, carbohydrate, and dietary fiber

Daily Value (DV) How a serving fits into the daily diet; it is expressed in a percent based on a daily diet of 2,000 calories

dandruff The excessive amount of dry, white flakes from the scalp

decubitus ulcer A pressure ulcer, pressure sore, or bedsore

defamation Injuring a person's name and reputation by making false statements to a third person

defecation The process of excreting feces from the rectum through the anus; a bowel movement

defense mechanism An unconscious reaction that blocks unpleasant or threatening feelings

dehiscence The separation of wound layers

dehydration The excessive loss of water from tissues; a decrease in the amount of water in body tissues

delegate To authorize another person to perform a task

delirium A state of temporary but acute mental confusion that comes on suddenly

delusion A false belief

delusion of grandeur An exaggerated belief about one's own importance, wealth, power, or talents

delusion of persecution A false belief that one is being mistreated, abused, or harassed

dementia The term used to describe the loss of cognitive function (thinking, remembering, and reasoning) caused by changes in the brain

development Changes in a person's psychological and social functioning

developmental disability A severe, permanent physical or mental disability that occurs before 22 years of age

developmental task That which the person must complete during a stage of development

dialysis Process of removing waste products from the blood

diarrhea The frequent passage of liquid stools

diastole The period of heart muscle relaxation

diastolic pressure The pressure in the arteries when the heart is at rest

digestion The process of physically and chemically breaking down food so that it can be absorbed for use by the cells

dilate To expand or open wider

diplegia Similar body parts are affected on both sides of the body; paralysis of both arms or both legs

dirty wound An infected wound

disability Any lost, absent, or impaired physical or mental function

disaster A sudden catastrophic event in which many people are injured and killed and property is destroyed

discharge Official departure of a person from an agency or nursing unit

discomfort To ache, hurt, or be sore; pain

disinfection The process of destroying pathogens

distal The part farthest from the center or from the point of attachment

distraction To change the person's center of attention

dorsal Located at or toward the back of the body or body part; posterior

dorsal recumbent position The back-lying examination position; the legs are together

dorsiflexion Bending backward

douche Vaginal irrigation

drawsheet A small sheet placed over the middle of the bottom sheet; it helps keep the mattress and bottom linens clean and dry; can be used to turn and move the person in bed; the cotton drawsheet

dysphagia Difficulty or discomfort *(dys)* in swallowing *(phagia)*

dyspnea Difficult, labored, or painful *(dys)* breathing *(pnea)*

dysuria Painful or difficult *(dys)* urination *(uria)*

early morning care AM care

edema The swelling of body tissues with water

ego The part of the personality dealing with reality; deals with thoughts, feelings, good sense, and problem solving

ejaculation The release of semen

elective surgery Scheduled surgery a person chooses to have at a certain time

embolus A blood clot (thrombus) that travels through the vascular system until it lodges in a distant blood vessel

emergency surgery Unscheduled surgery done immediately to save the person's life or limb

emotional illness Mental illness, mental disorder, psychiatric disorder

enema The introduction of fluid into the rectum and lower colon

enteral nutrition Giving nutrients through the gastrointestinal tract *(enteral)*

enuresis Urinary incontinence in bed at night

epidermal stripping Removing the epidermis (outer skin layer) with tape

epilepsy A condition that produces brief disturbances in the brain's normal electrical functions

episiotomy Incision *(otomy)* into the perineum

esteem The worth, value, or opinion one has of a person

ethics Knowledge of what is right conduct and wrong conduct

evaluation To measure if goals are met or if progress is made; a step in the nursing process

evening care HS care or PM care

evisceration The separation of the wound along with the protrusion of abdominal organs

expressive aphasia Difficulty expressing or sending out thoughts

expressive-receptive aphasia Difficulty expressing or sending out thoughts and difficulty receiving information

extension Straightening a body part

external rotation Turning the joint outward

fainting The sudden loss of consciousness from an inadequate blood supply to the brain

false imprisonment Unlawful restraint or restriction of a person's movement

fecal impaction The prolonged retention and accumulation of feces in the rectum

fecal incontinence Anal incontinence

feces The semisolid mass of waste products in the colon

first aid Emergency care given to an ill or injured person before medical help arrives

flatulence The excessive formation of gas in the stomach and intestines

flatus Gas or air passed through the anus

flexion Bending a body part

flow rate The number of drops per minutes (gtt/min)

Foley catheter A catheter that is left in place in the urinary bladder so urine drains constantly into a drainage bag; an indwelling or retention catheter

footdrop The foot falls down at the ankle (permanent plantar flexion)

Fowler's position A semisitting position; the head of the bed is elevated 45 to 60 degrees

fracture A broken bone

fraud Saying or doing something to trick, fool, or deceive another person

friction The rubbing of one surface against another

full-thickness wound The dermis, epidermis, and subcutaneous tissue are penetrated; muscle and bone may be involved

full visual privacy Having the means to be completely free from public view while occupying a bed

functional incontinence The involuntary, unpredicted loss of urine from the bladder

functional nursing A nursing care pattern focusing on tasks and jobs; nursing personnel have specific tasks to do

gait belt A transfer or safety belt

gangrene A condition in which there is death of tissue; tissues become black, cold, and shriveled

gastrostomy A surgically created opening *(stomy)* in the stomach *(gastro)*

gavage Tube feeding

general anesthesia Unconsciousness and the loss of feeling or sensation produced by a drug

geriatrics The branch of medicine concerned with the problems and diseases of old age and older persons; the care of aging people

gerontology The study of the aging process

glucosuria Sugar *(glucos)* in the urine *(uria)*; glycosuria

glycosuria Sugar *(glycos)* in the urine *(uria)*; glucosuria

goal That which is desired in or by the person as a result of nursing care

gossip To spread rumors or talk about the private matters of others

graduate A calibrated container used to measure fluid

ground That which carries leaking electricity to the earth and away from an electrical appliance

growth The physical changes that can be measured and that occur in a steady, orderly manner

guided imagery Creating and focusing on an image

hallucination Seeing, hearing, or feeling something that is not real

harassment To trouble, torment, offend, or worry a person by one's behavior or comments

hazardous substance Any chemical that presents a physical hazard or a health hazard in the workplace

health team Staff members who work together to provide health care

hematoma The collection of blood under the skin and tissues

hematuria Blood *(hemat)* in the urine *(uria)*

hemiplegia Paralysis on one side of the body

hemoglobin The substance in red blood cells that carries oxygen and gives blood its color

hemoptysis Bloody *(hemo)* sputum *(ptysis* meaning "to spit")

hemorrhage The excessive loss of blood in a short period of time

hemothorax The collection of blood *(hemo)* in the pleural space *(thorax)*

heterosexual A person who is attracted to people of the other sex

hirsutism Excessive body hair in women and children

holism A concept that considers the whole person; the whole person has physical, social, psychological, and spiritual parts that are woven together and cannot be separated

homosexual A person who is attracted to members of the same sex

horizontal recumbent position The dorsal recumbent position

hormone A chemical substance secreted by the glands into the bloodstream

hospice A health care agency or program for persons who are dying

hyperalimentation The intravenous administration of a solution highly concentrated with proteins, carbohydrates, vitamins, and minerals; fat also may be added

hyperextension Excessive straightening of a body part

hyperglycemia High *(hyper)* sugar *(glyc)* in the blood *(emia)*

hypertension Persistent blood pressure measurements above the normal systolic (140 mm Hg) or diastolic (90 mm Hg) pressures

hyperthermia A body temperature *(thermia)* that is much higher *(hyper)* than the person's normal range

hyperventilation Respirations that are rapid (hyper) and deeper than normal

hypoglycemia Low *(hypo)* sugar *(glyc)* in the blood *(emia)*

hypotension A condition in which the systolic blood pressure is below 90 mm Hg and the diastolic pressure is below 60 mm Hg

hypothermia A very low *(hypo)* body temperature *(thermia)*

hypoventilation Respirations that are slow *(hypo)*, shallow, and sometimes irregular

hypoxemia A reduced amount (hypo) of oxygen *(ox)* in the blood *(emia)*

hypoxia A deficiency *(hypo)* of oxygen in the cells *(oxia)*

HS care Care given in the evening at bedtime (hour of sleep [HS]); evening care or PM care

id The part of the personality at the unconscious level; concerned with pleasure

ileostomy An artificial opening *(stomy)* between the ileum (small intestine; *ileo*) and the abdominal wall

immunity Protection against a disease or condition; the person will not get or be affected by the disease

implementation To perform or carry out; a step in the nursing process

impotence The inability of the male to have an erection

incision An open wound with clean, straight edges; usually intentionally produced with a sharp instrument

indwelling catheter A retention or Foley catheter

infancy The first year of life

infected wound A wound containing large amounts of bacteria and that shows signs of infection; a dirty wound

infection A disease state resulting from the invasion and growth of microorganisms in the body

insomnia A chronic condition in which the person cannot sleep or stay asleep all night

intake The amount of fluids taken in by the body

intentional wound A wound created for therapy

internal rotation Turning the joint inward

intravenous therapy The administration of fluids into a vein; IV, IV therapy, and IV infusion

intubation The process of inserting an artificial airway

invasion of privacy Violating a person's right not to have his or her name, photograph, or private affairs exposed or made public without giving consent

involuntary seclusion Separating a person from others against his or her will; keeping the person confined to a certain area or away from his or her room without consent

jejunostomy A surgically created opening *(stomy)* into the middle part of the small intestine *(jejunum)*

Kardex A type of card file that summarizes information found in the medical record; includes drugs and treatments, diagnosis, routine care measures, and special equipment used by the person

ketone body Acetone

ketones Ketone bodies, acetone

knee-chest position The person kneels and rests the body on the knees and chest; the head is turned to one side, the arms are above the head or flexed at the elbows, the back is straight, and the body is flexed about 90 degrees at the hips

Kussmaul's respirations Very deep and rapid respirations; a sign of diabetic coma

laceration An open wound with torn tissues and jagged edges

laryngeal mirror An instrument used to examine the mouth, teeth, and throat

lateral Relating to or located at the side of the body or body part

lateral position The side-lying position

law A rule of conduct made by a government body

libel Defamation through written statements

licensed practical nurse (LPN) An individual who completed a 1-year nursing program and passed a state licensing examination; called licensed vocational nurse (LVN) in some states

lithotomy position The person is in a back-lying position, the hips are brought down to the edge of the examination table, the knees are flexed, the hips are externally rotated, and the feet are supported in stirrups

local anesthesia The loss of sensation in a small area, produced by a drug injected at the specific site

lochia The vaginal discharge that occurs during the postpartum period

logrolling Turning the person as a unit, in alignment, with one motion

malignant tumor A tumor that grows rapidly and invades other tissues; cancer

malpractice Negligence by a professional person

mechanical ventilation Using a machine to move air into and out of the lungs

medial Relating to or located at or near the middle or midline of the body or body part

medical asepsis The practices used to remove or destroy pathogens and to prevent their spread from one person or place to another person or place; clean technique

medical diagnosis The identification of a disease or condition by a doctor

medical record A written account of a person's illness and response to the treatment and care given by the health team; chart

melena A black, tarry stool

menarche The time when menstruation first begins

menopause The time when menstruation stops; it marks the end of the woman's reproductive years

menstruation The process in which the lining of the uterus breaks up and is discharged from the body through the vagina

mental Relating to the mind; something that exists in the mind or is performed by the mind

mental disorder Mental illness; emotional disorder, psychiatric disorder

mental health A state of mind in which the person copes with and adjusts to the stresses of everyday living in ways accepted by society

mental illness A disturbance in the person's ability to cope or adjust to stress; behavior and functioning are impaired; mental disorder, emotional illness, psychiatric disorder

metabolism The burning of food for heat and energy by the cells

metastasis The spread of cancer to other parts of the body

microbe A microorganism

microorganism A small *(micro)* living plant or animal *(organism)* seen only with a microscope; a microbe

micturition The process of emptying urine from the bladder; urination or voiding

middle-old Persons between 75 and 84 years of age

minimum data set (MDS) A form used by nurses in nursing centers to assess a resident's mental, physical, and psychosocial functioning

mixed incontinence A combination of urge and stress incontinence

morning care Care given after breakfast; cleanliness and skin care measures are more thorough at this time

nasal speculum An instrument used to examine the inside of the nose

nasogastric (NG) tube A tube inserted through the nose *(naso)* into the stomach *(gastro)*

nasointestinal tube A tube inserted through the nose into the duodenum or jejunum of the small intestine

need That which is necessary or desirable for maintaining life and mental well-being

negligence An unintentional wrong in which a person fails to act in a reasonable and careful manner and causes harm to a person or to the person's property

nocturia Frequent urination *(uria)* at night *(noct)*

nonpathogen A microbe that usually does not cause an infection

nonREM sleep NREM sleep

nonverbal communication Communication that does not involve words

normal flora Microbes that usually live and grow in a certain location

nosocomial infection An infection acquired during a stay in a health care agency

NREM sleep The stage of sleep when there is *no rapid eye movement;* nonREM sleep

nursing assistant An individual who gives basic nursing care under the supervision of an RN or LPN/LVN

nursing care plan A written guide giving direction about the nursing care a person should receive

nursing diagnosis A statement describing a health problem that is treated by nursing measures; a step in the nursing process

nursing intervention An action or measure taken by the nursing team to help the person reach a goal

nursing process The method used by RNs to plan and deliver nursing care; its five steps are assessment, nursing diagnosis, planning, implementation, and evaluation

nursing team Individuals who provide nursing care—RNs, LPNs/LVNs, and nursing assistants

nutrient A substance that is ingested, digested, absorbed, and used by the body

nutrition The many processes involved in the ingestion, digestion, absorption, and use of foods and fluids by the body

objective data Information that is seen, heard, felt, or smelled by another person; signs

observation Using the senses of sight, hearing, touch, and smell to collect information about a person

obsession A persistent thought or idea

obstetrics The branch of medicine concerned with the care of women during pregnancy, labor, and childbirth, and for the 6 to 8 weeks after birth

old-old Persons older than 85 years

oliguria Scant amount (*olig*) of urine (*uria*); usually less than 500 ml in 24 hours

open fracture Compound fracture

open wound The skin or mucous membrane is broken

ophthalmoscope A lighted instrument used to examine the internal structures of the eye

oral hygiene Measures performed to keep the mouth and teeth clean; mouth care

organ Groups of tissues with the same function

orthopnea Being able to breathe (*pnea*) deeply and comfortably only while sitting or standing (*ortho*)

orthopneic position Sitting up in bed (*ortho*) and leaning forward over the bedside table

orthostatic hypotension A drop in (*hypo*) blood pressure when the person stands (*ortho* and *static*); postural hypotension

ostomy The surgical creation of an artificial opening

otitis media Infection (*itis*) of the middle (*media*) ear (*ot*)

otoscope A lighted instrument used to examine the external ear and the eardrum (tympanic membrane)

output The amount of fluid lost by the body

overflow incontinence The loss of urine when the bladder is too full

oxygen concentration The amount of hemoglobin that contains oxygen (O_2)

pain Discomfort

panic An intense and sudden feeling of fear, anxiety, terror, or dread

paranoia A disorder (*para*) of the mind (*noia*); false beliefs (delusions) and suspicion about a person or situation

paraphrasing Restating the person's message in your own words

paraplegia Paralysis from the waist down; paralysis of the legs

partial-thickness wound A wound in which the dermis and epidermis of the skin are broken

passive physical restraint A restraint near but not directly attached to the person's body; it does not totally restrict freedom of movement and allows access to certain body parts

pathogen A microbe that is harmful and can cause an infection

patient-focused care A nursing care pattern; hospital services are moved from the departments to the bedside.

patient/resident pack Personal care equipment provided by the health care agency (wash basin, emesis or kidney basin, bedpan, urinal, water pitcher and glass, soap, and soap dish)

pediatrics The branch of medicine concerned with the growth, development, and care of children ranging in age from the newborn to the adolescent

pediculosis (lice) The infestation with lice

pediculosis capitis The infestation of the scalp (*capitis*) with lice

pediculosis corporis The infestation of the body (*corporis*) with lice

pediculosis pubis The infestation of the pubic (*pubis*) hair with lice

penetrating wound An open wound in which the skin and underlying tissues are pierced

percussion hammer An instrument used to tap body parts to test reflexes; reflex hammer

percutaneous endoscopic gastrostomy (PEG) tube A tube inserted into the stomach (*gastro*) through a stab or puncture wound (*stomy*) made through (*per*) the skin (*cutaneous*); a lighted instrument (*scope*) allows the doctor to see inside a body cavity or organ (*endo*)

pericare Perineal care

perineal care Cleansing the genital and anal areas

peristalsis Involuntary muscle contractions in the digestive system that move food through the alimentary canal; the alternating contraction and relaxation of intestinal muscles

personality The set of attitudes, values, behaviors, and traits of a particular person

personal protective equipment Special clothing or equipment worn to protect against a hazard

phantom pain Pain felt in a body part that is no longer there

phobia Fear, panic, or dread

planning Setting priorities and goals; a step in the nursing process

plantar flexion The foot (*plantar*) is bent (*flexion*)

plaque A thin film that sticks to the teeth; it contains saliva, microbes, and other substances

plastic drawsheet A drawsheet placed between the bottom sheet and the cotton drawsheet to keep the mattress and bottom linens clean and dry

pleural effusion The escape and collection of fluid (*effusion*) in the pleural space

PM care HS care or evening care

pneumothorax The collection of air (*pneumo*) in the pleural space (*thorax*)

pollutant A harmful chemical or substance in the air or water

polyuria The production of abnormally large amounts (*poly*) of urine (*uria*)

posterior Dorsal

postmortem After (*post*) death (*mortem*)

postoperative After surgery

postpartum After (*post*) childbirth (*partum*)

postural hypotension Orthostatic hypotension

posture The way in which body parts are aligned with one another; body alignment

preceptor A staff member who guides and teaches

prefix A word element placed at the beginning of a word to change the meaning of the word

preoperative Before surgery

pressure sore A bedsore, decubitus ulcer, or pressure ulcer

pressure ulcer Any injury caused by unrelieved pressure; a decubitus ulcer, bedsore, or pressure sore

primary caregiver The person in the child's environment who is mainly responsible for providing or assisting with the child's basic needs

primary nursing A nursing care pattern; an RN is responsible for patients' total care

pronation Turning downward

prone position Lying on the abdomen with the head turned to one side

prosthesis An artificial replacement for a missing body part

proximal The part nearest to the center or to the point of origin

pseudodementia False (*pseudo*) disorder of the mind (*dementia*)

psychiatric disorder Mental illness, mental disorder, emotional disorder

psychiatry The branch of medicine concerned with the diagnosis and treatment of people with mental health problems

psychosis A serious mental disorder; the person does not view or interpret reality correctly

puberty The period when the reproductive organs begin to function and secondary sex characteristics appear

pulse The beat of the heart felt at an artery as a wave of blood passes through the artery

pulse deficit The difference between the apical and radial pulse rates

pulse rate The number of heartbeats or pulses felt in 1 minute

puncture wound An open wound made by a sharp object; entry of the skin and underlying tissues may be intentional or unintentional

purulent drainage Thick green, yellow, or brown drainage

quadriplegia Paralysis from the neck down; paralysis of the arms, legs, and trunk

radiating pain Pain felt at the site of tissue damage and in nearby areas

range of motion (ROM) The movement of a joint to the extent possible without causing pain

receptive aphasia Difficulty receiving information

recording Writing or charting patient or resident care and observations

reflex An involuntary movement

reflex incontinence The loss of urine at predictable intervals; unconscious incontinence

regional anesthesia The loss of sensation or feeling in a large area of the body, produced by the injection of a drug; the person does not lose consciousness

registered nurse (RN) An individual who studied nursing for 2, 3, or 4 years and passed a state licensing examination

regurgitation The backward flow of food from the stomach into the mouth

rehabilitation The process of restoring the person to his or her highest possible level of physical, psychological, social, and economic functioning; restorative care

reincarnation The belief that the spirit or soul is reborn in another human body or in another form of life

relaxation To be free from mental or physical stress

religion Spiritual beliefs, needs, and practices

REM sleep The stage of sleep when there is *rapid eye movement*

reporting A verbal account of patient or resident care and observations

reservoir The environment in which a microbe lives and grows

resident assessment protocol (RAP) Triggers and guidelines used in developing the comprehensive care plan

respiration The process of supplying the cells with oxygen and removing carbon dioxide from them; the act of breathing air into (inhalation) and out of (exhalation) the lungs

respiratory arrest Breathing stops but the heart still pumps blood for several minutes

respiratory depression Slow, weak respirations that occur at a rate of fewer than 12 per minute; respirations are not deep enough to bring enough air into the lungs

responsibility The duty or obligation to perform some act or function

rest To be calm, at ease, and relaxed; to be free of anxiety and stress

restorative care Rehabilitation

restraint Any item, object, device, garment, material, or chemical that restricts a person's freedom of movement or access to one's body

retention catheter A Foley or indwelling catheter

reverse Trendelenburg's position The head of the bed is raised and the foot of the bed is lowered

rigor mortis The stiffness or rigidity (*rigor*) of skeletal muscles that occurs after death (*mortis*)

root A word element containing the basic meaning of the word

rotation Turning the joint

safety belt A transfer belt or gait belt

sanguineous drainage Bloody drainage (*sanguis*)

schizophrenia Split (*schizo*) mind (*phrenia*)

seizure The violent and sudden contractions or tremors of muscles; convulsion

self-actualization Experiencing one's potential

self-esteem Thinking well of yourself and being thought well of by others

semi-Fowler's position The head of the bed is raised 45 degrees, and the knee portion is raised 15 degrees; or the head of the bed is raised 30 degrees, and the knee portion is *not* raised

serosanguineous drainage Thin, watery drainage (*sero*) that is blood-tinged (*sanguineous*)

serous drainage Clear, watery fluid (*serum*)

sex The physical activities involving the organs of reproduction; the activities are done for pleasure or to produce children

sexuality The physical, psychological, social, cultural, and spiritual factors that affect a person's feelings and attitudes about his or her sex

shearing When skin sticks to a surface and muscles slide in the direction the body is moving

shock The condition that results when there is not enough blood supply to organs and tissues

side-lying position The lateral position

signs Objective data

simple fracture Closed fracture

Sims' position A left side-lying position in which the upper leg is sharply flexed so that it is not on the lower leg and the lower arm is behind the person

skin tear A break or rip in the skin that separates the epidermis from the underlying tissues

slander Defamation through oral statements

sleep A state of unconsciousness, reduced voluntary muscle activity, and lowered metabolism

spastic Uncontrolled contractions of skeletal muscles

sphygmomanometer The instrument used to measure blood pressure

spore A bacterium protected by a hard shell that forms around the microbe

sputum Expectorated mucus

stasis ulcer An open wound caused by poor blood return to the heart from the legs and feet; venous ulcer

sterile The absence of *all* microbes

sterile field A work area free of all pathogens and nonpathogens (including spores)

sterile technique Surgical asepsis

sterilization The process of destroying *all* microbes

stethoscope An instrument used to listen to the sounds produced by the heart, lungs, and other body organs

stoma An opening; see colostomy and ileostomy

stomatitis Inflammation *(itis)* of the mouth *(stomat)*

stool Excreted feces

straight catheter A catheter that drains the bladder and is removed

stress The response or change in the body caused by any emotional, physical, social, or economic factor

stress incontinence The loss of small amounts of urine with exercise and certain movements

stressor Any emotional, physical, social, or economic factor that causes stress

subconscious Memory, past experiences, and thoughts of which the person is not aware; they are easily recalled

subjective data That which is reported by a person and is not observed by others using the senses; symptoms

suction The process of withdrawing or sucking up fluid (secretions)

suffix A word element placed at the end of a root to change the meaning of the word

suffocation When breathing stops from the lack of oxygen

sundowning Increased signs, symptoms, and behaviors of Alzheimer's disease during hours of darkness

superego The part of the personality concerned with what is right and wrong

supination Turning upward

supine position The back-lying or dorsal recumbent position

suppository A cone-shaped solid medication that is inserted into a body opening; it melts at body temperature

surgical asepsis The practices that keep equipment and supplies free of all microbes; sterile technique

symptoms Subjective data

syncope A brief loss of consciousness; fainting

system Organs that work together to perform special functions

systole The period of heart muscle contraction

systolic pressure The amount of force it takes to pump blood out of the heart into the arterial circulation

tachycardia A rapid *(tachy)* heart rate *(cardia)*; the heart rate is over 100 beats per minute

tachypnea Rapid *(tachy)* breathing *(pnea)*; respirations are usually more than 24 per minute

tartar Hardened plaque on teeth

task A function, procedure, activity, or work that does not require an RN's professional knowledge or judgment

team nursing A nursing care pattern; the team leader (an RN) delegates the care of specific persons to RNs and LPNs/LVNs and delegates nursing tasks to nursing assistant

terminal illness An illness or injury for which there is no reasonable expectation of recovery

thrombus A blood clot

tinnitus Ringing in the ears

tissue A group of cells with similar function

tort A wrong committed against a person or the person's property

transfer Moving a person from one room, nursing unit, or agency to another

transfer belt A belt used to hold onto a person during a transfer or when walking with the person; a gait belt or safety belt

transsexual A person who believes that he or she is really a member of the other sex

transvestite A person who becomes sexually excited by dressing in the clothes of the other sex

trauma An accident or violent act that injures the skin, mucous membranes, bones, and internal organs

Trendelenburg's position The head of the bed is lowered, and the foot of the bed is raised

triggers Clues that direct the caregiver to the appropriate resident assessment protocol (RAP)

tumor A new growth of cells; tumors are benign or malignant

tuning fork An instrument used to test hearing

umbilical cord The structure that carries blood, oxygen, and nutrients from the mother to the fetus

unconscious Experiences and feelings that cannot be remembered

unconscious incontinence Reflex incontinence

unintentional wound A wound resulting from trauma

ureterostomy The surgical creation of an artificial opening *(stomy)* between the ureter *(uretero)* and the abdomen

urge incontinence The involuntary loss of urine after feeling a strong need to void

urgent surgery Surgery necessary for the person's health; it must be done soon to prevent further damage or disease

urinary frequency Voiding at frequent intervals

urinary incontinence The inability to control the loss of urine from the bladder

urinary urgency The need to void immediately

urination The process of emptying urine from the bladder; micturition or voiding

vaccination The administration of a vaccine to produce immunity

vaccine A preparation that contains dead or weakened microbes and is given to produce immunity against an infectious disease

vaginal irrigation The introduction of a fluid into the vagina and the immediate return of the fluid; douche

vaginal speculum An instrument used to open the vagina so that it and the cervix can be examined

vascular ulcer A circulatory ulcer

vein A blood vessel that carries blood back to the heart

venous ulcer A stasis ulcer

ventral Anterior

verbal communication Communication that uses the written or spoken word

vertigo Dizziness

vital signs Temperature, pulse, respirations, and blood pressure

voiding Urination or micturition

will A legal statement of how a person's property is to be distributed after the person's death

word element A part of a word

work ethics Behavior in the workplace

workplace violence Any physical assault or threatening behavior or verbal abuse that occurs in a work setting

wound A break in the skin or mucous membrane

young-old Persons between 60 and 74 years of age

INDEX